T0200432

CLINICAL AROMATHERAPY
Essential Oils in Healthcare
Third Edition

Jane Buckle, PhD, RN
London, UK

ELSEVIER

ELSEVIER

3251 Riverport Lane
St. Louis, MO 63043

CLINICAL AROMATHERAPY,
THIRD EDITION

ISBN: 978-0-7020-5440-2

Notice

Knowledge and best practice in this field are constantly changing. As new research and experience broaden our knowledge, changes in practice, treatment, and drug therapy may become necessary or appropriate. Readers are advised to check the most current information provided (i) on procedures featured or (ii) by the manufacturer of each product to be administered, to verify the recommended dose or formula, the method and duration of administration, and contraindications. It is the responsibility of the practitioner, relying on their own experience and knowledge of the patient, to make diagnoses, to determine dosages and the best treatment for each individual patient, and to take all appropriate safety precautions. To the fullest extent of the law, neither the Publisher nor the Editor assumes any liability for any injury and/or damage to persons or property arising out of or related to any use of the material contained in this book.

The Publisher

International Standard Book Number: 978-0-7020-5440-2

Senior Vice President, Content: Loren Wilson
Content Strategist: Shelly Stringer
Content Development Specialist: Brandi Graham
Publishing Services Manager: Julie Eddy
Project Manager: Sara Alsup
Designer: Reneé Duenow

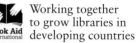

Working together
to grow libraries in
developing countries

www.elsevier.com • www.bookaid.org

Printed in Scotland

Last digit is the print number: 15 14 13 12 11 10 9 8

*This book is for those who want to push
the boundaries of clinical aromatherapy within healthcare.
Here is the evidence. Now, it's over to you.*

Foreword

Aromatherapy is possibly the simplest of all complementary therapies to integrate because when we inhale air, we inhale aroma, although we are usually unaware of it. However, aromatherapy is rarely presented in a cogent, scientific way; as a result, it has been difficult for physicians, nurses, and others in healthcare to take the field seriously or to understand how we could integrate it into our practice. Here is a book written by a PhD nurse with considerable research training and experience, who writes about aromatherapy in a way that we can identify.

As a small boy growing up in Turkey, I had my own special paradise—my grandfather's walled garden—where I became aware of the power of the senses; in particular, how the fragrance of plants made me feel good. Now, as a cardiovascular surgeon, I work on repairing the heart. I know the heart is perceived by many to be more than a pump, the epicenter of emotion, and I continue to be aware of how important our senses are to our well-being and how *feeling* good can help recovery. The very smell of many hospitals is unpleasant, alien, or distressing to our patients. Patients feel at their most vulnerable in a hospital's high-tech surroundings, so a familiar and comforting smell can do much to put them at their ease. In common with several forward-thinking hospitals in the United States, we now use aromatherapy at Columbia Presbyterian and we have worked with Jane Buckle on research since 1995.

Our sense of smell is located in the catacombs of the most primitive area of the brain and is extremely powerful. Smell can produce all sorts of physical reactions, ranging from nausea to napping. The amygdala, the brain's emotional center, is located in the limbic system and is directly connected to the olfactory bulb. Rage and fear are processed in the amygdala and both contribute to heart disease. Our studies at Columbia have found that diluted essential oils rubbed on the feet affected some volunteer's autonomic nervous system within minutes.

Clinical Aromatherapy, Third Edition, is presented logically, with some necessary background information given at the outset. I expect many readers will go straight to the clinical section to look at their own specialty. In each specialty, a few symptoms or problems have been explored and the way in which aromatherapy might help treat those symptoms or problems is clearly outlined. This third edition is greatly helped by the addition of many tables. There is also a huge increase in references. Although the clinical chapters will be of particular interest to readers working in that clinical specialty, I think the book will also be of great interest to those who want to know what clinical aromatherapy really is and how it can be used in a scientific way.

Jane Buckle has surpassed the excellence of the second edition and this does not surprise me. She was the first nurse to win a postdoctoral NIH-funded research fellowship to study an MSc in Epidemiology & Biostatistics in the School of Medicine at the University of Pennsylvania. No mean feat! She brings a wealth of knowledge and clinical experience acquired over 30 years in the field. With a PhD in health service management, a background in critical care nursing, a teaching degree, and a fistful of degrees from the world of alternative medicine, she writes authoritatively and she speaks from the heart. Jane was a co-presenter with me at The World Economic Forum in Davos, Switzerland, several years ago. We were invited to talk about the economics of alternative medicine and its affect on globalization. I was impressed by Jane's passion. An underlying question permeated all her presentations: What can we do to get the caring back into healthcare? When Jane speaks, people listen.

Jane Buckle is a pioneer and she uses writing, research, and teaching to get her message across. Her message is one of holism and she inspires those in healthcare to evaluate how they use simple things like smell and touch to help people heal. In the United States, many hospitals have integrated clinical aromatherapy and use Jane's program. She is still involved in numerous hospital research programs (apart from our own) and has been a reviewer for NIH grants in the USA and for the NHS in UK, where she currently lives.

Under her guidance, hundreds of students have carried out small pilot studies in American hospitals. She has written templates for aromatherapy policies and protocols that are used by hospitals. Jane Buckle works extraordinarily hard. More than anyone, she has labored to get the message of clinical aromatherapy across to health professionals globally, not as a possible add-on, but as a legitimate part of holistic care.

That achievement alone is remarkable; but she has another string to her bow. She has pioneered a registered method of touch, called the 'M' Technique®. Several years ago, the 'M' Technique was tested in our laboratory at Columbia Presbyterian and was found to have a pronounced parasympathetic response. While she was at the University of Pennsylvania, Jane conducted research to compare the effects of the 'M' Technique to conventional massage using brain imaging. The results showed that the 'M' Technique affected a different area of the brain to massage and the affects appeared to be more relaxing. Today the 'M' Technique is used in many hospitals, hospices, special needs schools, and long-term care facilities because it is so simple to learn and the effects are measurable in 5 minutes! The technique definitely is very relaxing (I have experienced it myself!) and eminently suitable for hospital patients (with or without the use of essential oils), so I am delighted to see that the 'M' Technique has a dedicated chapter in this third edition.

Essential oils offer extraordinary potential from a purely medicinal standpoint. The infection chapter highlighting studies on MRSA, MDRTB, and other resistant pathogens shows just how powerful they can be. I think this chapter will be of particular interest to pharmacists as well as those involved in infection control. When nausea is relieved through the inhalation of peppermint, insomnia is alleviated through the inhalation of lavender or rose, or *Candida albicans* is killed by tea tree, we are witnessing clinical results—not just the "feel-good" factor. Aromatherapy can work at a clinically significant level.

The subject of clinical aromatherapy is vast and will be of interest to anyone involved in healthcare as well as pharmaceutical companies and aromatherapists wanting to learn more. I share a goal with Jane Buckle—to enhance patient care and give the best of what we have to offer, whatever that may be. As a physician, I believe clinical aromatherapy has an important role to play in integrative medicine. Jane Buckle gives us a glimpse of the future and it smells good!

MEHMET OZ

Mehmet Oz, MD, is a cardiac surgeon. He is the Director of the Cardiovascular Institute and Vice Chairman of the Department of Surgery at Columbia Presbyterian Medical Center, New York, NY. He is the Emmy award-winning host of "The Dr. Oz Show."

Preface

"The biggest threats and dangers we face are the ones we don't see—not because they're secret or invisible, but because we're willfully blind."

Margaret Heffernan, 2011

This book is the first fully peer-reviewed, evidence-based book on clinical aromatherapy. The reviewers are professors and experts in their own field from Australia, Japan, The Netherlands, Turkey, UK, and USA. Their names and affiliations are listed with the chapter they reviewed. I am extremely grateful for their valued input and time, which has enabled this book to be truly ground-breaking.

Aromatherapy is a multifaceted therapy, so it is not surprising that many people do not know what it really is. The term "aromatherapy" was coined in France by a chemist (Gattefossé 1937) and then used by a nurse (Maury 1961) and a doctor (Valnet 1976). Thus, from the very beginning, the term "aromatherapy" was associated with healthcare. The definition "Aromatherapy is the use of essential oils" (Gattefossé 1937) is very specific. In 2013, the global market for essential oils was estimated to be worth $1000 million (Williamson 2013). Essential oils are used in household goods, cosmetics, by the food and drinks industry, the beauty world, and more recently in pharmaceutical production. Some essential oils are also used by the tobacco industry (Lawrence 1994).

Because my initial training was in nursing care, my focus has always been on the clinical aspects of aromatherapy. By calling it *clinical*, I strive to put aromatherapy back where I feel it belongs—in healthcare.

Mehmet Oz, MD, cardiothoracic surgeon at Columbia Presbyterian Medical Center and now famous for his "Dr. Oz Show," was one of the first doctors to realize the potential of aromatherapy. He wrote, "Aromatherapy appears to impact perceptions of pain" (Oz 1998). At the World Economic Forum at Davos (1999), I stated: "aromatherapy makes economic sense." What other complementary therapy can be used in so many different ways in healthcare, for so many different symptoms, is inexpensive, easy to use, and smells good?

Aromatherapy is better known for its soft side—for its caring. Florence Nightingale once said: "the cure is in the caring" (Dossey 2000). Clearly, relaxation and rest are important during illness and following surgery (Nightingale 1859), and the ability to relax can be greatly enhanced by aromatherapy. However, there is another side to aromatherapy—the curing side. Tea tree is not used to induce relaxation. It is used against bacterial, viral, and fungal infections (Carson et al 2006). Currently, the pharmaceutical industry is struggling to find new drugs to combat resistant infections and some drugs for chronic conditions are losing their potency. At the Gattefossé Foundation colloquium (2010) held in Gattefossé's family home, I introduced the concept of Evolutionary Pharmacology (Buckle 2010). Evolutionary Pharmacology (EP) blends a non-standardized essential oil with a conventional drug to create a medicine that is constantly evolving. I explain more about this in Chapter 7.

This book is about clinical aromatherapy in healthcare and is divided into three sections. Section I covers the basics of aromatherapy: the evolution of aromatherapy, how essential oils work, basic plant taxonomy, extraction, biosynthesis, chemistry, toxicity, and contraindications. This section also covers how clinical aromatherapy is already being used in integrative medicine and introduces the 'M' Technique ® as a method for relaxation (with or without essential oils). Sections II and III are both clinically focused. Section II, the General Clinical section, covers infection, insomnia, nausea and vomiting, pain and inflammation, plus stress and well-being. Section III covers nine key clinical specialties: Care of the Elderly; Critical Care; Dermatology; Mental Health; Oncology; Palliative, Hospice, and End-of-Life Care; Pediatrics; Respiratory Care; and Women's Health.

This book is intended to present an overview of what essential oils could do in healthcare. It is not meant to be a substitute for training. I believe strongly in education, preferably in a hands-on class where there can be face-to-face discussion and debate. There is a need for a clear clinical focus. Safety concerns need to be addressed and protocols and policies need to be written. With these guidelines in place, clinical aromatherapy can, I believe, enhance patient care and reduce costs.

"Willful blindness" is the legal term given to information that you should or could know, but disregard. It is estimated that 85% of companies have willful blindness (Heffernan 2011). Heffernan suggests that at a time when we are supposedly better informed than ever before, we are guilty of frequent and self-destructive acts of willful blindness. This includes the healthcare industry. Because we are living much longer and because there are no cures for most chronic illnesses, many healthcare systems are in crisis. Rahm Emanuel (former Chief of Staff at the White House) said: "Never let a serious crisis go to waste. It's an opportunity to do things you think you could not do before (2009)." I believe the healthcare crisis is aromatherapy's big opportunity. Healthcare can choose willful blindness. Or it can choose to evolve. Clinical aromatherapy could be part of that evolution.

REFERENCES

Buckle J. 2010. Is there a role for essential oils in current and future healthcare? *Bulletin Technique Fondation Gattefossé.* 103:95-110.

Carson C, Hammond K, Riley T. 2006. *Melaleuca alternifolia* (tea tree) oil: a review of antimicrobial and other medicinal properties. *Clin Microbiol Rev.* 19(1):50-62.

Dossy B. 2000. *Florence Nightingale: Mystic, Visionary, Healer.* Springhouse, PA: Springhouse.

Emanuel. R. 2009. www.youtube.com/watch?v=VjMTNPXYu-Y.

Gattefossé R-M. 1937. *Aromathérapie: Les Huiles Essentielles Hormones Végétales*. Ed. Librairie des Sciences Girardot.

Heffernan M. 2011. *Willful Blindness*. Walker & Company USA. Ted Talk.

Lawrence B. 1994. *Production of Clary Sage Oil and Sclareol in North America*. Emes Rencontres International. Nyon, France. December 5-7. http://legacy.library.ucsf.edu/documentStore/f/x/d/fxd13c00/Sfxd13c00.pdf. Accessed March 20, 2014.

Maury M. 1961. *Le Capital Jeunesse*. Editions de la Tables Rond, Paris.

Nightingale F. 1859. *Notes on Nursing: What It Is and What It Is Not*. London: Harrison & Sons.

Oz M. 1998. *Healing from the Heart*. Dutton: New York.

Valnet J. 1976. *Aromathérapie: Traitement des Maladies par les Essences des Plantes*. Robert Lafont. Paris.

Acknowledgments

First, I would like to give a huge thank you to the chapter reviewers who are listed on the following page. I would also like to give special thanks to the librarians at Panola College and Texas Health Harris Methodist Hospital, Fort Worth, Texas, who helped me with the initial literature searches. Thank you to Rhiannon Lewis, who sent me all the back copies of her excellent journal *International Journal of Clinical Aromatherapy* and to Bob Harris, whose aromatherapy database (http://quintessential.uk.com), helped me find relevant research papers that were not easily available elsewhere. Thank you to Elsevier for giving me access to the Science Direct database. Finally, thank you to my family and friends who waited for 18 months.

Reviewers

CHAPTER 1   Evolution of Aromatherapy
Martha Mathews Libster, PhD, MSN,
APRN-CNS, APHN-BC. Director Golden
Apple Healing Arts. Founding Director www.
BambooBridge.org. Professor of Nursing,
Governors State University, Il, USA

CHAPTER 2   How Essential Oils Work
Christine Carson, PhD. School of Medicine &
Pharmacology, University Western Australia,
Crawley & Harry Perkins Institute of Medical
Research, Nedlands, Australia.

**CHAPTER 3   Taxonomy, Extraction,
Biosynthesis, Analysis and Chemistry**
1) Taxonomy
Arthur Tucker. PhD. Emeritus Professor of
Agriculture & Natural Resources, Delaware
State University, Dover, DE, USA.
2) Extraction, Biosynthesis & Analysis
Stefan Gafner, PhD. Chief Science Officer,
American Botanical Council,
Austin, TX, USA.
3) Chemistry
K Husnu Can Baser. PhD. Professor Faculty
of Pharmacognosy, Anadolu University,
Eskisehir, Turkey

CHAPTER 4   Toxicity & Contraindications
Elizabeth M. Williamson, PhD, MRPharmS,
FLS. Director of Pharmacy Practice,
University of Reading, UK.

**CHAPTER 5   Aromatherapy in Integrative
Healthcare**
Mary Jo Assi DNP, RN, NEA-BC, FNP-BC,
AHN-BC. Director of Nursing Practice and
Work Environment at *American Nurses
Association*. Silver Spring, MD, USA.

CHAPTER 6   The 'M' Technique
Barbara Cordell PhD RN AHN-BCWil. Dean
of Nursing, Panola College, Carthage, Tx,
USA.

CHAPTER 7   Infection
Linda L. Halcon, PhD, MPH, RN, Associate
Professor. Chair, Population Health &
Systems Co-operative School of Nursing,
University of Minnesota, Minneapolis, MN,
USA.

CHAPTER 8   Insomnia
Dr George Lewith, MD, FRCP, MRCGP.
Professor of Health Research, University
of Southampton, UK.

CHAPTER 9   Nausea & Vomiting
Dr Ron Hunt, MD. Anesthesiologist
Carolinas Medical Center, Charlotte, NC,
USA.

CHAPTER 10   Pain & Inflammation
Dr Joyce Frye DO, MBA, MSCE, FACOG,
ABIHM, Formerly Clinical Assistant
Professor, Center for Integrative Medicine,
University of Maryland School of Medicine,
Baltimore, MD, USA.
and
Gloria Duke, PhD, RN. Professor and
Associate Dean, Office of Research &
Scholarship, College of Nursing & Health
Sciences. Chair, UT Tyler Institutional
Review Board Director, UT Tyler Center
for Ethics. The University of Texas at Tyler.
Tyler, Tx, USA.

CHAPTER 11   Stress & Wellbeing
Dr Kazuyo Yoshiyama, MD. Clinical
Psychiatrist. Director Association of
Complementary & Alternative Medicine for
IMMH (Association of Integrative Medicine
for Mental Health Care). Tokyo, Japan.

CHAPTER 12   Care of the Elderly
Dr Kazuhisa Maeda MD, PhD. Associate
Professor. Dept Complementary &
Alternative Medicine, Osaka University
Graduate School of Medicine, Osaka
University Hospital, Japan.

CHAPTER 13   Critical Care
Dr Stephen Rush, MD. Critical Care Surgery,
Texas Health Harris Methodist Medical
Center, Fort Worth, TX, USA
and
Diane M. Breckenridge, PhD, MSN, RN, ANEF
Chair and Professor
Department of Nursing
National University
San Diego, CA, USA.

CHAPTER 14   Dermatology
Dr Roberta A Lee, MD. Integrative Medicine/
Internal Medicine, Pantano Clinic, University
of Arizona Medical Center, Tucson, AZ., USA.

CHAPTER 15   Mental Health
Dr Wasyl Nimenko., GP,. Psychotherapist,
London UK
and
Elizabeth Wilde McCormick, MA.
Psychotherapist. Founder Member
Association for Cognitive Analytic Therapy,
UK.

CHAPTER 16   Oncology
Jacqui Stringer, PhD, RGN. Clinical Lead for
Supportive Care Services, The Christie NHS
Foundation Trust, Manchester, UK.

CHAPTER 17   Palliative, Hospice & End of Life Care
Carole Ann Drick, PhD, RN. President
American Holistic Nursing Association.
Director www.GoldenRoom Advocates.
USA.

CHAPTER 18   Pediatrics
Monique van Dijk. PhD RN. Associate
Professor Quality of Care, Dept of Pediatric
Surgery and Pediatrics. Erasmus MC-Sophia
Children's Hospital, Rotterdam, The
Netherlands. Honorary Associate Professor,
Dept Pediatric Surgery, University of Cape
Town, South Africa.

CHAPTER 19   Respiration
Dr Michael F. Roizen, MD. Chief Wellness
Officer (CWO) and Chair, Wellness Institute
of the Cleveland Clinic, Cleveland, OH, USA.

CHAPTER 20   Women's Health.
Dr E Joan Barice MD, MPH, FACP. Clinical
Associate Professor of Preventive Medicine
at Nova Southeastern University College of
Medicine, Ft Lauderdale, Affiliate Clinical
Associate Professor of Biomedical Science at
Florida Atlantic University, Boca Raton, FL,
USA.

Contents

Section I
OVERVIEW

Section I is an overview covering the basics of aromatherapy. This section opens with an overview of the history of aromatic medicine and the emergence of aromatherapy in the 1940s. How Essential Oils Work is self-explanatory—how and why essential oils affect us. Chapter 3 covers what an essential oil really is, from basic plant taxonomy, through extraction, biosynthesis, and analysis to the basic chemistry of essential oils. Chapter 4 covers toxicity and contraindications (the "when and why not" aspects of aromatherapy). Chapter 5 places aromatherapy within Integrative Medicine. Chapter 6 introduces the 'M' Technique®—a registered method of gentle structured touch that I have pioneered over the last 20 years or so, that is very easy to learn and has profound relaxation effects.

Chapter 1

The Evolution of Aromatherapy

"The fallen angel of the senses…a potent wizard that transports us across thousands of miles and all the years we have lived."

Helen Keller

ANCIENT HISTORY

The use of aromatic plants was originally part of herbal medicine. Herbal medicine dates back thousands of years and is not confined to any one geographical area. Residual patterns of use and trade in contemporary society suggest that nearly every part of the world has some history of the use of aromatic plants in its healthcare system. The use of technology in the distillation of essential oils from aromatic plants that forms the basis for contemporary "aromatherapy," as we know it, is much more recent. However, among the many countries that have a documented history of using aromatic plants in their healing traditions are China, Egypt, France, Greece, India, Iraq, Syria (was part of Mesopotamia), Switzerland, Tibet, UK, and the United States (Native Americans). Early aromatics were used in the form of steams, smokes, inhalants, fumigants, snuffs, salves, lotions, compresses, poultices, waters, colognes, perfumes, and baths.

EGYPT

One of the most famous manuscripts concerning aromatic medicines is the Papyrus Ebers manuscript written around 2800 BC. Another document, written about 800 years later, mentions "fine oils and choice perfumes." These manuscripts, written while the Great Pyramid was being built, show that frankincense, myrtle, galbanum, and eaglewood were used as medicines during the time of Moses (from the Old Testament) and myrrh was used to treat hay fever. When Tutankhamun's tomb was opened in 1922, thirty-five alabaster jars of perfume were found in his burial chamber and they were still faintly aromatic. All of them were broken or empty and the contents—frankincense and myrrh (highly valued commodities)—stolen (Steele 1992).

IRAQ, FRANCE, SYRIA

One of the earliest documented uses of aromatics dates back 60,000 years to the findings in a burial site of a Neanderthal skeleton found in the land that is now Iraq. The skeleton was found buried with concentrated extracts of yarrow, knapweed, grape hyacinth, mallow, and other plants (Erichsen-Brown 1979). Yarrow is an aromatic herb used in herbal medicine and the essential oil is used in aromatherapy. In France, drawings dating back 17,300 years found in a cave in Lascaux, France, showed medicinal herbs (Ryman 1991). Later, the Cathars would live in this region and become famous for their use of herbal remedies. The Sumerians, who lived in Syria, were sophisticated herbalists. There are records of them using caraway and thyme and pots that could have been used in plant distillation have been found. In the *Epic of Gilgamesh*, a Sumerian poet writes, "There is a plant whose thorns will prick your hand like a rose. If your hands reach that plant you will become a young man again" (Swerdlow 2000).

CHINA

The Great Herbal (Pen Ts'ao) was written by Shen Nung in 2800 BC. It lists 350 plants and many are still being used today. One of them is the herb *Ephedra sinica.* This was one of the herbs found in the Neanderthal grave in Iraq. Huang Ti (Yellow Emperor) wrote the *Huang Ti Nei Ching Su Wen.* The English translation is called *The Yellow Emperor's Classic of Internal Medicine* (Rose 1992). Today, a huge concrete statue of ginseng presides over the state-run herbal market in Anguo, China (3 hours south of Beijing), suggesting how important herbs are in Chinese culture today. The Chinese method of soaking a cloth in herbs (compress) and placing it on the skin indicates how the Chinese have always accepted transdermal delivery—something Western medicine denied for many years. There is a great similarity between Ayurvedic and Chinese medicine, and as early as 1000 BC, China was exchanging herbs with India (Swerdlow 2000).

INDIA

The first Sanskrit medical treatises, *Charaka Samhita* and *Sushrata Sambita,* date back to 2000 BC and describe the use of 700 plants, including aromatics such as ginger, coriander, myrrh, cinnamon, and sandalwood (Swerdlow 2000). The *Charaka Samhita* includes descriptions for the processes of distillation and condensation of volatile oils from plants (Ray & Gupta 1965). Ayurvedic medicine was pushed underground by the Muslim invasion of India in the eleventh and twelfth centuries, and later by the British occupation. The British prohibited the funding of Ayurvedic colleges and clinics. India fought back in 1921 with a document presented to the British government in Madras, India, stating that no Western scientist should think of criticizing Ayurveda until he had learned Sanskrit (Swerdlow 2000). In the last few decades Ayurveda has become popular again, in part because of the influence of Deepak Chopra, MD (Chopra 1991). Ayurveda has a strong spiritual base, and in northern India, Ayurvedic physicians are known as holy men. Interestingly, traditional Indian shamans were known as *perfumeros* and were healers who used the scents of aromatic plants (Steele 1991). Today, aromatics remain an important part of Ayurvedic medicine.

TIBET

Tibetan medicine is based on the *Four Tantras of Tibetan Medicine,* written in the eighth century. This whole medical system is similar to Chinese medicine and focuses on the relationship of the person with the environment and society in which the person lives, rather than the disease. Tibetan medicine has traditionally used aromatic herbs, often in steam. Prescriptions are usually complex mixtures such as *Aquilaria A* that contains clove, cardamom, sandalwood, and myrrh (Lawless 1992).

GREECE

Theophrastus was a pupil of Aristotle and inherited the botanical garden at Athens that Aristotle had planted (Stearn 1998). In 300 BC, Theophrastus wrote *Enquiry into Plants,* in which he described specific uses for aromatics. At that time doctors who used aromatic unctions were called iatralyptes. One aromatic formula, called *Kyphi,* contained 16 different ingredients. Kyphi was used as an antiseptic, an antidote to poison, soothed the skin and also "lulled one to sleep, allayed anxiety and brightened dreams." It was Theophrastus, later called the "father of botany" (Ryman 1991), who discovered the perfume of jasmine was stronger at night. Hippocrates (who lived around 460 BC) is recognized as the father of medicine. He wrote "aromatic baths are useful in the treatment of female disorders, and would often be useful for the other conditions too" (Chadwick & Mann 1983). He seemed to understand the principles of psychosomatic disorders when he wrote, "In order to cure the human body it is necessary to have knowledge of the whole" (Lawless 1994). Hippocrates also knew aromatics could have important antibacterial properties, and when an epidemic of plague broke out he urged the people to use aromatic plants to protect themselves and stop the spread of the disease. He also wrote, "the growth of plants forms an excellent parallel to the study of medicine" (Chadwick & Mann 1983).

Greek army doctors traveled with large supplies of herbal remedies. A manual written for the Emperor Claudius in 43 AD gives detailed instructions on how to recognize plants abroad, pick, and pack them.

Dioscorides (Pedanius Dioscorides) lived around 100 AD. He wrote *De Materia Medica.* This foundation of Western herbal medicine covers 700 plants that were in use including aromatics like basil, verbena, cardamom, rose, rosemary, and garlic (Holmes 1993). The plants are carefully drawn, described, and the contraindications listed (Griggs 1981). Dioscorides suggests that tarragon *(Artemesia dracunculus)* might be useful for cancer, for gangrene, to produce abortions, and to protect against viper bites. Tarragon was later used by a number of Native American tribes such as the Chippewa people, who decocted the leaf or root for "stoppage of periods…A decoction of the whole plant was taken as an aid in difficult labor (Moerman 1998, p. 95).

When Claudios Galenos (known in English as Galen) was appointed personal physician to Emperor Marcus (130 to 200 AD) he introduced a system for identifying plants (Griggs 1981). He also described a plant's energetic profile, which is similar to Chinese and Ayurvedic approaches. This approach is continued today with contemporary writers (Holmes 1993; Mojay 2000). Unfortunately, many of the 500 works he wrote were destroyed when his clinic in Rome burned down.

Galen described a disease in terms of temperature and moisture thus laying the cornerstone of modern pathophysiology (Lawless 1994).

During the immediate pre-Christian era, Jewish women in Essene communities infused wine with myrrh and frankincense (for their anesthetic effects) to offer those being tortured. The early Christian era considered aromatics to be pagan because they could heighten sensual pleasure. In 529 AD, Pope Gregory the Great passed a law banning all *Materia Medica*. The school of philosophy at Athens closed down, and the works of Galen and Hippocrates were smuggled to Syria. There the works of Galen, Hippocrates, and Dioscorides were translated into Arabic by Hunayn ibn Ishaq al'Ibadi. He was paid with his weight in gold.

ARABIA

In the prologue to *The Canterbury Tales,* Chaucer describes four Arabic physicians. Arabic doctors were considered the greatest medical authorities in the fourteenth century. One of Chaucer's physicians is an historical figure known as Ibn Sina—later called Avicenna (Tschanz 1997). New aromatics such as senna, camphor, tamarind, nutmeg, and cloves were introduced. Rose and orange-blossom water were used to make medicines taste more palatable. Arabic physicians were familiar with the anesthetic effect of inhaled henbane and they used topical sugar to staunch bleeding. (Sugar promotes new cell growth by drying the bed of the wound and dehydrating the bacteria there.) This practice is sometimes still used today (Swerdlow 2000).

By the third century AD, Alexandria had become a center for aromatic medicine. At the start of the ninth century, the first private apothecary shops opened in Baghdad. Medicines were manufactured and distributed commercially to physicians and pharmacists who dispensed them to the public as pills, tinctures, suppositories, and inhalants.

UZBEKISTAN

Abd Allah ibn Sina (980–1037) was born in what is now called Bukhara in Uzbekistan. His name was later westernized into Avicenna. Ibn Sina was to the Arabic world what Aristotle was to the Greeks. He was a child prodigy: a scholar who at the age of 10 could recite the entire Koran and who went on to excel in medicine, poetry, math, physics, and philosophy. When he was 20, ibn Sina was appointed court physician. He wrote more than 20 medical texts including the *Canon of Medicine,* which remained a standard medical textbook until the sixteenth century (Lawless 1994). The *Canon* lists 760 medicinal plants and the drugs that can be derived from them. Ibn Sina also laid out the basic rules of clinical drug trials, principles that are still followed today (Tschanz 1997).

Ibn Sina is thought to have invented an apparatus for distilling essential oils called an *alembic.* During the tenth century many classic texts were translated from Arabic to Latin, and ibn Sina's *Canon of Medicine* first appeared in Europe in the twelfth century. It is interesting that Constantinus Africus and Gerard of Cremorna (who translated the text together) came from two different worlds—Arabic and Christian. The joint project was possible because the two scholars lived in towns close to the border dividing the Arabic and Christian worlds at that time. Ibn Sina's portrait still hangs in the great hall of the School of Medicine at the University of Paris, and Dante Alighieri held him in the same regard as Hippocrates and Galen.

EUROPE

By the thirteenth century, "the perfumes of Arabia" mentioned by Shakespeare had spread to Europe. Bad odors were thought to harbor disease (interestingly *malaria* literally translated means *bad air*), and being surrounded by pleasant odors was supposed to give protection against disease, especially the plague. Physicians wore birdlike masks containing aromatics to protect themselves (Boeckl 2000). They also carried plague torches (fragrant herbs and aromatic resins burning in a tiny brazier at the top of a long stick) and sprinkled houses affected by disease with aromatic waters like eau de cologne (Stoddart 1990).

Glovemakers in London became licensed to impregnate their wares with essential oils, and legend has it this is why so many glovemakers and perfumers survived the Great Plague. Scent boxes and pomanders containing solid perfumes (which originated in the East) became popular among the aristocracy. During this time the Abbess of Bingen, St. Hildegarde, wrote four books on medicinal plants. By the sixteenth century, many Europeans had written their own collective works on herbs and aromatics. With the Renaissance and subsequent world exploration, many spices were added to Europe's knowledge of herbs. Cocoa *(Theobroma cacao)* was discovered in South America and tea tree *(Melalauca alternifolia)* in Australia.

NATIVE AMERICANS

Some tribes of Native Americans treated wounds with a tree gum, for example, from the fir tree *(Abies balsamea L.)*. They treated dysentery and other diseases with cedar leaves, and they used sweat lodges to promote spiritual healing. Native Americans also used narcotic plants such as water hemlock *(Cicuta maculata)* in topical applications, vigorously scratching the skin until it bled before applying the herb. Native American (NA) medicine has produced many plant remedies such as Black cohosh root *(Cimicifuga racemosa)* for musculoskeletal pain, headache and as an aid for labor and hormonal imbalances (Low Dog & Riley 2001) and witch hazel *(Hamamelis virginiana)* decoction of prepared twig bark for sore throat, colds, pain, dysentery and to purify blood (Liebster 2014). NA medicine is regaining the respect it held in the nineteenth century and NA traditional healers are becoming more respected for the depth, history, and sophistication of their medicine (Erichsen-Brown 1979). One of its advocates, Tieraona Low Dog, MD (Lakota tribe), an eminent physician and herbalist, served on the advisory Council for the National Institutes of Health National Center for Complementary and Alternative Medicine (NCCAM) until 2010.

FOURTEENTH CENTURY TO PRESENT DAY

Paracelsus was born Philippus Aureolus Theophrastus Bombast von Hohenheim in 1493 near Zurich, Switzerland. Although his father was a physician, it is unclear whether Paracelsus ever completed his medical training. He wandered from university to university and was something of a rebel. He learned herbal medicine from the Tartars in Asia and he learned anatomy from executioners. While he was on his travels he changed his name to Paracelsus. He was a controversial figure who angered the orthodox medical community by burning Avicenna's work at a public bonfire in Basel, Switzerland. Paracelsus was frustrated by what he felt were old principles. He questioned Galen's work and thought the plethora of herbal manuals in circulation were written by "quacks" who abused sick people's lack of knowledge, and were only after quick money. He wanted something innovative and new. He became the subject of legends, some suggesting he had magic powers and could conjure a hurricane with a twirl of his hat (Swerdlow 2000).

Paracelsus believed the way forward was to isolate an active ingredient from a plant. He believed isolating the active ingredient would enhance the medicine's strength and increase its safeness. He used mercury, iron, sulfur, and antimony as well as herbs. Although Paracelsus remained fascinated by alchemy all his life (Griggs 1981), he was also a strong believer in the doctrine of signatures: that plants indicate the organ or system of the body they can help by their shape or the place where they grow. Paracelsus wrote 14 books and was very successful.

Although a specific action of a plant may appear to depend on a single chemical constituent, isolating it may not make the effect more active or safer. However, plants have their own synergistic action that is irreplaceable. In the plant world, the sum of the parts really does add up to more than the total (Mills 1991). If the most active constituent is removed and applied in isolation, it may have a different effect or negative side effects. The ability of one part of a plant to "switch off" negative properties of another part is sometimes called *quenching* (Tisserand 2013). For example, isolated citral (an aldehyde found in lemongrass) produces a more severe sensitization reaction at a lower concentration than the complete essential oil, which contains a higher percentage of citral (Api & Isola 2000).

This concept is further demonstrated by separating all the active ingredients of an essential oil, then recombining them. They will not necessarily produce the same effect as the complete essential oil (or herb). Therefore, Paracelsus could be regarded as the first medical pharmacologist.

Descartes (1596–1650) declared that man was a machine thus mind and body had no relationship to each another. Descartes' philosophy was *"cognito, ergo sum,"* or "I think, therefore I am" (Cook 1978). The idea that an aromatic could have an effect on the body via the brain was discarded until the eighteenth century, when a physician called Gaub suggested that "bodily diseases may often be alleviated or cured by the mind and emotions" (Lawless 1994). Today we know that smell affects the mind (Littrell 2008). Also, the mind is not an isolated, single organ, but connected to every cell in our body and affects the way a person feels (Pert 1997). Today we know that how we feel in mind, body, and spirit has a direct impact on our health—our inner terrain is vital to our health (Libster 2009).

UNITED KINGDOM

William Turner (1520–1568) was one of the earliest documented male herbalists in England—prior to him there had been many women nurses and midwives who used herbs. A Cambridge graduate, he believed in the doctrine of signatures and named many plants, such as lungwort and liverwort, to indicate their use. At this time, qualifying to become a physician took 10 years. Shakespeare's son-in-law John Hall called himself a physician, although he had only a Master of Arts degree. However, this did not stop him from purchasing 300 plants, "practicing" medicine, and leaving notes from 178 different cases. One of his patients was the Earl of Compton who lived 40 miles away: several days' journey by horseback (Swerdlow 2000).

During Shakespeare's time, midwives, apothecaries (pharmacists), and physicians prescribed medicines. In an attempt to control the situation, the British Parliament introduced new laws in 1512 that controlled the prescription and sale of medicines. Six years later, the Royal College of Physicians was established in London.

However, the seventeenth century is remembered as the golden era for herbal medicine. Nicholas Culpeper published his *Complete Herbal* in 1660. Essential oils were widely used in "mainstream" medicine. In William Salmon's *The Compleat English Physician,* essential oils of cinnamon, lavender, lemon, clove, and rue are listed with others in a recipe to "cheer and comfort all the spirits, natural, vital and animal" (Tisserand 1979). In 1770, the British Parliament passed a law to protect men from the "guiles of perfumed women" who might trick them into matrimony as the "witchcraft of scent could manipulate their mind" (Watson 2000). The United States followed with a paper published in the *New York Medical Journal* on the "connections of the sexual apparatus with the ear, nose and throat" suggesting perfume was a conscious attempt to "stimulate lecherous thoughts" (Dabney 1913). I wonder what they would think of modern perfume advertising!

In 1992, the first scientific evaluation of essential oils was published in William Whitla's *Materia Medica and Therapeutics.* The industrial and scientific revolutions followed. During the next two centuries scores of essential oils were analyzed. It was thought important to identify and isolate therapeutic components of plants (just as Paracelsus had advocated). In the late 1890s specific components such as geraniol and citronellol were identified, and in 1868 William Henry Perkin announced the synthesis of coumarin.

MODERN DRUG DEVELOPMENT

Synthetic copies of perfumes and aromatics began to appear, and the era of modern drug development dawned. The salicylate in willow bark (*Salix alba*) became aspirin. Foxglove *(Digitalis purpurea)* became digoxin. Despite research on the therapeutic effects of essential oils by Cadeac and Meunier in France and Gatti and Cajola in Italy, essential oils and herbal medicine lost out to the profits of synthetic drugs. With the

1930 partnership of Rockefeller in the United States and Faben in Germany, the pet-rochemical pharmaceutical industry became a major economic and political force.

The 1910 Flexner report on the nation's medical schools (funded by the Carnegie Foundation) changed medical training in the United States and homeopathic and naturopathic medical schools in the United States were mostly eliminated. Herbal medicine, including the use of aromatics, was excluded from medical school curricula. Drug companies became major underwriters of medical colleges in the United States, the main funders of the American Medical Association and 90% of all medical research. It is encouraging that medical training in the United States is currently under review as it is thought to be 'incomplete' and does not produce a 'humane' physician (Doukas et al 2010).

RENAISSANCE OF AROMATHERAPY

The renaissance of aromatherapy began in France. It was a clinical affair and initially involved only three people: a chemist (Gattefossé), a physician (Valnet) and a nurse (Maury).

Rene-Maurice Gattefossé: Chemist

Gattefossé (1881–1950) discovered aromatherapy through an accident. In 1910, while working in his laboratory, he was burnt in an explosion. He ran outside and rolled on the grass to extinguish the flames. A few days later the wounds became infected with gas gangrene but "one rinse of essential oil of lavender (*Lavandula angustifolia*)" stopped the infection (Tisserand 1989). Impressed, Gattefossé dedicated his life to researching essential oils. Many of his patients were soldiers wounded in the trenches of World War I. He used essential oils such as thyme, chamomile, clove, and lemon. Until World War II, those essential oils were used to disinfect wounds and to sterilize surgical instruments (Ryman 1991). Gattefossé is thought to be one of the first people to use the word *aromatherapy*. He discovered that essential oils take between 30 minutes and 12 hours to be absorbed completely by the body after being applied topically. His work *Aromatherapie: The Essential Oils—Vegetable Hormones* (giving detailed medical case studies performed by various physicians) was published in France in 1937. The manuscript was discovered by Jeanne Rose, translated into English by Louise Davies, edited by Robert Tisserand and published in 1993.

Gattefossé's son, Henri-Marcel, took his father's interests into the pharmaceutical world and modern drug development. However, he himself self-medicated with essential oils (Moyrand 2010) and continued to research essential oils. In 2008, The Gateffossé Foundation was established by Sophie Gattefossé–Moyrand to pay tribute to her grandfather. In 2010, the 44th Journée Galéniques (annual meeting held at Gattefossé's home) was dedicated to the future of aromatherapy in healthcare. I was honored to be the closing speaker. My talk was entitled "Is there a role for essential oils in current and future healthcare?" (Buckle 2010).

Throughout World War II, French physicians used essential oils on infected wounds and as a treatment for gangrene. Perhaps the course of aromatic medicine would have been different if Alexander Fleming had not discovered a piece of moldy bread that led to the manufacture of penicillin. With the emergence of manufactured antibiotics—full of promise, profit, and easy availability—essential oils fell by the wayside.

JEAN VALNET: MEDICAL DOCTOR

Valnet (1920–1995), an army physician who was awarded the Légion d'Honneur for his bravery in the resistance in World War II and worked at the Military Special school of Saint-Cyr, spent much of his life researching aromatherapy. His publication *Aromatherapie* (Valnet 1969) was the first aromatherapy book written by a doctor: full of case studies and citing numerous references. During his time in Indochina, when he was commander of an advanced surgical unit, Valnet used essential oils with the full approval of his superiors. However, despite impressive results, when he returned to France he found the orthodox medical community unhappy with his use of "unconventional medicine" and they tried to strike him from the general medical list. Fortunately, some of his patients were high-ranking government officials, including the Minister of Health, so this did not happen (Scott 1993-1994). Valnet's book has been translated into many languages. It was translated into English *(The Practice of Aromatherapy)* by Libby Houston and Robin Campbell, edited by Robert Tisserand and published in 1982. When Valnet was interviewed by Christine Scott for the *International Journal of Aromatherapy* in 1993, he said "it is not necessary to be a doctor to use aromatherapy. But one has to know the power of essential oils in order to avoid accidents and incidents" (Scott 1993-1994).

MARGUERITE MAURY: NURSE

Marguerite Maury's life was initially one of tragedy. Born in Austria, she married and had her first child while still a teenager. Sadly her son died from meningitis when he was only 2 years old. Shortly afterward, her husband was killed in action, and his death was closely followed by her father's suicide. Keen to make a new start, Marguerite decided to move to France and train as a nurse. While working in France as a surgical assistant, she met and married Dr. Maury. He shared her fascination with alternative approaches to medicine, and together they formed a cohesive and inspirational team.

Marguerite Maury classified the use of essential oils into various clinical departments: surgery, radiology, dermatology, gynecology, general medicine, psychiatry, spa treatment, physiotherapy, sports, and cosmetics. She won two international prizes for her research on essential oils and the skin, and her book *Le Capital Jeunesse* was published in 1961 and translated into English three years later. She developed a unique method of applying essential oils to the skin with massage and established the first aromatherapy clinics in Paris, Great Britain, and Switzerland where she studied the rejuvenating properties of essential oils on the skin. Her students included Micheline Arcier and Daniel Ryman.

Gattefossé, Valnet, and Maury were pioneers of modern aromatherapy, and there were two now-famous names waiting in the wings to follow. Tisserand's ground-breaking work in translating the first two books on aromatherapy (and later writing his own books and establishing training) led the way. Shirley Price followed and her book *Aromatherapy for Health Professionals* helped to make aromatherapy into a recognized therapy in England and sparked the interest of the medical and nursing community. I remember reviewing parts of the first edition so many years ago now! Many researchers followed. Of particular note are Guenther, Duke, and Lawrence in the United States; Belaiche in France; Deans and Svoboda in the UK; and Penfold and Carson in Australia, all of whom wrote extensively about the clinical use of essential oils. Today, there is a wealth of information and sufficient evidence to suggest the medicine of the future could be a sweet-smelling one.

AROMATHERAPY TODAY

Some people believe aromatherapy means just inhalation. Others believe aromatherapy means aromatherapy massage. Physicians in France define aromatherapy to mean the inclusion of essential oils via oral, rectal, and vaginal routes. Clearly, different levels of types of training are required and need to be relevant to the student.

HERBAL MEDICINE

Although aromatherapy is a science and practice that is distinct from herbal medicine, the study and application of essential oils in herbal medicine is not. Essential oils are included in the botany curriculum in herbal medicine courses and programs. Most herbalists practice with whole plant applications rather than plant constituents, such as essential oils. However, it is not unusual for a medicinal grade essential oil to be produced or utilized in the practice of a traditional or medical herbalist. The herbalist who uses essential oils represents themselves as an herbalist rather than as an aromatherapist.

MIND-BODY MEDICINE

The fragrance of plants such as lemon balm (*Melissa officinalis*) holds, as Carl Jung knew, an important place in contemporary holistic mental health and mind-body care. Mind-body practitioners often partner with aromatherapists, or utilize simple applications of essential oils in practice in creating healing environments that demonstrate the ways plants can lift the spirits of their clients.

MASSAGE AND BODYWORK

Aromatherapy is not part of massage or bodywork training but the use of essential oils in the preparation of massage oils and lotions may be included in initial training programs and in continuing education courses.

ENERGY MEDICINE

Aromatherapy does not really fit here either, so it is hardly surprising that one of the largest surveys on integrative medicine in the United States (Horrigan et al 2012) did not include aromatherapy, even though aromatherapy is used in several of the participating centers. One of the authors explained that aromatherapy was not listed because "not enough centers were using it as an intervention in a clinical proto-col." However, the survey did find that aromatherapy products were sold in nearly 40% of centers surveyed.

Perhaps the many different methods of use and absorption and the wide span of symptoms that aromatherapy can address (depression to MRSA) have slowed the integration of aromatherapy into a clinical setting. Clearly, there is work to be done to get clinical aromatherapy accepted as a modality in its own right. Patients say it works. Nurses and doctors say it works. Other health professionals say it works. The clinical evidence may be mainly anecdotal, although the body of published research is growing rapidly. However, if something works, people use it. Good medicine is often based on practice-based evidence (PBE) rather than evidence-based practice (EBP). Published research is important, but it often lags behind practice. Clinical aromatherapy is effective, safe, and pleasant to use and receive; has few side effects; and is cost efficient. It also makes our hospitals nicer places to work in. A major collaborative effort is needed to bring together all clinical information so a "clinical pattern" can become clear. That pattern will be the basis for future research. The proposed template for such an effort is in the appendix.

Smell is now recognized as one of the most important senses in humans and a key determinant in behavior (Hoover 2010; Auffarth 2013; Croy et al 2013; Hoskison 2013). However, aromatherapy is not about smelling **anything**. The defi-nition of aromatherapy specifically states "the use of essential oils" (Tissserand & Young 2013, p. 2), (Price & Price 2012, p. 3). Plants can synthesize two types of oil: fixed oils—for example, olive or walnut oil, and essential oils—highly volatile from aromatic plants such as rose or lavender. Essential oils are either steam distillates from aromatic plants or obtained through expression (abrading) the peel of citrus fruit. Solvent extracted materials such as absolutes, resinoids, or carbon dioxide extracted oils are not classified as essential oils.

TYPES OF AROMATHERAPY

Gattefossé first coined the word *aromatherapy* and as seen above, the emergence of aromatherapy from France in the 1930s was clearly clinical. However, I think today there are three types of aromatherapy: aesthetic, clinical, and holistic.

AESTHETIC AROMATHERAPY

Aesthetic aromatherapy is about using an essential oil for the pleasure of its aroma. The beautiful smell of roses or orange blossom can make us all smile with delight. The Duchess of Cambridge chose orange blossom candles to perfume Westminster abbey on her wedding day (29 April 2011) and add olfactory pleasure to the occasion of her marriage to Prince William. Essential oils are still used in some expensive perfumes (such as Joy by Jean Patou) but many have been replaced by cheaper syn-thetics. A specific "British smell" was required for the bouquets of flowers handed to medalists at the 2012 London Olympic games. The bouquets chosen for the games included roses, lavender, rosemary, and mint (Cawley 2012).

CLINICAL AROMATHERAPY

Clinical aromatherapy is about targeting a specific clinical symptom (e.g., nausea) and measuring the outcome. French aromatherapists Gattefossé and Belaiche each wrote books about clinical aromatherapy from a pharmacist's and physician's point of view, respectively. Although aesthetic aromatherapy may not be part of the remit of a nurse, occupational therapist, physical therapist, or physician, clinical aromatherapy clearly is. Clinical aromatherapy can be subdivided into Medical aromatherapy (this includes oral use) and Nursing aromatherapy (this covers internal skin use but not oral use). In France, Germany, and Switzerland, the oral use of essential oils lies within the remit of physicians.

HOLISTIC AROMATHERAPY

Holistic aromatherapy is the term used by many aromatherapists the world over. Holistic means mind, body, and spirit. Holistic aromatherapy usually involves mixtures of essential oils. For many therapists, aromatherapy may be a simple add-on using a ready-made mixture to relax or energize their client. I have received aromatherapy massages myself in several different countries. The massage was usually great, but the aromatherapy mixture was often a purchased proprietary blend and the therapist knew little, if anything, about the individual essential oils in the mixture. However, there *are* holistic aromatherapists who know a great deal about the essential oils they use and who make up mixtures for individual clients based on the client's individual needs.

REFERENCES

Api A, Isola D. 2000. Quenching of citral sensitization demonstrated in a human repeated insult patch test. *Contact Dermatitis*. 46. (Suppl 4). p 37.

Auffarth B. 2013. Understanding smell. The olfactory stimulus problem. *Neuroscience and Biobehavioural Reviews*. 37(8): 1667–1679.

Boeckl C. 2000. *Images of Plague and Pestilence: Iconography and Iconology*. Truman State University Press. Kirksville, Missouri, USA.

Buckle J. 2010. Aromatherapy: is there a role for essential oils in current and future healthcare? *Bulletin Technique Gattefosse*. 103-2010. p 95–102.

Charaka Samhita: *A Scientific Synopsis*. Ed Ray, P. & Gupta, H. Indian National Science Academy, New Delhi. 1965

Cawley L. BBC News 2012. British smell is key to London 2012 Olympic victory bouquets. http://www.bbc.co.uk/news/uk-england-essex-19160168. Accessed January 8, 2013.

Chadwick J, Mann W (eds.). 1983. *Hippocratic Writings*. Harmondsworth, UK: Penguin Books.

Chopra D. 1991. *Perfect Health: The Complete Mind/Body Guide*. New York: Harmony Books.

Cook C (ed.). 1978. *Pears Cyclopedia*, 87th ed. London: Pelham, B19.

Croy I, Bojanowski V, Hummel T. 2013. Men without a sense of smell exhibit a strongly reduced number of sexual relationships, women exhibit reduced partnership security – a reanalysis of previously published data. *Biological Psychology*. 92(2): 292–294.

Dabney V. 1913. Connections of the sexual apparatus with the ear, nose and throat. *New York Journal of Medicine*. 97, 533.

Doukas D, McCullough L, Wear S. 2010. Re-visioning Flexner: educating physicians to be clinical scientists and humanists. *American Journal of Medicine*. 123(12):1155–1156.

Erichsen-Brown C. 1979. *Medicinal and Other Uses of North American Plants*. New York: Dover Publications.

Griggs B. 1981. *Green Pharmacy*. London: Jill Norman & Hobhouse.

Holmes P. 1993. *The Energetics of Western Herbs*. Vols. 1 and 2. Berkley, CA: Nattrop Publishing.

Hoover K. 2010. Smell with inspiration: the evolutionary significance of olfaction. *American Journal of Physical Anthropology* 143 Suppl 51:63–74.

Horrigan B, Abrams D, Pechura C, 2012. Integrative Medicine in America: How Integrative Medicine is being practices in clinical centers across the United States. *Global Advances in Health & Medicine.* 1(3):16-92.

Hoskison E. 2013. Olfaction, pheremones and life. *J Laryngol Otol.* 127(12):1156–1159.

Lawless J. 1992. *The Encyclopedia of Essential Oils*. Shaftesbury, UK: Element Books.

Lawless J. 1994. *Aromatherapy and the Mind*. London: Thorsons.

Libster M. 2009. Behind the Shield: A perspective on H1N1 from the inner terrain. *Journal of Holistic Nursing* 27: 218–221.

Liebster M. 2014. Personal communication.

Littrell J. 2008. The body-mind connection: not just a theory anymore. *Social Works Health Care.* 46(4):17–37.

Low Dog T, Riley D. 2001. An integrative approach to menopause. *Alternative Therapies in Health and Medicine.* 7(4) 45–55.

Mills S. 1991. *Out of the Earth*. London: Viking Arkana.

Moerman D. 1998. *Native American Ethnobotany*. Timber Press: Portland Oregon.

Mojay G. 2000. *Aromatherapy for Healing the Spirit*. London: Giai Books, Ltd.

Moyrand S. 2010. Foreword. *Bulletin Technique Gattefosse* 103-2010. P 4–5.

Pert C. 1997. *Molecules of Emotion*. New York: Scribner, 304.

Price S, Price L. 2012. *Aromatherapy for Health Professionals*. Churchill Livingstone. London.

Ray P., Gupta H (eds.). 1965. Charaka Samhita: *A Scientific Synopsis*. Indian National Science Academy, New Delhi.

Rose J. 1992. *A history of herbs and herbalism*. In Tierra M (ed.), American Herbalism. Freedom, CA: Crossing Press, 3–32.

Ryman D. 1991. *Aromatherapy*. London: Piatkus.

Scott C. 1993-1994. In profile with Valnet. *International Journal of Aromatherapy.* 5(4) 10–13.

Steele J. 1992. Anthropology of smell and scent in fragrance. In Van Toller S, Dodd G (eds.), *Fragrance: The Psychology and Biology of Perfume*. London: Elsevier Applied Science, 287–302.

Stearn W. 1998. *Botanical Latin*, 4th ed. Portland, OR: Timber Press.

Stoddart D. 1990. *The Scented Ape*. Cambridge, UK: Cambridge University Press, 5.

Swerdlow J. 2000. *Nature's Medicine: Plants That Heal*. Washington, DC: National Geographic Society.

Tisserand R. 1979. The Art of Aromatherapy. Saffron Walden, UK: CW Daniels.

Tisserand R, Young R. 2013. *Essential Oil Safety*. 2nd edition. Churchill Livingstone. P 73.

Tschanz D. 1997. *The Arab Roots of European Medicine*. Aramco World. May/June 20–31.

Valnet J. 1969. *Aromatherapie: Les huiles essentielles hormones vegetales*. Paris: Girardot.

Watson L. 2000. *Jacobson's Organ*. New York: Norton.

Chapter 2

How Essential Oils Work

"A mind that is stretched by a new experience can never go back to its old dimensions."
Oliver Wendell Holmes

CHAPTER ASSETS

HOW ESSENTIAL OILS WORK

The study of how essential oils are absorbed and excreted is called *pharmacokinetics*. Essential oils can be absorbed via olfaction, through the external skin, through the "internal skin" lining of orifices (mouth, vagina, and anus) and via ingestion (Jager et al 1992) (Figure 2-1 and Tables 2-1 and 2-2).

How Essential Oils Are Absorbed

There is published research to show inhaled essential oils can a) affect the human brain or lungs, b) be absorbed through the skin (both internal and external) and c) be absorbed by ingestion. Essential oils contain many different chemical components, and it is these components that are absorbed by the body. Lavender *(Lavandula angustifolia)* essential oil is not found in the bloodstream, but linalyl acetate and linalool (two major components in lavender essential oil) can be found in the bloodstream after inhalation, topical (internal or external) application, or ingestion (Kasper et al 2010).

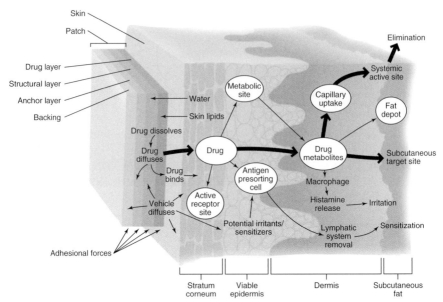

FIGURE 2-1 | How essential oils are absorbed through the skin. (From Clarke S. *Essential Chemistry for Safe Aromatherapy*. Churchill Livingstone. 2002.)

Essential oil components can be absorbed by four routes:
1. Topical: via external skin using massage, 'M' Technique, compress, or bath.
2. Inhaled: directly or indirectly, with or without steam using diffusers, aromastones, fans, humidifiers, aromasticks individual patches, individual packets or nostril clips.
3. Internal: via internal skin using mouthwashes, gargles, douches, pessaries or suppositories.
4. Oral: using gelatin capsules or diluted in honey, alcohol, or dispersant. Each method of application has its own physiologic process, advantages and disadvantages.

Topical Absorption
The Skin
The skin is the largest organ in the body and is a complex membrane, varying from less than a millimeter thick on the eyelid, to approximately 3-mm thick on the back. For many years the skin (stratum corneum) was thought to be a barrier that topically applied drugs, or essential oils, could not penetrate. Now we know that drugs such as acyclovir can reach the basal epidermal cells (Hasler-Nguyen et al 2009). Grégoire et al (2009) developed a model to predict the mass of a chemical absorbed into/through the skin from a cosmetic or dermatological formulation. Autoradiography has demonstrated both a) penetration to the dermis and b) deposition and retention sites within the epidermis, after topical application of drugs (Hayakawi et al 2004). When molecules are small enough, medicines (such as nitroglycerine,

TABLE 2-1 *Some Human Studies of Essential Oils Absorbed Into/Through the External Skin*

Author	Year	Essential Oil	Common Name	Condition
Ballard et al	2002	*Melissa officinalis*	Melissa	Agitation in dementia
Davies	2002	*Mentha × piperita*	Peppermint	Post-herpetic pain
Satchell et al	2002	*Melaleuca alternifolia*	Tea tree	Athletes foot
Dryden et al	2004	*Melaleuca alternifolia*	Tea tree	MRSA skin colonisation
Melli et al	2007	*Mentha × piperita*	Peppermint	Preventing nipple cracks in breast feeding
Matiz et al	2012	*Ocimum basilicum* *Citrus sinensis*	Basil Sweet orange	Acne
Kristiniak et al	2012	*Piper nigrum*	Black Pepper	Ease IV insertion
Hur et al	2012	Mixture*	Mixture*	Menstrual pain

*Clary sage *(Salvia sclarea)*, marjoram *(Origanum majoranum)*, cinnamon *(Cinnamomum zeylanicum)*, ginger *(Zingiber officialis)*, and geranium *(Pelargonium graveolens)*.

TABLE 2-2 *Some Human Studies of Essential Oils Absorbed Through the Internal Skin*

Author	Year	Essential Oil/ Component	Common Name	Condition
Jose et al	2002	*Melaleuca alternifolia*	Tea tree	Oropharyngeal candidiasis in AIDS
Soukoulis & Hirsch	2004	*Melaleuca alternifolia*	Tea tree	Gingivitis
Remberg et al	2004	*Artemisia abrotanum*	Southernwood	Allergic rhinitis
Khosravi et al	2008	*Zataria multiflora*	Iranian Thyme	Vaginal candidiasis
Solsto & Benvenuti	2011	Thymol and eugenol		Bacterial vaginitis Vaginal candidiasis
Joksimovic et al	2011	*Melaleuca alternifolia*	Tea tree	Hemorrhoids

estradiol, progesterone, testosterone, fentanyl, and scopolamine) can be administered transdermally on a continuous basis.

Skin Penetration and Permeation

Two processes are involved in topical absorption: penetration and permeation (Moser et al 2001). Penetration is the actual entry of a substance into and through the skin. Permeation is the subsequent absorption of the substance into the body. Obviously the former is more important if the skin is being treated and the latter if a systemic treatment is sought. The process of penetration and permeation is governed by Ficks First Law (Yu et al 2009). The amount of substance that permeates the skin is related to the a) skin permeability and b) concentration of the substance (Tisserand & Young 2013; Gabbanini et al 2009). If the essential oil is diluted in a substance with lower permeability, its absorption will be reduced. In other words, essential oils diluted in a fixed oil (carrier oil) are absorbed more slowly than undiluted essential oils (Cal 2006). The actual carrier medium can also affect (and to a certain extent inhibit) the concentration of the active ingredients of essential oils. For example, (Cross et al 2006) found the terpinen-4-ol absorption from a 20% solution of tea tree was smaller (1.1 to 1.9%) than from undiluted tea tree (2.4%). Occlusion will enhance penetration and prevent evaporation (Tisserand & Young 2013). Some essential oil components, such as +limonene, can enhance the absorption of other components like α-pinene and β-myrcene (Schmitt et al 2009).

Topical Absorption of Essential Oils

A search on PubMed using the words "essential oil topical absorption" produced 28 hits in January 2014. Essential oils are lipid soluble and many of the components can be absorbed through the skin rapidly. As early as 1997, Fuchs et al reported that carvone, a ketone in essential oils, was found in the bloodstream of a human subject within 10 minutes of a massage. Carvone was also found in the subject's urine. The subject, a 25-year-old woman, wore a mask to avoid inhaling the aroma. Since then, the dermal penetration and absorption of several essential oils such as lemon (Valgimigli et al 2012), eucalyptus (Karpanen et al 2010), rose (Schmitt et al 2010), tea tree (Reichling et al 2006), and juniper (Gavini et al 2005) have been published. Most essential oil constituents are able to cross the skin barrier (stratum corneum) to the epidermis (Tisserand & Young 2013). They can be stored in the epidermis for up to 72 hours, or reach the dermis and from there enter the blood supply. Recent published studies show how components within essential oils such as citronellol and geraniol (Gilpin et al 2010), linalool (Lapczynski et al 2008), and terpinen-4-ol (Cross et al 2006) are absorbed through the skin. A study by Nielsen & Nielsen (2006) found it was the least lipophilic components (i.e., most water soluble) of tea tree, such as terpinen-4-ol and a-terpineol, that most easily penetrated the skin. Bergapten—a component of bergamot *(Citrus bergamia)*—was found in the blood 4 hours after it had been applied to the skin diluted in jojoba oil (Wang & Tso 2002).

Although the topical use of tea tree over the last 80 years has found only mild side effects, tea tree can be toxic if taken orally in higher doses (Hammer et al 2006). This begins to explain the complexity of aromatherapy. Some essential oils are safe to use on the skin but not to take orally. Some essential oils need to be diluted and used with caution on the skin but are safe to inhale undiluted. Much depends on the chemistry of the essential oil. This will be covered in the chemistry chapter. As topically applied essential oil can affect the absorption of topically applied drugs including patch therapy, they should be used on separate parts of the body.

Polarity and Optical Activity

The exact time required for absorption depends on the weight of the molecule and certain physicochemical properties, such as polarity and optical activity

(Jager et al 1992). In simple terms, polarity refers to polar molecules, so called because they have a negative and positive "pole" that attract opposite charges (Bowles 2000). Optical properties refer to the ability of molecules to rotate in polarized light (Williams 1996). Differences in optical rotation may be the only way to differentiate between oils from two species that might otherwise be thought to be the same. For example, in *Boswellia carteri* and *Boswellia sacra*, the different optical rotation values, *B. sacra* (+30.1°) and *B. carterii* (−13.3°), demonstrate a significant difference between oils from the two species (Woolley et al 2012). Optical rotation can affect absorption. Naturally occurring menthol rotates to the left. That is, it is levorotatory (L-menthol or –menthol). Synthetic menthol is either racemic (equal quantities of left and right) or it rotates to the right, dextrorotatory (D-menthol or +menthol). Polarity and optical activity can affect how chemicals (including essential oil components) are absorbed into the body.

Friction, caused by stroking or massage, encourages dilation of blood vessels in the dermis and can increase the absorption of essential oil components (Tisserand & Young 2013). Essential oils are lipid soluble so components within them can gain access to lipid-rich areas of the body (Buchbauer 1993). This lipid solubility enables small molecules within essential oils to cross the blood-brain barrier (BBB) (Tisserand & Young 2013). The BBB contains capillary endothelial cells and astrocytes that prevent many substances in the blood accessing the brain (Brooker 2008). Although some areas of skin are more accessible, all skin is permeable (some more than others) so it is not necessary to give a full-body treatment. Applying essential oils to the feet requires no removal of clothes (apart from shoes and socks). Patients' feet may be more accessible than hands as they rarely have intravenous infusions attached to them. Feet are not highly innervated like the face, nor are they areas of low innervation like the back (Weiss 1979).

Damaged Skin
Caution should be taken when applying essential oils to damaged skin, because damaged skin can be more absorbent and more likely to have adverse reaction (Chiang et al 2012). Damaged skin includes skin affected by systemic disease, dermatological problems, injury, dehydration caused by a cold, dry environment, or the daily use of strong detergents. Stress (either physical or emotional) results in vascular shut-down. Psychologic stress also perturbs the epidermal permeability-barrier homeostasis (Garg et al 2001) suggesting that less essential oil is absorbed during periods of stress. Dilated blood vessels can increase penetration of essential oils except when a patient is sweating and the body is trying to lose heat. As skin ages it becomes thinner, its barrier function becomes diminished and therefore essential oils are absorbed faster.

Massage or The 'M' Technique
In an aromatherapy massage, or the 'M' Technique, most of the essential oil evaporates and is inhaled by the patient. Thus, any effect is from a combination of both the topically applied and the inhaled essential oils. These, plus gentle touch, may allow the patient to relax and breathe deeply. The amount of essential oil absorbed

from a full-body massage ranges between 0.01 and 0.15 mL (Tisserand & Young 2013). Topical absorption can be enhanced with an occlusive dressing. Lapczynski et al (2008) found that topical absorption of linalool increased three times when the skin was occluded. Covering the skin also increases its temperature, protects hydration and avoids evaporation. Topical application of essential oils has several advantages: the oils do not need to be digested, are simple to use, and are excreted slowly. This is the most direct way to treat skin problems, or muscle complaints. There are a few disadvantages. Some essential oils (those containing phenols) can be epidermal irritants. Some may cause sensitivity, or cross-sensitivity to cosmetics or perfumes (Tisserand & Young 2013). and some (those containing furocoumarins) may cause photosensitivity.

Epidermal absorption is an expanding new field and the use of essential oils to enhance or accelerate conventional drug absorption is increasing. Some drug companies are researching essential oils to enhance and/or to accelerate dermal absorption (Fang et al 2004). Other drug companies are researching how solid lipid microparticles (SLPs) can enhance dermal delivery of essential oils (Gavini et al 2005). Finally, many aromatic plants are grown with pesticides. Although gas chromatography might identify this, pesticides can also cause a reaction that has nothing to do with the essential oil. Expressed essential oils from citrus plants are most likely to have high levels of pesticides, so always use organic citrus peel oils.

Topical application of essential oils can be used for the following:
Relieving localized trauma such as bruising, sprains, stings, or burns
Relaxing and warming specific muscles
Cooling specific areas
Relieving neuralgic conditions
As an antiinflammatory
As an antispasmodic
As antiviral, antifungal, or antibacterial agents for skin infections
As a general body relaxant

Topical applications can be given in:
Carrier oil (cold-pressed vegetable oil)
Ointment
Gel
Undiluted in certain circumstances
Bath (sitz, hand, foot, or full)
Compress
Wound irrigation

The amount of an essential oil absorbed through the skin depends (not in any specific order) on the following:
Dilution used
Volume applied
Amount of skin surface covered
Chemistry of essential oil
Choice of carrier (lotion, oil, gel, cream, alcohol, water)

Part of the body used
Temperature of the skin
Integrity of the skin
Heat of the environment
Age of the skin

Inhalation

Inhaling essential oils is the fastest method of getting essential oils into the body. It may also be the oldest method. The word perfume is derived from the Latin *fume* meaning "to smoke." Perfume, spread by heat and smoke, was used in ancient rituals (Watson 2000). When we inhale essential oils, components can travel to the lungs, the brain, or both. Inhalation may be the oldest method of drug use, but it is also being rediscovered by the pharmaceutical industry. One of the latest drugs to be used via olfaction is insulin (Heinemann 2011).

Absorption to the Lungs

The nose has two distinct functions: to warm and filter incoming air and to act as the first part of the olfactory system (Brooker 2008). The lungs have a huge surface area that is intimately connected to the blood system via the alveoli. (Jori et al 1969) found inhaled 1,8-cineole (an oxide also known as eucalyptol found in many species of eucalyptus and several other essential oils) had a measurable effect on the lungs at very low concentrations. Inhaled 1,8-cineole is an effective antitussive (Takaishi et al 2012) and expectorant (Begrow 2012). Inhaled essential oils can be used to treat fungal, bacterial, and viral bronchial infections in situ (Ben-Ayre et al 2010).

Absorption to the Brain

Odors can affect our brains by influencing the production of endorphins and noradrenaline. Each species has an olfactory repertoire unique to the genetic makeup of that species (Hoover 2010). Olfaction is one of the most primal senses in the mammalian brain (Arisi et al 2012). The olfactory receptor gene family is the largest in the mammalian genome comprising 1% of all genes (Hoover 2010). Olfactory dysfunction has been pathologically linked to depression, neurodegenerative disorders and obesity (Hoover 2010) and sexual malfunction (Croy et al 2013).

Smell is a chemical reaction; receptors in the brain respond to chemicals (odor molecules) within the essential oil. As a person breathes in, these odor molecules move up behind the bridge of the nose and attach to the cilia of olfactory sensory receptor neurons within the olfactory epithelium (Figure 2-2 and Table 2-3). The olfactory epithelium sends axons through the olfactory nerve to the olfactory bulb (Arisi et al 2012). The olfactory bulb connects to brain structures such as the piriform cortex, amygdala, entorhinal cortex, striatum and hippocampus. These structures play an important part in odor recognition, social interaction, sexual behavior, emotional responses, learning, and memory (Arisi et al 2012).

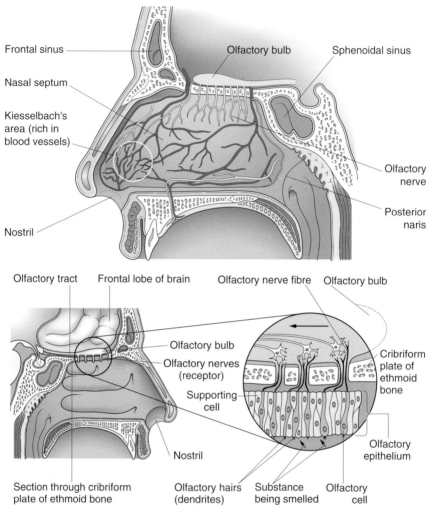

FIGURE 2-2 | How essential oils are absorbed through the nose.

Olfactory receptors are extremely sensitive and can be stimulated by very subtle (and sometimes subliminal) scents (Hummel et al 2013). Different odors bind to distinct arrays of receptors. This allows people to discriminate between more than 10,000 odors, even though there are only about 1000 odor receptors. Neurons in the olfactory epithelium are being constantly replaced (Nickell et al 2012) so it is surprising that olfactory receptors can become easily fatigued when odors seem less obvious. Air flows through the nostrils at different rates because of turbinate swelling (Sobel et al 2000). Every few hours, the nostril, taking in more air, switches to the other one. Odors breathed through the left or right nostril may have different effects because the nasal cavities and olfactory pathways up to the level of

TABLE 2-3 *Some Human Studies of Essential Oils Absorbed Through the Nose*

Author	Year	Essential Oil	Common Name	Condition
Norris & Dwyer	2005	*Mentha piperita*	Peppermint	Daytime sleepiness
Kritsidima et al	2008	*Lavandula angustifolia*	Lavender	Dental anxiety
Toda & Morimoto	2008	*Lavandula angustifolia*	Lavender	Salivary stress markers
Komori et al	2006	Mixture*	Mixture*	Drug addiction
Stringer & Donald	2011	*Mentha piperita* *Citrus limon*	Peppermint Lemon	Chemo-induced nausea
Jimbo et al	2012	*Commiphora myrrha* *Santalum album*	Myrrh Sandalwood	NIRS brain blood flow
Hunt et al	2012	Mixture[†]	Mixture[†]	Post op nausea
Varney & Buckle	2012	Mixture[‡]	Mixture[‡]	Burnout
Cordell & Buckle	2013	*Piper nigrum* *Angelica archangelica*	Black pepper Angelica	Nicotine withdrawal

*Sandalwood *(Santalum album)*, juniper *(Juniperus communis)*, rose *(Rosa damascena)*, and orris root.
[†]Aniseed *(Pimpinella anisum)*, fennel *(Foeniculum vulgare* var *dulce)*, Roman chamomile *(Anthemis nobilis)*, peppermint *(Mentha piperita)*.
NIRS, Near infrared spectroscopy.

the anterior commissure are completely separate. In one study, 17 out of 20 participants identified l-carvone differently, depending on which nostril was dominant (Walter et al 1964). Interestingly, sharks work out the direction of their prey by inter-nostril differences in odorant time of arrival (Arzi & Sobel 2010).

The Limbic System

The limbic system (LS) is the oldest part of the human brain, supposedly having evolved first, and is vital for normal human functioning. In lower vertebrates it is called the *smell brain,* because these animals depend on their sense of smell for survival. The LS is a complex inner ring of brain structures below the cerebral cortex, arranged into 53 regions and 35 associated tracts (Watts 1975). The main structures in the LS are the amygdala, hippocampus, anterior thalamus, and hypothalamus (Brooker 2008). As early as 1923, Gatti and Cajola noted that odors produced an immediate effect on respiration, pulse, and blood pressure, and concluded that odors had a profound effect on the central nervous system. Aromas have instant psychologic and physiologic effects (Hinton 2004), and sometimes just thinking about a smell can be as powerful as actually smelling it (Betts 1996). The amygdala and hippocampus are two of the most important parts of the limbic system associated with smell.

The Amygdala

The amygdala is an almond-shaped group of subcortical nuclei located under the surface of the front medial portion of the temporal lobe (Brooker 2008). It is thought to play a pivotal role in processing emotion, the formation of emotional memory and emotional response (Arisi 2012). In mammals, γ-aminobutyric acid (GABA) transmission in the amygdala is particularly important for controlling levels of fear and anxiety (Heldt et al 2012). People with obsessive compulsive disorder (OCD) have altered amygdala function, as shown by functional magnetic resonance imaging (fMRI) (Via et al 2014). The amygdala also plays an important role in controlling aggression (Pawliczek et al 2013). Some odors can arouse emotion (Kadohisa 2013). Inhaled lavender *(Lavandula angustifolia)* had a calming effect on the amygdala of rats, similar to chlordiazepoxide—a benzodiazepine, but weaker and more restricted (Shaw et al 2011).

The Hippocampus

The hippocampus is associated with learning and memory (Arisi 2012). There are three types of memory: semantic (facts and concepts), episodic (recollection of events), and spatial (recognition). The hippocampus is thought to be the storage area for new experiences before they become permanent memories stored in the cerebral cortex. The hippocampus is particularly vulnerable to ischemia, Alzheimer's disease, and epilepsy (Hatanpaa et al 2014). A stroke can affect memory, but only if it causes bilateral damage to the hippocampus. Some odors can help recall memories (Kadohisa 2013).

Smell and Brain Imaging

The effect of odors on the brain has been "mapped" using fMRI (Yousem et al 2013). This study found different responses to aromas between male and female subjects. fMRI has also shown that odors have an effect on the brain even if the person is anosmic or has congenital hyposmia, no or reduced ability to smell and detect odors, respectively (Henkin & Levy 2002). Odors can also have an effect even if they are subliminal (Hummel et al 2013; Lorig 2012). In earlier research Lorig et al (1990) first mapped the positive mood change effects of subliminal vanilla using EEG. Henkin & Levy (2001) later mapped the effect of imagined smell—in this case peppermint and banana—using fast low angle shot fMRI. Phantom smell (phantosmia) can also be revealed using fMRI (Henkin et al 2000).

Pheromones

Pheromones are subliminal odors that are detected by the vomeronasal organ (VNSO). The VNSO is connected through the vomeronasal nerve to the accessory olfactory bulb (AOB), from where information is sent mainly to amygdala (Arisi 2012). However, there is sufficient evidence that the olfactory epithelium can also respond to pheromones (Wysocki & Preti 2004; Hagino-Yamagishi 2008). This means the perception and interpretation of pheromones is far more complex than previously was thought because "second-messenger pathways" and neural circuits are used by each receptor family for pheromone perception (Hagino-Yamagishi 2008). Further research suggests male pheromones could play an important role in female reproductive success (Mak et al 2007).

APPLICATIONS

1) Inhalation
Inhalation can be direct (to a single patient) or indirect (to a room of people).

Direct Inhalation
No Steam *using aromasticks, aromapatches, aromapackets, cotton balls, aroma ribbons*

   Aromasticks. Drop four drops carrier oil (jojoba or grapeseed) to top, bottom and each side of wick to lock aroma.

   Drop 15 to 20 drops essential oil onto wick and insert wick into inhaler.

   Press flat plastic disc to seal and push firmly into place.

   Screw cap to secure inhaler for storage.

   Label contents with a small adhesive sticker.

   To use, unscrew and remove cover. Place top of inhaler just inside one nostril (blocking the other one) and inhale for sinus, nausea, insomnia problems etc. Repeat in other nostril. Alternatively, place in the mouth and inhale for sore throat and nicotine withdrawal. Use as needed. Replace cover when not in use. See the appendix for recommended suppliers.

   Aromapatches. These can be purchased blank so specific essential oil/s can be added. Or the patch can contain proprietary single essential oils or mixtures. Apply to skin of patient, preferably to collar bone so essential oils can evaporate upwards. See the appendix for recommended suppliers.

   Aromapackets. These can be purchased complete with tested mixtures for symptoms such as nausea, insomnia, curbing appetite, helping concentration. Open packet and breathe in several times holding small opening to nostrils. Close packet. See the appendix for recommended suppliers.

   Cotton balls. Add one to five drops of essential oil/s to a cotton ball and inhale for 5 to 10 minutes. Repeat as necessary.

   Aroma ribbons. This can be attached to the bedclothes of children or adults for an easily applied sleeping or comfort aroma. Cut off a 1-inch piece of ribbon and attach it to the mattress or pillow with a diaper pin. **Caution: Ensure that the pin is secure and that a child cannot put the ribbon in his or her mouth.**

Direct Inhalation with Steam
Add one to five drops of essential oil to a bowl of steaming water. Place a towel over the patient's head and ask him/her to inhale for 10 minutes. Remember to ask the patient to close his/her eyes and remove spectacles. Remove contact lenses before inhalation.

   Caution: Avoid this procedure with the elderly, confused, very young, or infirm.

Indirect Inhalation

1) Room Fresheners

Add one to five drops of essential oil to a bowl of hot water and place in a safe space. The warmth of the water gradually allows the essential oils to evaporate with the water. This is excellent in air-conditioned facilities where the atmosphere may be dry.

2) Burners

Burners usually have a small candle that heats a container suspended above. Fill container with water and float one to five drops of essential oil on top. The water stops the essential oil from burning and leaving a yellow, sticky residue. **Caution: Keep away from children and pets.**

3) Fans

Fans can be battery or electrically operated and come with a number of small, absorbent pads. Add one to five drops to the pad, place in the fan, and switch on. Inexpensive spare pads can be made by cutting incontinence pads or pantyliners into the correct small, square size.

4) Humidifiers

Humidifiers can be purchased in most drug stores. Fill the container with water. Place essential oils on a tissue and put the tissue in the direct pathway of the exiting steam. Do not float the essential oil on top of the water inside the humidifier because it will not come out with the steam, but will remain floating on the water. This is an excellent method for treating croup and asthma.

5) Diffusers

Diffusers are electric and some of the best are ultrasonic. They do not heat the essential oils and deliver micron-sized essential oil droplets. Please see the appendix for recommended supplier.

6) Nebulizers

Nebulizers are electrical units with small, glass attachments into which drops of undiluted essential oil are placed. Most nebulizers use no heat. They can be fragile and noisy. Avoid with thick, viscous essential oils like vetiver. **Caution: Avoid overdosing with essential oils.**

7) Spritzer Sprays (essential oils in water)

Spritzers are excellent for hot flashes or fatigue. Keep one in the fridge! **Caution: Remember to shake before you use and avoid spraying on plants.**

8) Aromastones

Aromastones are small ceramic holders (with an electric plug) that gently warm essential oil.

Inhaled Essential Oils Can Be Used For:

Upper and lower respiratory tract infections
Hay fever, sinusitis
Headache
Asthma
Prevention of cross-infection
Depression, fatigue, nausea
Insomnia
Nicotine or drug withdrawal
Posttraumatic stress

2) Internal

The internal skin route (using the inner skin of the mouth, throat, rectum, or vagina) is an extension of the external skin route and is very relevant to nursing or medical care. Mouthwashes, gargles, vaginal douches, creams, pessaries, and suppositories are excellent methods of getting essential oils directly to the problem area.

Mouthwashes and Gargles

Lister discovered thymol, a component found in essential oils, and a famous mouthwash was named after him—Listerine. Listerine contains several essential oil components: thymol, menthol, and eucalyptol. Mouthwashes and/or gargles containing essential oils or their components are excellent for dental issues (Sharma et al 2010), mouth or throat infections (Erriu et al 2013), gingivitis (Soukoulis & Hirsch 2004) or to help reduce radiation-induced oral mucositis (Buckingham 2010), (Maddocks-Jennings et al 2009). Gargles containing essential oils can also be very effective in treating oropharyngeal candidiasis in AIDS (Jose & Ahmad 2002), or a simple sore throat. For the latter, add three drops of an essential oil such as palma rosa *(Cymbopogon citratus)* in 15 mL of warm water for a soothing gargle that will also help to fight the infection. Repeat every 4 hours throughout the day for 3 days.

Vaginal Douches, Creams, and Tampons

Although the positive or negative effects of douching for "vaginal cleanliness" are debatable (Shaaban et al 2013), (Chu et al 2013), when there is a vaginal infection, such as *Candida albicans*, essential oils can be effective in a vaginal douche (Solsto et al 2011) or in a cream (Khosravi 2008). A tampon with three to five drops of tea tree *(Melaleuca alternifolia)* in 5 mL of carrier oil is superb against many recurrent (and resistant) vaginal infections. Repeat every 4 hours during the day (and replace every 8 hours at night) for 3 days (I have never known it to fail). Vaginal routes have a distinct advantage in the treatment of gynecological or urinary conditions because the essential oils are absorbed directly into the surrounding tissue.

Rectal Suppositories

Essential oils can be successfully used in rectal pessaries to treat infection and/or inflammation. Rectal suppositories have been used successfully to treat bronchitis

(Bardoux 2007) and an ointment applied rectally that contained tea tree was effective against hemorrhoids in a double-blind, randomized study (Joksimovic et al 2012). The usual concentrations are 10% essential oil per suppository—approximately 300 mg of essential oil per 3-g suppository. For children, use one drop of essential oil per 25-mg suppository. Cocoa butter is a good medium. Melt the cocoa butter, mix in essential oils, fill the suppository mold and store in refrigerator. Avoid using phenol-rich essential oils.

3) ORAL

There is a long history of essential oils being given to patients orally by doctors and nurses before the advent of modern pharmaceuticals. Several essential oils such as cinnamon, clove, peppermint, sandalwood, and eucalyptus are actually listed in the 1930 (8th edition) of *Useful Drugs,* published by the American Medical Association. Sandalwood was classically given for urinary infections. The oral route is an excellent one for treating gastrointestinal problems (Cappello et al 2007), (May et al 2000) or infections (Force 2000). Studies indicate it can also be useful for insomnia (Jahangir et al 2009) and anxiety (Kasper et al 2010). The oral route is perfectly safe and nontoxic provided the giver is trained appropriately and dosages are carefully measured. Not all essential oils are safe to use orally. Burfield (2000) and Tisserand & Young (2013) caution that certain essential oils such as hyssop, wormwood, and wintergreen should never be used orally. Essential oils that are high in phenols should be diluted and contained in gelatin capsules to avoid mucous irritation when administered orally. Others can be diluted in vegetable oil or aqueous alcohol (Tisserand & Young 2013). Essential oil components such as 1,8-cineole have also been used successfully by the oral route—in this instance for acute nonpurulent rhinosinusitis (Kehrl et al 2004).

Most insurance companies that cover aromatherapy do not include the oral use of essential oils. The Royal College of Nursing in UK accepts all other methods of aromatherapy as part of nursing care, apart from the oral use. Most State Boards of Nursing (BONs) in the United States now accept aromatherapy in nursing care but no state has yet accepted the oral route. In fact the Massachusetts BON 2012 revised Advisory Ruling on Nursing Practice to list aromatherapy and essential oils separately (2014). The fear of using essential oils orally is based on three things: a) a lack of knowledge, b) fear of poisoning and c) fear of litigation because the oral use of essential oils is perceived in many countries to be practicing medicine without a license. Clearly, education is vital. Tisserand & Young (2013) write "Medical practitioners who favor the oral route are frequently treating infectious diseases that require heavy dosing…. therefore only practitioners who are qualified to diagnose, trained to weigh risks against benefits and have knowledge of essential oil pharmacology should prescribe essential oils for oral administration." I agree.

As essential oils are very concentrated, doses are usually described in the number of drops given. However, drop sizes vary so it is safer to measure in milliliters. The recommended dose per 24 hours is 0.05 to 1.3 mL (Tisserand & Young 2013).

Method of Oral Use

Essential oils can be given orally in gelatin capsules, disper, or on vitamin C tablets (Table 2-4). Some essential oils can be taken in honey for occasional use—one drop of palma rosa in a teaspoon of honey can be excellent for a sore throat. Repeat every 2 hours for 1 day.

Gelatin Capsules

Size 00 capsules are filled with 20% essential oil(s) diluted in vegetable oil and poured into the capsules. Each capsule holds approximately 0.75 mL.

Disper

Disper is a lecithin-based emulsifier that holds the essential oils in a stable dispersion and is rapidly absorbed by the stomach. Mix 10 drops (or parts) of Disper to each drop (or part) of essential oil used, then add water to create a milky emulsion.

Honey

Essential oils can be blended with honey water. Mix the drops of essential oil in a teaspoon of honey, add warm water, and drink. Rose is an excellent antiviral oil to use in this way.

Enteric-Coated Gelatin Capsules

Enteric-coated gelatin capsules do not release the essential oil until they are in the small intestine (an environment of pH 6.8 or higher). This can be useful for irritable bowel syndrome (IBS) (Cappello et al 2007).

Human Studies on Oral Use

Pediatric physicians in the United States (Kline et al 2001) used enteric-coated capsules containing peppermint oil to treat IBS. Fifty children took part in a randomized, double-blind, controlled 2-week study. One or two capsules (each

TABLE 2-4 *Some Human Studies of Essential Oils Given Orally*

Author	Year	Essential Oil/Component	Common Name	Condition
Force et al	2000	*Oreganum vulgare*	Oregano	Enteric parasite
Kehrl et al	2005	1,8-Cineole		Acute nonpurulent rhinosinusitis
Cappello et al	2007	*Mentha piperita*	Peppermint	IBS
Jahangir et al	2009	*Rosa damascena*	Rose	Insomnia
Kasper et al	2010	*Lavandula angustifolia*	Lavender	Anxiety
Tayarani-Najaran et al	2013	*Mentha spicata* *Mentha × piperita*	Spearmint Peppermint	Chemo-induced nausea

IBS, Irritable bowel syndrome.

containing 187 mg) were given three times daily. The peppermint group showed a greater reduction in symptoms compared to the placebo group. No side effects were reported.

An Iranian medical study (Tayarani-Najaran 2013) explored the oral use of peppermint and spearmint for chemo-induced nausea. The four-arm study (peppermint, spearmint, control, and placebo) had 50 patients in each group. The aromatherapy groups received capsules containing either two drops of spearmint (*Mentha spicata*) or two drops of peppermint *(Mentha piperita)* oil and filled with sugar, every 4 hours. The capsules were given 30 minutes before chemotherapy treatment and then 4 and 8 hours later. There was a significant reduction in nausea for both the spearmint and the peppermint groups ($p < 0.05$) compared with control and placebo groups. No adverse effects were reported.

An Italian medical team (Cappello et al 2007) randomly allocated 57 patients with IBS to receive either enteric-coated peppermint oil *(Mentha piperita)* or placebo twice a day for 4 weeks. Symptoms measured included abdominal bloating, abdominal pain or discomfort, diarrhea, or constipation. Results showed 75% patients in the peppermint oil group had >50% reduction of symptoms compared to 38% in the placebo group ($p < 0.009$).

Belaiche (1985), a French physician, conducted a randomized, double-blind study to examine the effectiveness of *Melaleuca alternifolia* (tea tree) on 26 participants with chronic cystitis. The experimental group was given 24 mg of tea tree (3×8 mg in enteric-coated gelatin capsule). The control group was given a placebo that had the odor of tea tree. After 6 months, 60% of the aromatherapy group were completely cured. No one in the control group showed any improvement. There were no side effects to the treatment and liver function tests were normal. I hope this study will be replicated soon.

Finally, the trigeminal system also plays a role in the sensation of odors (Ishimaru et al 2011). The head-swiveling reflex, away from aggressive odors such as acetic acid and ammonia, is part of the trigeminal system and forms part of the fifth cranial nerve (Van Toller & Dodd 1991).

HOW ESSENTIAL OILS ARE EXCRETED

Essential oils are excreted through the kidney, lungs and skin (Tisserand & Young 2013) (Figure 2-3). Following oral administration, essential oil components are mainly excreted in the urine. However, components may also be excreted in the exhaled breath or in the feces. If the essential oil is inhaled, excretion is less likely to be through the urine. There is limited information about excretion of essential oils in humans. However, there are several studies on essential oil components found in the blood after topical application. Jager et al (1992) measured linalool and linalyl acetate. Wang & Tso (2002) measured 5-methoxypsoralen (bergapten). Nielsen & Nielsen (2006) measured γ-terpinene. Cross et al (2008) measured terpinen-4-ol. Lapczynski et al (2008) measured linalool. Gilpin et al (2010) measured citronellol and geraniol.

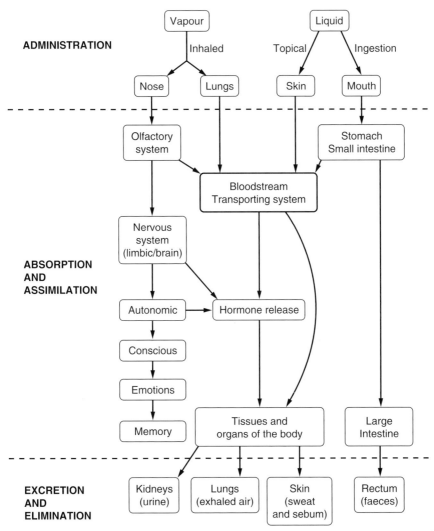

FIGURE 2-3 | How essential oils are absorbed and excreted. (From Clarke S. *Essential Chemistry for Safe Aromatherapy*. Churchill Livingstone. 2002.)

Thrall (2000) analyzed exhaled breath using an ion-trap mass spectrometer following dermal application of volatile chemicals (not essential oils).

REFERENCES

Arisi G, Foresti M, Mukherjee S, Shapiro L. 2012. The role of olfactory stimulus in adult mammalian neurogenesis. *Behav Brain Res.* 227(2):356-62.
Arzi A, Sobel N. 2010. Spatial perception: time tells where a smell comes from. *Curr Biol.* 20(13):R563-4.

Ballard C, O'Brien J, Reichelt K, Perry E. 2002. Aromatherapy as a safe and effective treatment for the management of agitation in severe dementia: the results of a double-blind, placebo-controlled trial with Melissa. *J Clin Psychiatry*. 63(7):553-8.

Bardoux F. 2007. Aromatology for respiratory pathologies. *Int J Clin Aromatherapy*. 4(1):34-39.

Begrow F, Bockenhold C, Ehmen M, Wittig T, Verspohl E. 2012. Effect of myrtol standardized and other substances on the respiratory tract: ciliary beat frequency and mucocilliary clearance as parameters. *Adv Ther*. 29(4):350-8.

Belaiche P. 1985. Germicidal properties of the essential oil of Melaleuca alternifolia related to urinary infections and chronic idiopathic Colibacillus. *Phytotherapie*. 15:9-11.

Ben-Ayre E, Dudai N, Eini A, Torem M, Schiff E, Rakover Y. 2010. Treatment of upper respiratory tract infections in primary care: a randomized study using aromatic herbs. *Evid Based Complement Altern Med*. 690346. Accessed October 17, 2013.

Betts T. 1996. The fragrant breeze: The role of aromatherapy in treating epilepsy. *Aromatherapy Quarterly*. 51(Winter):25-27.

Bowles J. 2000. *The Basic Chemistry of Aromatherapeutic Essential Oils*. Sydney, Australia: Pirie Printers.

Brooker C. 2008. *Medical Dictionary*. 16th Edition. Churchill Livingstone. London.

Buchbauer G. Molecular interaction. *International Journal of Aromatherapy* 5(1):11-14.

Buckingham L. 2010. Managing mucositis: a case study. *Internat J Clin Aromatherapy*. 7(2):31-33.

Burfield T. 2000. Safety of essential oils. *Int J Aromatherapy*. 19(1/2):16-29.

Cal K, 2006. How does the type of vehicle influence the in vitro absorption and elimination kinetics of terpenes? *Archives of Dermatological Research* 297(7):311-315

Cappello G, Spezzaferra M, Grossi L, Manzoli L, Marzio L. 2007. Peppermint oil (Mintoil) in the treatment of irritable bowel syndrome: a prospective double blind placebo-controlled randomized trial. *Dig Liver Dis*. 39(6):530-6.

Chiang A, Tudela E, Maibach H. 2012. Percutaneous absorption in diseased skin: an overview. *J Appl Toxicol*. 32(8):537-63.

Chu T, Chang Y, Ding D. 2013. Cervicovaginal secretions protect from human papillomavirus infection: effects of vaginal douching. *Taiwan J Obstet Gynecol*. 52(2):241-5.

Cordell B, Buckle J. 2013. The effects of aromatherapy on nicotine craving on a U.S. campus: a small comparison study. *J Alternet Complement Med*. 19(8):709-13.

Croy I, Bojanowski V, Hummel T. 2013. Men without a sense of smell exhibit a strongly reduced number of sexual relationships, women exhibit reduced partnership security – a reanalysis of previously published data. *Biological Psychology*. 92(2): 292-294.

Cross S, Russell M, Southwell I, Roberts M. 2006. Human skin penetration of the major components of Australian tea tree oil applied in its pure form and as a 20% solution in vitro. *Eur J Pharm Biopharm*. 69(1):214-22.

Davies S, Harding J, Baranowski A. 2002. A novel treatment of postherpetic neuralgia using peppermint oil. *Clin J Pain*. 18(3):200-2.

Dryden M, Dailly S, Crouch M. 2004. A randomized, controlled trial of tea tree topical preparations versus a standard topical regimen for the clearance of MRSA colonization. *J Hosp Infection*. 56(4):283-6.

Erriu M, Pilii F, Tuveri E, Pigliacampo D, Scano A et al. 2013. Oil essential mouthwashes antibacterial activity against *Aggregatibacter actinomycetemcomitans*: a comparison between antibiofilm and anti-planktonic effects. *Int J Dent*. doi: 10.1155/2013/164267. Accessed 12 January 2014.

Fang J, Leu Y, Hwang T, Cheng H. 2004. Essential oils from sweet basil *(Ocimum basilicum)* as novel enhancers to accelerate transdermal drug delivery. *Bio Pharm Bull*. 27(11):1819-25.

Force M, Sparks W, Ronzio R. 2000. Inhibition of enteric parasites by emulsified oil of oregano in vivo. *Phytother Research*. 14(3):213-4.

Gabbanini S, Lucchi E, Carli M. Minghetti A, Valgimigli L. 2009. In vitro evaluation of the permeation through reconstructed human epidermis of essentials oils from cosmetic formulations. *J Pharm Biomed Anal*. 50(3):370-6.

Garg A, Chren M, Sands L, Matsui M, Marenus K, Feingold K, Elias P: Psychological stress perturbs the epidermal permeability barrier homeostasis. *Archives of Dermatology* 137(1):53-59.

Gavini E, Sanna V, Sharma R, Juliano C, Usai M et al. 2005. Solid lipid microparticles (SLM) containing juniper oil as anti-acne topical carriers: preliminary studies. *Pharm Devel Technol.* 10(4):479-87.

Gilpin S, Hui X, Maibach H. 2010. In vitro human skin penetration of geraniol and citronellol. *Dermatitis.* 21(1):41-8.

Grégoire S, Riboud C, Benech F, Meunier J Garrigues-Mazert A et al. 2009. Prediction of chemical absorption into and through the skin from cosmetic and dermatological formulations. *Br J Dermatology.* 160(1):80-91.

Hagino-Yamagishi K. 2008. Diverse systems for pheromone perception: multiple receptor families in two olfactory systems. *Zoolog Sci.* 25(12):1179-89.

Hammer K, Carson C, Riley T, Nielson J. 2006. A review of the toxicity of *Melaleuca alternifolia* (tea tree) oil. *Food Chem Toxicol.* 44(5):616-25.

Hasler-Nguyen N, Shelton D, Ponard G, Bader M, Scaffrik M, Mallefet P. 2009. Evaluation of the in vitro skin permeation of antiviral drugs from penciclovir 1% cream and acyclovir 5% cream used to treat herpes simplex virus infection. *BMC Dermatology* 2009, 9(3): doi:10.1186/1471-5945-9-3. Accessed January 9, 2014.

Hatanpaa K, Raisanen J, Herndon E, Burns D, Foong C et al. 2014. Hippocampal sclerosis in dementia, epilepsy, and ischemic injury: differential vulnerability of hippocampal subfields. *J Neuropathol Exp Neurol.* 73(2):136-42.

Hayakawi N, Kubota N, Imai N, Stumpf W. 2004. Receptor microscopic autoradiography for the study of percutaneous absorption, in vivo skin penetration, and cellular-intercellular deposition. *J Pharmacol Toxicol Methods.* 50(2):131-7.

Heinemann L. 2011. New ways of insulin delivery. *Int J Clin Pract Suppl.* Feb;(170):31-46. doi: 10.1111/j.1742-1241.2010.02577.x. Accessed January 12, 2014.

Heldt S, Mou L, Ressler K. 2012. In vivo knockdown of GAD67 in the amygdala disrupts fear extinction and the anxiolytic-like effect of diazepam in mice. *Transl Psychiatry.* 13;2:e181. doi: 10.1038/tp.2012.101.

Henkin R, Levy L, Lin C. 2000. Taste and smell phantoms revealed by brain functional MRI (fMRI). *J Comput Assist Tomogr.* 24(1):106-23.

Henkin R, Levy L. 2001. Lateralization of brain activation to imagination and smell of odors using functional magnetic resonance imaging (fMRI): left hemispheric localization of pleasant and right hemispheric localization of unpleasant odors. *J Comput Assist Tomogr.* 25(4):493-514.

Henkin R, Levy L. 2002. Functional MRI of congenital hyposmia: brain activation to odors and imagination of odors and tastes. *J Comput Assist Tomogr.* 26(1):39-61.

Hinton D, Pich V, Chhean D, Pollack M, Barlow D. 2004. Ofactory-triggered panic attacks among Cambodian refugees attending a psychiatric clinic. *Gen Hosp Psychiatry.* 26(5):390-7.

Hoover K. 2010. Smell with inspiration: the evolutionary significance of olfaction. *Am J Phys Anthropol.* 143(Suppl 51):63-74.

Hummel T, Olgun S, Gerber J, Huchel U, Frasnelli J. 2013. Brain responses to odor mixtures with subthreshold components. *Front Psychol.* 24;4:786. doi: 10.3389/fpsyg.2013.00786. Accessed January 12, 2014.

Hunt R, Dienemann J, Norton J, Hartley W et al. 2012. Aromatherapy as treatment for postoperative nausea: a randomized trial. *Anesth Anal.* 117(3):597-604.

Hur M-H, Lee M, Seong K-Y, Lee M-K. 2012. Aromatherapy massage on the abdomen for alleviating menstrual pain in high school girls: a preliminary controlled clinical study. *Evid Based Compl Alt Med.* doi: 10.1155/2012/187163.

Ishimaru T, Reden J, Krone F, Scheibe M. 2011. Topographical differences in the sensitivity of the human nasal mucosa to olfactory and trigeminal stimuli. *Neurosci Lett.* 493(3):136-9.

Jager W, Buchbauer G, Jirovetz L, M. Fritzer M. 1992. Percutaneous absorption of lavender oil from a massage oil. *J Soc Cosmetic Chemists.* 43(1):49-54.

Jahangir U, Urooj S, Shah A, Ishaaq M, Habib A. 2009. A comparative clinical trial of rose petal (Gul gullab), rose hudrosol dilutd (Arq gulaab) and rose hdrosl (Rhu gulaab) in insomnia. *The Internet J Neurol.* 11(2):DOI:10.5580?22ec.

Jimbo D, Ichihashi K, Inoie M, Shioda S. 2012. Blood flow decrease by olfactory stimulations. Proceedings of 1st international congress of aromatherapy. *Journal of Japanese Society of Aromatherapy.* P 145.

Joksimovic N, Spasovski G, Joksimovic V, Zuccari C, Omini C. 2012. Efficacy and tolerability of hyaluronic acid, tea tree oil and methyl-sulfonyl-methane in a new gel medical device for treatment of haemorrhoids in a double-blind, placebo-controlled clinical trial. *Updates Surg.* 64(3):195-201.

Jose A, Ahmad A. 2002. Efficacy of alcohol-based and alcohol-free melaleuca oral solution for the treatment of fluconazole-refractory oropharyngeal candidiasis in patients with AIDS. *HIV Clin Trials.* 3(4): 379-385.

Jori A, Bianchelli A, Prestini P, 1969: Effects of essential oils on drug metabolism. *Biochemical Pharmacology* 19(9):2081-2095.

Kadohisa M. 2013. Effects of odor on emotion: with implications. *Front Syst Neurosci.* doi: 10.3389/fnsys.2013.00066. Accessed January 12, 2014.

Karpanen T, Conway B, Worthington T, Hilton A, Elliott T, Lambert P. 2010. Enhanced chlorhexidine skin penetration with eucalyptus oil. *BMC Infect Dis.* 10:278. doi: 10.1186/1471-2334-10-278. Accessed January 8, 2014.

Kasper S, Gastpar M, Muller W, Volz H, Moller H et al. 2010. Silexan, an orally administered lavandula oil preparation is effective in the treatment of subsyndromal anxiety disorder. A randomized, double-blind, placebo controlled trial. *Int Cl Psychopharmacology.* 15(5): 277-287.

Kehrl W, Sonnemann U, Dethlefsen U. 2004. Therapy for acute nonpurulent rhinosinusitis with cineole. Results of a double-blind, randomized, placebo-controlled trial. *Larngoscope.* 114(4): 738-742.

Khosravi A, Eslami A, Shokri H, Kashanian M. 2008. *Zataria multiflora* cream for the treatment of acute vaginal candidiasis. *Int J Gynaecol Obstet.* 101(2):201-2.

Kline R, Kline J, Di Palma J, Barbero G. 2001. Enteric-coated, pH-dependent peppermint oil capsules for the treatment of irritable bowel syndrome in children. *J Pediatr.* 138(1):125-8.

Komori T, Matsumoto T, Yamamoto M, Motomura E, Okazaki Y. 2006. Application of fragrance in discontinuing the long-term use of hypnotic benzodiazepines. *Int J Aroma.* 16(1):3-7.

Kristiniak S, Harpel J, Breckenridge D, Buckle J. 2012. Black pepper essential oil to enhance intravenous catheter insertion in patients with poor vein visibility: a controlled study. *J Altern Compl Med.* 18(11):1003-7.

Kritsidima M, Asimakopoulou K, Newton J. 2008. The influence of lavender scent on levels of dental anxiety: a randomized, controlled trial in a private dental setting. *Psychol Health* 23(Suppl 1):163-164.

Lapczynski A, Letizia CS, Api A. 2008. Addendum to Fragrance material review on linalool. *Food Chem Toxicol.* 46(Suppl 11):S190-S192. Review.

Lorig, T. 2012. Beyond self-report: Brain imaging at the threshold of odor perception. *Chemosensory Percept.* 5(1):46-54.

Lorig T, Herman K, Schwartz G et al. 1990. EEG activity during administration of low concentration odors. *Bull Psychonomic Soc.* 28:405-408.

Maddocks-Jennings W, Wilkinson J, Cavanagh M, Shillington D. 2009. Evaluation of the effects of the essential oils of *Leptospermum scoparium* (Manuka) and *Kunzea ericoides* (Kanuka) on radiotherapy-induced mucositis – a randomized, placebo-controlled feasibility study. *Eur J Oncol Nursing.* 13(2):87-93.

Mak G, Enwere E, Gregg C, Pakarainen T, Poutanen M, Huhtaniemi I. 2007. Male pheromone-stimulated neurogenesis in the adult female brain: possible role in mating behavior. *Nature Neuroscience.* 10(8): 1003-1011.

Matiz G, Osorio M, Camacho F, Atencia M, Herazo J. 2012. Effectiveness of antimicrobial formulations for acne based on orange *(Citrus sinensis)* and sweet basil *(Ocimum basilicum)* essential oils. *Biomedica.* 32(1):125-33.

Massachusetts State Board of Nursing. 2012. Advisory Ruling Number: 9801. Holistic Nursing and Complementary/AlternativeModalities. http://www.mass.gov/eohhs/gov/departments/dph/programs/hcq/dhpl/nursing/nursing-practice/advisory-rulings/holistic-nursing-and-complementary-therapies.html. Accessed January 13, 2014.

May B, Kohler S, Schneider B. 2000. Efficacy and tolerability of a fixed combination of peppermint oil and caraway oil in patients suffering from functional dyspepsia. *Aliment Pharmacol Ther.* 14(12):1671-7.

Melli M, Rashid M, Nokhoodchi A, Tagavi S, Farzadi L et al. 2007. A randomized trial of peppermint gel, lanolin ointment, and placebo gel to prevent nipple crack in primiparous breastfeeding women. *Med Sci Monit.* 13(9):CR406-411.

Moser K, Kriwet K, Froehlich C, Kalina Y, Guy H. 2001. Supersaturation: enhancement of skin penetration and permeation of lipophilic drug. *Pharmaceut Records.* 18(7): 1006-1011.

Nickell M, Breheny P, Stronberg A, McClintock T. 2012. Genomics of mature and immature olfactory sensory neurons. *J Comp Neurol.* 520(12):2608-29.

Nielsen J, Nielsen F. 2006. Topical use of tea tree oil reduces the dermal absorption of benzoic acid and methiocarb. *Arch Dermatol Res.* 297(9):395-402

Norris M, Dwyer K. 2005. Preliminary investigation of the effect of peppermint oil on an objective measure of daytime sleepiness. *Int J Psychophysiol.* 55(3): 291-298.

Pawliczek C, Derntl B, Kellermann T, Gur R, Schneider F, Habel U. 2013. Anger under control: neural correlates of frustration as a function of trait aggression. *PLoS one.* 8(10):e78503.

Reichling J, Landvatter U, Wagner H, Kostka K, Schaefer U. 2006. In vitro studies on release and human skin permeation of Australian tea tree oil (TTO) from topical formulations. *Eur J Pharm Biopharm.* 64(2):222-8.

Remberg B, Bjork L, Hedner T, Sterner O. 2004. Characteristics, clinical effect profile and tolerability of a nasal spray preparation of Artemisia abrotanum for allergic shinitis *Phytomedicine* 11(1): 36-42.

Satchell A, Sauragen A, Bell C, Barnetson R. 2002. Treatment of interdigital tinea pedis with 25% and 50% tea tree oil solution: a randomized, placebo-controlled, blinded study. *Austral J Dermatol.* 43(3):175-8.

Schmitt S, Schafer U, Dobler L, Reichling J. 2009. Cooperative interaction of monoterpenes and phenyl-propanoids on the in vitro human skin permeation of complex composed essential oils. *Planta Med.* 75(13):1381-5.

Schmitt S, Schäfer UF, Döbler L, Reichling J. 2010. Variation of in vitro human skin permeation of rose oil between different application sites. *Forsch Komplementmed.* 2010;17(3):126-31.

Shaaban O, Youseef A, Khodry M, Mostafa S. 2013. Vaginal douching by women with vulvovaginitis and relation to reproductive health hazards. *BMC Womens Health.* 2013 May 14;13:23. Accessed March 4, 2014.

Sharma N, Araujo M, Wu M, Quqish J, Charles C. 2010. Superiority of an essential oil mouthrinse when compared with a 0.05% cetylpyridinium chloride containing mouthrinse: a six-month study. *Int Dent J.* 60(3):175-80.

Shaw D, Norwood K, Leslie J. 2011. Chlordiazepoxide and lavender oil alter unconditioned anxiety-induced c-fos expression in the rat brain. *Behav Brain Res.* 224(1):1-7.

Sobel N, Khan R, Hartley C, Sullivan E, Gabrieli J. 2000. Sniffing longer rather than stronger to maintain olfactory detection threshold. *Chem Senses.* 25(1):1-8.

Solsto F, Benvenuti C. 2011. Controlled study on thymol + eugenol vaginal douche versus econazole in vaginal candidiasis and metronidazole in bacterial vaginosis. *Arzneimittelforschung.* 61(2):126-3.

Soukoulis S, Hirsch R. 2004. The effects of tea tree oil-containing gel on plaque and chronic gingivitis. *Australian Dental J.* 49(2): 78-83.

Stringer J, Donald G. 2011. Aromastix in cancer care. An innovation not to be sniffed at. *Complementary Therapies Clin Practice.* 17(2):116-121.

Takaishi M, Fujita F, Uchida K, Yamamoto S, Swafa Shimizu M et al 2012. 1,8 cineole, a TRPM8 agonist, is a novel natural antagonist of human TRPA1. *Mol Pain.* 29:8:86. Accessed October 17. 2013.

Tayarani-Najaran Z, Talasaz-Firoozi E, Nasiri R, Jalali N, Hassanzadeh M. 2013. Antiemetic activity of volatile oil from Mentha spicata and Mentha × piperita in chemotherapy-induced nausea and vomiting. *Ecancermedicalscience.* doi: 10.3332/ecancer.2013.290.

Thrall K, Poet T, Corley R, Tanajo H, Edwards J et al. 2000. A real-time in-vivo method for studying the percutaneous absorption of volatile chemicals. *Int J Occup Environ Health.* 6(2):96-103.

Tisserand R, Young R. 2013. *Essential Oils Safety.* 2nd edition. Churchill Livingstone. P 40-47.

Toda M, Morimoto K. 2008. Effect of lavender aroma on salivary endocrinological stress markers. *Arch Oral Biol.* 53(10): 964-968

Valgimigli L, Gabbanini S, Berlini E, Lucchi E, Beltramini C, Bertarelli Y. 2012. Lemon (Citrus limon, Burm.f.) essential oil enhances the trans-epidermal release of lipid-(A, E) and water-(B6, C) soluble vitamins from topical emulsions in reconstructed human epidermis. *Int J Cosmet Sci.* 34(4):347-56.

Van Toller S, Dodd G. 1991. Preface in Van Toller S, Dodd G (eds) *Perfumery: The pyschology and biology of fragrance.* Chapman & Hall, London.

Varney E, Buckle J. 2012. Effects of inhaled essential oils on mental exhaustion and moderate burnout: a pilot study. *J Alt Comp Med.* 18(12):69-71.

Via E, Cardoner N, Pujol J, Alonso P, Lopez-Sola M et al 2014. Amygdala activation and symptom dimensions in obsessive-compulsive disorder. *Br J Psychiatry.* 204:61-8. doi: 10.1192/bjp.bp.112.123364. Accessed January 12, 2014.

Walter R, Cooper R, Aldridge V, McCallum W, Winter A: Contingent negative variation: an electric sign of sensorimotor association and expectancy in the human brain. *Nature.* 203:380-384.

Wang L, Tso M. 2002. Determination of 5-methoxypsoralen in human serum. *J Pharm Biomed Anal.* 15;30(3):593-600.

Watson L. 2000. *Jacobson's Organ.* New York: Norton.

Watts G, 1975: *Dynamic Neuroscience: Its application to Brain Disorders,* Harper & Row, New York.

Weiss S. 1979. The language of touch. *Nursing Res.* 28, 76-79.

Williams D. 1996. *The Chemistry of Essential Oils.* Weymouth, Dorset, England: Michelle Press.

Woolley C, Suhail M, Smith B, Boren K, Taylor L et al 2012. Chemical differentiation of Boswellia sacra and Boswellia carterii essential oils by gas chromatography and chiral gas chromatography-mass spectrometry. *J Chromatogr A.* 1261:158-63. doi: 10.1016/j.chroma.2012.06.073. Accessed Jan 2014.

Wysocki C, Preti G. 2004. Facts, fallacies, fears, and frustrations with human pheromones. *Anat Rec A Discov Moll Cell Evol Biol.* 281(1):1201-11.

Yousem D, Malidijan J, Siddiqi F, Hummel T, Alsop D et al. 2013. Gender effects of odor-stimulated functional magnetic resonance imaging. *Brain Res.* 818(2):480-487.

Yu Y, Zhou L, Li X. 2009. Studies of in vitro releasing properties on cyclovirobuxine D matrix-type patch. *Zhongguo Zhong Yao Za Zhi.* 34(7):825-8.

Chapter 3

Basic Plant Taxonomy, Basic Essential Oil Chemistry, Extraction, Biosynthesis, and Analysis

"A weed is a flower in the wrong place, a flower is a weed in the right place, if you were a weed in the right place you would be a flower; but seeing as you're a weed in the wrong place you're only a weed—it's high time someone pulled you out."

Ian Emberson

CHAPTER ASSETS

BASIC PLANT TAXONOMY

Learning how and why a plant manufactures an essential oil is relevant to understanding aromatherapy. The way plants make essential oils gives some insight into their complexity. Traditionally, biochemists have studied primary metabolism and organic chemists have studied secondary metabolism. In aromatherapy, it is useful to have an overall picture of both metabolic processes. Why some plants make essential oils is the subject of ongoing scientific debate and is relevant to the therapeutic potential of using essential oils in healthcare.

The process of extraction clarifies the need for unadulterated essential oils. Unadulterated essential oils are required for clinical use to prevent possible side effects from solvents or residues. The process of steam distillation or expression produces an essential oil with no residue. CO_2 extraction (supercritical carbon dioxide) does not produce a residue but it does produce a different extract. Steam-distilled German chamomile *(Matricaria recutita)* is dark blue due to the high content of chamazulene. CO_2 extract is green—no chamazulene.

The Latin names of plants can seem a bit intimidating initially, but they are the best way of being sure you have the correct essential oil. Carl Linnaeus (1707–1778) established the basis for naming plants in Latin (Stearn 1998). Today, botanical (Latin) names are recognized globally by gardeners, botanists, herbalists, and aromatherapists. A plant may have many common names, but it only has one Latin name and the common names may mean completely different plants. For example, in aromatherapy, bergamot means the essential oil extracted from the peel of the citrus fruit *Citrus bergamia*. To a gardener, bergamot means the plant *Monarda didyma*. In aromatherapy, *geranium* means *Pelargonium* "Graveolens" [the plant cultivated today is actually a cultivar group involving hybrids of *P. capitatum*, *P. radens*, and *P. graveolens* (Tucker 2014)]. To a gardener, *geranium* means the plant *Pelargonium* sp., although a medicinal plant person might assume geranium means *Geranium maculatum*.

Plant taxonomy, by its simplest definition, includes (1) naming and describing, (2) identifying, and (3) classifying of plants. The botanical name for each plant is composed of two words. The first word is the name of the genus. The second word is the name of the species. All plants can be grouped into categories. For plants to be properly identified they are divided into division, class, order, family, genus, and species. This process takes into account the number, shape and position of leaves on the stem; the shape and position of the flowers; the number and shape of the petals; whether the plant is hairy, prickly, or smooth; whether the stem is ridged; and so on.

EXAMPLES OF WHY THE BOTANICAL NAME IS IMPORTANT

LAVENDER

Lavender belongs to a plant family called Lamiaceae (previously Labiatae): the mint family. This family includes many species and some are used in aromatherapy. Plants in this family usually have five united petals with two lobes on the top and three on the bottom forming lips (labia). The leaves are usually directly opposite each other on the stem and often the stem is square. The Latin name for the lavender genus is *Lavandula,* so all lavenders begin with *Lavandula.* (See Table 3-1.) Two of the most commonly used "lavenders" are *Lavandula angustifolia* and *Lavandula latifolia.*

Lavandula angustifolia is sometimes called *L. vera* or *L. officinalis,* although the correct name is *L. angustifolia* (Lawrence 1989). This plant also has several common names: English lavender, French lavender, and true lavender.

Lavandula latifolia is sometimes called *L. spica,* and its common name is spike lavender or spike. Spike is completely different from spikenard *(Nardostachys jatamansi),* which is closely related to valerian and belongs to the family Valerianaceae.

Lavandula angustifolia and *Lavandula latifolia* were both listed in the *British Pharmacopoeia* and supplied to hospitals in vats labeled simply "lavender." However, the two plants have very different therapeutic properties. *L. angustifolia* is a sedative, relaxant, and hypotensor. *L. latifolia* is a stimulant and expectorant.

Another commonly used "lavender" is *Lavandula × intermedia* (older synonym *L. hybrida*). This is a naturally occurring hybrid that was first observed in 1828 (Tucker 2014). Today, *Lavandula × intermedia* tends to be a manufactured cultivar with a trade name Lavandin. It is a cross (hence the multiplication sign between the genus and the species) between two *Lavandula* species: *L. angustifolia* and *L. latifolia.* Because Lavandin belongs to the *Lavandula* genus, it can legitimately be called a "lavender." This can cause confusion when people think they have true lavender (*L. angustifolia*) when in fact they have Lavandin. There is a third less-commonly used species of lavender, *L. stoechas,* that can also be used clinically.

TABLE 3-1 *Lavenders and Some of Their Properties*

Latin Name	Common Name	Properties
Lavandula angustifolia *Lavandula vera* *Lavandula officinalis*	True lavender	Calming, sedative, good for burns, analgesic, antibacterial, immune-system enhancer
Lavandula latifolia *Lavandula spica*	Spike lavender	Expectorant, mucolytic, possible stimulant
Lavandula stoechas	Stoechas	Useful against *Pseudomonas* spp., high in ketones

Chamomile

Chamomile can also cause confusion initially. There are three main types of chamomile used in aromatherapy: German, Roman, and Moroccan (Table 3-2). They are quite different and produce different-colored essential oils that have different properties, but they all belong to the same family: Asteraceae or Compositae—the daisy family.

German chamomile *(Matricaria recutita)* is a smoky smelling, dark-blue oil that contains chamazulene. The oil's color is related to the amount of chamazulene present and the method of extraction. Chamazulene is not present in the fresh flower (or in its CO_2 extract) but is produced during distillation (Lawless 1992). It is possible to obtain a green or yellow German chamomile oil that has less than 3% chamazulene, but the dark-blue variety always has more than 7%. The price of German chamomile oil is usually related to the amount of chamazulene it contains. Chamazulene is an antiinflammatory with a history of use in the treatment of skin problems (Jakovlev et al 1983), (Ramadan et al 2006). German chamomile also contains a second antiinflammatory compound called (−)-alpha-bisabolol that is a sesquiterpene alcohol (Alves Ade et al 2010). In addition, this species has antibacterial properties (Salehi et al 2005) and is effective against *Staphylococcus aureus, Streptococcus,* and *Candida albicans* (Khezri et al 2013). CO_2-extracted German chamomile is dark green, or brownish green, and semi-solid at room temperature. It smells of sweet apples with an earthy undertone.

Roman chamomile (*Chamaemelum nobile* or *Anthemis nobilis*) is commonly known as English chamomile or garden chamomile, is colorless to pale blue that turns yellow with storage. Listed in the *British Herbal Pharmacopoeia,* it contains up to 80% esters. Esters have antispasmodic properties, and essential oil of Roman chamomile is traditionally used topically as an antispasmodic and inhaled as a relaxant, while the herbal extract is used as a carminative. Roman chamomile also has mild antiinflammatory properties (Franchomme & Penoel 1990). Recent research suggests it may have antitumoral properties (Guimaraes et al 2013).

Moroccan chamomile (*Ormenis multicaulis* or *O. mixta*) is a relative newcomer to the aromatherapy world. The main component in the essential oil is santolina alcohol (Zrira et al 2007). It does not contain chamazulene. However, it does have some antibacterial properties (Darriet et al 2012). Adding further confusion is Chamomile Blue Tansy—*Tanacetum annum.* This is not a true chamomile—its genus is not *Chamaemelum* or *Ormenis*—but it is blue and it does contain chamazulene.

TABLE 3-2 *Chamomiles and Some of Their Properties*

Latin Name	Common Name	Properties
Matricaria recutita	German chamomile	Dark blue, useful for skin complaints and inflammation
Chamaemelum nobile	Roman chamomile	Pale blue or yellow, sedative, useful for spasms
Ormenis mixta	Moroccan chamomile	Mainly used by perfume industry, some antibacterial activity

DIFFERENT ESSENTIAL OILS FROM DIFFERENT PARTS OF THE PLANT

Occasionally, different parts of the same plant can produce different essential oils. In the case of the bitter orange plant (*Citrus × aurantium* var. *amara*), three different types of essential oils can be obtained: petitgrain from the stems and leaves, neroli from the petals, and bitter orange from the fruit. Neroli-like and petitgrain-like essential oils can be obtained from the petals and leaves of other citrus species. Bergamot essential oil is obtained from the rind of a fruit that is a subspecies of the bittersweet orange. The shorthand for *Citrus aurantium* var. *bergamia* (bergamot) is *Citrus bergamia* (Guenther 1976).

Sometimes just the part of the plant is listed (e.g., cinnamon bark or cinnamon leaf). Cinnamon bark contains approximately 50% eugenol (a phenol). Cinnamon leaf contains 80 to 96% eugenol. Eugenol is strongly antimicrobial (Kamatou et al 2012). However, it can cause sensitization (Svedman et al 2012) and if used in high concentrations can burn the skin. It can also dissolve metal, false teeth, and pearls (Ryman 1991). Cinnamon bark and cinnamon leaf are used by the fragrance and pharmaceutical industries in very low dilutions.

CLONES AND CHEMOTYPES

To complicate the situation a bit more, some plants have clones or cultivars. These will have different chemistries (Table 3-3). Clones or cultivars are manufactured and the essential oil has a specific chemical profile. This might make it more suitable for treating a particular ailment, or make it safer to use. Common thyme *(Thymus vulgaris)* has several chemotypes: linalol, geraniol, α-terpineol, thujanol-4, carvacrol, and thymol (Vernet & Gouyon 1976). The first four are all safe to use on the skin, because they are high in alcohols. However, thymol and carvacrol are phenols and can cause skin irritation. There are four different chemotypes of Lavandin (*Lavandula × intermedia* or *Lavandula hybrida*)—each with a different chemistry. Tea tree, eucalyptus, rosemary, and German chamomile are other essential oils that

TABLE 3-3 *Some Examples of Essential Oil Chemotypes*

Latin Name	Chemical Constituents	Research Paper
Achillea millefolium	Caryophyllene, farnesene, azulene-free	Hethelyi et al 1988 Oswiecimska 1974
Artemesia dracunculus	Methyl chavicol, sabinene	Tucker and Maciarello 1987
Ocimum basilicum	Linalool, methyl chavicol, eugenol	Sobti et al 1978
Matricaria recutita	Bisabolone oxide, bisabolol, chamazulene, chamazulene-free	Frantz 1993
Salvia officinalis	α- and β-thujone, cineole, thuhone-free	Tucker and Maciarello 1990

have commercial chemotypes. Chemotypes will become more common as aromatic plants are grown for the pharmaceutical or food industry.

REFERENCES

Alves Ade M, Goncalves J, Cruz J, Araujo D. 2010. Evaluation of the sesquiterpene (−)-alpha-bisabolol as a novel peripheral nervous blocker. *Neurosci Lett.* 12;472(1):11-5.

Darriet F, Bendahou M, Costa J, Muselli A. 2012. Chemical compositions of the essential oils of the aerial parts of Chamaemelum mixtum. *J Agriculture Food Chem.* 60(6):1494-502.

Franchomme P, Penoel D. 1990. *Aromatherapie Exactement.* Limoges, France: Jollois.

Frantz C. 1993. Genetics. In Hay R, Waterman P (eds). Volatile Oil Crops: Their Biology, Biochemistry and Production. *Longman Scientific & Technical.* Essex, UK. 63-96.

Guenther E. 1976. *The Essential Oils,* Vol. III. Malaber, FL: Krieger.

Guimaraes R, Barros L, Duenas M, Calhelha R, Calvalho A et al. 2013. Nutrients, phytochemicals and bioactivity of wild Roman chamomile: a comparison between the herb and its preparations. *Food Chem.* 15;136(2):718-25.

Hethelyi E, Danos B, Tetenyi P. 1988. Investigation of the essential oils of the Achillea genus. 1. The essential oils composition of Achillea distans. *Herba Hungarica.* 27:35-42.

Jakovlev V, Isaac C, Flaskamp E. 1983. Pharmacological investigations with compounds of chamomile. VI. Investigations on the antiphlogistic effects of chamazulene and matricin. *Planta Medica.* 49(2) 67-73.

Kamatou G, Vermaak I, Viljoen A. 2012. Eugenol—From the Remote Maluku Islands to the International Market Place: A Review of a Remarkable and Versatile Molecule. *Molecules,* 17, 6953-6981. doi:10.3390/molecules17066953. Accessed Jan 24, 2014.

Khezri H, Gorji M, Morad A, Gorji H. 2013. Comparison of the antibacterial effects of matrica & Persica™ and chlorhexidine gluconate mouthwashes in mechanically ventilated ICU patients: a double blind randomized clinical trial. *Rev Chil Infectol.* 30(4). http://dx.doi:10.4067/S0716-10182013000400003. Accessed Jan 22, 2014.

Lawless J. 1992. *Encyclopedia of Essential Oils.* Shaftesbury, UK: Element Books.

Lawrence B. 1989. *Essential Oils: 1981-1987.* Wheaton, IL: Allured Publishing.

Oswiecimska M. 1974. Correlation between number of chromatosomes and prochamazuelene in East European Achillea. *Planta Medica.* 25(4):389-395.

Ramadan M, Goeters S, Watzer B, Krause E, Lohmann K et al. 2006. Chamazulene carboxylic acid and matricin: a natural profen and its natural prodrug, identified through similarity to synthetic drug substances. *J Nat Prod.* 69(7):1041-5.

Ryman D. 1991. *Aromatherapy.* London: Piatkus.

Salehi P, Kohanteb G, Momeni Danaei Sh, Vahedi R. 2005. Comparison of the antibacterial effects of Persica and Matrica, two herbal mouthwashes with chlorhexidine mouthwash. *Shiraz Univ Dental J.* 6 (1,2): 63-72.

Sobti S, Pushpangadan P, Thapa R. 1979. Chemical and genetic investigations in essential oils of some Ocimum species, their FI hybrids and synthesized allopolyploids. *Lloydia.* 4: 50-55.

Stearn W. 1998. *Botanical Latin, 4th ed.* Portland, OR: Timber Press.

Svedman C, Engfeldt M, Api A, Politano V, Belsito D, et al. 2012. A pilot study aimed at finding a suitable eugenol concentration for a leave-on product for use in a repeated open application test. *Contact Dermatitis.* 66(3):137-9.

Tucker A. 2014. Personal communication.

Tucker A, Maciarello M. 1987. Plant identification. In Simon J Grant (ed) *Proceedings of the 1st National Herb Growing and Marketing Conference.* West Lafayette IN. Purdue University Press. 341-372.

Tucker A, Maciarello M. 1990. Essential Oils of Cultivars of Dalmation safe (Salvia officinalis). *Journal of Essential Oil Research.* 2:139-144.

Vernet P, Gouyon D. 1976. Le polymorphisme chimique de *Thymus vulgaris.* Parfums, Cosmetiques, Aromes. 30:31-45.

Zrira S, Menut C, Bessiere J, Benjilali B. 2007. Chemical Composition of the Essential Oils of Moroccan *Ormenis mixta* (L.) Dumort. ssp. *Multicaulis. J Essential Oil Bearing Plants.* 10(5): 378-85.

BASIC ESSENTIAL OIL CHEMISTRY

Chemistry makes an excellent handmaid but the worst possible mistress. Buhner 2012.

For this section, I am grateful to Professor K. Hüsnü Can Başer for his essential oil chemistry chapters plus numerous papers and to Ian Cambray-Smith for his chemistry course notes and creating most of the chemical drawings. I have tried to make what is an extremely complicated subject as simple and as relevant to aromatherapists, as possible. I have selected research papers to illustrate the wide range of potential properties of essential oil components. My intention is that the reader will look anew at essential oils they may have used previously for other outcomes. It is worth remembering that sometimes the minor components of essential oils can be important in aromatherapy. For example, the strong, sweet, floral smell of rose *(Rosa damascena)* is created by the high content of citronellol, geraniol modified by nerol (5 to 11%) and farnesol (0.2 to 1.4%) (Başer et al 2012). For possible toxicity and side effects please see Chapter 4.

ESSENTIAL OILS COMPONENTS

Essential oils are made up of terpenoids and nonterpenoid volatile hydrocarbons (Baser & Demirci 2011). These constituents contain a basic frame of carbon and hydrogen to which a "functional group" is added (Tisserand & Young 2013). A functional group is a term familiar to aromatherapists and means "a group of atoms the shape of which determines the characteristic chemical properties of the molecule" (Tisserand & Young 2013). There are six classes (functional groups) of organic compound that are important to aromatherapists (Cambray-Smith 2013). In alphabetical order, they are: alcohols, aldehydes, esters, ethers, ketones, and phenols.

Simple hydrocarbons such as alkanes, alkenes, and benzenoids are called nonterpenoid hydrocarbons due to the fact that their biosynthesis is not due to mevalonate or nonmevalonate (D-erythritol 4-phosphate [MEP]) pathways. Phenylpropanoids are synthesized through the Shikimic acid pathway (Tisserand & Young 2013). For more information, please see the biosynthesis section of this chapter. Please see Figure 3-1 for chemical drawings.

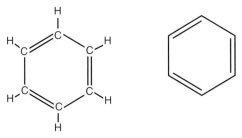

FIGURE 3-1 | Benzene rings (aromatic ring).

NONTERPENOID HYDROCARBONS

TERPENES

Terpenes—the largest single class of compounds found in essential oils, also called isoprenoids (Baser & Demirci 2011)—are made up of isoprene molecules. Each isoprene molecule (sometimes called isoprene unit) contains five carbon atoms with double bonds. The simplest terpenes are monoterpenes that contain two isoprene molecules. Sesquiterpenes have three isoprene molecules and diterpenes have four (Table 3-4). Because each isoprene molecule has five carbon atoms, it is easy to calculate the number of carbon atoms per molecule (Table 3-5). Terpenes can be subdivided into groups *acyclic* or *cyclic* which indicate their structure. Acyclic terpenes are linear, like the monoterpene β-myrcene. Cyclic terpenes form a ring, like the monoterpene *p*-cymene. Monocyclic, bicyclic, and tricyclic monoterpenes (meaning one, two, or three nonaromatic rings) occur in essential oils (Baser & Demirci 2007). All terpenes end in *-ene*.

MONOTERPENES

Monoterpenes are light molecules that evaporate quickly and are called "top notes" by the perfume industry. Citrus oils, with the exception of bergamot, contain a high proportion of monoterpenes, in particular the optical isomer D-limonene, a cyclic form (Cambray-Smith 2013). D-Limonene is the most commonly found optical isomer or enantiomer of limonene and it is generally called limonene alone without mentioning its D-enantiomer. All monoterpenes have antiseptic properties and they are thought to be psychologically uplifting. Ocimene, α-pinene and limonene are monoterpenes. Some monoterpenes such as limonene and α-pinene have antitumoral properties (Rabi & Bishayee 2009), (Bhattacharjee & Chatterjee 2013). Please see Table 3-6 for some chemical structures. Limonene also is effective for relief of heartburn and gastroesophageal reflux (GERD) due to its gastric acid neutralizing effect and its support

TABLE 3-4 *Structure of Terpenes*

Molecular Structure	Name	Example
Chain, no ring	Acyclic	α-Myrcene
One ring	Cyclic	D-Limonene
Two rings	Bicyclic	Thujane

TABLE 3-5 *Isoprene Units in Terpenes*

Chemical Constituent	Number of Isoprene Units	Number of Carbon Atoms
Monoterpene	2 isoprene units	10 carbon atoms
Sesquiterpene	3 isoprene units	15 carbon atoms
Diterpene	4 isoprene units	20 carbon atoms

of normal peristalsis (Sun 2007). Limonene occurs in most citrus oils and in dill *(Anethum graveolens)*. L-Limonene is present in spearmint oil and pine oil. Limonene oxidizes on air-exposure. Oxidized D-limonene can cause skin irritation (Christensson et al 2009). Because terpenes are insoluble in water, the perfume industry frequently removes them to produce "terpeneless" essential oils (Guenther 1972).

SESQUITERPENES

Sesquiterpenes are less volatile than terpenes, have a greater potential for stereochemical diversity (Waterman 1993) and have stronger odors. They are antiinflammatory (Jeena et al 2013) and have bactericidal properties (Ishnava et al 2013). Please see Table 3-7 for some chemical structures. Sesquiterpenes oxidize over time into sesquiterpenols. In patchouli oil, this oxidation is thought to improve the odor. One of the most antiinflammatory sesquiterpenes, chamazulene, only has 14 carbon atoms but is usually included with sesquiterpenes. Chamazulene and caryophyllene have strong antioxidant (Ornano et al 2013) and antitumor activity (Feraz et al 2013; Park et al 2011). Chamazulene is found in German chamomile. Sesquiterpenes can be monocyclic, bicyclic or tricyclic and are a very diverse group (Baser & Demirci 2007). Examples include α-bisabolene in black pepper *(Piper nigrum)* and β-caryophyllene in ylang ylang *(Cananga odorata)* (Cambray-Smith 2013). Some sesquiterpenes such as α-farnesene can be effective against the bacteria that cause tooth decay (Ishnava et al 2013).

DITERPENES

There are very few diterpenes in essential oils because they are big, heavy molecules with correspondingly high boiling points, so very few are present following the steam distillation process (Cambray-Smith 2013). Diterpenes are generally found in resins (Baser & Demirci 2007). An example is α-camphorene (Cambray-Smith 2013). Diterpenes can occur in solvent extracts.

TABLE 3-6 *Some Monoterpenes and Their Properties*

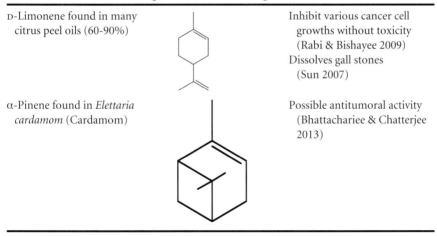

D-Limonene found in many citrus peel oils (60-90%)		Inhibit various cancer cell growths without toxicity (Rabi & Bishayee 2009) Dissolves gall stones (Sun 2007)
α-Pinene found in *Elettaria cardamom* (Cardamom)		Possible antitumoral activity (Bhattachariee & Chatterjee 2013)

TABLE 3-7 *Some Sesquiterpenes and Their Properties*

α-Zingiberene found in *Zingiber officinalis* (ginger)		Antioxidant, increases glutathione production and reduces inflammation (Jeena et al 2013)
α-Farnesene in *Eucalyptus globulus* (blue gum eucalyptus)		Effective against cariogenic bacteria that cause tooth decay (Ishnava et al 2013)

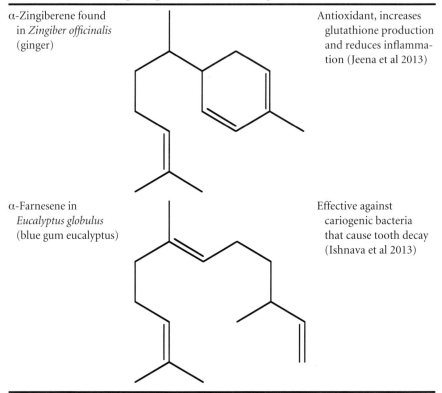

ALCOHOLS

Terpenic alcohols (terpenols) are found in many essential oils. Their names all end in *-ol*. Structurally, they have a hydroxyl group attached to one of their carbon atoms (Table 3-8). Monoterpenols are thought to be good antiseptics with some antibacterial, antifungal, and antiviral properties (Opaichenova & Obreshkova 2003), (Chiang et al 2005). Some alcohols, such as terpinen-4-ol, are uplifting; others like linalool are thought to be sedative (Yamamoto et al 2013). Usually essential oils with a high percentage of monoterpenols, for example, palma rosa *(Cymbopogon martini)*, are safe to use undiluted on the skin. Geraniol in *Cymbopogon martini* (palma rosa) is effective against *Escherichia coli* (Duarte et al 2007) and has antitumor and anticancer activity (Madankumur et al 2013). Terpinen-4-ol in *Melaleuca alternifolia* (tea tree) is effective against multidrug-resistant *Staphylococcus aureus* (MRSA) (Thomsen et al 2013), (Loughlin et al 2008) and also has antitumor properties (Calcabrini et al 2004). Terpinen-4-ol was also found to prevent the influenza virus from entering host cells by disturbing the normal viral membrane fusion procedure (Li et al 2013).

TABLE 3-8 *Some Monoterpenols and Their Properties*

Linalool in *Ocimum basilicum* (basil) Linalool in *Lavandula angustifolia* (lavender)	OH	Effective against MRSA and resistant *Pseudomonas* (Opaichenova & Obreshkova 2003); antiviral (Chiang et al 2005) Inhaled linalool altered hypothalamic gene expression in rats under stress (Yamamoto et al 2013)
Geraniol in *Cymbopogon martini* (palma rosa)	CH₂OH	Antitumor and anticancer activity (Madankumur et al 2013) Antimicrobial against *E. Coli* (Duarte et al 2007)
Terpinen-4-ol in *Melaleuca alternifolia* (tea tree)	OH	Effective against MRSA (Loughlin et al 2008) Antitumor and anticancer activity (Madankumur et al 2013); inhibits growth of melanoma cells (Calcabrini et al 2004)

SESQUITERPENOLS

Sesquiterpenols have 15 carbon atoms and a variety of therapeutic effects (Table 3-9). Farnesol found in Australian sandalwood *(Santalum spicatum)* enhanced amphotericin B and caspofungin activity against *Candida* (Cordeiro et al 2013). It also appeared to protect lungs from the damage of cigarette smoke (Wajhul & Sarwat 2008). Patchoulol found in *Patchouli cablin* (patchouli) is effective against influenza (Kiyohara et al 2012) and also has antiinflammatory properties (Li 2011). α-Bisabolol found in *Matricaria recutita* (German chamomile) has its own antiinflammatory (Kamatou et al 2010) and antinociceptive-like action (de Miranda et al 2010). Nerolidol, found in *Melaleuca quinquenervia*, enhanced the insecticidal and ovicidal effect of 0.5% tea tree against hair nits (Di Campli et al 2012). The Amazonian Waiapi tribe treat malaria by inhaling the essential oil from the leaf of *Virola surinamensis*. Nerolidol is one of the active components of *Virola surinamensis* (Lopes et al 1999). Sclareol has shown significant cytotoxic activity against both human leukemic and breast cell lines

TABLE 3-9 *Some Sesquiterpenols and Their Properties*

Farnesol found in *Santalum spicatum* (Australian sandalwood)	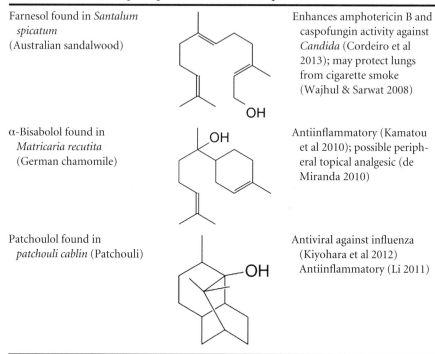	Enhances amphotericin B and caspofungin activity against *Candida* (Cordeiro et al 2013); may protect lungs from cigarette smoke (Wajhul & Sarwat 2008)
α-Bisabolol found in *Matricaria recutita* (German chamomile)		Antiinflammatory (Kamatou et al 2010); possible peripheral topical analgesic (de Miranda 2010)
Patchoulol found in *patchouli cablin* (Patchouli)		Antiviral against influenza (Kiyohara et al 2012) Antiinflammatory (Li 2011)

and also enhances the effect of anticancer drugs (doxorubicin, etoposide, and cisplatinum) against MDD2 breast cancer cell lines (Dimas et al 2006).

PHENOLIC TERPENES

A phenol is a hydroxyl group that is bonded directly to one of the six carbon atoms in a benzene ring (Table 3-10). Like alcohols, phenol names end in *-ol*, but they should not be mistaken for the much gentler alcohols. Benzene (aromatic) rings can easily be formed from aliphatic (nonbenzene) rings, but the reverse reaction rarely occurs (Guenther 1972). Phenols are widespread in nature, for example, adrenaline and tetrahydrocannabinol (the hallucinogenic ingredient in marijuana) (Cambray-Smith 2013). There are two principal phenols found in essential oils: carvacrol and thymol. Carvacrol and thymol of oregano, satureja, thyme, etc., are isomeric monoterpenic phenols.

Phenols need to be treated with care because they are irritating to the skin and mucous membrane (Tisserand & Young 2013). Most have very strong antibacterial properties, with a stimulating effect on both the nervous system and the immune system. Thymol (from *Thymus vulgaris CT thymol*) has antimicrobial, antioxidant, and antitumoral properties (Nikolić et al 2014). It is effective against *Pseudomonas* and may be useful in cystic fibrosis (Helenicy et al 2012). Eugenol, found in *Syzygium aromaticum* (clove bud) and *Ocimum sanctum* (holy basil), is

TABLE 3-10 *Some Phenols and Their Properties*

Thymol found in *Thymus vulgaris,* common thyme Thymol found in *Lippia sidoides* (pepper-rosmarin)		Antimicrobial, antioxidant, and antitumoral (Nikolić et al 2014) Effective against *Pseudomonas* and may be useful in cystic fibrosis (Helenicy et al 2012)
Eugenol found in *Syzygium aromaticum* (clove bud) Eugenol found in *Ocimum sanctum* (holy basil)		Vasorelaxant (Damiani et al 2003) Antimicrobial against *E. coli, S. aureus* (Walsh et al 2003) Antifungal against *Aspergillus* (Kumar et al 2010)
Carvacrol found in *Zataria multiflora* (Iranian thyme) Carvacrol found in *Origanum bilgeri* (Turkish oregano)		Effective against bacterial vaginosis (Simar et al 2008), vaginal candida (Islami et al 2004) Acaricidal against ticks (Koc et al 2013)

a vasorelaxant (Damiani et al 2003). It has antimicrobial properties, particularly against *E. coli* and *S. aureus* (Walsh et al 2003) and is also antifungal (Kumar et al 2010). Carvacrol found in *Zataria multiflora* (Iranian thyme), *Origanum vulgare* (oregano) and *Thymus vulgaris CT carvacrol* (thyme) is effective against bacterial vaginosis (Simar et al 2008) and vaginal candida (Islami et al 2004). Carvacrol is also acaricidal and effective against ticks (Koc et al 2013). Carvacrol also has anticarcinogenic effects (Baser 2008). The compound phenol (carbolic acid) is a disinfectant derived from coal tar and not found in essential oils (Tisserand & Young 2013).

ETHERS (PHENOLIC) OR PHENYLPROPANOIDS

Ethers found in essential oils are phenylmethyl ethers or phenolic ethers or, more scientifically, alkenylbenzenes (Cambray-Smith 2013). Ethers occur when a methyl or ethyl group is attached to a benzene ring via an oxygen molecule (Table 3-11). Examples (in alphabetical order) are anethole, apiol, eugenol, estragole, myristicin, and safrole (Tisserand & Young 2013). Estragole is sometimes called

TABLE 3-11 *An Ether and Its Properties*

trans-Anethole in *Foeniculum* *vulgare* (fennel)	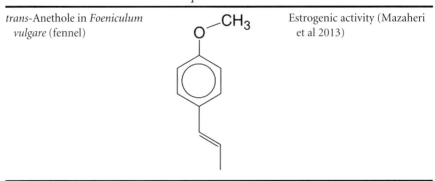	Estrogenic activity (Mazaheri et al 2013)

methyl-chavicol (Tisserand & Young 2013). Ethers are not widely distributed but are found in some common essential oils, for example: anise, basil, cinnamon leaf, and fennel. Ethers are less aggressive on the skin than phenols. However, some ethers like myristicin have hallucinogenic properties when taken orally (Ehrenpreis et al 2014). Myristicin (found in nutmeg) has a similar structure to MMDA a precursor to MDMA (ecstasy). *trans*-Anethole in *Foeniculum vulgare* (fennel) has estrogenic activity (Mazaheri et al 2013) as does anethole from several *Pimpinella* species (Baser et al 2007).

ALDEHYDES

An aldehyde is a partially oxidized primary alcohol (Tisserand & Young 2013). Structurally, it has an oxygen atom double bonded to a carbon atom at the end of a carbon chain (Table 3-12). The fourth bond is always a hydrogen atom (Bowles 2000). Aldehydes usually end in -*al* and often have sedative, calming effects, as well as being important to the aroma of the plant. Examples include citral in lemon balm *(Melissa officinalis)*, β-citronellal in lemongrass *(Cymbopogon citratus)*, geranial in lemon eucalyptus *(Eucalyptus citriodora)*, and neral in lemon verbena *(Aloysia triphylla)*. Geranial and neral are isomers. This means they have the same molecular make-up but the carboxyl molecule is in a different place. Geranial (α-citral) and neral (β-citral) occur naturally as a mixture of the two isomers in citral (Tisserand & Young 2013). Citral has strong antiseptic and antibacterial properties and is effective against MRSA (Saddiq & Khayyat 2010). It also has antiinflammatory properties and enhances the effect of naproxen (Ortiz et al 2010). Citronellal has antifungal properties (Mimica-Dukic et al 2004) especially against *Candida* (Zore et al 2011). In some interesting new research, citronellal may increase olfactory sensitivity in patients with Parkinson-impaired olfaction (Haehner et al 2013). Cinnamaldehyde found in *Cinnamomum zeylanicum* (cinnamon) has antimicrobial and antifungal properties (Unlu et al 2010). It is a potential antidiabetic agent (Subash et al 2007) and has been found to decrease muscle soreness after exercise (Mashhadi et al 2013). Isolated aldehydes can be

TABLE 3-12 *Some Aldehydes and Their Properties*

Citronellal found in *Eucalyptus citriodora* Citronellal found in *Melissa officinalis* (melissa)		Antifungal especially *Candida* (Zore et al 2011) Antifungal (Mimica-Dukic et al 2004) May increase olfactory sensitivity in patients with Parkinson-impaired olfaction (Haehner et al 2013)
Neral & geranial (citral) in *Cymbopogon citratus* (lemongrass)		Antibacterial against MRSA (Saddiq & Khayyat 2010) Enhances antiinflammatory effect of naproxen (Ortiz et al 2010)
Cinnamaldehyde in *Cinnamomum zeylanticum* (cinnamon)		Antimicrobial, antifungal (Unlu et al 2010) Potential antidiabetic agent (Subash et al 2007) Decreases muscle soreness after exercise (Mashhadi et al 2013)

dermal irritants, but when the whole essential oil is used the irritating effect of aldehydes appears to be ameliorated by the presence of terpenes, such as limonene or α-pinene (Opdyke & Letizia 1982).

ESTERS

Esters are a combination of an acid and an alcohol and take their name from the acid and alcohol (Table 3-13). Hence, acetic acid and linalool produce linalyl acetate. Acids do not occur in essential oils but can be found in floral waters. Esters end in –*ate* and have antispasmodic (Ou et al 2012) and calming properties (Igarashi 2013). Some are also antifungal. They often smell very fruity. Examples include linalyl acetate in lavender *(Lavandula angustifolia)*, clary sage *(Salvia sclarea)* and bergamot *(Citrus aurantium* subsp. *bergamia)*, and geranyl acetate in sweet marjoram *(Origanum majorana)*. An essential oil with a very high ester content (85%) is Roman chamomile *(Chamaemelum/Anthemis nobilis)*. Esters are usually safe in high amounts except for methyl salicylate. Methyl salicylate occurs at approximately 98% in sweet birch (*Betula lenta*) and wintergreen (*Gaultheria procumbens*) essential oils. Methyl anthranilate found in mandarin (*Citrus reticulata*) has antiandrogenic potential that could be useful in prostate cancer (Roell et al 2011). Bornyl

TABLE 3-13 *Some Esters and Their Properties*

Linalyl acetate found in *Lavandula angustifolia* (lavender)		Reduces stress in pregnant women (Igarashi 2013) Pain relief in primary dys-menorrhea (Ou et al 2012) Reduce serum cortisol in healthy men (Shiina et al 2008)
Methyl anthranilate found in *Citrus reticulata* (mandarin)	NH_2 $COOCH_3$	Antiandrogenic potential for prostate cancer (Roell et al 2011)
Bornyl acetate found in *Picea mariana* (black spruce)	$OCOCH_3$	Possible preventive agent for lung inflammatory diseases (Chen et al 2014)

acetate found in *Picea mariana* (black spruce) is a possible preventive agent for lung inflammatory diseases (Chen et al 2014). Linalyl acetate found in lavender (*Lavandula angustifolia*) reduced serum cortisol in healthy men (Shiina et al 2008).

KETONES

Ketones contain the carbonyl group (–C=O) and so are related to the aldehydes. Ketones and aldehydes are both found in biological molecules, e.g., progesterone and testosterone (Cambray-Smith 2013). A ketone is derived from an alcohol by oxygenation and has an oxygen atom double bonded to a carbon atom that is also bonded to two other carbon atoms (Table 3-14) (Bowles 2000). Ketones end in -*one* with a single exception: camphor. This substance has no relation to the plant camphor. Some ketones can produce adverse effects when taken orally and, because ketones are resistant to metabolism, this adverse effect can build up in the liver. The most cited toxic ketone is D-pulegone (found in pennyroyal), which caused the death of a 23-year-old woman in 1897 after she drank 15 mL of undiluted essential oil (Allen 1897). That is a large amount to swallow. A child who developed hepatic malfunction and severe epileptic encephalopathy after swallowing a large amount of unknown essential oil tested positive for pulegone (Bakerink et al 1996).

Examples of essential oils that contain large amounts of ketones (in alphabetical order) are: caraway, frankincense, hyssop, peppermint, rosemary, sage, and spearmint (Cambray-Smith 20130. Clearly caution should be used when these

TABLE 3-14 *A Ketone and Its Properties*

L-Carvone found in *Mentha ×* *spicata* (spearmint)	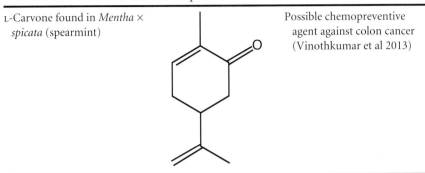	Possible chemopreventive agent against colon cancer (Vinothkumar et al 2013)

are ingested. Ketones that are beneficial to the skin include jasmone in jasmine *(Jasminum officinale)* and isomenthone in geranium *(Pelargonium graveolens).* Other useful ketones are D-carvone in spearmint *(Mentha × spicata),* fenchone in fennel *(Foeniculum vulgare* var. *dulce)* and verbenone in rosemary *(Rosmarinus officinalis).* D-Carvone is a possible chemopreventive agent against colon cancer (Vinothkumar et al 2013). Carvone occurs in two mirror images or enantiomers: R(–)-carvone (or L(-)carvone) smells like spearmint. Its mirror image, S-(+)-carvone (or D-carvone), smells like caraway.

Two unusual ketones (italidione and beta-diketone) are found only in "everlasting" (sometimes called "immortelle")—*Helichrysum italicum* (Stewart 2005). A diketone contains two ketone groups. Both italidione and beta-diketone contribute to the unusual fragrance of *Helichrysum* and its remarkable antihematoma properties. I have used *Helichrysum* occasionally undiluted on the skin for bruises and contusions with excellent results, but I could find no published research, which is rather surprising.

OXIDES

In chemical terminology, an oxide is called an ether or a peroxide. However, using the term *ether* might be confusing because there is group of phenolic ethers in aromatherapy that have different properties. The use of the term *oxide* in aromatherapy is a little more general because the carbons are not neighbors. (Oxides in organic chemistry typically involve an oxygen bridge between two neighboring carbon atoms.) In aromatherapy, an 'oxide' has an oxygen atom in a chain of carbons, that forms a non aromatic ring (Table 3-15). The most common oxide is cineole—a strong expectorant. Both 1,4-cineole and 1,8-cineole occur in essential oils (Tisserand & Young 2014). 1,8 cineole is sometimes called eucalyptol and is found in blue gum *(Eucalyptus globulus),* rosemary *(Rosmarinus officinalis CT cineole),* and bay laurel *(Laurus nobilis).* Research indicates that 1,8-cineole, found in *Eucalyptus globulus* (blue gum) is a possible antiinflammatory agent for neurodegenerative disease (Khan et al 2014). Other oxides are ascaridole found

TABLE 3-15 *An Oxide and Its Properties*

1,8-Cineole found in *Eucalyptus globulus* (blue gum)		Possible antiinflammatory agent in neurodegenerative disease (Khan et al 2014)

TABLE 3-16 *Lactones and Their Properties*

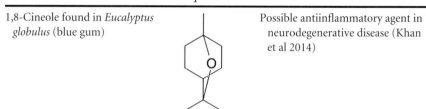

Nepetalactone found in *Nepeta parnassica* (giant catnip) Alantolactone found in *Inula helenium* root (elecampane)		Mosquito repellant (Gkinis et al 2014) Antimicrobial against *Staphylococcus aureus* (Stojanović-Radić et al 2012) Anticancer activity in some cancer lines (Khan et al 2013)

in wormseed *(Chenopodium ambrosioides* var. *anthelminticum)* and rose oxide found in both geranium *(Pelargonium graveolens)* and rose *(Rosa damascena).* Ascaridole shows interesting antitumor activity in sarcoma cells (Bezerra 2009).

LACTONES

Lactones are mainly found in expressed oils and some absolutes like jasmine (Clarke 2002). They are cyclic esters derived from lactic acid (Baser & Demirci 2007) and have an oxygen atom double bonded to a carbon atom. The carbon atom is attached to another oxygen atom that is part of a closed ring (Table 3-16). Lactones tend to end in *-lactone* or *-ine.* The percentage of lactones present may be low, but they are traditionally thought to play an important role as mucolytics (Clarke 2002; Schnaubelt 2011; Rhind 2012). Alantolactone is present in elecampane *(Inula helenium)* and is effective against *Staphylococcus aureus* (Stojanović-Radić et al 2012). It also has anticancer activity in some cancer lines (Khan et al 2013). However, elecampane is linked to skin sensitization, as are many lactones (Tisserand & Young 2013). Nepetalactone, found in catnip *(Nepeta cataria),* is a mosquito repellant (Gkinis et al 2014). It is also feline attractant.

COUMARINS

Coumarins are a subgroup of lactones. They have an oxygen atom double bonded to a carbon atom. That carbon atom is attached to another oxygen (that is part of a closed ring) and they also have a benzene ring attached (Table 3-17). Coumarins usually end in *-one* (pronounced *own*), as in umbelliferone, or

TABLE 3-17 *Structural Similarities between Coumarin and Warfarin*

Coumarin		May have potential use in Alzheimer's (Huang et al 2013)
Warfarin		Anticoagulant (Cavallari et al 2011)

with -*in*, as in coumarin. Coumarins are present in very small amounts in essential oils. There is sometimes confusion between the functional group, coumarin, and the chemical dicoumarol (Mills 1991). Dicoumarol is created naturally by the breakdown of the sweet clover plant. Synthetic dicoumarol is the basis of the anticoagulant drug warfarin (Cavallari et al 2011). The chemical drawing (see Figure 3-18) shows a coumarin structure within warfarin. Some coumarins may reduce clotting time if taken internally. Ramesh & Pugalendi (2007) found that umbelliferone normalized prothrombin, clotting and bleeding time in diabetic rats. Previously, they had found umbelliferone to be antihyperglycemic (Ramesh et al 2006) and antidiabetic (Ramesh et al 2005). Coumarins may have a future role to play in Alzheimer's disease as coumarins are important acetylcholinesterase (AChE) inhibitors. Chinese research found a coumarin derivative was a 100 times better than the conventional drug donepezil (Huang et al 2013).

FURANOCOUMARINS

Furanocoumarins (FCs) are present (<2%) in citrus-peel oils and a few other essential oils, for example: angelica *(Angelica archangelica)* root and rue *(Ruta graveolens)*. FCs react in the presence of ultraviolet light to produce a phototoxic effect, resulting in burns or erythema. Even small dilutions (0.03%) applied to the skin can result in phototoxicity (Tisserand & Young 2013). A phototoxic effect was also produced with a 2.4% concentration on pale skin and 15% concentration on dark brown or black skin. Sometimes, the pigmentation can remain for life. Extensive burns can also result from oral ingestion of FCs in combination of UV exposure (Tisserand & Young 2013). Common FCs include bergapten (found in expressed bergamot, bitter orange, grapefruit, lemon, lime (and in steam distilled angelica root), and bergamottin (found in expressed bergamot, grapefruit, lemon and lime). Bergamottin is antitumoral in human fibrosarcoma HT-1080 cells (Hwang et al 2012).

APART FROM CHEMISTRY

Some people believe there is more to an essential oil than the sum of its parts: that there is a synergy of all those parts working together. Some people believe there is an energy or vibration to an essential oil and this plays a major role in healing. Some people think essential oils have yin- and yang-like qualities. Others think the effect of essential oils is purely chemical so by isolating the part, the effect will be grasped. Whatever your view, I hope this short overview of chemistry for aromatherapists, has been useful. There are some excellent chemistry chapters, books, and courses relevant to aromatherapy available for those wanting to delve further.

REFERENCES

Allen W. 1897. Note on a case of supposed poisoning by pennyroyal. *Lancet.* 1:1022-1023.

Bakerink J, Gospe S, Dimand R et al. 1996. Multiple organ failure after ingestion of pennyroyal oil from herbal tea in two infants. *Pediatrics.* 98(5) 944-947.

Baser K. H. C., Demirci F. 2007. In Flavours and Fragrances: *Chemistry, Bioprocessing and Sustainability.* Berger RG. Ed. Springer, Berlin. P 43-86.

Baser K. H. C., Tabanca N, Kirimer N, Bedir E, Khan I, Wedge D. 2007. Recent advances in the chemistry and biological activities of the Pimpinella species of Turkey. *Pure Appl Chem.* 79(4):539-556.

Başer K. H. C. 2008. Biological and Pharmacological Activities of Carvacrol and Carvacrol Bearing Essential Oils. *Current Pharmaceutical Design.* 14, 3106-3120.

Baser K. H. C., Demirci F. 2011. *Kirk-Othmer Encyclopedia of Chemical Technology.* 4th edition. Wiley. P 1-37.

Başer K. H. C., Altintas A, Kürkçüoglu M. 2012. A Review of the History, Ethnobotany, and Modern Uses of Rose Petals, Rose Oil, Rose Water, and Other Rose Products. *Herbalgram.* 96:41-53.

Bezerra D, Marinho Filho B, Alves A, Pessoa C, De Moraes M et al. 2009. Antitumor activity of the essential oil from the leaves of *Croton regelianus* and its component ascaridole. *Chem Biodivers.* 6(8): 1224-1231.

Bhattacharjee B, Chatterjee J. 2013. Identification of proapoptopic, anti-inflammatory, anti- proliferative, anti-invasive and anti-angiogenic targets of essential oils in cardamom by dual reverse virtual screening and binding pose analysis. *Asian Pac J Cancer Prev.* 14(6):3735-42.

Bowles J. 2000. *The Basic Chemistry of Chemotherapeutic Essential Oils.* Sydney, Australia: Pirie Printers.

Buhner S H. 2012. *Herbal Antibiotics.* Storey Publishing. p 381.

Calcabrini A, Stringaro A, Toccacieli L, Meschini S, Marra M, Colone M et al. 2004. Terpinen-4-ol, the main component of *Melaleuca alternifolia* (Tea tree) oil inhibits the in vitro growth of human melanoma cells. *J Invest Dermatol.* 122: 349-360.

Cambray-Smith I. 2013. *Essential Chemistry Course Notes.* Natural Science. Malmsbury, UK.

Cavallari L, Shin J, Perera M. 2011. Role of Pharmacogenomics in the Management of Traditional and Novel Oral Anticoagulants. *Pharmacotherapy.* 31(12): 10.1592/phco.31.12.1192. Accessed January 27, 2014.

Chen N, Sun G, Yuan X, Hou J, Wu Q et al. 2014. Inhibition of lung inflammatory responses by bornyl acetate is correlated with regulation of myeloperoxidase activity. *J Surg Res.* 186(1):436-45.

Chiang L-C, Ng L-T, Cheng P-W, Chiang W, Lin C-C. 2005. Antiviral activities of extracts and selected constituents of Ocimum Basilicum. *Clin Exp Pharmacol Phys.* 32(10): 811-816.

Christensson J, Forsström P, Wennberg A-M, Karlberg A-T, Matura M. 2009. Air oxidation increases skin irritation from fragrance terpenes. *Contact Dermatitis.* 60(1): 32-40.

Clarke S. 2002. *Essential Chemistry for Safe Aromatherapy.* Churchill Livingstone. London.

Cordeiro R, Teixerira C, Brilhante R, Casteol-Branco D, Paiva M et al. 2013. Minimum inhibitory concentrations of amphotericin B, azoles and caspofungin against Candida species are reduced by farnesol. *Med Mycol.* 51(1):53-9.

Damiani C, Rossoni L, Vassallo D. 2003. Vasorelaxant effects of eugenol on rat thoracic aorta. *Vascular Pharmacol.* 40(1):59-66.

de Miranda A, Alves H, Carolos J, Gonçalves R, Santos Cruz G et al. 2010. Evaluation of the sequiterpene (-) a-bisabolol as a novel peripheral nervous blocker. *Neurosci Lett.* 472(1):11-15.

Di Campli E, Di Bartolomeo S, Delli Pizzi P, Di Giulio M, Grande R et al. 2012. Activity of tea tree oil and nerolidol alone or in combination against *Pediculus capitis* (head lice) and its eggs. *Parasitol Res.* 111(5):1985-1992.

Dimas K, Papadaki M, Tsimplouli C, Hatziantoniou S, Alevizopoulos K et al. 2006. Labd-14-ene-8,13-diol (sclareol) induces cell cycle arrest and apoptosis in human breast cancer cells and enhances the activity of anticancer drugs. *Biomed Pharmacol.* 60(3):127-133.

Duarte M, Leme E, Delarmelina C, Soares A, Figueira G et al. 2007. Activity of essential oils from Brazilian medicinal plants on Escherichia coli. *J Ethnopharmacol.* 111(2):197-201.

Ehrenpreis J, DesLauriers C, Lank P, Armstrong K, Leikin J. 2014. Nutmeg Poisonings: A Retrospective Review of 10 Years Experience from the Illinois Poison Center, 2001-2011. *J Med Toxicol.* Jan 23. [Epub ahead of print]. Accessed 31/1/2014.

Feraz R, Cardozo G, da Silva T, Fontes J, Prata A et al. 2013. Antitumour properties of the leaf essential oil of *Xylopia frutescens. Food Chem.* 141(1):196-200.

Gkinis G, Michaelakis A, Koliopoulos G, Ioannou E, Tzakou O, Roussis V. 2014. Evaluation of the repellent effects of Nepeta parnassica extract, essential oil, and its major nepetalactone metabolite against mosquitoes. *Parasitol Res.* PMID: 24449446. Accessed January 29 2014.

Evaluation of the repellent effects of Nepeta parnassica extract, essential oil, and its major nepetalactone metabolite against mosquitoes. *Parasitol Res.* PMID:24449446. Accessed January 28 2014.

Guenther E. 1972. *The Essential Oils, Vol. I.* Malabar, FL: Krieger.

Guenther E. 1976. *The Essential Oils, Vol. III.* Malaber, FL: Krieger.

Haehner A, Tosch C, Wolz M, Klingelhoefer L, Fauser M et al. 2013. Olfactory training in patients with Parkinson's Disease. *PLoS One.* 8(3):e61680. Accessed January 28/1/2014.

Helenicy N, Veras F, Rodrigques A, Colares I, Menez H et al 2012. Synergistic antibiotic activity of volatile compounds from the essential oil of *Lippia sidoides* and thymol. *Fitoterapia.* 83(3): 508-512.

Huang L, Su T, Li X. 2013. Natural products as sources of new lead compounds for the treatment of Alzheimer's disease. *Curr Top Med Chem.* 13(15):1864-78.

Hwang Y, Yun H, Choi J, Kang K, Jeong H. 2012. Suppression of phorbol-12-myristate-13-acetate-induced tumor cell invasion by bergamottin via the inhibition of protein kinase Cdelta/p38 mitogen-activated protein kinase and JNK/nuclear factor-kappaB-dependent matrix metalloproteinase-9 expression. *Mol Nutr Food Res.* 54(7):977-90.

Igarashi T. 2013. Physical and psychologic effects of aromatherapy inhalation on pregnant women: a randomized controlled trial. *J Altern Complement Med.* 19(10):805-10.

Ishnava K, Chauhan J, Barad M. 2013. Anticariogenic and phytochemical evaluation of *Eucalyptus globulus. Saudi J Biol Science.* 20(1): PMCID: PMC3730900. Accessed 24/1/2014.

Islami, A Ansari A, Kashanian M, Bekhradi R, Akbari M et al. 2004. *Zataria multiflora* vaginal cream compared with clotrimazole vaginal cream in the treatment of candida vaginitis. *Iran. J. Pharm. Res.* Suppl2. 36-37.

Jeena K, Liju V, Kuttan R. 2013. Antioxidant, anti-inflammatory and antinociceptive activities of essential oil from ginger. *Indian J Physiol Pharmacol.* 57(1):51-62.

Kamatou G, Viljoen A. 2010. A review of the application and pharmacological properties of a-bisabolol and a-bisabolol-rich oils. *J Am Oil Chem Soc.* 87(1): 1-7.

Khan M, Li T, Ahmad Khan MK, Rasul A, Nawaz F et al. 2013. Alantolactone induces apoptosis in HepG2 cells through GSH depletion, inhibition of STAT3 activation, and mitochondrial dysfunction. *Biomed Res Int.* 2013;2013:719858. Accessed 31/1/2013.

Khan A, Vaibhav K, Javed H, Tabassum R, Ahmed ME et al. 2014. 1,8-cineole (eucalyptol) mitigates inflammation in amyloid Beta toxicated PC12 cells: relevance to Alzheimer's disease. *Neurochem Res.* 39(2):344-52.

Kiyohara H, Ichino C, Kawamura Y, Nagai T, Sato N, Yamada H. 2012. Patchouli alcohol: in vitro direct anti-influenza virus sesquiterpene in *Pogostemon cablin* Benth. *J Nat Med-Tokyo*, 66 (2012): 55-61.

Koc S, Oz E, Cinbilgel I, Aydin L, Cetin H. 2013. Acaricidal activity of *Origanum bilgeri* P.H. Davis (Lamiaceae) essential oil and its major component, carvacrol against adults *Rhipicephalus turanicus*. *Vet Parasitol.* 193(1-3):316-9.

Kumar A, Sukia R, Singh P, Dubey N. 2010. Chemical composition, antifungal and antiaflatoxigenic activities of *Ocimum sanctum* L. essential oil and its safety assessment as plant based antimicrobial. *Food Chem Toxicol.* 48(2):539-543.

Li X, Duan S, Chu C, Xu J, Zeng G et al. 2013. Melaleuca alternifolia concentrate inhibits in vitro entry of influenza virus into host cells. *Molecules.* 8(8):9550-66.

Li Y, Xian Y, Ip, S, Su Z, Su, J, He J et al. 2011. Anti-inflammatory activity of patchouli alcohol isolated from Pogostemonis Herba in animal models. *Fitoterapia*, 82(8): 1295-1301.

Lopes N, Kato M, Andrade E et al. 1999. Antimalarial use of volatile oil from the leaves of *Virola surinamensis* by Waiapi Amazon Indians. *J Ethnopharmacol.* 67(3): 313-319.

Loughlin R, Gilmore B, McCarron P, Tunney M. 2008. Comparison of the cidal activity of tea tree oil and terpinen-4-ol against clinical bacterial skin isolates and human fibroblast cells. *Lett Appl Microbiol.* 46(4):428-33.

Madankumur A, Jayakumar S, Gokuladhas K, Rajan B, Radhunandhakumar S. et al. 2013. Geraniol modulates tongue and hepatic phase I and phase II conjugation activities and may contribute directly to the chemopreventive activity against experimental oral carcinogenesis. *Eur J Pharmacol.* 705(1-3):148-55.

Mashhadi N, Ghiasvand R, Askari G, Feizi A, Hariri M et al. 2013. Influence of ginger and cinnamon intake on inflammation and muscle soreness ensued by exercise in Iranian female athletes. *Int J Prev Med.* 4(suppl 1): S11-15.

Mazaheri S, Nematbakhsh M, Bahadorani M, Peseshki Z, Talebi A et al. 2013. Effects of fennel essential oil on cisplatin-induced nephrotoxicity in ovariectomized rats. *Toxicol Int.* 20(2): 138-145.

Mimica-Dukic N, Bozin N, Sokovic M, Simin N. 2004. Antimicrobial and antioxidant activities of *Melissa officinalis* L. (Lamiaceae) essential oil. *J Agricult Food Chem.* 52(9): 2485-2489.

Mills S. 1991. *Out of the Earth.* London: Viking Arkana, 295.

Nikolić M, Glamočlija J, Isabel C, Ferreira I, Ricardo C. 2014. Chemical composition, antimicrobial, antioxidant, antitumor activity of *Thymus serpyllum, Thymus algeriensis, Thymus vulgaris* essential oils. *Industrial Crops Products.* 52:183-190.

Opaichenova G, Obreshkova D. 2003. Comparative studies on the activity of basil—an essential oil from *Ocimum basilicum* L. against multidrug resistant clinical isolates of the genera Staphylococcus, Enterococcus and Pseudomonas by using different test methods. *J Microbiol Methods.* 54(1):105-10.

Opdyke D, Letizia C 1982. Monographs on fragrance raw materials. *Food Cosmet Toxicol.* 20. (Suppl).

Ornano L, Venditti A, Ballero M, Sanna C, Quassinti L et al. 2013. Chemopreventive and antioxidant activity of the chamazulene-rich essential oil obtained from *Artemisia arborescens* L. growing on the Isle of La Maddalena, Sardinia, Italy. *Chem Biodivers.* 10(8):1464-74.

Ortiz M, Gonzalex-Garcia M, Ponce-Monter H, Castaneda-Hernandez G, Arguilar-Robles P. 2010. Synergistic effect of the interaction between naproxen and citral on inflammation in rats. *Phytomedicine.* 18(1):74-79.

Ou M, Hsu T, Lai A, Lin Y, Lin C. 2012. Pain relief assessment by aromatic essential oil massage on outpatients with primary dysmenorrhea: a randomized, double-blind clinical trial. *J Obstet Gynaecol Res.* 38(5):817-22.

Park K, Nam D, Hun H, Le S, Jang H et al 2011. β-Caryophyllene oxide inhibits growth and induces apoptosis through the suppression of PI3K/AKT/mTOR/S6K1 pathways and ROS-mediated MAPKs activation. *Cancer Lett.* 312(2):178-88.

Rabi T, Bayashee A. 2009. d-Limonene sensitizes docetaxel-induced cytotoxicity in human prostate cancer cells: Generation of reactive oxygen species and induction of apoptosis. *J Carcinog.* 8:9. doi: 10.4103/1477-3163.51368. Accessed 24.1.2014.

Ramesh B, Pugalendi KV. 2005. Antihyperlipidemic and antidiabetic effects of Umbelliferone in streptozotocin diabetic rats. *Yale J Biol Med.* 78:189-96.

Ramesh B, Pugalendi KV. 2006. Antihyperglycaemic effect of Umbelliferone in STZ-diabetic rats. *J Med Food.* 562-6.

Ramesh B, Pugalendi K. 2007, Effect of umbelliferone on tail tendon collagen and haemostatic function in streptozotocin-diabetic rats. *Basic Clin Pharmacol Toxicol.* 101(2):73-7.

Rhind J. 2012. *Essential Oils.* 2nd edition. Singing Dragon. London. UK.

Roell D, Rosler T, Degen S, Matusch R, Baniahmad A. 2011. Antiandrogenic activity of anthranilic acid ester derivatives as novel lead structures to inhibit prostate cancer cell proliferation. *Chem Biol Drug Des.* 77(6):450-9.

Saddiq A, Khayyat S. 2010. Chemical and antimicrobial studies of monoterpene: Citral. *Pesticide Biochem Physiol.* 98(1):89-93.

Schnaubelt K. 2011. *The Healing Intelligence of Essential Oils.* Healing Arts Press. Rochester, Vermont, USA.

Shiina Y, Funabashi N, Lee K, Toyoda T, Sekine T et al 2008. Relaxation effects of lavender aromatherapy improve coronary flow velocity reserve in healthy men evaluated by transthoracic Doppler echocardiography. *Int J Cardiol.* 129(2):193-197.

Simar M, Azarbad Z, Mojab F, Alavi Majd H. 2008. A comparative study of the therapeutic effects of the *Zataria multiflora* vaginal cream and metronidazole vaginal gel on bacterial vaginosis. *Phytomedicine.* 15(12):1025-1031.

Stewart D. 2005. *The Chemistry of Essential Oils.* Care publishing. Marble Hill. Missouri, USA. Page 53.

Stojanović-Radić Z, Comić Lj, Radulović N, Blagojević P, Denić M et al. 2012. Antistaphylococcal activity of Inula helenium L. root essential oil: eudesmane sesquiterpene lactones induce cell membrane damage. *Eur J Clin Microbiol Infect Dis.* 31(6):1015-25.

Subash Babu P, Prabuseenivasan S, Ignacimuthu S. 2007. Cinnamaldehyde—a potential antidiabetic agent. *Phytomedicine.* 14(1): 15-22.

Sun J. 2007. D-Limonene: safety and clinical applications. *Alter Med Review.* 12(3):259-64.

Thomsen N, Hammer K, Riley T, Van Belkum A, Carson C. 2013. Effect of habituation to tea tree (*Melaleuca alternifolia*) oil on the subsequent susceptibility of Staphylococcus spp. to antimicrobials, triclosan, tea tree oil, terpinen-4-ol and carvacrol. *Int J Antimicrob Agents.* 41(4):343-51.

Tisserand R, Young R. 2014. *Essential Oil Safety.* 2nd edition. London: Churchill Livingstone.

Unlu M, Ergene E, Unlu G, Zeytinoglu H, Vural N et al. 2010. Composition, antimicrobial activity and in vitro cytotoxicity of essential oil from *Cinnamomum zeylanicum*. *Food Chem Toxicol.* 48(11): 3274-80.

Vinothkumar R, Sudha M, Viswanathan P, Kabalimoorthy J, Balasubramanian T, Nalini N. 2013. Modulating effect of d-carvone on 1,2-dimethylhydrazine-induced pre-neoplastic lesions, oxidative stress and biotransforming enzymes, in an experimental model of rat colon carcinogenesis. *Cell Prolif.* 46(6):705-20.

Wajhul K, Sarwat S. 2008. Farnesol ameliorates massive inflammation, oxidative stress and lung injury induced by intratracheal instillation of cigarette smoke extract in rats: An initial step in lung chemoprevention. *Chemico-Biol Interact.* 176(2-3):79-87.

Walsh S, Maillard J-Y, Russell A, Catrenich C, Charbonneau D et al. 2003. Activity and mechanisms of action of selected biocidal agents on Gram-positive and -negative bacteria. *J Appl Microbiol.* 94(2):240-247

Waterman P. 1993. *The chemistry of volatile oils.* In Hay R, Waterman P (eds.), Volatile Oil Crops: Their Biology, Biochemistry and Production. Essex, UK: Longman Scientific and Technical, 47-61.

Yamamoto N, Fujiwara S, Saito-Lizumi K, Kamei A, Shinozaki F et al. 2013. Effects of Inhaled (S)-Linalool on Hypothalamic Gene Expression in Rats under Restraint Stress. *Biosc Biotechnol Biochem.* 77(12):2413-8.

Zore G, Thakre A, Jadhav S, Karuppayil S. 2011. Terpenoids inhibit *Candida albicans* growth by affecting membrane integrity and arrest of cell cycle. *Phytomedicine.* 18(13) 1181-1190.

EXTRACTION, BIOSYNTHESIS, AND ANALYSIS

"All we have yet discovered is but a trifle in comparison with what still lies hid in the great treasury of nature." Anton von Leeuwenhoek. 1679.

EXTRACTION

There are several ways of extracting volatile components from plants. Some methods produce classic essential oils, others produce extracts. See Figure 3-2 and Table 3-18 for comparisons of the extraction procedures used for aromatic extracts and essential oils. Traditionally aromatherapy has specified only the use of essential oils (from distillation or expression), but some extracts are now becoming acceptable.

Essential oils are either distilled or expressed (Arctander 1960). Distillation can mean water distillation, water-and-steam distillation, steam distillation, or steam-and-vacuum distillation (Arctander 1960). To give some idea of yield, 200 kg of *Lavandula angustifolia* flowers will produce 1 kg of essential oil. However, between 2 and 5 metric tons of rose petals are needed to produce the same amount of rose oil.

DISTILLATION (STEAM)

The design of the distillation plants varies from region to region. Traditional and sometimes rather simple methods are still being used in some developing countries. Industrialized nations tend to use more technologically advanced equipment that

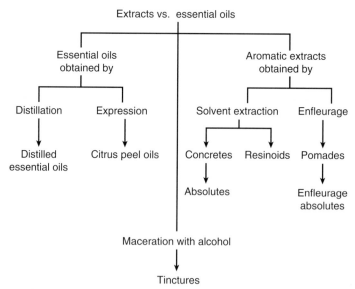

FIGURE 3-2 | Essential oils versus extracts. (Adapted from Williams D. Lecture Notes on Essential Oils. With kind permission of Eve Taylor, London. 1989.)

is computer-controlled with software that can monitor the product throughout the distillation process. Nevertheless, excellent quality oils can be obtained even with a basic distillation apparatus. The aromatic plant material is placed on a grid through which steam passes, usually at a temperature not above 100° C (Bowles 2000). See Figure 3-3 for more details. The water boils at temperatures between 88° C and 100° C depending on the altitude at the distillation site.

High-pressure steam is the fastest way of distilling essential oils with high-boiling constituents like vetiver, sandalwood, and clove. The steam loosens the volatile non-polar constituents of the plant and they pass, with the steam, into a condenser that cools the mixture. Steam also alters some of the components within an essential oil, for example, turning matricin to chamazulene. Some of the polar components from the plant dissolve in the water, producing floral water. The mixture of floral water and essential oil is cooled and becomes liquid. As essential oils and floral water do not mix, they quickly separate—the majority of essential oils float above the floral water, but some sink, depending on their specific gravity.

The degree of heat and the amount of time are vital parts of the distillation process as some components of plants are very sensitive to heat and others take much longer to distill (Guenther 1974). The distillation process for *Lavandula angustifolia* is approximately one hour, but it is considerably longer for sandal-wood or vetiver. The length of the distillation process will affect the chemical composition of the essential oil (Guenther 1976). Steam distillation is suitable for the highly volatile components such as the monoterpenes, but heavier molecules like di or sesquiterpenes take longer. Some floral waters (hydrolats) can also be used therapeutically. Portable distillation equipment is simple to make and can

TABLE 3-18 *Advantages and Disadvantages of Various Extraction Processes*

Extraction Process	Advantages	Disadvantages
Distillation	Economical	Changing constituents
	Large quantities can be processed	Depending on time/temp
	Little labor needed	
Expression	No heat required	Some flavoring left
	Simple apparatus	Only citrus peel oils
		Oxidize quickly
Enfleurage	Low temperature needed	Time consuming
		Labor intensive
		Expensive
CO_2 extraction	Constant product	Expensive
	No heat used	Different chemistry to essential oil
Solvent extraction	Constant product	Solvent residues
		Different chemistry to essential oil

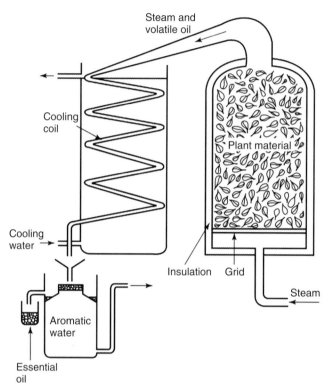

FIGURE 3-3 | Steam distillation. (Reproduced from Price S. Practical Aromatherapy, with the kind permission of Harper Collins, London. 1983.)

be used for small quantities of plants when essential oils must be distilled on site (Alkaire & Simon 1992).

Variations of Steam Distillation

1) **Cohobation:** The water used in the distillation process is reused (Guenther 1974).
2) **Fractional distillation:** The essential oil is distilled at specific temperatures for specific lengths of time to collect different factions (or functional groups) within the essential oil. For example, peppermint contains menthol (a monoterpene) that is less volatile than other peppermint monoterpenes (e.g., α-pinene, β-pinene, sabinene and limonene) and other low boiling hydrocarbons. Monoterpenes evaporate at different temperatures, but many of the peppermint monoterpenes evaporate below 150° to 185° C, so this temperature can be used to "get rid" of lower boiling monoterpenes in order to obtain a high-quality peppermint flavor (Gafner 2014). Nowadays, fractional distillation is often done at reduced pressure in order to lower the boiling temperature.
3) **Rectification:** This aims to separate the volatile and nonvolatile components of an essential oil. If an essential oil contains impurities, it can be purified by

redistillation. This process is called rectification. Sometimes peppermint and caraway seed oils can take on an unpleasant odor if they have been in contact with the wall of a hot still. This aroma can be removed through rectification (Guenther 1974).

4) **Steam-plus-vacuum distillation:** This method uses steam with partial vacuum (Arctander 1960). The pressure used is typically 100 to 200 mm Hg. The advantage of this method is speed. The disadvantage is a fast method of cooling is required.

EXPRESSION

In expression, the production of essential oils (by mechanically pressing the product) involves mainly the peel of citrus plants, like oranges, lemons, or grapefruit. The peel of the fruit is racked or abraded by mechanical scrapers, and the essence collected by centrifugal separation. Sometimes the whole fruit is crushed before the essential oil is separated from the juice and peel. Expressed oils will naturally contain a proportion of waxes, and citrus oils may include other components such as bergapten, a coumarin that can cause phototoxicity (Tisserand & Young 2013).

METHODS FOR PRODUCING AROMATIC EXTRACTS (NOT ESSENTIAL OILS)

There are other methods of extraction that produce compounds called *absolutes*. These are mainly used by the fragrance and cosmetics industry. Rose absolute is yellow, viscous, and sticky. Rose essential oil is clear and solid at room temperature. The essential oil is ten times the price of the absolute. Residual solvents in extracts can produce adverse reactions.

Enfleurage

This method was used on fragile blossoms like jasmine and tuberose. It is rarely used today as it is very labor intensive. I watched this process in Grasse, France. Animal fat is pounded until soft, then glass plates are coated with the fat. Each fat-covered glass plate is called a *chassis*. Fresh blossoms are placed close together on the *chassis* and left until the fat becomes saturated with essential oil. The chassis are constantly being replenished with fresh blossoms, and the old blossoms discarded. This process can take days or even weeks. The resulting oil/fat mixture is called a *pomade*. The *pomade* is washed with alcohol to remove the fat. The remaining extract is called an absolute. However, 99% of jasmine and tuberose extract is now produced by solvent extraction.

Supercritical Fluid Extraction

Supercritical fluid extraction (SFE) with carbon dioxide has been available since the 1980s. When the temperature of CO_2 is maintained at approximately 31° C, under pressure, it acts like a fluid and dissolves the CO_2-soluble constituents of an herb. The interest in SFE has increased in recent years because of legal limitations of solvent residues and solvents (Vagi et al 2005). However, the chemistry of the resulting extract is different to a steam-distilled essential oil because (a) less heat is used and (b) some different components are absorbed by CO_2 extraction (Guan Hou et al 2007). For example, steam-distilled German chamomile *(Matricaria recutita)* essential oil is dark blue because heat converts matricine (found in the plant) to chamazulene—a sesquiterpene. However, matricine is present in the SFE extract. SFE extracts are not available for every plant used in aromatherapy but there is no reason not to use them, provided the chemistry is known and the components are relevant to the clinical goal being targeted. Volatile oils can also be extracted with other solvents. The use of benzene has declined but it is still used (Tisserand & Young 2013). Hexane is commonly used [cyclohexane and *n*-hexane (Tisserand & Young 2013)]. Such extracts are called "volatile oils" to differentiate them from essential oils (Coelho et al 2012).

Resinoids

Resinoids are obtained from resins (amber and mastic), balsams (benzoin) or gum-like exudates (frankincense and myrrh). Frequently resinoids are extracted by solvents. However, frankincense and myrrh can also be obtained by steam distillation or SFE. Resins are soluble in alcohol but not in water. Gums are soluble in water but not in alcohol.

Notes (Aroma Intensities)

The aromas of essential oils have variable intensities, and these may last for different periods of time. The perfume industry calls these properties "notes" (Teixeiry et al 2013). Poucher developed a classification method based on a perfume's evaporation rate (1 to 100) that is still used today (Poucher 1993). Scents that evaporate quickly (1 to 15) are called top notes, for example, mandarin (2) and nutmeg (11). Middle notes (16 to 69) include marjoram (18), ylang ylang (24), and rose (43). Base notes last the longest (70 to 100), for example, angelica (94). Perfumes with the highest ratings last the longest and evaporate the slowest, for example, frankincense, patchouli, sandalwood, and vetiver). A top note might last for a few hours, a middle note for a couple of days, and a base note may last for several weeks.

Oxidation

The odor of an essential oil deteriorates as a result of oxidation. When an essential oil has contact with air, certain components within it react with the oxygen. For example, alcohols can react with oxygen to become aldehydes (Bowles 2000).The rate of oxidation is dependent on the exposure to oxygen and the reactivity of each individual component of the essential oil. Heat and sunlight can speed up oxidation. The oxidization of an essential oil will affect its chemistry and thus its therapeutic potential.

TERPENE BIOSYNTHESIS: HOW AND WHY PLANTS MAKE ESSENTIAL OILS

Biosynthesis is the production of all plant secondary metabolites: alkaloids, bitters, glycosides, gums, saponins, steroids, and essential oil components. Only 1% of flowering plants produce an essential oil in any significant amount, and for a long time essential oils were thought to be unimportant to the plant. The number of identified volatile chemicals synthesized by various plants exceeds 1000 and is likely to grow as more plants are examined (Pichersky et al 2006). The largest class of essential oil components is derived from isoprenoid pathways. The two basic pathways are called the malonic acid pathway and the shikimic acid pathway (Taiz & Zeiger 2014). Terpenoids are formed by malonic pathways and most phenylpropanoids and benzenoids derive from the shikimic acid pathway (Yang et al 2009).

Mevalonic Acid Pathway

Aromatic plants contain enzymes called terpene synthases (TPSs). These enzymes: dimethylallyl pyrophosphate (DMAPP), geranyl pyrophosphate (GPP), farnesyl pyrophosphate (FPP) and geranyl pyrophosphate (GPP), act as catalysts in the formation of mono-, sesqui-, and diterpene essential oil components (Pichersky et al 2006). The plant first converts mevalonic acid to a 5-carbon structure called isoprene. Isoprene, known as methylbuta-1,3-diene to chemists, is a branched chain hydrocarbon containing five carbon atoms and two double bonds. Isoprene is then converted with GPP—an enzyme catalyst—to a 10-carbon molecule like a terpene (Cambray-Smith 2013). This process can continue with another enzyme catalyst, FPP, to produce a 15-carbon molecule like a sesquiterpene. Once the plant has formed GPP, the substance can be converted into alcohols or aldehydes as well as terpenes.

Shikimic Acid Pathway

Shikimic acid (3,4,5-trihydroxy-1-cyclohexene-1-carboxylic acid), another enzyme, is an important catalyst in this second pathway of biosynthesis. This enzyme is proceeded by another enzyme, phenylalanine ammonia lyase (PAL). The pathway is complex, but ultimately leads to the second largest class of essential oil components that contain an aromatic ring, such as phenols (Mann 2001a). Please see Figure 3-4.

Storage of Essential Oils in Plants

Essential oils are stored in specific parts of a plant (Table 3-19). For example, rose essential oil is found in the petals of the flowers, not the roots, leaves, or stem. However, sometimes an essential oil is found in different parts of the same plant, as in the case of angelica *(Angelica archangelica)* root and angelica seed, when the chemistry of each essential oil is different. The essential oil from the root of angelica can cause a skin reaction when ultraviolet light is used on the skin within 24 hours of applying topically, but the essential oil from the seed does not.

Secretory and Storage Structures of Essential Oils in Plants

Essential oils are stored in special secretory structures (Table 3-20). These can be on the surface of the plant or within the plant tissue, and are found in many kinds of plant: perennial, annual, biennial, evergreen and deciduous (Svoboda & Svoboda 2001). Secretory structures vary and include oils cells, secretory ducts or cavities and glandular hairs (Baser & Demirci 2007). Often the whole

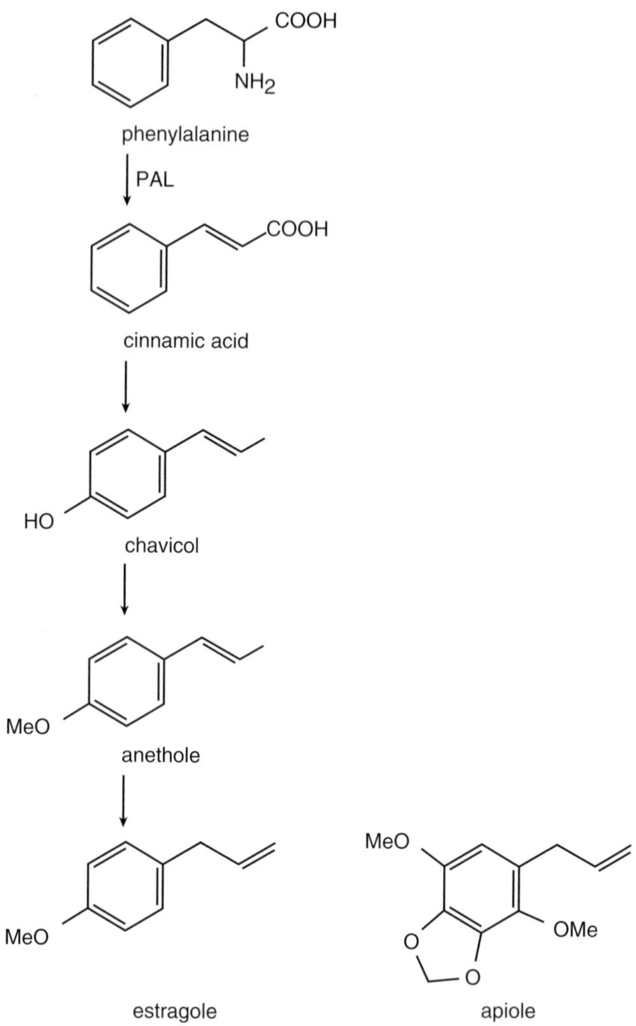

FIGURE 3-4 | Biosynthesis. (Adapted from Waterman P. 1993. The Chemistry of volatile oils. In Hay R, Waterman P (eds.), Volatile Oil Crops: Their Biology, Biochemistry and Production. Essex, UK: Longman Scientific and Technical, 47-61.)

family, or genus, of a plant will have a similar secretory system. This can be useful in plant identification.

Single, secretion-containing cells are common in many aromatic plants like the leaves of lemongrass, rhizome of ginger, seed coat of cardamom, fruit wall of black pepper, bark of cinnamon, and root of valerian. Secretory ducts are elongated cavities found in plants like coriander, cumin, angelica, dill, anise, and fennel (all members of the Umbelliferae family). Secretory cavities are prevalent in the fruit and leaves of lemon, orange and bergamot in the Citrus

TABLE 3-19 *Parts of Plant Where Essential Oils Are Stored*

Plant	Location Where Oil Is Stored
Angelica	Root, seed
Black pepper	Seed
Cinnamon	Bark, leaf
Clove	Leaf, bud
Eucalyptus	Leaf
Juniper	Berry
Mandarin	Fruit peel
Myrrh	Resin
Pine	Needles
Rose	Flower
Rosemary	Whole herb
Sandalwood	Wood

TABLE 3-20 *Secretory Parts of Plants*

Part	Plant
Single secretion cells	Ginger, black pepper, cardamom, valerian, lemongrass
Secretory cavities	Citrus fruits, clove, myrrh, frankincense
Secretory ducts	Tarragon, angelica, aniseed, pine
Secretory hairs	Many plants in the Lamiaceae and Geraniaceae families

family. They are also found in the bark of myrrh, frankincense and in clove buds. Glandular hairs are found on leaves and stems of plants such as basil, lavender, and marjoram in the Lamiaceae family. Epidermal cells diffuse essential oil directly through the cytoplasm and cell wall to the outside, and the amount of essential oil diffused is very low. Examples of aromatics with epidermal cells are rose and jasmine.

The function of essential oils in plants is not fully understood. Some may protect a plant from being eaten by plant-eating animals or insects by repelling them (Pichersky & Gershenzon 2002). For example, wild tobacco (*Nicotiania sylvestris*) can increase its production of nicotine by three or four times when under attack, and the bitter taste deters predators (Mann 2001b). Sometimes an essential oil component can reduce the growth, or maturation, of an insect that is eating the plant. Grasshoppers eating *Cyperus iria* become sterile. Tenulin (a sesquiterpene lactone) in *Helenium amarum* disrupts the growth and development of insect larvae (Mann 2001b). Many animals find the aroma (and taste) of essential oil components repellent and will not eat aromatic plants. Voles (a small rodent common in Europe) will not eat pine needles. However, there are exceptions. Australian possums and kangaroos are two mammals that have adapted to live off a diet of Eucalyptus leaves. I saw this personally when I visited Australia in 2013.

Certain plants exude aromas that deter insects. The Lamiaceae family has two well-known plants, pennyroyal and peppermint, that deter insects. The mosquito that carries yellow fever is repelled by mugwort *(Artemisia vulgaris)*. Clinical studies found that mosquitoes carrying malaria or Dengue fever are repelled by *Artemisia annua* (Sharma et al 2014).

Other essential oils are thought to increase pollination by attracting insects. Many chemical compounds found in the odor glands of insects are also found in flower fragrances. Usually it is a mixture of compounds that generates the aroma the insect is seeking. Each part of the fragrant area of the plant may present a different volatile profile. The rose, for example, produces different aromas in its petals than in the sepals and stamens. Odor is thought to be more important to a pollinating insect than color. This is obvious with night-flying creatures as some flowers are pollinated by bats or moths. Insects can discern a scent at 1/100 the level compared with a human. Floral fragrances such as monoterpenes are important insect attractants. Some plants, such as *Datura innoxia*, produce a narcotic, so the hawkmoth becomes addicted and returns regularly for "fixes" (Mann 2001a). Insects live in a world where actions are triggered by smell, rather than noise or light.

Plants may produce secondary metabolites to protect them from bacteria, viruses and fungi. Plants respond to attack by producing stress metabolites called phytoalexins. Some synthetically produced phytoalexins are now used to protect crops from parasites (Holscher et al 2014).

Allelopathy

Allelopathy is the ability of a plant to prevent other plants from growing too close to it. Bracken and ferns leach germinating inhibitors (usually phenols) into the ground to deter other species from germinating or growing too close. Aromatic plants can use essential oils such as camphor to protect the land around them from other plants. Terpenes are the largest group of chemical components found in aromatic plants, and many terpenes can inhibit the respiration of other plants (Mann 2001b). The sage bush *(Salvia leucophylla)*, which is prolific in the near-desert terrain of southern California, contains chemical compounds 1,8-cineole and camphor that deter other plants from germinating.

One of the other ideas suggested or why plants make essential oils is their antitranspirant activity. Essential oils aid survival in difficult climatic conditions when a haze of volatile oils may influence stomatal closure, and thus prevents excess water loss from the leaves.

Quality of Essential Oils

There are many factors that can affect the quality of an essential oil (Box 3-1). The chemical make-up of all living plants depends on climate and environmental conditions (such as rainfall, sunlight, soil acidity, altitude and pollution) (Guenther 1972). The chemistry of the same species of rose grown in Bulgaria will be subtly

BOX 3-1 *Factors Affecting Quality of Essential Oil*

Age of plant
Altitude
Climate
Genetics
Geography
Length of time essential oil is distilled
Number of times essential oil is distilled
Soil type
Temperature at which essential oil is distilled
Time of harvest (including both time of year and time of day)
Use of fertilizers and pesticides

different from the same one grown in England. Similarly, *Lavandula angustifolia* grown high in the mountains will contain more esters, which are thought to have a greater antispasmodic effect, than *Lavandula angustifolia* grown closer to sea level. If *Lavandula angustifolia* is distilled at a high altitude this will also increase the amount of esters. *Lavandula angustifolia* essential oil with a higher percentage of esters will have an aroma that is softer and fruitier. There are so many variables that the simplest way to be sure of the composition of the essential oil is to use modern analytical methods as well as the nose.

ANALYSIS TESTS FOR PURITY IN ESSENTIAL OILS

There are several methods that are used to analyze the composition of an essential oil: the most frequently used is gas chromatography (GC). Other important analytical methods include high-performance liquid chromatography (HPLC) and nuclear magnetic resonance (NMR) (Tisserand & Young 2013).

GAS CHROMATOGRAPHY

GC is a technique to separate the individual components in the essential oil (e.g., α-pinene, β-myrcene and linalyl acetate). The instrument is linked to a detector, most often a flame ionization detector (FID) or a mass spectrometer (MS). The individual constituents are shown in a computerized printout as a succession of peaks, and the peak size can be correlated to the amount of the constituent in the oil. The lighter molecules will show up first. The MS detector can be used to identify the peaks based on a comparison of the mass spectrum with data from a library. This is particularly useful for the detection and identification of pesticides. Although using a GC/MS will allow identifying and quantifying most of the chemical components, it may not always identify synthetic chemicals that have been added to extend, or alter the essential oil. Two-dimensional gas chromatographs (GC × GC) can show which way molecules rotate (Tisserand & Young 2013). This can help detect synthetic additives.

HPLC

HPLC is another separation technique, which can be used to analyze a much wider range of components, including nonvolatile molecules which cannot be analyzed by GC. HPLC is most often connected to an ultraviolet/visible (UV/Vis) detector, but MS detectors have become more and more popular due to the additional information that can be obtained.

NMR

The NMR is a high-end technique that is mainly used to determine the structure of pure compounds, but can also be used to get a view of the totality of the essential oil (fingerprint). Comparing such NMR fingerprints to fingerprints of authentic essential oils by statistical means can be a good way to detect adulteration of essential oils.

Optical Rotation

Molecules within essential oils have the ability to rotate a plane of polarized light. Molecules that rotate counterclockwise are called levorotatory, or L for short. Those that rotate clockwise are called dextrorotatory, or D. This ability is indicated in the name of the molecule, for example, D-limonene. Almost all essential oils show optical activity. Optical rotation can reveal synthetic compounds that alter the optical rotation. Synthetic menthol rotates in a different way to menthol from the mint plant (Stewart 2005).

Refractive Index

When light passes through a liquid it is refracted. This refraction can be measured and is consistent for a given essential oil. In scientific terms, it is the ratio of the speed of light of a given frequency in a vacuum to the speed of light in a medium of some kind, at a specified temperature. It is important that the test be carried out at the same temperature as the reference (the standard).

Infrared Spectroscopy

When infrared light is passed through an essential oil it produces a spectrum that is like the fingerprint of the essential oil. Similar to NMR, a comparison of the fingerprint to authentic materials will help to detect adulteration of the oil.

The Nose (Organoleptic Evaluation)

This is an underestimated but important part of analysis. When you first start you may find it hard to notice differences between synthetic and real essential oils, or pure and adulterated ones. However, with patience the nose does learn. Never smell directly from the bottle. Put one or two drops on to a special smell strip (made from paper a little like blotting paper). Recap the bottle. Hold the smell strip approximately 6 inches in front of your face. The sense of smell may be different from one nostril to the other as the aroma reaches different parts in the brain, so move the strip back and forth several times. One nostril may detect a sweeter smell than the other. Close your eyes and concentrate. Rate the aroma on a scale of 0 to 10: when 0 means you dislike the odor intensely, and 10 means the odor is very pleasant. Write down a word that describes the aroma. When testing essential oils from an unknown source, first try one known to be authentic to "fix" the smell imprint in your brain. Then try the new one. Also, since the sense of smell adapts quickly to an odor, care should be taken to allow for sufficient time in between smelling consecutive samples in order to avoid olfactory fatigue. The trained human nose plays an important role in analysis. If your nose says the oil doesn't smell quite right, pay attention!

BUYING ESSENTIAL OILS

Essential oils can be purchased in a great many places, as well as online. Just remember that essential oils are easy to dilute or adulterate, and if the price sounds too good to be true, it probably is. The most common method of dilution is by adding vegetable oil or alcohol. The most common adulteration is adding a small amount of a cheaper oil, for example, adding geranium to rose, or petitgrain to neroli. Real melissa oil is very difficult to find, because it is frequently adulterated with lemongrass or citral. Sometimes particular components are added, such as citronella, geraniol, or linalool. Sometimes individual components are mixed in a test tube and the result is labeled "natural essential oil." Several countries can produce the same essential oil but they may be of varying quality. For example, rose is grown (and distilled) in France, Bulgaria, Turkey, China, and Morocco. Some essential oils may not be suitable for clinical use because they have been grown with pesticides.

If essential oils are being used clinically, they should be from a reputable supplier who can state the following: country of origin, botanical name, part of the plant, wild-crafted or organic, method of extraction, batch number, expiry date and the chemotype (when relevant). Reputable suppliers are happy to provide gas-chromatography/mass spectrometry (GCMS) information and material safety data sheets (MSDS).

Bottles should contain integral droppers and be made of colored glass. "Pure 100 percent essential oil" should be clearly marked. Basic safety precautions such as "do not take by mouth," "keep away from children," and "avoid contact with eyes" should be on the label. Apart from the product description, label and price, use your common sense and your nose. Long established, reputable companies would lose too much by compromising themselves on quality and are usually proud they can prove the authenticity of their oils. I have used the same small group of companies for 20 years. They are listed at the back of the book and also on www.rjbuckle.com. I have never sold essential oils. I do not have my own brand (although I have been asked to create one many times) so I can be completely independent. I dislike the cult-like behavior that some multilevel marketing seems to produce.

REFERENCES

Arctander S. 1960. *Perfume and Flavor Materials of Natural Origin.* Wheaton, IL: Allured Publishing, 13.

Alkaire B, Simon J. 1992. A portable steam distillation unit for essential oil crops. *Hort-Technology* 2(4) 473-476.

Baser KHC, Demirci F. 2007. Chemistry of Essential Oils. *In Flavours and Fragrances: Chemistry. Bioprocessing and Sustainability.* RG Berger (Ed). Springer. Berlin. P 43-86.

Bowles J. 2000. *The Basic Chemistry of Aromatherapeutic Essential Oils.* Sydney, Australia: Pirie Printers.

Cambray-Smith I. 2013. Essential Chemistry. Natural Science Course Notes.

Coelho J, Cristino A, Matos P, Rauter A, Nobre B et al. 2012. Extraction of Volatile Oil from Aromatic Plants with Supercritical Carbon Dioxide: Experiments and Modeling. *Molecules.* 17, 10550-10573. Accessed 5/2/2014.

Gafner S. 2014. Personal communication.

Guenther E. 1972. *The Essential Oils, Vol. I.* Melbourne, FL: Krieger Publishing.

Guenther E. 1974. *The Essential Oils: Individual Essential Oils of the Plant Families.* Melbourne, FL: Krieger Publishing.

Guenther E. 1976. *The Essential Oils, Vol. V.* Melbourne, FL: Krieger Publishing.

Holscher D, Dhakshinamoorthy S, Alexandrov T, Becker M, Bretschneider T et al. 2014. Phenalenone-type phytoalexins mediate resistance of banana plants (Musa spp.) to the burrowing nematode Radopholus similis. *Proc Natl Acad Sci USA.* 11(1):105-10.

Hou C, Li S, Guan W, Wang J, Yan R. 2007, Simulation of supercritical CO_2 extraction of clove oil. *Journal of Chemical Industry & Engineering*(China).

Mann J. 2001a. *Chemical Aspects of Biosynthesis.* Oxford, UK: Oxford Science Publications, 2.

Mann J. 2001b. *Secondary Metabolism.* Oxford, UK: Oxford Science Publications, 7.

Pichersky E, Gershenzon J. 2002. The formation and function of plant volatiles: perfumes for pollinator attraction and defense. *Curr Opin Plant Biol.* 5(3):237-43.

Pichersky E, Noel J, Dudareva N. 2006. Biosynthesis of Plant Volatiles: Nature's Diversity and Ingenuity. *Science.* 10: 311(5762):808-811.

Poucher W. 1993. *Poucher's Perfumes, Cosmetics and Soaps*, Vol 2, 9th ed. Chapman & Hall.

Sharma G, Kapoor H, Chopra M, Kumar K, Agrawal V. 2014. Strong larvicidal potential of Artemisia annua leaf extract against malaria (Anopheles stephensi Liston) and dengue (Aedes aegypti L.) vectors and bioassay-driven isolation of the marker compound. *Parasitol Res.* 113(1):197-209.

Taiz L, Zeiger E. 2014. Plant Physiology Onlone. 5th edition. Accessed 7/2/2014. http://5e.plantphys.net/article.php?ch=t&id=23.

Teixeiry M, Rodriquez O, Gomez P, Mata V, Rodriges B. 2013. Design of Perfumes. in *Perfume Engineering: Design, Performance & Classification.* Butterworth Heinemann.

Tisserand R, Young R. 2013. *Essential Oil Safety.* 2nd ed. London: Churchill Livingstone.

Svoboda K, Svoboda T. 2001. *Secretory Structures of Aromatic and Medicinal Plants.* Wales, UK: Microscopix Publications.

Vagi E, Simandi B, Suhajda A, Hethely E. 2005. Essential oil composition and antimicrobial activity of *Origanum majorana* L. extracts obtained with ethyl alcohol and supercritical carbon dioxide. *Food Research International.* 38(1):51-57.

von Leeuwenhoek A. 1679. *In Medicine Quest* by Plotkin M. 2000. Viking.

Yang Z, Sakai M, Sayama H, Shimeno T, Yamaguchi K et al. 2009. Elucidation of the biochemical pathway of 2-phenylethanol from shikimic acid using isolated protoplasts of rose flowers. *J Plant Physiology.* 166(8):887-891

Chapter 4

Essential Oil Toxicity and Contraindications

"The difference between a deadly poison and a lifesaving medicine can be very small; in fact, it is sometimes merely a question of dosage."

Dr. Richard Evans Schultes, 1980

CHAPTER ASSETS

Just because essential oils are natural does not mean they do not have potential risks, or hazards if used inappropriately. This chapter addresses toxicity and contraindications. Put in context, essential oils, as used in aromatherapy, are extremely safe and carry few of the risks of many modern medicines. However, it is pertinent to the increasingly high profile of aromatherapy that those using essential oils clinically should be aware of their potential toxicity, possible side effects, and interactions. This chapter is a short synopsis of an extensive subject. The author is extremely grateful for reference to the second edition of *Essential Oil Safety* (Tisserand & Young 2013) and strongly recommends this for further reading.

This chapter is divided into two parts: **Part 1: Essential Oil Toxicity and Toxicology**

This covers dermal toxicity, skin irritants, allergens, phototoxins, chemical burns. Oral toxicity, nephrotoxins, neurotoxins, hepatotoxins, psychotropics, measuring toxicity. Inhaled toxicity.

Part 2: Contraindications and Safety
This covers possible drug interactions, essential oils to avoid in epilepsy, pregnancy, oncology. General contraindications and general safety rules.

PART 1: ESSENTIAL OIL TOXICITY AND TOXICOLOGY
Toxicity
Toxicity is defined as the amount or degree of a substance needed to be poisonous (Brooker 2008). Toxicity is dependent on the amount and concentration used, frequency of use, interactions of the person receiving the substance, and individual reaction of the person (Dybing et al 2002; Tisserand & Young 2013). Toxicity can be systemic or local. It can be reversible or nonreversible. It can be acute, subacute, or subchronic. Systemic toxicity means toxicity at a cell level that causes the organ to fail with the possible death of the organism. Local toxicity means the organ responsible for absorption and elimination may be severely affected, for example, stomach, liver, skin, lungs, or kidney. The effects may be reversible (when the toxic agent has been removed) or irreversible. The effects may also be acute, subacute, or subchronic.

Toxicology
Toxicology is the study of harmful interactions between xenobiotics and living systems. Xenobiotics are substances, such as drugs, that are foreign to the human body (Brooker 2008) or to an ecological system (Oxford English Dictionary 2005). For the purpose of this chapter, xenobiotics are the chemical constituents found in essential oils that have a negative effect on humans. Toxicology covers areas such a dermal toxicity and skin irritants, allergens, phototoxins, and chemical burns. It also covers nephrotoxins, hepatotoxins, neurotoxins, and psychotropics.

Essential Oils are Complex Compounds
Because essential oils are made up of many different chemical compounds, it is more difficult to extrapolate their toxicity from data of one of the supposed toxic compounds. When mixtures or blends of essential oils are used, this complicates matters even further because mixed components can interact to produce an additive, synergistic, or antagonistic effect. For example, citral is found in several essential oils. If two essential oils containing citral were added together, the concentration of citral would double, and thus double the possibility of a skin sensitivity reaction (Tisserand & Young 2013). Some essential oil components appear to have a synergistic reaction. This is when the effect of the sum of the components is greater than the effect of a single component. Itani et al (2008) found that combining three components (linalyl acetate, terpineo, and camphor) from Lebanese sage (*Salvia fruticosa* or *Salvia libanotica*) caused synergistic inhibition of the growth of two human colon cancer cell lines. Individually, the components did not have that effect. Sometimes there is an antagonistic effect when one component appears to "quench" the negative effect of another. For example, D-limonene and eugenol had a "quenching" effect on cinnamaldehyde contact sensitization in human studies (Guin et al 1984).

The wide range and complexity of components in essential oils suggests that nature is offering a "balanced menu," so the receiver can take the parts of the meal the body needs and leave the rest. This may be why the effect of an isolated ingredient can be much stronger: it is no longer part of the "balanced menu."

OVERVIEW

Essential oils have been in the public domain for over a hundred years. They are traded globally and, in 2013, the market trade was worth over $1000 million (Williamson 2013). Essential oils are used in cosmetics, pharmaceuticals, food, beverages, cleaning materials, and in the perfume industry. Approximately 400 essential oils are in use (Tisserand & Young 2013). Of these, approximately 100 essential oils are used regularly in aromatherapy. The number of toxicity problems reported is very small, leading to the conclusion that most essential oils are safe. This may change as essential oils become more easily obtainable and people push the boundaries and become more adventurous with dilutions and applications.

DIFFERENT APPROACHES

There is a certain amount of controversy about the potential toxicity of essential oils. Some aromatherapists feel essential oils should never be taken orally. Some people take essential oils orally or recommend their oral use and see no problem. Some use essential oils every day: others feel using an essential oil for longer than 3 weeks could lead to liver damage. A person's point of view is usually based on their background and training.

The British approach to aromatherapy has focused (until recently) on using diluted essential oils (up to 5%) applied to the skin, usually in a massage. An aromatherapy massage is solely intended to improve relaxation and help stress management. There are no reports of toxic effects from using essential oils in this way. Recently, aromasticks have become an attractive alternative to topical use, particularly in cancer care. Please see Chapter 2, How Essential Oils Work: Applications.

The French approach to aromatherapy may use several milliliters of undiluted essential oil on the skin at a time, sometimes several times a day—usually to combat an infection. Physicians may also give gelatin capsules (each containing three or four drops of essential oils, diluted in a carrier oil or gel) to be taken orally, three or four times a day. In France, essential oils are used to treat infection, or a chronic condition, and are rarely used just for relaxation. There is more chance of toxicity from the oral route, although there have been virtually no cases recorded. The majority of French physicians who use essential oils in this way are working alongside bacteriologists and pharmacists and are well aware of toxicity issues. A potential toxicity hazard could occur when untrained people use essential oils orally and ingest too much.

Some aromatherapists (including myself) are trained in both British and French approaches to aromatherapy. Clearly there is a place for both. However, each approach is relevant to the experience, training, and expectations of the person using the essential oils. The oral use of essential oils can be seen as using them as

medicines. This is outside the remit of many health professionals in many countries, including the United States. Using essential oils orally increases the possibility
of overdosing and the risk of a toxic reaction. "Virtually all cases of serious poisoning from essential oils are the consequence of oral ingestion of an undiluted oil in
amounts much higher than the therapeutic dose" (Tisserand & Young 2013, p. 25).
However, there is a place for the oral use of certain essential oils in certain circumstances. Recent research indicates that drug companies are looking at this emerging
market with increasing interest (Kasper et al 2014).

DERMAL TOXICITY

Because essential oils are often applied to the skin (albeit usually diluted), it is
important to know about adverse skin reactions. Tisserand & Young (2013) write
that when there are no established recommendations, diluted essential oils are safe
to use on the skin. So far, there has not been a recorded fatality from the topical
absorption of essential oils. However, there are adverse skin reactions that can be
caused by skin irritants or allergens within an essential oil, or a combined reaction
of phototoxins and sunlight. (Patch testing to avoid skin irritation or sensitivity is
covered in Chapter 4.)

SKIN IRRITANTS

Essential oils are complex mixtures of chemical compounds, any of which (singly
or together) may irritate the skin. Primary irritation (contact dermatitis) occurs
rapidly the first time an essential oil is used, manifesting as a red wheal or burn.
Primary irritation is more likely to occur when essential oils are used that contain large amounts of phenols, e.g., carvacrol and thymol, or aromatic aldehydes,
e.g., cinnamaldehyde. Examples are oregano *(Origanum vulgare)*, thyme *(Thymus
vulgaris* CT thymol), and cinnamon bark *(Cinnamomum verum)*. Cinnamon bark
oil caused burning (Sparks 1985) and blistering (Perry et al 1990). Cinnamaldehyde is a dose-dependent skin irritant and sensitizer (Decapite & Anderson 2004;
Tisserand & Young 2013). Skin reaction is usually limited to the area where the
essential oil is applied. Immediate dilution with a vegetable oil or milk (to dilute the
essential oil) is required, followed by washing with warm water and nonperfumed
soap. This kind of instant irritation is more likely to occur with concentrations
above 5% and/or on abraded skin. Guba (2000) suggests using 90% nonirritant
essential oil with 10% phenolic oil if high concentrations or undiluted essential oils
are required. There has only been one recorded instance of anaphylactic shock. This
followed the topical application of cinnamaldehyde (Diba & Statham 2003).

SKIN ALLERGENS

Allergic contact dermatitis (ACD) is a clinical response to delayed hypersensitivity,
and occurs when an essential oil containing allergens is used over a period of time.
Symptoms are a bright red rash. ACD can also sometimes occur from an inhaled
or ingested essential oil (Salam & Fowler 2001; Trattner & David 2003). Sometimes

ACD includes pigmentation of skin—usually Asian skin (Yu et al 2007). Examples of essential oils that can cause skin sensitivity include melissa *(Melissa officinalis)* and lemon verbena *(Aloysia citriodora)* where the maximum recommended concentration for dermal application is 0.9% (Tisserand & Young 2013). Sensitivity can build up to any essential oil. It is encouraging that despite the popularity of lavender *(Lavandula angustifolia)* and Lavandin *(Lavandula × intermedia)*, there have been very few reported incidences of sensitivities. However, this may only be a question of time. Juniper took 25 years to produce sensitivity in the case of a lady who sold food smoked and spiced in juniper oils. Eventually she developed a dry cough and asthma. Skin tests showed sensitivity to juniper, although it was not established whether the wood resin or the berries were to blame (Roethe et al 1973).

A florist who presented with an allergic reaction to Roman chamomile *(Chamaemelum nobile)* was found to have a prior sensitivity to chamomile herbal teas and ointments (Van Ketel 1982). Another florist, with dermatitis of the face for 1 year, was found to be allergic to the sesquiterpenes in German chamomile *(Matricaria chamomilla)* (Van Ketel 1987). I have found that patients taking multiple medications are more prone to essential oil sensitivities, especially those patients who also have an allergy-like illness such as asthma, eczema, or hay fever.

PHOTOTOXINS

Photosensitization is a reaction between a phototoxin in an essential oil that is applied to the skin in the presence of sunlight or ultraviolet A (UVA) light (this includes sun beds). Furanocoumarins (FCs) are phototoxins. They occur mainly in expressed citrus peel oils, although they are also found in angelica root *(Angelica archangelica)*, rue *(Ruta graveolens)*, parsley leaf *(Petroselinum crispum)*, and marigold *(Tagetes minuta)* essential oils. FCs are not found in distilled citrus peel oils. The most common FCs are bergapten and psoralen. When an essential oil containing FCs is applied to the skin and the skin is exposed to UVA light, an inflammatory skin reaction occurs. Reactions can vary from pigmentation, blistering, to severe full-thickness burns. Some foods such as parsnips, celery, and grapefruit juice contain FCs. Consuming large amounts of these can increase total FC load and thus the phototoxic effect of essential oils containing FCs (Tisserand & Young 2013). There is no risk of photosensitization if the skin is covered to prevent exposure to UVA light for at least 2 hours (Dubertret et al 1990) or preferably 8 hours (Tisserand & Young 2013). There is no photosensitivity risk if furanocoumarin-free (FCF) essential oils are used. Deterpenated citrus oils (often used in the perfume industry) contain disproportionately higher concentrations of FCs and are best avoided.

CHEMICAL BURNS

Parys (1983) reported on undiluted peppermint oil inadvertently spilled on skin that had already been traumatized by skin grafts. The area necrosed and required excision and further surgery. Multiple chemical burns to the entire oral cavity, pharynx, and soft palate occurred when a 49-year-old woman ingested 40 drops of undiluted peppermint to treat a cold. She also had respiratory stridor, tachycardia

(132 beats/min) and required emergency nasal intubation. Intravenous (IV) steroids and antibiotics were given and she survived (Tamir et al 2005).

Overview

Skin reactions are dose-dependent on the dilution of essential oils. Although I agree mostly with Tisserand & Young (2013), I think the maximum dermal application of certain essential oils could be higher in specific limited instances. For example, their suggested limit of 15% for the dermal application of tea tree *(Melaleuca alternifolia)* could be higher for spider bites, warts, nail fungus, and herpes. Having said that, tea tree is now used in so many proprietary products that sensitization may become a problem if undiluted tea tree is used repeatedly over time. There have already been several cases of skin allergy from using undiluted tea tree. However, for the specific limited examples listed above, the advantages outweigh the disadvantages. The European Union (EU) labeling for allergens lists 16 essential oil components. However, the possibility of reaction is very low—ranging from 0.03% (benzyl benzoate) to 1.15% (cinnamaldehyde)—and the data supporting it is questionable (Tisserand & Young 2013).

ORAL TOXICITY

Symptoms of oral poisoning can occur rapidly and include a burning sensation in the mouth and throat, abdominal pain, and spontaneous vomiting, although the latter may be delayed by up to 4 hours. "Death from essential oils is slow — 15 minutes — 3 days" (Tisserand & Young 2013, p. 26). Dangerous respiratory depression also can occur with deep coma. Convulsions may occur in children but are rare in adults. The dose range within which an essential oil becomes lethal is wide. For example, the safe dose for internal use of eucalyptus is 0.006 to 0.2 mL (Martindale 1977). Death in adults has occurred after ingestion of as little as 4 to 5 mL (MacPherson 1925). However, some people have recovered after ingesting up to 220 mL of eucalyptus essential oil with emergency medical intervention (Gurr & Scroggie 1965).

Nephrotoxins

There are very few known cases of essential oils adversely affecting the urinary system, and these are all in cases of oral overdose. Overdoses of wintergreen *(Gaultheria fragrantissima)*, wormseed oil *(Chenopodium ambrosioides)*, and pennyroyal *(Mentha pulegium)* have caused nephrotoxicity (Table 4-1). Kidney damage showed in the autopsies of children who had mistakenly been given wintergreen or wormseed oil (Kloss & Boeckmans 1967; Opdyke 1976, p. 713-715). The kidney tubules of a woman were destroyed after ingesting pennyroyal and she died (Vallance 1955). Renal failure after ingesting 10 mL of wormseed oil caused hospitalization of a 31-year-old man. The man had been looking at the liqueur absinthe on the internet and discovered that wormseed oil was an ingredient. He purchased wormseed oil electronically from a commercial provider of essential oils used in

TABLE 4-1 *Reported Cases of Overdose with Common Essential Oils*

Essential Oil	Amount (mL or Drops)	Symptoms	Author
Cinnamon *Cinnamomum verum*	60 mL	Dizziness, double vision, nausea, vomiting, collapse.	Pilapil 1989
Citronella *Cymbopogon nardus*	15 mL 25 mL	12-month-old girl: vomiting, shock, frothing at the mouth, deep rapid respiration, cyanosis, convulsions, brain hemorrhage. Died. 16-month-old boy: gastric lavage. Survived.	Mant 1961 Temple et al 1991
Clove *Syzygium aromaticum*	5 mL 5–10 mL 10 mL 8 mL	7-month-old child: severe acidosis, central nervous system depression, ketones in urine; gastric lavage. Survived. 2-year-old boy: clove plus paracetamol; acidosis, deteriorating liver function, extremely low blood glucose, generalized seizure, deep coma; given heparin; conscious after 6 days. Survived. 15-month-old boy: liver failure; given intravenous injection of N-acetylcysteine; liver function returned within 4 days. Survived. 32-year-old woman: self-injected intravenously; acute respiratory distress, noncardiogenic pulmonary oedema; abnormal chest X-ray; medical intervention for 7 days. Survived. 3-month-old girl: fulminant hepatic failure; gastric lavage; intravenous injection of N-acetylcysteine. Survived.	Lane et al 1991 Hartnoll et al 1993 Janes et al 2005 Kirsch et al 1990 Eisen et al 2004
Eucalyptus (cineole-rich species)	5 mL	Vertigo, loss of coordination, abnormal respiration, epigastric pain, cold sweats. Lesser amounts = excess respiratory tract mucus; greater amounts = decreased respiratory tract mucus, pinpoint pupils, rapid drowsiness, unconsciousness. 109 children (mean age 23 months) over 10 years; gastric lavage, naso-gastric charcoal and medical intervention. All survived.	Craig 1953 Patel & Wiggins 1980 Tibballs 1995

continued

TABLE 4-1 *Reported Cases of Overdose with Common Essential Oils—cont'd*

Essential Oil	Amount (mL or Drops)	Symptoms	Author
Hyssop *Hyssopus officinalis*	10-20 drops 30 drops 10 drops	6-year-old boy: convulsions, hospitalized. Survived. 18-year-old girl: unconscious, seizure. Survived. 26-year-old girl: seizure. Survived.	O'Mullane et al 1982 O'Mullane et al 1982 Millet et al 1981
Pennyroyal *Mentha pulegium*	10 mL	4 case studies including 1 death. Review of 18 cases in adult women with moderate to severe toxicity. One death.	Anderson et al 1996
Pine *Pinus sylvestris*	400-500 mL	Suicide attempt; hospitalization; hemoperfusion with activated charcoal plus Amberlite and hemodialysis. Patient survived.	Koppel et al 1982
Dalmation sage *Salvia officinalis*	7 mL Unspecified 5 mL	44-year-old woman took sage for asthma: convulsions, dyspnea, cardiac failure, death. 33-day-old baby boy: accidentally given sage oil for colic; seizures, nys-tagmus, hyperreflexia, and irritability; hospitalization; IV diazepam and midazolam. Survived. 5-year-old girl: given sage oil for colic; seizures; hospitalized; gastric lavage and active charcoal treatment. Survived.	Whitling 1908 Halicioglu et al 2011 Halicioglu et al 2011
Tea tree *Melaleuca alternifolia*	15 mL 10 mL "Small amount"	17-month-old boy: ataxia, drowsiness; recovered within 8 hours. 23-month-old boy. 4-year-old boy: ataxic, non-responsive, intubated. Survived.	Del Beccaro 1995 Jacobs & Hornfeldt 1994 Morris et al 2003
Wintergreen *Gaultheria fragrantissima*	1 oz	5 mL of wintergreen is equivalent to 22 adult aspirin tablets. Wintergreen is 98% methyl salicylate. 44-year-old man: seizure; hospitalized. Died 18 hours later.	Botma et al 2001 Davis 2007 Cauthen & Hester 1989

aromatherapy, mistakenly thinking he was buying absinthe (Weisbord et al 1997). He survived. Absinthe is banned in the EU and United States. Tisserand & Young (2013) suggest caution when using aniseed oil *(Pimpinella anisum)* orally by people who are taking diuretics, or who have renal insufficiency. No evidence was found that juniper *(Juniperus communis)* caused nephrotoxicity.

HEPATOTOXINS

Liver damage caused by essential oils (or their components) in humans is rare. However, the liver is the main organ that detoxifies the body of essential oils and autopsy results for oral overdose have shown liver damage (Siegel & Wason 1986). Two children who had ingested clove *(Syzygium aromaticum)* essential oil presented with deteriorating liver function (Hartnoll et al 1993; Janes et al 2005). Both survived with medical intervention. Massive hepatic necrosis was part of the clinical picture of an 18-year-old girl who had swallowed 30 mL of pennyroyal *(Mentha pulegium)*. She died 6 days later as a result of liver damage. Tisserand & Young (2013) suggest avoiding the oral use of essential oils that contain β-pulegone in patients who are taking paracetamol or alcohol regularly because β-pulegone depletes hepatic glutathione. This would include essential oils such as pennyroyal *(Mentha pulegium)*, buchu *(Agathosma betulina)*, and calamint *(Calamintha nepeta)*.

Coumarin was once thought to be useful in lymphedema following breast cancer. Several studies explored the potential nephrotoxic effect of coumarin (taken orally over a period of weeks) (Cox et al 1989; Loprinzi et al 1999; Schmeck-Lindenau et al 2003; Vanscheidt et al 2002). There were very few incidences of liver damage. As an example, in the study by Cox et al (1989), 0.37% of 2173 patients developed liver problems. The authors conclude "this hepatitis was probably a form of idiosyncratic hepatotoxicity and may have been immune in origin."

Menthol has caused liver problems in people who are deficient of the enzyme glucose-6-phosphate dehydrogenase (G6PD). This enzyme is involved in the metabolism of menthol. G6PD deficiency occurs in the blood cells of Africans, their descendants, those from the Mediterranean region and those from the Middle East (Brooker 2006). G6PD deficiency is more frequent in men. Usually people are aware of their condition because they are intolerant to aspirin and antimalarial drugs. (They are also intolerant to henna.) Jaundice-like symptoms have also been seen after oral administration of estragole and isosafrole (Tisserand & Young 2013).

NEUROTOXINS

Neurotoxins cause reversible or irreversible effects on behavior, cognitive, functional, and motor coordination. Wormseed *(Chenopodium ambrosioides)* and wintergreen *(Gaultheria fragrantissima)* essential oils are known neurotoxins (Kloss & Boeckmans 1967; Cauthen & Hester 1989). Wormseed oil should never be used in any application (Tisserand & Young 2013). Eucalyptus has caused seizures in a few young children who have taken large amounts orally (Craig 1953; Wilkinson 1991). Pinocamphone, found in hyssop *(Hyssopus officinalis)* essential oil, has convulsant effects (O'Mullane et al 1982; Millet et al 1981). Thujone (both α and β) has both convulsant and neurotoxic effects in rats (Millet et al 1981). Several essential oils such as sage *(Salvia officinalis)*, thuja *(Thuja occidentalis)*, and tansy *(Tanacetum vulgare)* contain >25% thujone (Tisserand & Young 2013). Camphor is another essential oil component with potential neurotoxicity (Kopelman et al 1979). The toxicity of an essential oil depends on the amount of neurotoxic component present in the essential oil and the method of application. Children and infants are particularly susceptible to neurotoxicity and to convulsants (Tisserand & Young 2013).

Craig (1953) discusses the case of a 3-year-old who consumed 10 mL of eucalyptus (two teaspoons). The child became deeply unconscious; his pupils constricted, muscle tone was markedly reduced, and there were no tendon reflexes. His breathing was shallow and irregular at a rate of 10 breaths per minute. Insertion of an endotracheal tube produced no gag reflex. His pulse was 70 beats per minute, and blood pressure was 75/40 mm Hg. The child's serum urea was 6.3 µmol/L (38 mg/100 mL) with normal electrolytes. He was given gastric lavage with sodium bicarbonate solution. Sodium sulfate (100 mL) was administered as a cathartic. After 2 hours, his pulse, blood pressure, and respiration were normal. He was discharged from hospital after 48 hours.

Wilkinson (1991) discusses the toxic effect of ingested essential oils on three children admitted to an emergency room in Australia. Their ages were 19 months, 23 months, and 25 months. The 19-month-old infant ingested an indeterminate amount of lavender. The type of lavender was not specified, but the chemistry of *Lavandula angustifolia*, *Lavandula latifolia*, and *Lavandula stoechas* are very different and therefore their toxicities are different. *L. stoechas*, which contains ketones, would be more toxic than *L. angustifolia*, which contains mainly linalyl acetate or linalool. The 25-month-old child took an unknown amount of tea tree oil, and the 23-month-old child ingested 40 mL of eucalyptus oil. All three children were ataxic. All three were anesthetized and given gastric lavage, and two were intubated. Charcoal was given in all cases and sorbitol in one. All three children recovered fully in the hospital. Lethal doses of essential oils for children under 6 years are given in Table 4-2.

PSYCHOTROPIC ACTIVITY

A psychotropic effect is a substance that exerts a specific effect on the brain (Brooker 2008). Nutmeg *(Myristica fragrans)* essential oil has psychotropic effects. The psychotropic effects are attributed to the presence of myristicin. Nutmeg had demonstrable anticonvulsant effect in animal models and the authors suggest it "may be effective against grand mal and partial seizures" (Wahab et al 2009). Inhaled nutmeg oil also reduced locomotion in mice by <60% (Muchtaridi et al 2010).

ESSENTIAL OILS USED IN SUPPOSITORIES

The European Medicines Agency state there is a risk of neurological disorders, especially convulsions, in infants and small children under 30 months old with the use of suppositories containing essential oils. Therefore, their use is contraindicated within EU countries (Kolassa 2013).

TABLE 4-2 *Potentially Lethal Oral Doses of Essential Oil for a Child Under 6 Years*

Common Name	Botanical Name	Oral Lethal Dose for a Child (mL)
Basil	*Ocimum basilicum* (estragole above 55%)	8
Aniseed	*Pimpinella anisum*	25
Clove	*Syzygium aromaticum*	19
Eucalyptus	*Eucalyptus globulus*	5
Hyssop	*Hyssopus officinalis*	19
German spearmint	*Mentha longifolia*	6.5
Egyptian round leaf	*Mentha rotundifolia*	10
Oregano	*Oreganum vulgare*	21
Parsley seed oil	*Petroselinum sativum*	21
Pennyroyal	*Mentha pulegium*	3
Sage	*Salvia officinalis*	26
Savory, Summer	*Satureja hortensis*	19
Tansy	*Tanacetum vulgare*	5
Tarragon	*Artemesia dracunculus*	26
Thuja	*Thuja occidentalis*	10
Wintergreen	*Gaultheria fragrantissima*	5

Adapted from Watt M. 1991. Essex, UK: Witham. This book discusses adverse reactions and toxicity in greater detail. Not all the botanical names are given.

MEASURING TOXICITY

Much of the information available on toxicity is based on animal studies. (This is also true of conventional drugs.) Most essential oils have had extensive toxicologic studies carried out by the fragrance industry (for inhaled and topically applied essential oils) and the flavor industry (for ingested essential oils). In animal toxicology studies, a very large amount of essential oil is given to the test animal in a very short period. This is totally unlike the human situation where small amounts of essential oils are given over a longer period. The huge amounts given in animal testing are never given to humans all at once, nor are such large amounts given during an extended period. In 2008, 18 pharmaceutical companies petitioned to have animal toxicity studies removed as a requirement for drug approval (Tisserand & Young 2013) because they felt that animal toxicity tests had limited relevance to human toxicity.

Oral Lethal Dose

Oral lethal dose is usually tested on laboratory mice or rats. The animals are force-fed essential oils until 50% of them die. The amount the test group has ingested when death occurs is the median lethal dose, which is known as LD50; this is the number of milligrams or grams of essential oil per kilogram of animal body weight that is required to kill half of the animals.

Dermal Lethal Dose

The LD50 dermal lethal dose is determined via a test on a shaved area of the skin of animals, usually rabbits. The dose at which 50% of the test subjects die is the dermal LD50. Human skin is less permeable than rabbit skin. There have been very few clinical tests on human skin. Those that have been done involved volunteers who were given a patch test for a 24-hour period (Watt 1991).

Simple math can demonstrate how distant a 5% solution of an essential oil used as topical application is from a toxic level. If the dermal LD50 of *Eucalyptus globulus* is 5 g/kg (actually it is more than 10% according to Kligman), then the following equations determine toxicity:

An average woman weighs 150 lbs = approximately 75 kg.

$5 \times 75 = 375$ g = approximately 400 mL (allowing for specific gravity).

If the solution is 5%, 8000 mL are required = 8 L.

It is unknown exactly how much of the eucalyptus is absorbed through the skin—certainly not 100%. Much depends on the skin's integrity, its temperature, and whether it is covered after application of the oil. Let us allow for 50% absorption (which is generous). It is impossible for 4 L of essential oil to be absorbed by the skin all at once. (However, there would be considerable effects from inhaling the essential oil as well.)

Oral LD50 of *Eucalyptus globulus* is 2.48 g/kg.

Average woman of 150 lbs = approximately 75 kg.

$2.48 \times 75 = 186$ g = approximately 200 mL (allowing for specific gravity).

INHALATION TOXICITY

Inhaled essential oils are unlikely to produce a toxic reaction. Hypothetically, a toxic reaction could occur if a person was confined in a nonventilated room, the temperature was very high, and there was a constant diffusion of essential oil until the air was saturated. This would be more akin to suffocation than a reaction to the essential oil. However, the effects of long-term environmental fragrancing with essential oils is not known and could lead to sensitivity. Some chemotypes of perilla *(Perilla frutescens)* contain perilla ketone—a potent lung toxin to animals that may cause pulmonary toxicity in humans (Tisserand & Young 2013). This is relevant because perillyl alcohol, another component of perilla *(Perilla frutescens)*, is used for the treatment of advanced ovarian cancer (Bailey et al 2002). More recent studies have explored the use of inhaling perillyl alcohol for neoplasms of the central nervous system (Peterson 2014) and to enhance the effect of other anticancer medications in pancreatic cancer (Sarkar et al 2014).

There have been several accidental toxic events in young children when essential oils have been placed inside their nasal cavities (Melis et al 1989; Crandon & Thompson 2006). This is different from inhaling essential oils.

CONCLUSION

This has been a very brief overview of toxicology. Put into context, our world is full of toxic substances, but this only becomes a problem if exposure to the toxic substance poses a risk. Coffee, bananas, glyoxal, and hydrogen peroxide are potentially hazardous but we use them in sufficiently small amounts for them not to harm us. The same applies to essential oils. This is why training in the use of essential oils is so important. Often the chemical structure of the components within an essential oil can give a general indication of its potential toxicity (Tisserand & Young 2013). Keeping essential oils away from children and preventing oral use among those who mistake essential oils for something else will help prevent more accidents. Lachenmeier (2012) writes in his response to a report of sage poisoning "We do not want to belittle the tragedy of such cases if they occur, especially in children because of the ignorance of their parents. However, overall, these rare and exceptional cases certainly do not constitute a major public health threat, globally or in any region." Finally, it is interesting that anethole (an essential oil component) now plays a role in forensic toxicology. It is used in blood sampling for suspected alcoholic consumption (Dawidowicz & Dybowski 2014).

PART 2. CONTRAINDICATIONS & SAFETY

Possible Drug Interactions

Some essential oils have the potential to alter the effectiveness of certain drugs (Tisserand & Young 2013) because they can compete at a plasma, cellular, or receptor level. This can reduce the drug's effectiveness, or it could enhance it. The degree of change depends on the amount of essential oil used, the percentage strength, and the method of use. Interdrug interactions are frequent (Luna et al 2007; Duke et al 2013; Strasberg et al 2013). Although some interdrug reactions are known and flagged, individual patients can respond in different ways to the same dose of the same drug. This variation is related to individual pharmacokinetics: the rate and extent of absorption, distribution, and elimination of drugs in the person's body (Brooker 2008). For more about pharmacokinetics, see Chapter 2. In the same way, a patient may respond to a drug–essential oil combination idiosyncratically.

Cytochrome P450

Certain essential oils and their components induce and/or inhibit cytochrome P450 enzymes. This family of liver enzymes is important in the oxidation and clearance of lipid-soluble drugs by making them more water-soluble, so they can be safely excreted via the kidneys (Brooker 2008). In vitro data showed that high amounts of citral and geraniol strongly inhibited CYP2B6 hydroxylase activity in a competitive manner, and this might interact with drugs that are metabolized by CYP2B6 (Seo et al 2008). Lemongrass (*Cymbopogon citratus*), lemon myrtle (*Backhousia citriodora*), and lemon-scented tea tree (*Leptospermum petersonii*) are examples of essential oils high in citral. Palmarosa (*Cymbopogon martini*) is high in geraniol (<85%).

German chamomile *(Matricaria chamomilla)* and its major component, chamazulene, were found to be major inhibitors of CYP1A2, another of the human cytochrome P450 enzymes (Ganzara et al 2006). Chamazulene (up to 35%) is also found
in blue tansy *(Tanacetum annum)* and (up to 19%) in yarrow *(Achillea millefolium)*.
This is a small selection that suggests the oral use of essential oils has the potential
to affect cytochrome P450 in certain circumstances.

Platelet Aggregation

Some essential oils and their components inhibit blood clotting and could increase
the activity of warfarin, heparin, or aspirin. The strong platelet activating factor (PAF)
antagonistic activity of some oils is related to their high content of sesquiterpenes
and sesquiterpenoids (Moharam et al 2010). Star anise *(Illicium verum)*, holy basil
(Ocimum tenuiflorum), sweet fennel *(Foeniculum vulgare)*, and oregano *(Origanum
vulgare)* are a few examples of essential oils that affect PAF (Tsai et al 2007). Animal studies show that fennel *(Foeniculum vulgare)* essential oil, and its main component, anethole, has antithrombotic activity and broad-spectrum antiplatelet activity
(Tognolini et al 2007). Lavandin *(Lavandula × hybrida* CT grosso) was found to have
antiplatelet activity in animal studies (Ballabeni et al 2004). However, 100 mg/kg/day
orally for 5 days was required to significantly reduce the thrombotic events.

Monoamine Oxidase Inhibitors

Monoamine oxidase inhibitors (MAOIs) are a group of antidepressant drugs that
inhibit the action of monoamine oxidase (Brooker 2008). Monoamine oxidase is an
enzyme that breaks down neurotransmitters such as adrenaline, dopamine, norepinephrine, and serotonin.

Oral doses of essential oils increase the potential for an essential oil to have an
effect on MAOIs (Tisserand & Young 2013). Eugenol inhibits monoamine oxidase
A (MAOA) and there is a potential link between the antidepressant activity of eugenol and its MAOA inhibitory activity (Tao et al 2005). Large amounts (>50%) of
eugenol are found in the essential oils from bud, leaf, and stem of clove *(Syzygium
aromaticum)* and from cinnamon leaf *(Cinnamomum verum)*. Therefore, these
essential oils could affect MAOIs if taken orally.

Antidiabetic Effects

Korean research found lemon balm *(Melissa officinalis)* essential oil given orally to
mice for 6 weeks significantly reduced their blood glucose (65%; $p < 0.05$) (Chung
et al 2010). Chinese cinnamon *(Cinnamomum cassia)* had a regulative role in the
blood glucose level and lipids of mice, and improved the function of pancreatic
islets (Ping et al 2010). Tunisian research found that fenugreek *(Trigonella foenum-
graecum)* essential oil considerably inhibited key enzymes that were related to diabetes, such as α-amylase activity (by 46% and 52%) and maltase activity (by 37% and
35%) in the pancreas and plasma of rats (Hamden et al 2011). In an Indian study,
turmeric *(Curcuma longa)* essential oil inhibited glucosidase enzymes more effectively than the reference standard drug acarbose, which is used in type 2 diabetes

(Lekshmi et al 2012). Geranium *(Pelargonium graveolens)* essential oil was found to have a significantly better (*p* < 0.05) hypoglycemic effect at the dose of 150 mg/kg body weight than the standard diabetic drug glibenclamide (Boukhris et al 2012). This is just a small selection of research studies that suggest that the oral use of certain essential oils on a regular basis might interfere with diabetic drugs in humans.

Diuretics

When aniseed *(Pimpinella anisum)* was added to the drinking water of rats, it reduced the volume of the urine produced and increased the activity of renal Na$^+$-K$^+$ ATPase even at extremely low concentrations (Kreydiyyeh et al 2003).

Enhancing Drug Delivery/Absorption

Some essential oils, and the isolated components from essential oils (such as nerolidol, limonene, cineole, pinene, and carvone), are used to enhance drug delivery (Krishnaiah et al 2006; Krishnaiah et al 2008; Ahad et al 2011; Valgimigli et al 2012; Shen et al 2013). Essential oil components appear to enhance drug absorption by interacting with the polar domain of the skin lipids (Chen et al 2013). Some components, such as carvone, can also reverse the permeation enhancement effect so that vital skin barrier function is restored and not permanently changed after the application of dermal enhancers (Kang et al 2007; Aggarwal et al 2012). Some components enhance the permeation of other components; for example, limonene enhances the absorption of citronellol and eugenol (Schmitt et al 2009) via the skin. Therefore, it is recommended that essential oils are not used on the skin close to conventional drug patch therapy.

Epilepsy

Some essential oils, when taken orally, can cause convulsions. Therefore, it is sensible to avoid those essential oils in people who are vulnerable to epileptic fits. Please see Table 4-3. (For a more extensive list, please see Tisserand & Young 2013.) Personally, I would avoid using hyssop (*Hyssopus officinalis* CT pinocamphone), fennel *(Foeniculum vulgare)*, peppermint *(Mentha piperita)*, and rosemary *(Rosmarinus officinalis)*, although there is no published report of any of these triggering a seizure. I would also ask people who are prone to fitting episodes what smells they disliked!

TABLE 4-3 *Examples of Commonly Used Essential Oils to Avoid in Patients with Epilepsy (in Alphabetical Order)*

Birch	Betula Lenta
Pennyroyal	Mentha pulegium
Rosemary	Rosmarinus officinalis CT verbenone
Spanish lavender	Lavandula stoechas
Tansy	Tanacetum vulgare
Yarrow	Achillea millefolium
Wintergreen	Gaultheria fragrantissima

Pregnancy

Essential oils should not be used in pregnancy (or breastfeeding) if they contain large amounts (above 40%) of the following components: (*E*)-anethole, apiol, β-eudesmol, camphor, methyl salicylate, pinocamphone, or thujone (Tisserand & Young 2013) (Table 4-4). Of the more commonly used essential oils, this would rule out: aniseed (*Pimpinella anisum*), star anise (*Illicium verum*), cypress (*Cupressus sempervirens*), dill (*Anethum graveolens*), fennel (*Foeniculum vulgare*), hyssop (*Hyssopus officinalis*), and Spanish lavender (*Lavandula stoechas*). For a more inclusive list, please see Tisserand & Young (2013). Although there has been much hype surrounding pennyroyal (*Mentha pulegium*) as an abortifacient, Tisserand & Young (2013, p 383) state that it is not an abortifacient "unless taken in such massive quantities that it causes acute hepatotoxicity in the mother." There have been no recorded instances of pennyroyal toxicity following dermal application. Pregnancy should be a time to enjoy aromatherapy. Using essential oils to combat nausea in early pregnancy, to help relaxation during labor, or having an aromatic bath at the end of the day are some safe suggestions. Please see Chapter 20 on Women's Health.

Hormone Replacement Therapy

Hormone replacement therapy (HRT) is not adversely affected by aromatherapy because any hormonal effect of the essential oil would be considerably weaker than the effect of the HRT (Tisserand & Young 2013).

Oncology

Some malignant growths depend on estrogen, so perhaps the use of essential oils that are thought to have mildly phytoestrogen-like activity should be avoided, although there is very little published literature to substantiate this. Tisserand & Young (2013) include the following essential oils to avoid in oncology: aniseed (*Pimpinella anisum*), star anise (*Illicium verum*), bitter fennel (*Foeniculum vulgare* var. *amara*), sweet fennel (*Foeniculum vulgare* var. *dulce*), and myrtle (*Myrtus communis*) (Table 4-5). I would add clary sage (*Salvia sclarea*) because I think it has mild estrogenic activity based on my clinical experience of its ability to regulate irregular periods and reduce premenstrual syndrome (PMS). Clary sage contains approximately 2.5% sclareol— thought by Franchomme and Penoel (1990) to have estrogen-like properties.

TABLE 4-4 *Selection of Common Essential Oils to Avoid During Pregnancy*

Common Name	Essential Oil	Toxic Component	%
Aniseed	*Pimpinella anisum*	(*E*)-Anethole	<96
Cypress	*Cupressus sempervirens*	β-Eudesmol	14
Dill	*Anethum graveolens*	Apiole	<52
Hyssop	*Hyssopus officinalis*	Pinocamphone	<80
Spanish lavender	*Lavandula stoechas*	Camphor	<56
Star anise	*Illicium verum*	(*E*)-Anethole	92

However, there is a counter-argument. Soy products (that contain phytoestrogens) are not contraindicated in estrogen-dependent breast cancer. Recent research has found that soy isoflavones are structurally similar to the steroid hormone 17β-estradiol (Virk-Baker et al 2014) and may protect against both breast cancer (Prietsch et al 2014) and prostate cancer (Mahmoud et al 2014). In a similar way, perhaps clary sage could also be of benefit in some breast cancer. Sclareol (found in clary sage) showed cytotoxic activity against breast cell lines and appeared to enhance the effect of some cancer drugs used in breast cancer (doxorubicin, etoposide and cisplatinum) in vitro (Dimas et al 2006).

GENERAL CONTRAINDICATIONS

Some essential oils are generally contraindicated for all therapeutic uses. These include boldo leaf, calamus, cassia, bitter fennel, mugwort, mustard, rue, sassafras, tansy, wintergreen, and wormwood. These oils all contain toxic constituents. The essential oils contraindicated for undiluted topical application include oregano, clove bud and leaf, cinnamon bark, camphor, and red thyme. Essential oils that I would use with caution in patients with hypertension include rosemary, spike lavender, hyssop, juniper, thyme, and clove, although there is no published report of blood pressure being substantially raised by essential oils (Table 4-6).

TABLE 4-5 *Essential Oils Thought to Have Mild Estrogenic Activity that Might Be Best Avoided in Some Estrogen-Dependent Tumors*

Common Name	Essential Oil
Aniseed	*Pimpinella anisum*
Clary sage	*Salvia sclarea*
Fennel (bitter)	*Foeniculum vulgare* var. *amara*
Fennel (sweet)	*Foeniculum vulgare* var. *dulce*
Myrtle	*Myrtus communis*
Star anise	*Illicium verum*

TABLE 4-6 *Essential Oils to Avoid with Hypertension*

Common Name	Essential Oil
Clove	*Syzygium aromaticum*
Juniper	*Juniperus communis*
Hyssop	*Hyssopus officinalis*
Rosemary	*Rosmarinus officinalis*
Spike lavender	*Lavandula latifolia*
Thyme	*Thymus vulgaris* CT thymol

SAFETY AND STORAGE OF ESSENTIAL OILS

SAFETY

Aromatherapy requires knowledge, and yes, in the wrong hands, essential oils can be hazardous. Just like paracetamol (acetaminophen) and aspirin, which can be bought over the counter almost everywhere, essential oils should always be kept out of the reach of children. See Table 4-2 for potentially lethal dosages in children.

If a child appears to have drunk several spoonfuls of essential oil, contact the nearest poison unit (often listed at the front of a telephone directory). Keep the bottle for identification and encourage the child to drink whole milk. Do not try to induce vomiting. If essential oils (diluted or not) get into the eyes it is important to irrigate the eyes as rapidly as possible with whole milk or vegetable oil. This will dilute the essential oil. Then rinse with water and seek medical help. If there is a skin reaction to an essential oil, dilute the essential oil with vegetable oil, then wash the area with a nonperfumed soap. The majority of the components found in essential oils are nonpolar; therefore essential oils do not mix well or dissolve in water.

STORAGE

Essential oils are powerful, and it is important that they are stored away from children, people who have diminished ability to think clearly, or those unaware of what essential oils are. Essential oils kept in a hospital should be stored in a locked container. If stored in a cool, dry, dark place, undiluted essential oils can stay fresh for several years. Citrus peel oils have the shortest shelf life, both opened and unopened. All essential oils should be kept in colored (blue or amber) glass bottles to protect them from ultraviolet light, with the bottles sealed. Bottles should have an integral dropper contained in the lid to prevent spillage. All opened bottles should be stored away from heat and sunlight (ideally in a refrigerator, similar to the storage of heparin). All bottles should carry a firmly attached label, stating the botanical name, the supplier's name, and the use-by date. Most reputable companies also include a label warning that the oils should be kept away from the eyes, out of reach of children, and not be taken by mouth. It is helpful to keep a record of when each essential oil was purchased, the supplier's name, and the price. A separate list should be kept with the patient's name, the name of the physician, the dates the patient received aromatherapy, and any therapeutic (or adverse) results. Recording this information makes a portfolio on the use of essential oils easily available.

Essential oils are highly flammable, so they must be stored away from open flames such as those from candles, fire, matches, cigarettes, and gas cookers. Sprinkling them on top of light bulbs is not a good idea!

Patch testing can do much to detect and avoid skin reactions. The amount of essential oil used is usually measured in drops or percentage. On average there are 20 drops of essential oil in 1 mL. Patch tests can be used to test for irritation and are suggested for all potential-risk patients. Dilute the essential oil to double the concentration to be used regularly, and put it on an adhesive bandage. Place the bandage on the patient's forearm. If irritation is going to occur, it will do so quickly.

REFERENCES

Aggarwal G, Dhawan S, HariKumar S. 2012. Natural oils as skin permeation enhancers for transdermal delivery of olanzipine: in vitro and in vivo evaluation. *Curr Drug Deliv.* 9(2):172-81.

Ahad A, Aqil M, Kohli K, Sultana Y, Mujeeb M, Ali A. 2011. Interactions between novel terpenes and main components of rat and human skin: mechanistic view for transdermal delivery of propranolol hydrochloride. *Curr Drug Deliv.* 8(2):213-24.

Anderson I, Mullen W, Meeker J. Khojasteh-Bakht S, Oishi S. 1996. Pennyroyal toxicity: measurement of toxic metabolite levels in two cases and review of the literature. *Ann Intern Med.* 124(8):726-734.

Bailey H, Levy D, Harris L, Schink J, Foss F et al. 2002. A Phase II trial of daily perillyl alcohol in patients with advanced ovarian cancer. Eastern Cooperative Oncology Group Study E2E96. *Gynecol Oncol.* 85(3):464-468.

Ballabeni V, Tognolini M, Chiavarini M, Impicciatore M, Bruni R et al. 2004. Novel antiplatelet and antithrombotic activities of essential oil from Lavandula hybrida Reverchon "grosso." *Phytomedicine.* 11(7-8):596-601.

Botma M, Colquhoun-Flannery W, Leighton S. 2001. Laryngeal oedema caused by accidental ingestion of oil of wintergreen. *Int J Ped Otorhinolaryngology.* 58(3):229-232.

Boukhris M, Bouaziz M, Feki I, Jemai H, Feki A et al. 2012. Hypoglycemic and antioxidant effects of leaf essential oil of Pelargonium graveolens L'Hér. in alloxan induced diabetic rats. *Lipids Health Dis.* 26;11:81. doi: 10.1186/1476-511X-11-81.

Brooker C. 2008. *Medical Dictionary.* 16th edition. Churchill Livingstone. Edinburgh, Scotland.

Cauthen W, Hester W. 1989. Accidental ingestion of oil of wintergreen. *J Fam Pract.* 29(6):680-681.

Chen Y, Wang J, Cun D, Wang M, Jiang J et al. 2013. Effect of unsaturated menthol analogues on the in vitro penetration of 5-fluorouracil through rat skin. *Int J Pharm.* A 16;443(1-2).

Chung M, Cho S, Bhuiyan M, Kim K, Lee S. 2010. Anti-diabetic effects of lemon balm (*Melissa officinalis*) essential oil on glucose- and lipid-regulating enzymes in type 2 diabetic mice. *Br J Nutrition.* 104(2):180-8.

Cox D, O'Kennedy R, Thornes R. 1989. The rarity of liver toxicity in patients treated with coumarin. *Hum Toxicol.* 8(6):501-506.

Craig J. 1953. Poisoning by the volatile oils in children. *Archives of Disease in Childhood.* 55(5):475-483.

Crandon K, Thompson J. 2006. Olbas oil and respiratory arrest in a child. *Clin Toxicol.* 44:568.

Davis J. 2007. Are one or two dangerous? Methyl salicylate exposure in toddlers. *J Emergency Medicine.* 32(1):63-69.

Dawidowicz A, Dybowski M. 2014. Simple SPE-GC method for anethole determination in human serum. *J Sep Sci.* 37(4):393-7.

Decapite T, Anderson B. 2004. Allergic contact dermatitis from cinnamic aldehyde found in an industrial odour-masking agent. *Contact Dermatitis.* 51(5-6):312-313.

Del Beccaro M. 1995. Melaleuca oil poisoning in a 17 month old. *Vet Human Toxicol.* 37(6):557-8.

Diba V, Statham B. 2003. Contact urticaria from cinnamon leading to anaphylaxis. *Contact Dermatitis.* 48(2):119.

Dimas K, Papadaki M, Tsimplouli C, Hatziantoniou S, Alevizopoulos K et al. 2006. Labd-14-ene-8, 13-diol (sclareol) induces cell cycle arrest and apoptosis in human breast cancer cells and enhances the activity of anticancer drugs. *Biomed Pharmacol.* 60(3):127-133.

Dubertret L, Serraf-Tircazes D, Jeanmougin M, Morliere P, Averbeck D et al. 1990. Photoxic properties of perfumes containing bergamot oil on human skin: photoprotective effect of UVA and UVB suncreams. *J Photochem Photobiol B.* 7(204):251-259.

Duke J, Li X, Dexter P. 2013. Adherence to drug-drug interaction alerts in high-risk patients: a trial of context-enhanced alerting. *J Am Med Inform Assoc.* 20(3):494-8.

Dybing E, Doe J, Groten J, Kleiner J, O'Brien J et al. 2002. Hazard characterisation of chemicals in food and diet. Dose response, mechanisms and extrapolation issues. *Food Chem Toxicol.* 40(2-3):237-82.

Eisen J, Koren G, Juurlink D, Ng V. 2004. N−Acetylcysteine for the treatment of clove oil induced fulminant hepatic failure: Case report and review of the literature. *Clin Toxicol.* 42(1):89-92.

Franchomme P, Peneol D. *Aromathérapie Exactement.* Roger Jollois. Limoge, France.

Ganzara M, Schneider P, Stuppner H. 2006. Inhibitory effects of the essential oil of chamomile (*Matricaria recutita*) and its major constituents on human cytochrome P450 enzymes. *Life Science.* 78(8):856-861.

Guba R. 2000. Toxicity myths: The actual risks of essential oil use. *International Journal of Aromatherapy.* 10(1/2):37-49.

Guin J, Meye B, Drake D, Haffley P. 1984. The effect of quenching agents on contact urticaria caused by cinnamic aldehyde. *J Am Acad Dermatol.* 10(1):45-51.

Gurr F, Scroggie J. 1965. Eucalyptus poisoning treated by dialysis and mannitol infusion with an appendix on the analysis of biological fluids for alcohol and eucalyptol. *Australasian Annals of Medicine.* 14(3):238-249.

Halicioglu O, Astarcioglu G, Yaprak I, Aydinlioglu H. 2011. Toxicity of Salvia officinalis in a newborn and a child: an alarming report. *Pediatr Neurol.* 45(4):259-60.

Hamden K, Keskes H, Belhaj S, Mnafgui K, Feki A et al. 2011. Inhibitory potential of omega-3 fatty and fenugreek essential oil on key enzymes of carbohydrate-digestion and hypertension in diabetes rats. *Lipids Health Dis.* 10:226. doi: 10.1186/1476-511X-10-226.

Hartnoll G, Moore D, Douek D. 1993. Near fatal ingestion of oil of cloves. *Archives of Disease in Childhood.* 69:392-393.

Itani W, El-Banna S, Hussan S, Larsson R, Bazarbachi A et al. 2008. Anti colon cancer components from Lebanese sage (Salvia libanotica) essential oil: Mechanistic basis. *Cancer Bio Ther.* 7(11):1765-73.

Jacobs M, Hornfeldt C. 1994. Melaleuca oil poisoning. *Clinical Toxicology (New York).*

Janes S, Price C, Thomas D. 2005. Essential oils poisoning: N-acetylcysteine for eugenol-induced hepatic failure and analysis of a national database. *Eur J Pediatr.* 164(8):520-2.

Kang L, Poh A, Fan S, Ho P, Chan Y, Chan S. 2007. Reversible effects of permeation enhancers on human skin. *Eur J Pharm Biopharm.* 67(1):149-55.

Kasper S, Gastpar M, Müller W, Volz H, Möller H et al. 2014. Lavender oil preparation Silexan is effective in generalized anxiety disorder - a randomized, double-blind comparison to placebo and paroxetine. *Int J Neuropsychopharmacol.* 2014 Jan 23:1-11. [Epub ahead of print].

Kirsch C, Yenokida G, Jenson W, Wendland R, Suh H et al. 1990. Non-cardiogenic pulmonary oedema due to the intravenous administration of clove oil. *Thorax.* 45(3):235-6.

Kligman A. 1996. The identification of contact allergens by human assay. *J Invest Derm.* 47(5):393-409.

Kloss J, Boeckmans C. 1967. Methyl salicylate poisoning. *Ohio State Med J.* 63(8):1064-1065.

Kolassa N. 2013. Menthol differs from other terpenic essential oil constituents. *Regulatory Toxicology and Pharmacology.* 65(1):115-118.

Kopelman R, Miller S, Kelly R, Sunshine I. 1979. Camphor intoxication treated by resin hemoperfusion. *JAMA.*16,241(7):727-8.

Koppel C, Tenczer J, Tonnesmann U, Schirop T, Ibe K. 1982. Acute poisoning with pine oil – metabolism of monoterpenes. *Arch Toxicol.* 49(1):73-78.

Kreydiyyeh S, Usta J, Knio K, Markossian S, Dagher S. 2003. Aniseed oil increases glucose absorption and reduces urine output in the rat. *Life Sci.* 74(5):663-73.

Krishnaiah Y, Al-Saidan S, Jayaram B. 2006. Effect of nerodilol, carvone and anethole on the in vitro transdermal delivery of selegiline hydrochloride. *Pharmazie.* 61(1):46-53.

Krishnaiah Y, Raju V, Shiva Kumar M, Rama B, Raghumurthy V et al. 2008. Studies on optimizing in vitro transdermal permeation of ondansetron hydrochloride using nerodiol, carvone and limonene as penetration enhances. *Pharm Dev Technol.* 2008;13(3):177-85.

Lachenmeier D. 2012. Epileptic seizures caused by accidental ingestion of sage (*Salvia officinalis* L.) oil in children: a rare, exceptional case or a threat to public health? *Pediatric Neurology.* 46(3):201.

Lane B, Ellenhorn MJ, Hulbert TV et al. 1991. Clove ingestion in an infant. *Human Exp Toxicol.* 10(4):291-294.

Lekshmi P, Arimboor R, Indulekha P, Menon A. 2012. Turmeric (*Curcuma longa* L.) volatile oil inhibits key enzymes linked to type 2 diabetes. *Int J Food Sci Nutr.* 63(7):832-4.

Loprinzi C, Kugler J, Sloan J, Rooke T, Quella S et al. 1999. Lack of effect of coumarin in women with lymphoedema after treatment for breast cancer. *N Engl J Med.* 340(5):346-350.

Luna D, Otero V, Canosa D, Montenegro S, Otero P, de Quirós FG. 2007. Analysis and redesign of a knowledge database for a drug-drug interactions alert system. *Stud Health Technol Inform.* 129(Pt 2):885-9.

MacPherson J. 1925. The toxicology of eucalyptus oil. *Med J Australia.* 2:108-110.

Mahmoud A, Yang W, Bosland M. 2014. Soy isoflavones and prostate cancer: a review of molecular mechanisms. *J Steroid Biochem Mol Biol.* 140:116-32.

Mant A. 1961. A case of poisoning by oil of citronella. Association Proceeding VI. *Medicine, Science, and the Law.* 1, 170-171.

Martindale W. 1977. *The Extra Pharmacopoeia*, 27th ed. London: Pharmaceutical Press.

Melis K, Bochner A, Janssens G. 1989. Accidental nasal eucalyptol and menthol instillation. *Eur J Pediatr.* 148(8):786-788.

Millet Y. 1981. Toxicity of some essential plant oils. Clinical and experimental study. *Clin Toxicol.* 18(12):1485-1498.

Moharam B, Jantan I, Ahmed F, Jalil J. 2010. Antiplatelet aggregation and platelet activating factor (PAF) receptor antagonistic activities of the essential oils of five *Goniothalamus* species. *Molecules.* 15(8):5124-38.

Morris M, Donaghue A, Marovitw J. 2003. Ingestion of tea tree oils (Melaeuca oil) by a 4-year-old boy. *Pediatr Emerg Care.* 19 (3):169-171.

Muchtaridi I, Subarnas A, Apriyantono A, Mustarichie, R. 2010. Identification of compounds in the essential oil of nutmeg seeds (*Myristica fragrans* Houtt.) that inhibit locomotor activity in mice. *Int J Mol Sci.* 11(11):4771-81.

O'Mullane N, Joyce P, Kamath S, Tham M, Knass D. 1982. Adverse CNS effects of menthol-containing Olibas oil. *Lancet.* 1(8281):1121.

Opdyke D. 1976. Monograph on fragrance raw materials. *Food Cosmet Toxicol.* 14 Suppl. 713-715.

Oxford English Dictionary. 2005. Oxford University Press. UK.

Parys B. 1983. Chemical Burns resulting from contact with peppermint oil: a case report. *Burns.* 9(5):374-375.

Patel S, Wiggins J. 1980. Eucalyptus poisoning. *Arch Disease Childhood.* 55(5):405-406.

Perry P, Dean B, Krenzelok E. 1990. Cinnamon oil abuse by adolescents. *Vet Hum Toxicol.* 32(2):162-164.

Peterson A, Bansal A, Hofman F, Chen T, Zada G. 2014. A systematic review of inhaled intranasal therapy for central nervous system neoplasms: an emerging therapeutic option. *J Neurooncol.* 116(3):437-46.

Pilapil V. 1989. Toxic manifestations of cinnamon oil ingestion in a child. *Clin Pediatrics.* 28(6):276.

Ping H, Zhang G, Ren G. 2010. Antidiabetic effects of cinnamon oil in diabetic KK-Ay mice. *Food Chem Toxicol.* 48(8-9):2344-9.

Prietsch R, Monte L, da Silva F, Beira F, Del Pino F. 2014. Genistein induces apoptosis and autophagy in human breast MCF-7 cells by modulating the expression of proapoptotic factors and oxidative stress enzymes. *Mol Cell Biochem.* 2014 Feb 27. [Epub]. Accessed March 14, 2014.

Roethe A, Heine A, Rebohie E. 1973. Oils from juniper berries as an occupational allergen for the skin and the respiratory tract. *Berufs-Dermatosen.* 21(1):11-16.

Salam T, Fowler J. 2001. Balsam-related systemic contact dermatitis. *Am J Dermatol.* 45(3):377-381.

Sarkar S, Azab B, Quinn BA, Shen X, Dent P et al. 2014. Chemoprevention gene therapy (CGT) of pancreatic cancer using perillyl alcohol and a novel chimeric serotype cancer terminator virus. *Curr Mol Med.* 4(1):125-40.

Schmeck-Lindenau H, Naser-Hijazi B, Becker E, Henneicke-von Zepelin H, Schnitker J. 2003. Safety aspects of a coumarin-trozerutin combination regarding liver function in a double-blind, placebo-controlled study. *Int J Clin Pharmacol Ther.* 41(5):193-199.

Schmitt S, Schaefer U, Doebler L, Reichling J. 2009. Cooperative interaction of monoterpenes and phenylpropanoids on the in vitro human skin permeation of complex composed essential oils. *Planta Med.* 75(13):1381-5.

Schultes R. 1980. *In Medicine Quest* by Mark Plotkin. 2000. Viking.

Seo K, Kim H, Ku H, Ahn H, Park S et al. 2008. The monoterpenoids citral and geraniol are moderate inhibitors of CYP2B9 hydroxylase activity. *Chem Biol Interact.* 174(3):141-146.

Shen T, Zu H, Went W, Zhang J. 2013. Development of a reservoir-type transdermal delivery system containing eucalyptus oil for tetramethylpyrazine. *Drug Delivery.* 20(1):19-24.

Siegel E, Wason S. 1986. Camphor toxicity. *Pediatric Clin North Am.* 33(2):375-379.

Sparks T. 1985. Cinnamon oil burn. *West J Med.* 142(6):835.

Strasberg H, Chan A, Sklar S. 2013. Inter-rater agreement among physicians on the clinical significance of drug-drug interactions. *AMIA Annual Conf Proc.* 2013:1325-8. eCollection 2013.

Tamir S, Davidovitch Z, Attal P, Aliashar R. 2005. Peppermint oil chemical burn. *Otolaryngol - Head Neck Surg.* 133(5):801-802.

Tao G, Irie Y, Li D, Keung. 2005. Eugenol and its structural analogs inhibit monoamine oxidase A and exhibit antidepressant-like activity. *Bioorg Med Chem* 13(15):4777-47788.

Temple W, Nerida A, Beasley M, et al. 1991. Management of oil of citronella poisoning. *Clin Toxicol.* 29(2):257-262.

Tibballs J. 1995. Clinical effects and management of eucalyptus oil ingestion in infants and young children. *Med J Aust.* 163(4):177-180.

Tisserand R, Young R. 2013. *Essential Oil Safety.* London: Churchill Livingstone.

Tognolini M, Ballabeni V, Beroni S, Bruni R, Impicciatore M, Barocelli E. 2007. Protective effect of *Foeniculum vulgare* essential oil and anethole in an experimental model of thrombosis. *Pharmacol Res.* 56(3):254-60.

Trattner A, David M. 2003. Patch testing with fine fragrances: comparison with fragrance mix, balsam of Peru and a fragrance series. *Contact Dermatitis.* 49(6):287-9.

Tsai T, Hsu H, Yang W. 2007. A-Bulnesene, a PAF inhibitor isolated from the essential oil of *Pogostemon cablin.* *Fitoterapia.* 78:7-11.

Valgimigli L, Gabbanini S, Berlini E, Lucchi E, Beltramini C, Bertarelli Y. 2012. Lemon (*Citrus limon*, Burm.f.) essential oil enhances the trans-epidermal release of lipid-(A, E) and water-(B6, C) soluble vitamins from topical emulsions in reconstructed human epidermis. *Int J Cosmet Sci.* 34(4):347-56.

Vallance W. 1955. Pennyroyal poisoning – a fatal case. *Lancet.* 269(6895):850-851.

Van Ketel W. 1982. Allergy to *Matricaria chamomilla.* *Contact Dermatitis.* 8(2):143.

Van Ketel W. 1987. Allergy to *Matricaria chamomilla.* *Contact Dermatitis.* 16(1):50-51.

Vanscheidt W, Rabe E, Naser-Hijazi B, Ramelet A, Partsch H et al. 2002. The efficacy and safety of a coumarin/troxerutin combination (SB-LOT) in patients with chronic venous insufficiency: a double-blind placebo controlled randomized study. *Vasa.* 31(3):185-190.

Virk-Baker M, Barnes S, Krontiras H, Nagy T. 2014. S-(-)equol producing status not associated with breast cancer risk among low isoflavone-consuming US postmenopausal women undergoing a physician-recommended breast biopsy. *Nutr Res.* 34(2):116-25.

Wahab A, Ul Haq R, Ahmed A, Khan R, Razza M. 2009. Anticonvulsant activities of nutmeg oil of *Myristica fragrans.* *Phytother Res.* 23(2):153-8.

Watt M. 1991. *Plant Aromatics.* Essex, UK: Witham.

Weisbord S, Soule J, Kimmel P. 1997. Poison on line – acute renal failure caused by oil of wormwood purchased through the internet. *N Engl J Med.* 337(12):825-827.

Whitling H. 1908. "Cures" for asthma: fatal case from an overdose of oil of sage. *Lancet.* 171(4415):1074-75.

Wilkinson H. 1991. Childhood ingestion of volatile oils. *Med J Australia.* 154:430-431.

Williamson E. (2013). Foreword in *Essential Oil Safety.* 2nd edition. Tisserand R, Young R. Churchill Livingstone. Page vii.

Yu S, Pai S, Neyhaus I, Grekin R. 2007. Diagnosis and treatment of pigmentary disorders in Asian skin. *Facial Plast Surg Clin Am.* 15:367-380.

Chapter 5

Aromatherapy and Integrative Healthcare

"Character is like a tree and reputation like a shadow. The shadow is what we think of it, the tree is the real thing."

Abraham Lincoln

CHAPTER ASSETS

This chapter has replaced Evidence-Based Aromatherapy in Nursing Practice because many different health professionals use aromatherapy, not just nurses. To discover who was integrating aromatherapy, I contacted a selection of hospitals in the United States, where my Certified Clinical Aromatherapy Practitioner (CCAP) and Clinical Aromatherapy for Hospitals (CAH) courses have been taught, plus a hospital in South Africa, and a few hospitals in the UK, where I now live. The aim of this chapter is to inspire health professionals to consider integrating clinical aromatherapy into their facility. A list of the hospitals approached can be found in Box 5-1.

INTEGRATIVE HEALTHCARE—WHAT'S IN A NAME?

Over the last 10 years, the terms *integrative medicine* (IM), *integrative therapies*, or *integrative healthcare* (IH) have emerged to describe a new alliance that combines Complementary and Alternative Medicine (CAM) with conventional medicine.

95

BOX 5-1 *Hospitals Consulted for this Chapter*

Aurora Healthcare, Wisconsin and Illinois, USA
Beth Israel Center for Health and Healing, New York, USA
Carolinas Medical Center University, North Carolina, USA
Huntington Hospital, New York, USA
Penny George Institute for Health and Healing (PGIHH), Minneapolis, USA
Primary Children's Hospital, Utah, USA
Red Cross Memorial Children's Hospital, Cape Town, South Africa
Texas Health Harris Methodist Hospital, Texas, USA
The Christie Hospital, Manchester, UK
The Royal Marsden Hospital, London, UK
University College London Hospital, London, UK

This has happened because patients want both CAM and conventional medicine. The word *integrative* suggests sharing and partnership, rather than the "them" and "us" of the past. Kreitzer (2013), who spoke at the *Integrative Medicine and the Health of the Public* (US) summit sponsored by the Institute of Medicine (IOM) and the Bravewell Collaboration, points out that the word *integrate* means to "put things together to form something new." Boon et al (2004) suggest that IH should be nonhierarchical and different to parallel, consultative, collaborative, coordinated, multidisciplinary, and interdisciplinary.

In 2012, David Eisenberg, MD, (founding Chief of the Division for Research and Education in Complementary and Integrative Medical Therapies at Harvard Medical School and lead author of the 1991 study on the use of complementary medicine in the United States), Wayne Jonas (current president and CEO of the Samueli Institute who was also one of the early directors of the Office of Alternative Medicine) and Ian Coulter (Samueli Institute Chair in Policy for Integrative Medicine) debated multiple aspects of IH including its effectiveness, utility, and the future of IH at University of California (UCLA, Los Angeles, CA). A podcast on this debate was available from the Samueli Institute in 2013 (https://www.samueliinstitute.org). During the podcast, the three men suggested that IH was a combination the "best of orthodox medicine with the best of evidence-based CAM."

This may be so, however, "evidence-based CAM" usually means CAM that has research-based evidence. Mariano (2013), a nursing professor at New York University, writes "although research evidence is important it is not enough, particularly when the evidence is limited mostly to what is funded by private interest, or grounded in the pharmacologic treatment of disease." Also, research is an expensive enterprise and most research into CAM is funded by the pharmaceutical industry with a vested interest. A great deal of CAM is based on practice-based evidence, sometimes gleaned over many years of clinical practice. Perhaps the very best kind of IH would combine not just CAM and conventional medicine, but evidence-based practice with practice-based evidence.

In Japan, *integrative medicine* is the title used to describe a "fusion of experience-backed traditional medicine and CAM with science-backed Western medicine"

(Atsumi 2012). The term *integrative medicine* (IM) is preferred to *integrative health-care* (IH) in Japan. IM is seen as a "combination of modern medicine with CAM therapies" (Imanishi & Kishida (2012). At Meiji University of Integrative Medicine, Japan (where I had the pleasure of presenting an overview of clinical aromatherapy in 2012), IM means a blend of Oriental and Western medicine (in a spectacular setting!). Here, evidence-based practice and centuries of clinical expertise provide a solid foundation while recognizing that research can, and does, add to the body of knowledge.

WHY DO WE NEED IH?

Ralph Snyderman, Chancellor Emeritus, Duke University (Durham, NC, USA) said in his keynote address (Snyderman 2009) that "the disease-driven approach to care has resulted in spiraling costs as well as a fragmented health system that is reactive, episodic, inefficient and impersonal." Harold Walach, Research Professor in Psychology, University of Nottingham, UK, suggests that CAM and its subsequent acceptance as part of IH are patient-led. Patients do not "experience the benefits promised by biomedicines: medications don't work for everyone, some have deeply unpleasant side effects, some may produce only short-term relief or lead to other problems that need more medication" (Walach 2009) so patients turn to CAM. If CAM is part of IH, patients will be better served as they will receive the benefit of both approaches.

WHERE DOES AROMATHERAPY FIT IN AN INTEGRATIVE MODEL OF HEALTHCARE?

There are many kinds of aromatherapy and many ways of using essential oils. This can lead to confusion as to what the practice of aromatherapy entails. Essential oils come from botanicals and they are natural products. Essential oils can have mind–body effects and they are sometimes used in massage and/or meditation.

In the United States, the National Center for Complementary and Alternative Medicine (NCCAM) divides CAM into three groups (http://nccam.nih.gov/health/whatiscam):

(1) **Natural products:** includes herbs (also known as botanicals), vitamins and minerals, and *probiotics*.
(2) **Mind and body practices:** includes acupuncture, healing touch, guided imagery, massage, meditation, relaxation, tai chi, and yoga.
(3) **Other health approaches:** includes Ayurvedic medicine, Chinese medicine, homeopathy, naturopathy, and traditional healing.

Although aromatherapy is not listed individually, it could fit into either Group 1 or Group 2.

MODELS OF INTEGRATION

In the United States, 30% of academic medical establishments have IH centers (Jonas 2013). However, each IH or IM clinic/program is different. Each has its own approach, offering services that are relevant to their patient population (Bravewell Best Practice 2007). For example, The Jefferson–Myrna Brind Center for Integrative Medicine in Philadelphia has a fee structure that reflects a mix of insurance reimbursement (physicians) and fee-for-service (nonphysician providers and some services provided by physicians) (Bravewell Best Practice 2007). Space is rented by therapists who charge a fee to patients. The most commonly treated conditions are cancer care, cardiovascular issues, menopause, pain management, and osteoporosis. The Consortium of Academic Health Centers for Integrative Medicine lists 57 academic medical centers and affiliate institutions that have used IM (http://www.imconsortium.org/).

As for the integration of aromatherapy, some hospitals pay their aromatherapists a fee-for-service, some include it as part of holistic nursing care, and some institutions have unpaid volunteers. These are all methods of integrating aromatherapy into clinical practice.

BUILDING THE FOUNDATION: INTEGRATION OF CLINICAL AROMATHERAPY IN THE PRACTICE SETTING

I created the first clinical aromatherapy course for nurses and doctors in the United States and began teaching it in 1995. Since then, the CCAP course has been taught in 27 US states. Please see Box 5-2 and Box 5-3. The course initially comprised five

BOX 5-2 *Initial Hospital Locations for the Certified Clinical Aromatherapy Practitioner (CCAP) Course Taught by Dr. Buckle (in Alphabetical Order of State)*

AK. Anchorage
FL. West Palm Beach
GA. Atlanta
ID. Boise
IN. Indianapolis
KA. Wichita
LO. Shreveport
MA. New Bedford
MI. Detroit, Lansing
MN. Minneapolis, St. Paul
NH. Manchester
NJ. Dover, Ridgewood
NM. Albuquerque
NY. New York City, Yonkers
PA. Scranton, Reading
TX. Houston, Fort Worth
VA. Suffolk
WA. Anacortes, Seattle
WI. Wauwatosa, Milwaukee

BOX 5-3 *Hospitals Where the (CCAP) Course Has Been Taught by RJBA Instructors (in Alphabetic Order of State)*

AZ. Desert Samaritan Hospital, Mesa
CT. Stamford Hospital, Stamford
IL. Infinity Foundation, Chicago
IN. Deaconess Hospital, Evansville
MA. Boston Medical Center, Boston
MA. Boston Children's Hospital, Boston
MA. Mercy Medical Center, Springfield
MA. Franklin Medical Center, Greenfield
MA. Cooley Dickenson Hospital, Northampton
MA. The VA Medical Center, Leeds
MA. Woodlands Hospital, Woodbury
MI. Ingham Regional Medical Center, Lansing
MI. Integrated Health Professionals, Montague
MI. Visiting Nurse Services, Muskegon
MI. Samaritan Hospital, Troy
MN. Children's Hospital, St. Paul
MN. Herrepin County Medical Center, Minneapolis
MN. United Hospital, St. Paul
MN. St John's Hospital, Maplewood
MN. St Joseph's Hospital, St. Paul
MN. Woodwinds Hospital, St. Paul
NC. Mission Hospital, Asheville
NC. Western Carolina University, Asheville
NE. Good Samaritan Hospital, Kearney
NJ. Shore Memorial Hospital, Somers Point
NJ. St. Clare's Hospital, Dover
NJ. The Valley Hospital, Ridgewood
NY. Beth Israel Continuum Center, New York City
NY. Northern Westchester Hospital, Mount Krisco
NY. Highlands Hospital, Rochester
NY. Good Samaritan Hospital, Suffern
NY. St. John's Riverside Medical Center, Yonkers
OH. Heather Hill Hospital, Chardon, OH
OH. Four Winds Academy, Cincinnati, OH
OH. Insight Learning and Wellness Center, Cleveland
OK. Mercy Hospital, Edmund
PA. Fredericksen Outpatient Center, Mechanicsburg
PA. Pinnacle Health Polyclinic Hospital, Harrisburg
TN. Holistic Alternative Wellness Clinic, Clarkson
TX. Harris Methodist Fort Worth Hospital, Fort Worth
TX. Panola College, Carthage
VA. Sentara Obici Hospital, Suffolk.
WA. Highline Community Hospital, Burien
WI. Beaver Dam Community Hospital, Beaver Dam

Continued

BOX 5-3 *Hospitals Where the (CCAP) Course Has Been Taught by RJBA Instructors (in Alphabetic Order of State)—cont'd*

WI. St Clare's Hospital, Baraboo
WI. Aurora Sinai Medical Center, Milwaukee
WI. Aurora Medical Center, Oshkosh
WI. Aurora Medical Center, Grafton
WI. Aurora Healthcare System, Wauwatosa
WI. St. Luke's South Shore Hospital, Milwaukee
WI. Shawno Medical Center, Shawno
WI. West Allis Memorial Hospital, West Allis

weekends plus one weekend of testing, spread out over 18 months, so it meant a lot of travelling for me. The course is now four weekends plus the weekend test since the 'M' Technique became a separate course, although parts of the 'M' Technique are still included in the CCAP course. It was obvious from the start that progress would be slow because the concept was so new. For aromatherapy to be accepted clinically, it needed to be clinically focused. This meant targeting symptom management (reduced nausea, improved sleep, reduced perception of pain, infection control) or achievement of optimal outcomes (such as improved patient satisfaction, retention of clinical staff, or cost reduction). The CCAP course was endorsed by the American Nurses Association (AHNA) in 1999—the first aromatherapy course to be endorsed by a national nursing organization. I realized I could not do it all myself and invited other nurses to help me teach the course. I also set up a database to track students, instructors, co-ordinators and student research projects. Many small pilot studies were carried out, each targeting a specific clinical outcome in one department of a hospital. The studies were mainly carried out by nurses and doctors as part of their course. For transparency, the study results were presented to an outside examiner in both a written paper (all read and critiqued by me) and for an oral defense in front of an external examiner.

The CCAP external examiner was usually a hospital physician, or a nurse who also had a PhD. It helped if they knew nothing, or very little, about aromatherapy so they could come with an open mind. During the pilot studies, interest from work colleagues often spread to other hospital departments. If the study worked, the hospital was often keen to adopt clinical aromatherapy. If the targeted outcome was not achieved, the study might be repeated using a different percentage. An example was the topical use of black pepper *(Piper nigrum)* to help access veins before intravenous insertion in patients with difficult veins. Several RJ Buckle student studies were completed (Ballard 2004; Story 2005; Carter 2005) before an effective percentage was found. This led to the controlled study that was published in the *Journal of Alternative & Complementary Medicine* (Kristiniak et al 2012).

Some students published their findings, but most did not have the time, or expertise. Therefore, I am keen (and very proud) to mention some RJBA studies

BOX 5-4 *Clinical Aromatherapy for Hospitals (CAH) Courses*

> Carolinas Medical University, Charlotte, NC
> Danbury Hospital, Danbury, CT
> Minneapolis VA Healthcare System, Minneapolis, MN
> Mission Hospital, Asheville, NC
> St. Francis Hospital, Hartford, CT
> Westerly Hospital, Westerly, RI

in this third edition. In integration, training is key. The results will only be as good as the training given. Sometimes, online training is acceptable; however, classroom courses allow plenty of time for dialogue and discussion that is hard to emulate online. In either case, evidence of knowledge, skill acquisition, and competency are required before state Board of Nursing (BON) acknowledgment is granted. Some state BONs, such as Massachusetts, list "aromatherapy" and "use of essential oils" separately (MA BON Advisory Ruling 9801, 2012). Today, clinical aromatherapy is available as part of CAM and as part of IH in many hospitals in the United States.

I introduced a much shorter course (14 hours over 2 days), Clinical Aromatherapy for Hospitals (CAH), several years ago. This was intended for hospitals wanting to integrate aromatherapy initially in a very small way. Please see Box 5-4 for hospitals where this course has been taught.

EXAMPLES OF INTEGRATION

The next part of this chapter examines different ways of integrating aromatherapy in different countries.

UNITED STATES—ALL GREAT THINGS BEGIN WITH SMALL BEGINNINGS

North Carolina

Ron Hunt, MD, an anesthesiologist, set up an IH clinic in Charlotte, NC, in 2000. Staffed by a physician, a chiropractor, a massage therapist (MT), a physical therapist (PT), and an acupuncturist, they used herbs and aromatherapy in a multidisciplinary approach (Hunt 2014) to patient care. The clinic was geared toward treating patients with chronic pain who had exhausted traditional medical therapies and interventions (Hunt 2014). Hunt was so impressed with aromatherapy that he set up a clinical trial ($N = 303$) at Carolinas Medical Center University (Charlotte, NC) to explore the effect of inhaled essential oils for postoperative nausea. The positive results (Hunt et al 2013) impressed the nursing staff and other medics. Aromatherapy is now used regularly in the Post Anesthesia Care Unit (PACU) by RNs, and there is a hospital aromatherapy policy in place. In spite of this very encouraging advance, integrating aromatherapy in other areas of the hospital is proving slow (Hunt 2013). Dr. Hunt completed the RJBA CAH course in 2012.

New York
Huntington Hospital

Judy Dibartolo, RN was one of the pioneers who helped integrate aromatherapy into Huntington Hospital, NY, and created a whole new Complementary Care Center. Today, aromatherapy treatments are available to patients throughout the hospital. An aromatherapy hospital policy is in place. There is no additional fee to the patients. Nurses who use aromatherapy complete a mandatory in-service training. Six single essential oils—eucalyptus *(Eucalyptus globulus)*, frankincense *(Boswellia carteri)*, ginger *(Zingiber officinalis)*, lavender *(Lavandula angustifolia)*, mandarin *(Citrus reticulata)*, and peppermint *(Mentha × piperita)*—are used topically in the 'M' Technique, or inhaled using aromastix (Dibartolo 2014). Nursing staff also use an essential oil "purification spray." Judy received the 2006 Magnet Nursing Award for setting up the Complementary Care Center. It is hoped the use of essential oils will be extended to include infection control in the future. Judy completed the RJBA CCAP course in 2011.

The Center for Health and Healing

At Beth Israel Hospital, New York City, integration means taking care of staff as well as patients. The Center for Health and Healing (previously called Continuum Center for Health and Healing) Department of Integrative Medicine is an initiative of Mount Sinai Beth Israel that started in 2000 (http://www.healthandhealingny.org). Today, 75% of the nursing staff have learned basic information on a small set of essential oils via funding from the Evans Foundation (Lee 2014). The funding covers an integrative stress management program for staff and patients. Grounded in holistic nursing, the program includes aromatherapy as well as yoga and breathing exercises (CIRE-IM 2014). The center also has a special DK aromatherapy cancer project funded by Donna Karan (Ocampo 2014). This project trains staff to use four essential oils—lavender *(Lavandula angustifolia)*, ginger *(Zingiber officinalis)*, peppermint *(Mentha × piperita)*, and ylang ylang *(Canaga odorata)*—to relieve anxiety, pain, and nausea. Aurora Ocampo, BS, RN, heads the 2-day training for the DK project and is clinical aromatherapy lead for integration. Aurora completed the RJBA CCAP training in 2000 and became both a CCAP and an 'M' Technique instructor in 2003.

Minnesota

An example of successful integration is the oncology inpatient care provided through the Penny George Institute for Health and Healing (PGIHH) in Minneapolis (Kinney 2012). PGIHH is the integrative arm of Allina Health, one of the largest healthcare systems in the United States with 11 hospitals, 90 clinics, and more than 23,000 employees. A small number (began with four) of single essential oils are used. All 6000 Allina Health nurses have access to an online aromatherapy education course that enables them to use aromatherapy at the bedside (Kinney 2014). The clinically focused and research-backed course was created by two nurses who had completed the RJBA training. Between 2003 and 2012, more than 10,000 aromatherapy treatments were offered for symptoms such as nausea, pain, and anxiety and this was documented in patient electronic medical records (Kinney 2012). Mary-Ellen Kinney, RN, completed her RJBA CCAP training in 2005.

Texas

Carol Scheidel, RN, BSN, is the clinical aromatherapy lead instructor for Texas Health Harris Methodist Hospital, Fort Worth, TX, as well as being the hospital Ethics Manager. The hospital started training its staff via the RJBA CCAP course in 2004 and has graduated 130 healthcare professionals, including nurses, physical therapists, and pharmacists. Currently, there are 28 CCAPs on staff (Scheidel 2014). The course is currently taught by five RJBA-certified CCAP instructors, led by Carol Scheidel. A choice of 33 essential oils are used, individually or in mixtures, either topically (in the 'M' Technique) or inhaled. There is a hospital policy and protocol in place. Examples of use in the med-surgical unit are: topical black pepper to help intravenous insertion, ginger or peppermint for nausea, and sweet marjoram for gut motility following abdominal surgery (Scheidel 2014). Essential oils are also used in the midwifery clinic, intensive care unit (ICU), and many other areas of the hospital. The hospital has been featured in the national press for its pioneering stance on integrating clinical aromatherapy. Carol Scheidel completed her RJBA CCAP training in 2004.

Utah

Dr. Lynn Gershan, Medical Director of Pediatric Integrative Medicine, began integrating aromatherapy into the Integrative Medicine program at Primary Children's Hospital, Salt Lake City, UT, just over 3 years ago. Her overall aim is that everyone on staff will be able to use a few selected essential oils (Gershan 2014). For nurse education, Dr. Gershan is assisted by Jody Osteyee, DNP, APRN, CPNP. By October 2013, hospital policies and protocols were in place and a 15-minute computer-based training module had been created with the assistance of Jaclyn White, RN. This was followed with a home package that nurses and Child Life Specialists could use to try out the essential oils at home (Osteyee 2014). Higher levels of training will be created for those overseeing the integration and, as the program expands, so the level of training will increase. Currently, the four oils in use are lavender *(Lavandula angustifolia)*, peppermint *(Mentha × piperita)*, spearmint *(Mentha × spicata)*, and mandarin *(Citrus reticulata)*. These are provided on cotton balls for inhalation or in personal inhalers (aromastix). Symptoms targeted are anxiety, pain, nausea, and insomnia. Response to treatment is recorded in the patient's electronic medical record (Gershan 2014).

The clinical aromatherapy integration program is currently used in both the inpatient and the outpatient pediatric oncology setting. It will gradually expand to include the whole hospital system, starting with the Intermountain Healthcare (IHC) system's Maternity Suite in Logan, and both the inpatient and the Same Day Surgery units at Riverton Hospital (Gershan 2014).

There is no additional charge to the patient because each hospital unit pays for the essential oils out of its budget. Essential oils are purchased from a group of different companies known to Dr. Gershan. A small pilot study was conducted in the outpatient oncology clinic targeting nausea using aromastix. The study was recently completed and has been submitted for publication. Therapeutic use of essential oils is also taught to rotating pediatric residents by the IM team that includes Dr. Gershan and Malinda Horton, NP (Nurse Practitioner). Diagnoses treated include dermatologic side effects of chemotherapy, wounds, snake bites, dysmenorrhea, abdominal and muscle pain, and migraines (Gershan 2014). Patient education is an important facet of this service. Dr. Gershan completed the RJBA clinical aromatherapy home study course in 2010.

HOSPITAL SYSTEMS
AURORA HEALTHCARE

Founded in 1984, Aurora Healthcare (AHC) has 15 hospitals and 185 clinics as well as home care, hospices, and pharmacies in eastern Wisconsin and northern Illinois. AHC employs approximately 6300 registered nurses, 1500 physicians, and is one of Wisconsin's largest private-sector employers. The use of clinical aromatherapy began approximately 10 years ago via RJBA's CCAP training program (Conway 2014). To date, 50 staff members have completed the training. Integration varies at each site location. Specific departments that request greater knowledge or expertise are led by CCAPs who are also nurses, nurse practitioners, or physician assistants (Conway 2014). There is no patient charge for aromatherapy. The hospital policy states that board of nursing approval, CCAP training, and physician approval are required for nurses to administer essential oil treatments. (The CCAP training covers 33 essential oils. These can be used either singly or in mixtures, topically or inhaled; therefore, there is a wide choice.)

Aurora has created two separate training programs for other staff so they can use aromatherapy via diffusers or topically. The first provides patients with the choice to use essential oils to scent their room during their inpatient stay. The second provides night nurses with a lavender (*Lavandula angustifolia*)-scented cream that they can apply to patients at bedtime. An informal survey (subjective) found both programs were popular. The older nurses particularly liked the chance to put "back in touch" with the patients, because many had practiced back rubs in their training. Anecdotal feedback found patients needed less sleep or anxiety medication and staff felt empowered (Conway 2014).

Patients can also use personal inhalers (aromastix) for specific conditions such as reduction of chemo-induced nausea (Conway 2014). Diane Ames, MSN, NP, CCAP, has led the integration of clinical aromatherapy into Aurora Healthcare. She completed her CCAP training in 2004 and became a CCAP instructor in 2006. Diane also consults throughout the hospital on the use of essential oils for methicillin-resistant *Staphylococcus aureus* (MRSA) and wound infections, under the direction of Nancy Conway, MS, Director Integrative Medicine. Aromatherapy is listed on the Aurora Healthcare website under patient services (Aurora 2014).

Veterans Affairs System: Minneapolis

The Minneapolis Veterans Affairs (VA) system has been using essential oils for about 4 years in the hospice/palliative care program. This was expanded to a few other units as interest expanded and education was made available to staff (Katseres 2014). By early 2014, all nursing staff had received 4 hours of integrative therapy education. This includes the hand 'M' Technique, information on some essential oils, and aspects of holistic nursing. Integrative therapy will shortly be available to all patients (both inpatient and outpatient), and in the community-based outreach clinics (Katseres 2014). Essential oils are available at no extra cost to patients through the hospital supply distribution center. However, if patients need a refill, they can order directly from Plant Extracts International—a local essential oil company that has worked with the VA to develop and provide the six different essential oil mixtures in current use. Applications are either topical, inhalation via cotton ball, diffusers, and the 'M' Technique, or direct application to the affected site. Aromastix are particularly popular for patients undergoing chemotherapy and radiotherapy (Katseres 2014). The clinical aromatherapy nurse lead is Julie Katseres who completed her CCAP training in 2011.

Planetree Organization

Griffin Hospital is a 160-bed acute care community hospital serving more than 100,000 residents of the Lower Naugatuck Valley Region (http://www.griffinhealth.org). Griffin Hospital is the flagship for the Planetree organization—arguably where patient-centered care began 36 years ago—and is affiliated to Yale School of Medicine. Planetree's international membership of approved hospitals comprises more than 500 organizations from eight countries. The Planetree model is designed to ensure that patients' well-being, comfort, and dignity are central to patient care. Planetree offers a viable and effective option because it helps hospitals to balance this sharpened focus on the patient experience within the context of day-to-day demands including budget concerns, regulatory pressures, staffing shortages, and growing consumer and media interest in hospital performance outcomes (http://www.planetree.org).

Aromatherapy was introduced at Griffin Hospital in the early 2000s (Stumpo 2014) and is currently used as part of integrative care throughout the hospital (med/surgical, critical care, inpatient psychiatry, same-day surgery, gastrointestinal [GI] department, and childbirth center). All new staff attend a 2-day/overnight retreat where they are introduced to the Planetree philosophy and integrative therapies including aromatherapy. Each hospital department has a basket containing four single essential oils: lavender *(Lavandula angustifolia)*, bergamot *(Citrus bergamia)*, mandarin *(Citrus reticulata)*, and peppermint *(Mentha piperita)* (Carino 2014). Essential oils are used via inhalation only: either one or two drops on cotton balls, on a tissue, or used in a personal inhaler (aromastick). There is no extra charge to the patient for any integrative therapy. Essential oils are purchased from a variety of essential oil companies known to the clinical aromatherapy nurse lead, Eileen Carino. Essential oils are used daily in the psych department to help detoxification.

Eileen completed her CCAP training in 2003 and her research project focused on aiding detoxification in a psych unit using inhaled bergamot.

It is amazing what one person can achieve. Kathy Duffy, LPN, MH, CCAP, is an RJBA aromatherapy instructor who needs special mention, because single-handedly she has managed to integrate clinical aromatherapy into 14 hospitals throughout the United States! Since I relocated back to the UK in 2005, Kathy has taken on the mantle of travelling most weekends to spread the word. She is a great instructor, her evaluations are excellent, and her student research projects have opened the doors to integration in a big way. The courses in Valley Hospital, Stamford and Boston Medical Center have been running every year for 10, 8, and 4 years, respectively. All the hospitals are still using clinical aromatherapy. Thank you, Kathy!

UNITED KINGDOM
Manchester
Clinical aromatherapy is part of an integrative approach at The Christie Hospital, the largest cancer hospital in Europe. The Christie registers around 12,500 new patients and treats about 40,000 patients every year. It is the lead cancer center for the Greater Manchester and Cheshire Cancer Network, covering a population of 3.2 million, and runs clinics at 16 other general hospitals (http://www.christie.nhs.uk). The Christie is a National Health Service (NHS) Foundation Trust hospital. Aromatherapy is offered for symptom control of nausea, depression, and insomnia as well as for infection control (Stringer 2014). The Christie was one of the first hospitals to publish its use of aromastix (Stringer & Donald 2011). Aromatherapy is also used in massage, gargles, mouthwashes, and to enable wounds to heal (Stringer et al 2008). Specific blends are used in aromastix and mixtures of essential oils (rather than single essential oils) are used for massage in the units and for clinical work (Stringer 2014). There are currently two nurse/aromatherapists on staff and three other aromatherapists are brought in from outside. Jacqui Stringer PhD, RGN is the clinical nurse aromatherapy lead.

London
The Royal Marsden Hospital
The Royal Marsden Hospital, London, is an NHS Hospital Trust and was the first hospital in the world to be dedicated solely to cancer care (http://www.nhs.uk). It has been integrating aromatherapy throughout the hospital for over 20 years (Lewis 2014). Aromatherapy treatments generally involve massage; however, personal inhalers (aromastix) are also used and the hospital has, to date, conducted and published three service evaluations (audits) of aromastix use. The Royal Marsden has two hospital sites (Sutton and Chelsea). Aromatherapists are brought in from outside and are salaried (Lewis 2014). Rhi Lewis (previously Rhi Harris) is a British trained nurse and editor of the *International Journal of Clinical Aromatherapy*. She has led the advanced clinical aromatherapy training at the Royal Marsden for the past 11 years. She also teaches therapists outside the hospital who are working in cancer and/or palliative care.

University College Hospital

University College Hospital (UCH) (NHS Hospital Trust) has used aromatherapy for over 15 years. Aromatherapists are part of the Support and Information Team based in the Macmillan UCH Cancer Center (UCLH 2014). Aromatherapy is given via massages. Aromastix, room diffusers, aromastones, and aromastreams are also used in therapy rooms and on the inpatient wards (Charlesworth 2014). Between 2012 and 2013, 500 aromastix were given to patients and 1200 aromatherapy massages were given to cancer patients and their relatives (Charlesworth 2014). Treatments are given in the outpatient department, but also to inpatients. Essential oils are used as preprepared mixtures in aromastones on the wards via the nursing staff, and are also given to patients with general advice. There is a hospital policy that covers all complementary therapists. Essential oils are given to reduce the side effects of radiotherapy and chemotherapy and are mixed to suit individual patient needs. Elaine Charlesworth is the senior complementary therapist for UCH Macmillan Cancer Center. Although the team is employed by the NHS, much of their funding is through charitable donations (UCLH 2014).

Leeds

Marianne Tavares was a nurse for 30 years in England. Between 1999 and 2009 she worked at St. Gemma's Hospice, Leeds, where she led the complementary therapy program and chaired the Association of Complementary Therapists in Hospice and Palliative Care. Before moving to Canada, Marianne wrote a guide to integrating clinical aromatherapy into a palliative care program (Tavares 2011). In it she includes aromatherapy protocols for wound care, skin care, and mouth care, based on her clinical experience.

SOUTH AFRICA

Linda-Anne O'Flaherty began working as an aromatherapist volunteer at Red Cross Memorial Children's Hospital in Cape Town, South Africa, 10 years ago. Currently, there are eight volunteer aromatherapists working in the hospital and Linda-Anne is part of the pain team. The wards covered are Oncology, Trauma, Medical, Burns, ICU, Surgical, Renal/Transplant, and Cardiac/Tracheostomy (O'Flaherty 2014). Volunteers visit once a week. Initially the response from the medical staff was quite patronizing. However, the majority of the medical staff have now witnessed the effects of the treatments and are very supportive and positive. Currently, the aromatherapist volunteers receive requests and referrals from doctors, nurses, physical therapists, occupational therapists, and social workers. Aromatherapy is mainly administered by the 'M' Technique or massage (O'Flaherty 2014). Linda-Anne completed her 'M' Technique practitioner training in 2008 and instructor training in 2009.

SUMMARY

Although the above examples are encouraging, clinical aromatherapy still has some way to go before it is accepted in every medical establishment. One of the major studies carried out on integrative medicine in the United States was sponsored by The

Bravewell Collaboration. However, this study did not include aromatherapy (Horrigan et al 2012). When asked why not, the primary investigator replied "not enough centers were using it as an intervention in a clinical protocol" (Horrigan 2014). This was surprising because out of the 29 integrative medicine centers interviewed for the study, several were known to be using aromatherapy. This could be because aromatherapy is often used as part of holistic nursing. For example, Kligler et al (2011) examined the cost-effectiveness of integrative medicine using a program called Urban Zen in the oncology department at Beth Israel. Urban Zen uses a combination of "yoga therapy, holistic nursing techniques, and a healing environment." On further inspection, the holistic nursing techniques used included aromatherapy. Specifically, essential oils such as lavender and ylang ylang were incorporated into treatment to address common inpatient complaints including insomnia and anxiety. So sometimes it looks as if aromatherapy is not being used, when in fact it is.

Aromatherapy is recognized as part of holistic nursing by the American Holistic Nurses Association (AHNA) and by most State Boards of Nursing in the United States. Complementary therapies (including aromatherapy) are "a necessary curriculum content of baccalaureate nursing education" (AACN 2008; Santangelo 2013)— although students are not required to be trained in complementary therapies. One of the most interesting parts of the study by Horrigan et al (2012) was Appendix 7 (p 88-91). This section asked what were the factors driving the success of integration. Each facility gave its own reply. Many cited the importance of strong leadership, a sincere belief in integration, good practitioner skills, and patient satisfaction.

EXAMPLES OF HOW AROMATHERAPY CAN BE USED IN HOSPITALS

There are many ways to use essential oils in hospitals. They range from the simple mood-enhancing effects of smelling something pleasant (Dobetsberger & Buchbauer 2011) to the use of an essential oil to reduce anxiety (van der Watt & Janca 2008). Essential oils with antimicrobial properties can reduce infections (Garozzo et al 2009; Tohidpour et al 2010; Warnke et al 2013). Essential oils can also reduce postoperative nausea (Hunt et al 2013) and perception of pain (Kim et al 2006). Aromatherapy can be cost-saving—reducing the need for antiemetic, anxiolytic, and hypnotic medications (Kligler et al 2011).

Dobetsberger & Buchbauer (2011) reviewed the action of essential oils on the central nervous system (CNS) and demonstrated that some inhaled essential oils can affect mood. A lot of hospitals or long-term care facilities do not smell nice. Yet, how we feel affects how we are, and how we heal (Littrell 2008). If it is possible to positively alter the environment to promote healing and improve overall well-being through the use of essential oils, this is a goal worth pursuing.

Patients undergoing radiotherapy or computer-assisted tomography scans are isolated in a room during treatment and have to lie absolutely still for lengthy periods of time. Many find this experience stressful. Wearing an aromapatch, an aromapacket or an aromastix with a soothing mix of essential oils may help

(Stringer & Donald 2011). These are inexpensive to purchase and can be filled with a customized mixture.

Residential care homes often have unpleasant smells: a mixture of incontinent patients, hospital food, and lavatory cleaner. This was obvious when I recently visited a friend with Parkinson's disease. The home was lovely, the care was great, but the smell was not.

Sixty percent of patients in ICUs gain a hospital-acquired infection (HAI) and this is a strong predictor for mortality (Vincent et al 2009; Kaye et al 2010). Many essential oils have antibacterial (Roller et al 2009; Tohidpour et al 2010; Warnke et al 2013) and antiviral properties (Loizzo et al 2008; Garozzo et al 2009). Using essential oils that are effective against HAIs such as MRSA (Warnke 2013) or *Acinetobacter baumannii* (Duarte et al 2012) can reduce additional hospital inpatient days and associated costs. Essential oils can reduce the work-induced stress of hospital staff (Pemberton & Turpin 2008). Aromatherapy can also help visitors cope with the trauma and emotion of visiting their hospitalized loved one. Learning how to give their loved one a 5-minute hand 'M' Technique with relaxing essential oils has been demonstrated to empower visitors and soothe, their loved ones (Pritchard 2012). Happier patients and visitors can reduce the stress of nursing and medical staff.

HOW TO BEGIN INTEGRATION

Integration takes time. Be realistic. People are busy. Many people still think aromatherapy is massage with a nice smell. Target one department—it is probably the one where you work or feel most comfortable. It is a good idea to target one symptom that could be problematic/costly/time consuming. Nausea? Insomnia? Infection? Make a short (10 minutes) factual presentation to key personnel such as the unit manager and the staff who would be administering essential oils. Conduct a review of the literature and have relevant references and research citations on hand. As you move further into this process, consider developing a feasibility study with cost analysis. Your aim is to show that aromatherapy is a viable, cost-effective, safe, and simple therapy for symptom management with both qualitative and quantitative benefits. Once approval has been received to either pilot or institute aromatherapy, all potential stakeholders should be engaged in the process (Box 5-5), and a policy or protocol will need to be developed. In a nutshell, this means answering several questions such as who is permitted to administer aromatherapy treatments, what is the training and education required, what safety requirements are needed for storage and administration of aromatherapy, and so on (Box 5-6).

CONDUCTING A PILOT STUDY

When an integrative modality such as aromatherapy is new to a facility, it may be helpful to start any program of research with a small pilot study (N = 10) targeting one symptom. The study should include a specific measurable outcome using

BOX 5-5 *Suggested Order of Integration*

Select Target Department
    Eg: Critical care, dermatology, care of elderly, hospice, labor and delivery, long-term care, mental health, oncology, palliative, pediatrics, recovery room, well-being, women's health, etc.
    Things to Consider
    Administrative Support
    In small facilities, the support of one key administrator may be enough. Often the nursing executive can champion the cause. Other times you will also need the support of the chief executive officer (CEO). Make sure you know where the 'permission' resides in your facility before you proceed. Ask yourself, who is the gate-keeper?
    General Support
    In larger facilities, try to cultivate support from a major department, for example, nursing, physical therapy, social work, or pharmacy. The majority of staff will be supportive, interested, or neutral. If someone expresses overt negativity, try gently educating that person.
    Physician Support
    Physicians are important to the acceptance of clinical aromatherapy into the facility. Try to get support from at least one physician. It takes time to develop trust and it is important to be able to present credible research. Hopefully, some of the references in this book will help.
    Therapeutics Committee
    Most healthcare facilities have a therapeutics committee or a mechanism for approving new modalities to be used by staff. (Even the lotion provided at the bedside will need to be approved.) Start with a few, well-chosen essential oils.
    Policy and Procedure
    A policy states *who* and *how*. It is important that staff know who is allowed to use essential oils and how they are to be used. Make sure you follow the requirements for new policy development.
    Training of Staff
    Facilities that support the integration of clinical aromatherapy will need to be reassured on the quality and relevance of training. Generally, we have found that the 10.5-hour Clinical Aromatherapy for Hospitals (CAH) classroom-taught course is enough to begin with. This enables staff to use six essential oils safely. Several staff can then take the Certified Clinical Aromatherapy Practitioner (CCAP) course (250 hours) that enables them to mentor and lead the therapeutic use of essential oils throughout the facility.
    Creation of a Policy
    Buy in from all areas (representatives who support aromatherapy). Medical therapeutics should be involved in policy creation. MSDS (Material Safety Data Sheets) must be available for use of any substance in a healthcare facility.

BOX 5-6 *Sample Hospital Clinical Aromatherapy Policy*

Purpose
To outline the management of patients receiving aromatherapy treatment.

Scope
This guideline applies to hospital inpatient and outpatient services.

Goals
To promote physical, emotional, or spiritual well-being.
To promote relaxation and reduction of stress.

Guideline
Certified Clinical Aromatherapy Practitioners (CCAPs) will supervise the use of essential oils for therapeutic purposes at the hospital.

Definitions
Clinical aromatherapy is the controlled use of essential oils to enhance health and well-being by alleviating specific symptoms or reaching specified outcome targets.

Topical application refers to the 'M' Technique a compress with water, carrier oil, or gel (spore- and bacteria-free) directly over the affected area, or a bath (hand, foot, sitz, or full).

Direct inhalation is targeted to a single individual. Examples include:
- Applying 2-5 drops of essential oil to a tissue and breathing normally for up to 15 minutes.
- Applying 2-5 drops of essential oil on a cotton ball/tissue placed under the pillow case.
- Using 6-12 drops of essential oil in an aromastix as required.
- Using ready-made aromapatches or adding 2-3 drops of essential oil to an aromapatch.
- Using 2-4 drops of essential oil in an electrically operated aromastone.
- Using proprietary aromapatches or aromapackets.

Indirect inhalation may affect multiple individuals. Examples include:
- Using an electric nebulizer or battery-operated diffuser to diffuse fine particles of essential oil within a room.
- Applying 2-5 drops of essential oil to a cotton ball or paper towel and placing it on a surface in a patient room where diffuse particles of essential oil can be inhaled by anyone in the room.

Carrier oil is a fixed oil used to "carry" or act as a vehicle for administering essential oils to the body. Carrier oils have specific properties. The most frequently used is sweet almond oil. Culinary oils are not suitable.

Patch testing is the process used to determine if a person reacts negatively to an essential oil before topical applications (see Section 6.3.3).

Procedure
Assess Patient
History:
- Allergies
- Skin integrity, sensitivities
- Aroma likes/dislikes

Continued

BOX 5-6 *Sample Hospital Clinical Aromatherapy Policy—cont'd*

- Chronic diseases: seizure disorder, hypertension
- Estrogen-dependent tumors

Physical Assessment:
Include pregnancy and vital signs

Current Problem:
What symptom needs to be addressed:
- Patient evaluation of intensity 0-10 scale
- Degree of impact on life/activities/recovery

Discuss Treatment
- Possible choice of oils, if applicable
- Method
- Safety measures for all essential oils

Patient Agreement
- Oil selection
- Verbal consent
- Patch Testing, if indicated, for any topical use:
  - Two drops of mixture at **double** the concentration to be used are put on an adhesive bandage, attached to the patients' upper arm, and left for 15 minutes. (Assess first for allergy to adhesives: if allergic to adhesive, use cotton ball with paper or nonadhesive tape.) This is particularly important if the essential oil contains high amounts of phenols or oxides.

Perform Treatment
Evaluate
- Immediate effect
- Follow-up effect

Document
- Assessment
- Essential oil(s) used
- Method of use
- Outcome or effect

Safety Considerations
Practitioner related, when applicable:
- Maintain good ventilation in treatment area
- Open door to ventilate room after treatment
- Allow a minimum of 5 minutes breathing "fresh air" between treatments
- Wash hands before and after applying essential oils

Patient related. Examples of situational responses:
- Essential oil in the eye:
  - Irrigate the eye with milk, or carrier oil, then with water
  - Keep the bottle to show which essential oil was being used
  - Notify physician, if patient involved
  - Report to employee health, if staff involved

BOX 5-6 *Sample Hospital Clinical Aromatherapy Policy—cont'd*

- Undiluted essential oil (high phenol variety) on the skin, skin burned:
  - Dilute with carrier oil
  - Wash with nonperfumed soap and water and dry
  - Notify physician, if patient involved
  - Report to employee health, if staff involved
- 5 mL (or more) essential oil taken orally:
  - Give milk to drink
  - Keep the bottle to show which essential oil was being used
  - Essential oils when taken in amounts greater than 5 mL by mouth should be treated as poisons

Notify physician, if patient involved
Report to employee health, if staff involved
- Broken bottle with essential oil and glass on floor:
  - Use paper towels to soak up oil and collect glass
  - Put mixture in paper and dispose in double-sealed plastic bag

General Safety with Essential Oils
- MSDS (Material Safety Data Sheets) will be available in areas where essential oils are used

Storage
- Out of reach of children
- Cool area
- In tightly closed containers
- Away from foods or drink

Labeling
- All bottles containing essential oils should be clearly marked with indelible labels that include the following:
  - Full botanical names
  - Relevant safety information
  - Quantity of oil(s)
  - Expiration date

Packaging
All pure essential oils should be packaged in colored glass bottles that may include an integral dropper of standard (20 drops per mL) size

Procedures
- Whenever possible, essential oils should be used in enclosed areas to prevent the aromas from spreading
- All essential oils used should be documented in the patient record
- The positive and negative effects (outcomes) of essential oils should be evaluated and documented
- Use topically in 1% to 5% dilution, except in specific situations as recommended by safety guidelines
- Mixtures of essential oils plus carrier oil for single patient use may be stored in a plastic bottle for up to 2 weeks (see Labeling 7.3.3)

Continued

BOX 5-6 *Sample Hospital Clinical Aromatherapy Policy—cont'd*

Clothing
- No special clothing is required, but some essential oils such as German chamomile and mandarin may leave a stain

Disposal
- They should be disposed of in a sealed plastic bag

Contraindications
Use with caution in pregnancy, epilepsy, hypertension, estrogen-dependent tumors, and patients with sensitivities and allergies

---

a published tool, for example, the visual analog scale (VAS) or numerical scale (0-10). If possible, seek help from an experienced research scientist to consult with you on the design of the study and the study proposal. There are also some excellent easy-to-read research books that can be very useful. A proposal of this type must go to the Institutional Review Board or the Ethics Committee for approval before you can begin the study. Although embarking on a new research study may create a little anxiety, particularly to the novice researcher, keep in mind that a pilot study need not be complicated to provide findings that are very useful in the clinical setting. When the study has been completed, it is important to disseminate the findings internally to key stakeholders within the organization, and externally so that all clinicians have access to what was learned from the study.

Take one step at a time. One small step for integrative medicine, one huge leap for clinical aromatherapy! If RJBA students have been able to do this, then you can too.

REFERENCES

American Association of Colleges of Nursing (AACN). 2008. The essentials of baccalaureate education for professional nursing practice. http://www.aacn.nche.edu/education-resources/baccessentials08.pdf. Accessed February 22, 2014.

Aurora Healthcare. 2014. http://www.aurorahealthcare.org/services/integrative-medicine/patient-services/aromatherapy. Accessed March 4, 2014.

Atsumi K. 2012. Integrative Medicine in the 21st Century. Conference Proceedings from the 1st International Congress of Aromatherapy, Kyoto, Japan. Japanese Society of Aromatherapy. p 71.

Ballard M. 2004. Topical use of 5% black pepper prior to phlebotomy. Unpublished RJBA dissertation.

Boon H, Verhoef M, O'Hara D, Findlay B. 2004. From parallel practice to integrative healthcare: a conceptual framework. *BMC Health Services Res.* 4(1):15.

Bravewell Collaborative Best Practice Report. 2007. Integrative Medicine best practices.

Carino E. 2014. Personal communication.

Carter S. 2005. Topical use of 10% black pepper prior to phlebotomy. Unpublished RJBA dissertation.

Charlesworth E. 2014. Personal communication.

Center Institute for Research & Education in Integrative Medicine (CIRE-IM). 2014. http://healthandhealingny.org/Institute/educational-programs/nursing-research-and-education.aspx Accessed February 21, 2014

Conway N. 2014. Personal communication.

Dibartolo J. 2014. Personal communication.

Dobetsberger C, Buchbauer G. 2011. Actions of essential oils on the central nervous system: an updated review. *Flavour Fragr.* 26(5):300–316.

Duarte M, Ferriera S, Silva F, Dominigues F. 2012. Synergistic effect of coriander oil and conventional antibiotics against *Acinetobacter baumannii*. *Phytomedicine.* 19(3):236–238.

Garozzo A, Timpanaro R, Bisignano B, Furneri P, Bisignano G et al. 2009. In vitro antiviral activity of *Melaleuca alternifolia* essential oil. *Lett Appl Microbiol.* 49(6):806–808.

Gershan L. 2014. Personal communication.

Horrigan B, Lewis S, Abrams D, Pechura C. 2012. Integrative medicine in America – how integrative medicine is being practiced in clinical centers across the USA. *Global Adv Health Med.* 1(3):16–67.

Horrigan B. 2014. Personal communication.

Hunt R, Dienemann J, Norton H, Hartley W, Hudgens H et al. 2013. Aromatherapy as treatment for postoperative nausea: a randomized trial. *Anesth Analg.* 117(3):597–604.

Hunt R. 2014. Personal communication.

Imanishi J, Kishia S. 2012. Usefulness of integrative medicine including aromatherapy in cancer care. Conference Proceedings from the 1st International Congress of Aromatherapy, Kyoto, Japan. Japanese Society of Aromatherapy. p 62.

Jonas W. 2013. The Summit on Integrative Medicine and the Health of the Public. http://www.bravewell.org/integrative_medicine/national_summit/. Accessed February 17, 2014.

Katseres K. 2014. Personal communication.

Kaye K, Marchaim D, Smialowicz C, Bentley L. 2010. Suction regulators: a potential vector for hospital acquired pathogens. *Infect Control Hosp Epidemiol.* 31(7):772–4.

Kim J, Wajda M, Cuff G, Serota D, Schlame M et al. 2006. Evaluation of aromatherapy in treating postoperative pain: a pilot study. *Pain Pract.* 6(4):273–277.

Kinney M-E. 2012. Clinical Aromatherapy and Inpatient Oncology: Insights on Integrative Health in a large United States Health Care System. Conference Proceedings from the 1st International Congress of Aromatherapy, Kyoto, Japan. Japanese Society of Aromatherapy. P 59.

Kinney M-E. 2014. Personal communication.

Kligler B, Homel P, Harrison L, Levenson H, Kenney J, Merrell W. 2011. Cost savings in inpatient oncology through an integrative medicine approach. *Am J Managed Care.* 16(12):779–84.

Kreitzer M-J. 2013. Nursing at the forefront of integrative health care. *AHNA Beginnings.* 33(4):8–10.

Kristiniak S, Harpel J, Breckenridge D, Buckle J. 2012. Black pepper essential oil to enhance intravenous catheter insertion in patients with poor vein visibility. A controlled study. *J Alt Cam Medicine.* 18(11):1003–7.

Lee R. 2014. Personal communication.

Lewis R. 2014. Personal communication.

Littrell J. 2008. The body-mind connection: not just a theory anymore. *Soc Works Health Care.* 46(4):17–37.

Loizzo M, Saab A, Tundis R. 2008. Phytochemical analysis and in vitro antiviral activities of the essential oils of seven Lebanon species. *Chem Biodivers.* 5:461–70.

Mariano C. 2013. Current trends and issues in holistic nursing. In *Holistic Nursing: A Handbook for Practice.* 6th Edition. Jones & Bartlett. Burlington, Massachusetts. USA. pp 85–106.

Massachusetts State Board of Nursing. *Holistic Nursing and Complementary/Alternative Modalities Advisory Ruling 9801* (updated 2012). http://www.mass.gov/eohhs/gov/departments/dph/programs/hcq/dhpl/nursing/nursing-practice/advisory-rulings/holistic-nursing-and-complementary-therapies.html. Accessed February 17, 2014.

Ocampo A. 2014. Personal communication.

O'Flaherty L-A. 2014. Personal communication.

Osteyee J. 2014. Personal communication.

Pemberton E, Turpin P. 2008. The effect of essential oils on work-related stress in intensive care nurses. *Holistic Nurse Practice.* 22(2):97–102.

Price S, Price L. 2011. *Aromatherapy for Health Professionals,* 4th Edition, Churchill Livingstone, Edinburgh, Scotland.

Pritchard C. 2012. Aromatherapy intervention to reduce the anxiety and depression levels of family members and friends of patients with traumatic injury. Unpublished RJBA dissertation.

Roller S, Ernest N, Buckle J. 2009. The antimicrobial activity of nigh-necrodane and other lavender oils on methicillin-sensitive and resistant *Staphylococcus aureus* (MSSRA and MRSA). *J Altern Comp Med.* 15(3):275–9.

Samueli Institute (2013). Podcast. Integrative Healthcare and Medicine. http://www.rand.org/multimedia/audio/2012/07/18/integrative-health-care-medicine.html. Accessed February 3, 2014.

Santangelo L. 2013. Bridging the gap: an overview of CAM education in Nursing. *Beginnings.* American Holistic Nurses Association. 33(2):18–21.

Scheidel C. 2014. Personal communication.

Story L. 2005. Topical use of 20% black pepper prior to phlebotomy. Unpublished RJBA dissertation.

Stringer J, Swindell R, Dennis M. 2008. Massage in patients undergoing intensive chemotherapy reduces serum cortisol and prolactin. *Psychooncology.* 7(10):1024–31.

Stringer J, Donald G. 2011. Aromastix in cancer care: an innovation not to be sniffed at. *Comp Ther Clin Practice.* 17(2):116–21.

Stringer J. 2014. Personal communication.

Stumpo B. 2014. President Patient Care Services at Griffin Hospital. Personal communication

Snyderman R. 2009. The Summit on Integrative Medicine and the Health of the Public. http://www.bravewell.org/integrative_medicine/national_summit/. Accessed February 17, 2014.

Tavares M. 2011. Integrating Clinical Aromatherapy in Specialist Palliative Care. The use of essential oil for symptom management. Available at: www.clinicalaromapac.ca.

Tohidpour A, Sattari M, Omidbaigi R, Yadegar A, Nazemi J. 2010. Antibacterial effect of essential oils from two medicinal plants against methicillin-resistant Staphylococcus aureus (MRSA). *Phytomedicine.* 17(2):142–5.

UCLH. University College London Hospital. 2014. http://www.uclh.org/OurServices/ServiceA-Z/Cancer/CSS/CCT/Pages/Home.aspx. Accessed March 2, 2014.

van der Watt G, Janca A. 2008. Aromatherapy in nursing and mental health care. *Contemporary Nurse.* 30(1):69–75.

Vincent J, Rello J, Marchall J, Silva E, Anzueto A et al. 2009. International study of the prevalence and outcomes of infection in intensive care units. *JAMA.* 302(21):2323–9.

Walach H. 2009. The campaign against CAM - a reason to be proud. *J Holistic Med.* 6(1):8–13.

Warnke P, Lott A, Sherry E, Podschun R. 2013. The ongoing battle against multi-resistant strains: in vitro inhibition of hospital-acquired MRSA, VRE, *Pseudomonas*, ESBL *E coli* and *Klebsiella* species in the presence of plant derived antiseptic oils. *J Cranio-Maxillofacial Surg.* 41(4):321–6.

Chapter 6

The 'M' Technique®

"And I realized that all the world wants to be held in spite of it all."

Jack Kornfield

After the Ecstasy, the Laundry

CHAPTER ASSETS

WHAT IS IT?

The 'M' Technique® is a registered method of gentle, structured touch suitable for the very fragile, actively dying, or stressed individual. It is also useful for those who would like to soothe someone with gentle touch, but are not trained in massage. Anyone can learn the 'M' Technique—it is suitable for caregivers, family members, volunteers, patient ambassadors and friends, as well as nurses and other health professionals.

WHY IS IT RELEVANT TO A BOOK ON CLINICAL AROMATHERAPY?

The combination of essential oils with touch is a powerful mix to relieve stress and anxiety. However, touch is rarely included in nursing, medical, or other health trainings, so many health professionals do not know how to touch their patients and do not have the time, money, or inclination to take a massage therapy training course. Massage training in the United States takes 500 to 1000 hours; in the UK, Australia, Canada, and many other countries it takes 60 to 100 hours.

Because the 'M' Technique is simple, it can be learned quickly (4 hours for a hand and foot course, 2 days for a full body course). Because the 'M' Technique is gentle, it can be used when conventional massage would be inappropriate, i.e., for those at the end of life (Roberts & Campbell 2011), sick children in hospital (Daniels & O'Flaherty 2010), or premature babies (Smith et al 2012).

Because the 'M' Technique is repetitive, it can be helpful to soothe children with special needs (Breen Rickerby & Cordell 2012) or patients with dementia (Tappin 2010). The repetitive strokes have been called "physical hypnotherapy (Buckle 2002)." Brain imaging research found the effect of the 'M' Technique on the brain was different to that of conventional massage (Buckle et al 2008) and was more akin to meditation. Also, the 'M' Technique appeared to have a cumulative effect, possibly because the patient quickly recognized the repetitive strokes and began to relax deeply, knowing what was coming next (Hunter 2012; Clayton 2014).

Because the 'M' Technique is structured and never changes, it is useful for research (Quate 2002; Richardson 2008; de Jong et al 2011). The possible variables of pressure, number of strokes, and sequence of strokes are fixed and repetitive. Everyone receives the same 'M' Technique whether they are young or old, sick or healthy, regardless of their size. It is like learning the steps of a dance; the steps remain the same.

The 'M' Technique is also a useful tool for caregivers. Amanda Richardson, a community nurse for 22 years, did her BSc (Honors) in Complementary Therapies at the University of Wales. Her dissertation explored the effectiveness of the 'M' Technique to reduce stress and improve the physical and psychological well-being of nonprofessional caregivers of clients with dementia. Measurements were objective (pulse and blood pressure) as well as self-recorded: stress using VAS (0-10) and perceived well-being using Measure Your Medical Outcome Profile (MYMOP). Results across all measurements found that the 'M' Technique reduced caregiver stress and improved their physical and psychological well-being (Richardson 2009). Amanda won first prize for her dissertation from Elsevier.

WHAT IS THE RELEVANCE OF THE 'M' TECHNIQUE IN HEALTHCARE?

Hippocrates described the importance of touch in the 5th century BC and declared it his favorite of all health essentials. Touch is as an integral part of health and social care (Chang 2001; Rombalski 2003; Rousseau & Blackburn 2008; Roberts & Campbell 2011; Breen Rickerby & Cordell 2012). However, touch is not taught as part of nursing or medical care.

WHERE DID THE 'M' TECHNIQUE COME FROM?

After I had completed my nursing training, I specialized in critical care. Many of my patients could hear me, but they could not communicate with me because they were intubated. I found myself patting them gently to try and reassure them and gradually realized what I really wanted was a non-verbal method of communication. Touch seemed the answer. I wanted to be sure what I was doing was right, so I completed a massage training course. This gave me confidence to touch, but much of what I learned was completely inappropriate for such fragile patients. So I started to devise my own method of gentle, structured touch. It was easy to see what worked and what did not by watching the monitors. Over the years, distinctive patterns emerged that differentiated it from massage: the pressure was much lighter, the strokes were repeated a set number of times, and the sequence never altered. This combination seemed to really relax my patients. I named it the 'M' Technique—the 'M' stands for manual, although over the years, people have also called it *Magic* and *Mesmerizing*. I moved to the United States in 1994. The 'M' Technique® was registered with the United States Patent and Trademark Office (Registration No. 2,203,159) in 1998 and is protected. Copyright laws apply.

WHERE IS THE RESEARCH?

The first informal piece of research was carried out in 1996 at Columbia Presbyterian Medical Center, New York (sponsored by Dr. Oz). The 'M' Technique was applied to the legs of volunteer medical students who were connected to an eight-lead electrocardiogram (ECG) monitor to measure the parasympathetic response. The ECG showed a positive parasympathetic response within 5 minutes. Several pilot studies on end-of-life agitation were subsequently carried out using the 'M' Technique: at Scranton Hospice, Pennsylvania (Katz 1999); Beth Israel Hospice, New York (Ocampo 2001); and Harris Methodist hospice unit, Fort Worth, Texas (O'Keefe 2001; Anderson 2004). In each case, the 'M' Technique reduced terminal agitation.

Hundreds of case studies and case series followed. Here is just a small selection. Lori Mitchell, a critical care nurse in Kalispell Hospital, Kalispell, Montana, found that the hand 'M' Technique calmed patients in intensive care before extubation (1999). Aileen Nathan, a midwife on Long Island, used the hand 'M' Technique to help a patient with pregnancy-induced hypertension to relax and it reduced her blood pressure (2000). Dawn Marino, another midwife, used the foot 'M' technique to help her laboring mothers (2004). In 2004, a small randomized, controlled pilot study (n = 10) was carried out in the pediatric unit at Harris Methodist Medical Center, Fort Worth, TX. The 'M' Technique appeared to reduce perception of pain in infants following circumcision (Raquepo 2004). Measuring tools were a cardiorespiratory monitor, a blood pressure monitor, an O_2 saturation monitor, and the Neonatal Infant Pain Scale (NIPS). The 'M' Technique was performed 2 hours after circumcision using Eucerin cream. The babies receiving the 'M' Technique appeared to be in less pain and had increased O_2 saturation (three babies had a 5% increase in O_2, two babies had a 20-50% decrease on the NIPS). All babies in the control group had increased heart rate and their pain scale increased. The pilot study was followed from 2006 to 2008 with a larger randomized, controlled trial that replicated the original findings. Sadly, the PI never found the time to publish the results.

The year 2005 brought an amazing opportunity and, with it, a breakthrough. I was awarded a government-funded scholarship to attend a full-time, 2-year post-doctoral Master of Science (MSc) training in Epidemiology and Biostatistics within the School of Medicine at the University of Pennsylvania. As part of my MSc,

I was able to conduct research that would otherwise have been beyond my reach. With help from a government grant, and partially funded by the American Massage Foundation, we carried out a case series and longitudinal study, comparing the 'M' Technique to conventional Swedish massage using brain imaging. We used single photon emission computed tomography (SPECT). A radiopharmaceutical was injected intravenously into subjects before and after SPECT and the scans compared across 65 areas of the brain.

The results were very interesting. Compared with conventional massage, the effect of the 'M' Technique lit up different areas of the brain and the effect appeared to be more profound. We repeated the study after 10 weeks of once-weekly massage or 10 weeks of once-weekly 'M' Technique. The results were similar, and this time there was a bonus. The effects of the "Technique appeared to be cumulative—much more than conventional massage. Also, the 'M' Technique participant stated that "'time disappeared' as she 'drifted in and out of wakefullness.'" The participant who received conventional Swedish massage did not experience the same feeling. This appeared to give credence to what so many people had said over the years—that the 'M' Technique was different to massage and its effects were different. The research findings were presented at the American Massage Therapy conference in Cincinnati, Ohio, USA, in September 2007 and later published in the *Journal of Alternative and Complementary Medicine* (Buckle et al 2008).

WHERE IS IT USED?

In 2014, the use of the 'M' Technique is documented in the UK, United States, The Netherlands, South Africa, Japan, and Australia.

UNITED KINGDOM

Hospitals and Hospices

The 'M' Technique is used in over 40 hospices in the UK (Table 6-1) and it is beginning to be integrated into the National Health System (NHS), beginning with University Hospitals Coventry and Warwickshire of the NHS Trust. This is one of the largest acute teaching hospitals in the UK, with 1250 beds and 27 operating rooms. The special Hospital (hand and foot) 'M' Technique course has been taught to several groups of staff and a special 'M' Technique trainer course will allow hospital trainers to teach the 'M' Technique to staff throughout the entire hospital. It is hoped that other hospitals will follow. See Table 6-2 for some hospitals that use the 'M' Technique. In 2014, just over 600 people had taken the 'M' Technique practitioner course in the UK. Many others have taken the 4-hour course for use in hospices, hospitals, long-term care facilities, and special needs schools. There are 10 UK-based instructors.

SPECIAL NEEDS

The 'M' Technique is useful for patients with special needs as the repetitive nature of the technique is very soothing. Breen Rickerby and Cordell (2012) wrote about

TABLE 6-1   *A Selection of UK Hospices using the 'M' Technique (in Alphabetical Order)*

Hospice	Town	County
Acorns Children's Hospice	Birmingham	West Midlands
Bury St. Edmunds Hospice	Bury St. Edmunds	Suffolk
Deans Forest Hospice	Coleford	Gloucestershire
Dorothy Hospice	Bradford Upon Avon	Wiltshire
Eden Vale Hospice	Carlisle	Cumbria
Farleigh Hospice	Chelmsford	Essex
John Eastwood Hospice	Sutton-in-Ashfield	Nottingham
John Taylor Hospice	Birmingham	West Midlands
Kemp Hospice	Kidderminster	Worcestershire
Leckhampton Court Hospice	Cheltenham	Gloucestershire
Mary Anne Evans Hospice	Nuneaton	Warwickshire
Myrton Hospice	Warwick	Warwickshire
Peace Hospice	North Harrow	Middlesex
Pendleside Hospice	Burnley	Lancashire
Primrose Hospice	Bromsgrove	Warwickshire
Shakespeare Hospice	Stratford Upon Avon	Warwickshire
Shalom House	St. Davids	Pembrokeshire, Wales
St. Christopher's House	Penge	London
St. Elizabeth Hospice	Ipswich	Suffolk
St. Francis Hospice	Romford	Essex
St. Francis Hospice	Dublin	Ireland*
St. Giles Hospice	Litchfield	Staffordshire
St. Giles Hospice	Sutton Coldfield	West Midlands
St. Helena's Hospice	Colchester	Essex
St. Luke's Hospice	Harrow	Middlesex
St. Michael's Hospice	Bartestree	Hereford
St. Peter's Hospice	Bristol	Avon
St. Richard's Hospice	Worcester	Worcestershire
Trinity Hospice	Clapham	London
Wakefield Hospice	York	Yorkshire

*The name of one hospice in Dublin, Ireland, is included.

using the 'M' Technique at an orphanage in Belarus. The children were severely disabled from the Chernobyl disaster and had been abandoned by their families. In one case, the sensory interpretation of touch appeared to change after a 10-year-old boy (E) with cerebral palsy received the 'M' Technique on his back every day for 1 week. Each session lasted only 8 minutes. During the first 'M' Technique session,

TABLE 6-2 *A Selection of UK Hospitals using the 'M' Technique*
             (in Alphabetical Order)

Hospital	Town	County
Addenbrooks Hospital (Wallace Cancer Care)	Cambridge	Cambridgeshire
Cheltenham General Hospital	Cheltenham	Gloucestershire
Hornsea Palliative Day Care Hospital	Hornsea	Yorkshire
University Hospitals Coventry and Warwickshire NHS Trust	Coventry	West Midlands
Whipps Cross Hospital	Leytonstone	London

E hardly stopped moving around his cot. However, after the first few strokes of the second 'M' Technique, E stopped moving around and lay quietly on his stomach until the session was completed. He appeared less agitated for the rest of the afternoon. He was more content in himself—no longer grabbing at toys and then immediately discarding them. In another case, a 12-year-old girl with cerebral palsy, microcephaly, autism, and a history of self-harming received the 'M' Technique to her feet for 4 minutes every day for 1 week. After the first session she stopped self-harming. She was unable to speak, but after the first session of the 'M' Technique, she began making sounds, and tried to interact with her caregivers for the very first time (Breen Rickerby & Cordell 2012).

Mary Bolton, a nurse, used the 'M' Technique on a 7-year-old girl (A) with severe metabolic disorder that resulted in complex seizures and severe learning disabilities. Because many of the little girl's seizures happened at night, disrupting A's sleep, both she and her parents were very tired. Mary used the 'M' Technique on A. This took some time, because A would keep wandering off to play. However, over the space of 1 hour, Mary managed to do the 'M' Technique on A's face, back, hands, and feet while A's mother and aunt watched. Mary repeated the 'M' Technique sessions on A's mother and then her aunt as they each watched, so they themselves would be able to do the 'M' Technique on A. While Mary pointed out that the 'M' Technique was not going to change A's diagnosis or prognosis, she felt it was a valuable tool that empowered A's family, calmed A so she could sleep, and thus gave the family some respite. Mary wrote: "Now, I understand why this is a *technique* rather than a *massage*" (Bolton 2014).

THE ELDERLY

Barbara Probert (2014) wrote about her work in a residential home for the elderly in Dorset. One patient was a 91-year-old lady (T) with many medical problems. She was still grieving for her husband who had died 4 years previously. Her only daughter lived abroad and she had no other living relatives. Barbara started using the 'M' Technique on her hands, feet, and on her clothed back as T leaned forward against a table with cushions to support her. Over the weeks, Barbara progressed to using the 'M' Technique on T's bare back. T said no other person had touched her except her husband. When Barbara began the 'M' Technique back sequence, T relaxed and afterward said she felt comforted. Barbara's comment was that it was a privilege to be able to give T a better quality of life. Christiane Mills (2014) wrote about 'M'ing her 93-year-old mother. Christiane is also trained in massage and wrote an interesting observation in her case study. She felt the 'M' Technique was "a more loving way of touching" than massage.

END OF LIFE

Roberts and Campbell (2011) wrote about using the 'M' Technique as therapy for patients at the end of life in St. Richard's Hospice, Worcestershire. One of the patients was a 45-year-old woman (S) with end-stage multiple sclerosis (MS). S had decided against treatment with percutaneous endoscopic gastrostomy (PEG) feeding, a urinary catheter, or intravenous antibiotics. She was receiving morphine for the pain in her legs and hyoscine for her abdominal discomfort, both via a syringe driver. Despite an additional bolus of morphine, she was groaning in pain. While the nurses prepared IV midazolam to help relax her, S received the hand 'M' Technique. By the time the midazolam was given, her pain had been reduced from 10 to 5 (scale 0-10). S drifted into a light sleep and died peacefully the following day.

CANCER CARE

Danielle Webster (2014) wrote of her work with Macmillan Cancer Complementary Therapy Services at her local hospital. Danielle was assigned to a woman (D) with bowel cancer and metastases who had previously received conventional massage. Her understanding of English was limited. She had been very anxious throughout the massage and had been unable to relax. She appeared very frail and she had extensive arthritis. Danielle did a full body 'M' Technique on D, and by the end of it D was asleep. At the second session, her daughter said that following the 'M' Technique her mother had slept very well (unusual for her), and after awakening, her mother had wanted to go out. Her mother had not had the energy or inclination to go out for some time and Danielle was delighted with the change.

THE NETHERLANDS

The 'M' Technique is used on children and infants in the intensive care unit (ICU) of the Erasmus Medical Center, Rotterdam (van Dijk 2013). The Erasmus Medical center is the largest, and one of the most authoritative, scientific university medical centers in Europe (Erasmus 2014). Marjan de Jong was the first nurse who integrated the 'M' Technique into the hospital in 2008. Since then, over 30 staff members have been trained in the 'M' Technique. Marjan also conducted research using the 'M' Technique on infants immediately following major craniofacial surgery (de Jong 2011). Although the study found that the 'M' Technique did not benefit children in this category, the author does write that the 'M' Technique was, and is, of great value for patients suffering from other conditions because it gives the opportunity to touch patients in a positive way. It can also be a comforting mechanism for patients with withdrawal symptoms (i.e., "crack babies"). By 2014,

55 people had taken the 'M' Technique practitioner training course in The Netherlands. This number does not include those who have taken the Hospital (hand and foot) course, or those using the hand 'M' Technique as part of nursing care. There are currently five instructors in The Netherlands.

JAPAN

By 2014, 60 people had taken the 'M' Technique practitioner course in Japan. Practitioner courses were held in Osaka and Kobe and several 4-hour hand and foot 'M' Technique courses have also been held. I taught the first group of courses myself; now the 'M' Technique training is being continued by the Holistic Care Professional School (HCPS) in Kobe. The 'M' Technique is used on patients in the palliative care department of Himeji Medical Center (Himeji City, Hyogo) and for elderly care in Meikai hospital (Akashi City, Hyogo) by Masumi Kanagawa (an aromatherapist). Junko Masuda uses the 'M' Technique on patients in the palliative care department of Senri Chuo hospital. Masumi says the patients like the light touch very much. Yukiko Shibata uses the 'M' Technique in the care of the elderly department at Meikai Hospital (Akashi City, Hyogo). She also uses the 'M' Technique in the palliative care department of Senri Chuo Hospital (Toyonaka City, Osaka) and Okubo Hospital (Akashi City, Hyogo). Yukiko says she uses the 'M' Technique for pain relief and relaxation in patients who have bony metastasis or systemic metastasis and for those who are very anxious. There are currently eight instructors with another instructor course planned for late 2014 to be held at HCPS in Kobe.

SOUTH AFRICA

In Cape Town, there is one instructor, Linda-Anne O'Flaherty, and by 2014, there were 18 'M' Technique practitioners in South Africa. Linda-Anne uses the 'M' Technique in the Red Cross Memorial Hospital, particularly in the burns unit (Daniels & O'Flaherty 2010). Linda-Anne works at relaxing the children before having their burn dressings removed. This is a very stressful time for the children. Linda is now part of the hospital pain team and uses the 'M' Technique wherever it is required (O'Flaherty 2014).

Carol Swanepoel wrote very movingly of her work with a 52-year-old recovering alcoholic lady who had been divorced for many years and lived alone. After starting the 12-step program, her life became a bit more manageable. However, several bouts of bronchitis made her try to give up smoking. This was unsuccessful and pushed her back into drinking. She was filled with self-loathing. A diagnosis of advanced metastatic brain cancer resulted in her being referred to palliative care. During counseling she refused all offers of comfort. However, slowly she accepted the idea that the 'M' Technique might be a treatment rather than, what she perceived was, an indulgence. Rather grudgingly she allowed Carol to use the 'M' Technique on her hands and feet. Her comment afterward was "well, that wasn't too bad!" As her cancer progressed her headaches worsened, and morphine no longer seemed to help. In desperation, she decided to accept a full body 'M' Technique treatment from Carol. Afterward, she lay very still (unusual for her) before she began crying silently. Then she asked if Carol could repeat the 'M' Technique again the next day. Carol did so and then visited her daily, doing whatever part of the 'M' Technique she preferred. The patient died 2 weeks later with Carol 'M'ing her feet. Carol wrote: "what greater gift can one receive than to be allowed into another's private world of chaos and see it transformed into the peace of acceptance that becomes holy ground?" (Swanepoel 2014).

UNITED STATES

The 'M' Technique is used in many hospitals in the United States and is accepted as part of *holistic* nursing care (American Holistic Nurses Association 2014). One of the earliest hospitals to train its nurses in the 'M' Technique was The Valley Hospital, Ridgewood, New Jersey (2001). Since then, nurses from every department have received training in the 'M' Technique. Currently, approximately 40% of nurses use the hand 'M' Technique as part of their daily nursing care (Mazzer 2014). In the Neonatal Intensive Care Unit (NICU), Baby 'M' is being studied. Initial signs are good—premature babies are responding well to this nurturing, positive touch by the nursing staff, and their parents are enjoying learning something to soothe their baby (Bischoff 2012). Peg Bischoff, who is conducting the research, presented her initial findings at the 6th Annual Meeting of the National Association of Neonatal Nurses in 2013 and won first prize for the Best Neonatal Nursing Abstract submission from Elsevier (publisher of the *Journal of Neonatal Nursing*).

Baby 'M' research is also being carried out at the Children's Hospital, St Louis, MO. Dr. Joan Smith PhD, RN presented her findings at the St. Louis Children's Hospital's 8th Annual Multidisciplinary Research/EBP Conference in 2011 and published them in 2012 (Smith et al 2012). Baby 'M' training is only available to experienced NICU personnel because it is important that the caregiver can understand premature infant cues (Smith 2014). However, certified baby 'M' practitioners can show parents of infants in the NICU how to soothe their infants.

As of 2014, there were 16 certified 'M' Technique instructors in the United States. They are located in CT, MA, MI, NJ, NY, OK, PA, SD, TX, and WA. After myself, Kathy Duffy has probably taught the most 'M' Technique courses. Because the 'M' Technique was originally part of the Certified Clinical Aromatherapy Practitioner (CCAP) course, those graduating before 2004 are 'M' Technique practitioners as well as CCAPs. 'M' Technique courses have been taught in almost every state in the United States.

THE 'M' TECHNIQUE AS PART OF NURSING CARE

Nursing practice developed from the care of people's bodies using touch (Atkinson et al 2010). Yet today nurses seem apprehensive and unwilling to touch patients. Instrumental or procedural touch is taught in nursing school as part of assessment and procedures, but expressive or comfort touch is rarely taught as part of nursing care. This is a great pity because knowing *how* to touch patients in a way that can reassure them is a very useful tool that can empower nurses and enable them to do what they became nurses to do—make people *feel* better. Not every patient wants to be touched, but a great many really appreciate the comfort of touch (O'Lynn & Krautscheid 2011). Research shows that touch can also emphasize the patient's belief in treatment (Guengen & Vion 2009).

Today, many nurses struggle with an overload of paperwork and computer work. Nurses spend as much time (if not more) watching monitor screens as they do watching patients. Compassion fatigue is a phenomenon commonly experienced by nurses (Romano et al 2013). Do nurses even have time to feel compassion? And when they do, how can nurses show compassion in an acceptable way? How can compassion be shown in a simple way that does not take too much time, but makes the nurse feel better, as well as the patient? The 'M' Technique may be the answer. The practice of touch is a tool that Dr. Jean Watson, a nursing theorist, placed within a caring–healing model (Watson 2006; Watson 2008; Watson 2009). The very act of touching can show caring (Gale & Hegerty 2000) and the very act of touching can empower the caregiver (Buckle 2013). As it is accepted as part of holistic nursing, why not use the 'M' Technique (Jackson & Latini 2013)?

I had a hip replacement a few years ago—major surgery that necessitated several days in hospital because things did not go to plan. During the first 4 days I was an inpatient, no one touched me. I felt horribly miserable and depressed—very unusual for me. On the fifth day, a young male nurse put a hand on my shoulder and asked "Are you OK?" I burst into tears with gratitude that someone cared enough to touch me. I told him, I felt so down and that was very unlike me. The nurse listened carefully. A subsequent blood test showed a previously over-looked very low hemoglobin. (After three pints of blood, I felt much more like me.) That hand-on-the-shoulder experience confirmed what I had been teaching for so many years—how comforting it is to be touched. And how it then becomes possible to say how you really feel.

When people are deprived of touch for a period of time, they suffer from *skin hunger* (Montagu 1986). I remember doing the hand 'M' Technique on an elderly gentleman in a long-term care facility many years ago. Silent tears began to pour down his face. "Am I hurting you?" I asked. He shook his head. "Shall I stop?" I inquired. He shook his head again. I finished the 5-minute hand 'M' Technique. After a few minutes, he swallowed and then said, "You are the first person to touch me since my wife died." "When did she die?" I asked. He replied, "3 years ago."

Today, healthcare is a business where every intervention has a price tag. But what about an intervention that has no price tag and yet is priceless? So let's start a revolution. Next time, you see a patient, put your hand on their arm, or their shoulder and see how they respond. Then go and learn the 'M' Technique!

Twelve years ago I wrote the following, and I still feel the same way: "The 'M' Technique is my life's work. It is what I am meant to do and what I hope to do for as long as I can." Being really present with a frightened, critically ill or dying person is at the very heart of being human. We are human beings, not human doings. But sometimes, it is hard to just "be." It can be uncomfortable "being" with someone you care about when you cannot fix the problem. The 'M' Technique is a tool that gives you something to do when nothing else can be done. It allows you to speak with your hands and "be" the best you can be under the circumstances. Mary Mazzer, a nurse at The Valley Hospital and one of the first to train in the 'M' Technique, wrote "the 'M' Technique enables you to enter a spiritual dance with the strokes as the music." It is my dream that the 'M' Technique will one day become part of standard nursing care everywhere. It is my dream that no one will die in a hospital or a hospice without being comforted by their relatives using the 'M' Technique. Being able to share the 'M' Technique has been a real privilege. Thank you for reading this chapter.

REFERENCES

American Holistic Nurses Association (AHNA). 2014. http://www.ahna.org/Home/For-Consumers/Holistic-Modalities. Accessed March 18, 2014.

Anderson C. 2004. Hand 'M' Technique at end of life. Unpublished RJBA dissertation.

Atkinson S, Macnaughton J, Saunders C. 2010. Cool intimacies of care for contemporary clinical practice. *Lancet.* 14(12):1732-3.

Bischoff M. 2012. Personal communication.

Bolton M. 2014. Case-studies for 'M' Technique practitioner certification.

Breen Rickerby C, Cordell B. 2012. Application of the 'M' Technique to two severely disabled children in Belarus. *Int J Palliative Nursing.* 18(7):355-9.

Buckle J. 2002. The 'M' Technique. Physical hypnotherapy for the critically ill. *Massage Bodywork.* 15(1):52-5, 58-9, 64.

Buckle J, Newberg A, Wintering N, Hutton E, Lido C, Farrar J. 2008. Measurement of regional cerebral blood flow associated with the 'M' Technique-light massage therapy: a case series and longitudinal study using SPECT. *J Alt Complement Med.* 14(8):903-10.

Buckle J. 2013. Touch for fragile clients. *In Essence.* 12(2):14-18.

Chang SO. 2001. The conceptual structure of physical touch in caring. *J Adv Nurs.* 33(6):820-7.

Clayton S. 2014. Calming touch. *In Essence.* 11(3):14.

Daniels R, O'Flaherty L-A. 2010. Aromatherapy at the Red Cross War Memorial Children's Hospital. *Int J Clin Aroma.* 7(2):1-4.

De Jong M, Lucas C, Bredero H, van Adrichem L, Tobboel D, van Dijk M. 2011. Does postoperative 'M' Technique massage with or without mandarin oil reduce infant's distress after major craniofacial surgery? *J Adv Nursing.* 68(8):1748-57.

Erasmus. 2014. http://www.erasmusmc.nl/411667/840872/mtechniek?lang=en

Gale E, Hegerty J. 2000. The use of touch in caring for people with learning disabilities. *Br J Dev Disabl.* 46(91):97-108.

Guenguen N, Vion M. 2009. The effect of a practitioner's touch on a patient's medication compliance. *Psychol Health Med.* 15(6):689-94.

Hunter P. 2012. Different strokes. *In Essence.* 11(3):9.

Jackson C, Latini C. 2013. Touch and hand-mediated therapies. In *Holistic Nursing: A Handbook for Practice.* 6th edition. Ed. Montgomery Dossey B, Keegan L. pp 417-437.

Katz J. 1999. Hand & Foot 'M' Technique at end of life. Unpublished RJBA dissertation.

Kornfield J. 2000. *After the Ecstasy, the Laundry.* London: Rider, 223.

Marino D. 2004. The 'M' Technique in labor. Unpublished RJBA dissertation.

Mazzer M. Valley Hospital. Ridgewood. NJ. Personal communication. 2005.

Montagu A. 1986. *Touching: The Human Significance of the Skin.* Harper & Row. NY, USA.

Mills C. 2014. Case-studies for 'M' Technique Practitioner certification.

Mitchell L. 1999. Aromatherapy and the 'M' Technique in ICU. Unpublished RJBA dissertation.

Nathan A. 2000. Aromatherapy and the 'M' Technique in pregnancy-induced hypertension. Unpublished RJBA dissertation.

Ocampo A. 2001. Hand 'M' Technique at end of life. Unpublished RJBA dissertation.

O'Keefe M-L. 2001. Foot 'M' Technique at end of life. Unpublished RJBA dissertation.

O'Lynn C, Krautscheid L. 2011. "How should I touch you?": A qualitative study of attitudes on intimate touch in nursing care. *AJN*. 111(3):24-31.

Probert B. 2014. 'M' Technique case-study for practitioner certification.

Quate D. 2002. 'M' Technique in dementia. Unpublished RJBA dissertation.

Raquepo F. 2004. The 'M' for infants following circumcision. Unpublished RJBA dissertation.

Richardson A. 2008. Can the 'M' Technique reduce stress and improve physical and psychological well-being of non-professionals carers of clients with dementia? BSc(Hons) Dissertation. University of Wales. Cardiff School of Health Sciences.

Richardson A. 2009. Personal communication.

Roberts K, Campbell H. 2011. Using the 'M' Technique as therapy for patients at the end of life. *Int J Palliat Nurs*. 17(3):114-8.

Romano J, Trotta R, Rich V. 2013. Combating compassion fatigue: an exemplar of an approach to nursing renewal. *Nurs Adm Q*. 37(4):333-6.

Rombalski J. 2003 A personal journey in understanding physical touch as a nursing intervention. *J Holist Nurs*. 21(1): 73-80

Roquepo F. 2004. The 'M' Technique for children post elected circumcision. Unpublished RJBA dissertation.

Rousseau PC, Blackburn G. 2008. The touch of empathy. *J Palliat Med*. 11(10):1299-300.

Smith J, Raney M, Conner S, Coffelt P, McGrath J, et al. 2012. Application of the "M" Technique in hospitalized very preterm babies. *Adv Neonatal Care*. 12(5S):S10-S17.

Smith J. 2014. Personal communication.

Swanepoel C. 2014. 'M' Technique case-study for practitioner certification.

Tappin P. 2010. My Work. Milford War Memorial Hospital. Pier Professional Ltd. *Working with Older People*. 14(1):34-36.

van Dijk M. 2013. Personal communication.

Watson J. 2006. Caring theory as ethical guide to administrative and clinical practices. *Nurse Adm Q*. 30(1):48-55.

Watson J. 2008. *Nursing. The Philosophy and Science of Care*. Revised Edition. University Press of Colorado, Boulder, CO.

Watson J. 2009. Caring science and human caring theory: transforming personal/professional practices in nursing and health care. *J Health Hum Serv Adm*. 31(4):466-82.

Webster D. 'M' Technique case-study for practitioner certification.

Section II

CLINICAL USE OF AROMATHERAPY

This part of the book focuses on how aromatherapy could be used clinically. It is divided into two sections: Section 2: a general section and Section 3: a specialized section.

In this general clinical section, I have focused on five main symptom areas. In alphabetic order they are: infection, insomnia, nausea and vomiting, pain and inflammation, stress and well-being. These symptoms have far-reaching effects on the quality and cost of healthcare, and are of interest to a wide range of readers. With Western medicine at a breaking point, clinical aromatherapy might relieve some of the pressure. For example, Zofran is a powerful drug for nausea. But, sometimes it is worth trying an anti-emetic essential oil first. Please see Chapter 9.

The chapter on infection was an exciting one to update, because there is now much more published evidence on the effectiveness of essential oils against all kinds of infection, as well as against hospital-acquired infection (HAI) and drug-resistant pathogens. This chapter discusses each pathogen individually, and a table of published studies on the antimicrobial effect of essential oils against that specific pathogen is presented. These studies are encouraging, particularly as the power of conventional antibiotics appears to be waning.

The chapters on insomnia and on nausea and vomiting are arranged by essential oil. However, the chapter on pain covers a much larger area and so it is arranged differently. It begins by looking at conventional approaches to pain and then looks at different ways of using essential oils for pain. The stress and well-being chapter concentrates on stress for patients, staff and visitors, with separate sections on burnout and posttraumatic stress.

Chapter 7

Infection

Microbes maketh man. People are not just people. They are an awful lot of microbes too.

The Economist, August 19, 2012

CHAPTER ASSETS

INFECTION

For the number of articles on specific pathogens and essential oils consulted for this chapter please see Table 7-1. Infection is the successful invasion, establishment and growth of a micro-organism, on the body surface or in the tissue of the host that results in a tissue reaction (Brooker 2008). Infection is mainly caused by a pathogenic organism such as a bacteria, virus, or fungus. There are other infections caused by disease-carrying insects or parasites, but these will not be covered in this chapter. Infectious diseases used to be the most common cause of death

TABLE 7-1 *Databases Searched for Specific Pathogens and Essential Oils*

Pathogen	Number of articles found in 2013		
	PubMed	ScienceDirect	Quintessential
Acinetobacter B	4	205	3
Clostridium difficile	3	76	1
E. coli	515	3462	54
E. faecalis	27	486	3
Klebsiella pneumoniae	97	163	4
MRSA	67	345	7
Proteus mirabilis	29	199	2
Pseudomonas aeruginosa	284	1262	16
Serratia marcescens	10	160	0
Staphylococcus aureus	476	2394	58
Streptococcus	115	1126	10
Tuberculosis	31	793	3

(MacSween & Whaley 1992). With the advent of new infectious diseases, and the reoccurrence of diseases that are now resistant to conventional medicines, perhaps infectious diseases will again become the most common cause of death. Since the second edition of this book, the world has seen bird-flu in 2003 (still occurring in China and a few other parts of the world), the H1N1 virus and the norovirus—a nasty vomiting bug that spreads within hours. Smallpox may have been eradicated, and the incidence of diphtheria and polio greatly reduced, but the emergence of mutated and drug-resistant pathogens is worrying. According to the World Health Organization, tuberculosis (TB) is second only to HIV/AIDS as the greatest killer worldwide that is caused by a single pathogen. In 2011, nearly 9 million people fell ill with TB and 1.4 million people died from it (http://www.who.int/mediacentre/factsheets/fs104/en/). Multiple-drug-resistant TB was present in 80% of those infected. Several essential oils are effective against TB in vitro (Machan 2006; Başer et al 2009; Crandall 2012) and in vivo (Sherry et al 2004). Some are effective against MRTB (Bueno et al 2011) and others may enhance the effect of antibiotics and perhaps make them effective once more.

Antibiotic resistance is rapidly becoming the new norm for all classes of microorganisms (Ena et al., 1993). For example, resistant gonorrhea, a sexually transmitted bacteria, has emerged in several countries, which is resistant to ciprofloxacin, penicillin, and tetracycline (Tsai et al 2013). Cholera, once killed by chlorine, has re-emerged resistant to many antibiotics (Chomvarin et al 2012; Waturangi et al 2013). Malaria, spread by mosquitoes in the tropics, had mutated to become drug-resistant (Ndiaye et al 2013) and malaria-bearing mosquitoes have been found in Greece (Zeller et al 2013). The incidence of West Nile fever—also carried by mosquitos—is increasing in the United States and South Africa. It has also been found in Israel, Italy, and Greece (Arnold 2012). Essential oil of spearmint *(Mentha spicata)* has a significant toxic effect against early third-stage larvae of three types of mosquito: *C. quinquefasciatus, A. aegypti*, and *A. stephensi* (Govindarajan et al 2012). The drug artemisinin (made from the plant *Artemisia annua*) contains the antimalarial sesquiterpene lactone. Artemisinin combination treatment (ACT) is the recommended treatment of choice in Indonesia (where resistant malaria is rampant) (Harijanto, 2010) and is consistent with the WHO (World Health Organization) recommendation (Greenwood et al 2008). It would be interesting to see some research on essential oil of *Artemisia annua* (sweet wormwood) for malaria. However, research found *Anethum graveolens, Apium graveolens, Carum carvi, Curcuma longa, Cyminum cyminum, Foeniculum vulgare, Melia azedarach, Petroselium crispum* and *Piper nigrum* enhanced conventional insecticides against mosquitoes (Mansour et al 2012).

The number of people infected with the virus herpes (HSV1 and HSV2) worldwide has reached more than 500 million (http://www.who.int/en/). Now there is a drug-resistant strain of HSV1 and 2 (Krawczyk 2013). Despite improved living conditions in many countries, viral infections like the common cold and influenza are still major causes of working days lost. Indeed, influenza appears to be growing ever more virulent with the emergence of A/H1N1 and its declared global pandemic (Lapidus et al 2013; Kandel et al 2012; Gupta et al 2013).

Drug-resistant *Candida albicans*, a fungal infection, has spread worldwide as fluconazole, the drug of choice, has become ineffective (Oliveira et al 2013). *Candida* is a real challenge to immune-compromised patients (Chien et al 2013).

Many common parasites are becoming resistant to pharmaceutical products—for example, malaria, head lice, and scabies. Parasites affecting non-human species have also demonstrated resistance, for example, the varroa mite that attacks honeybees. In the United States, 90% of wild honeybees have been killed following an infestation of varroa mites that had become resistant to conventional pesticides. It is thought the mites came on illegally imported bees several years ago. Honeybees have been dying off in many countries, although it is disputed by some whether the loss is due to mites or the extensive use of pesticides in farming, particularly nicotine-based pesticides such as clothianidin and thiamethoxam (Badiou-Bénéteau et al 2012). Although this is a book on clinical aromatherapy, readers might be interested to hear of a study conducted by one of my students, Brock (2004), a nurse and beekeeper. Fifty hives were selected from five farms (10 hives each). Treatment was randomized to one of three groups: 2.5% tea tree *(Melaleuca alternfolia)*, 2.5% spearmint *(Mentha spicata)*, or the control (CheckMite). A white paper towel was placed on top of the main chamber below the inner cover. The diluted essential oil was applied to four lines. Hives were marked with the water-resistant letters, S, T, or C. The results showed only 1 hive out of 10 treated with tea tree had mites when the hives were reopened a month later. This was better than the hives treated with CheckMite or spearmint where mites remained in two hives.

Hospital-Acquired Infections

Being a hospital patient brings with it an increased threat of HAI. The incidence of HAI has risen substantially over the last 10 years and with it, the incidence of multiple-drug-resistant HAI. Hospital-acquired resistant infections (HARI) are now the fourth leading cause of death in the United States (Buhner 2013). There is now a specific journal on this topic *(Journal of Hospital Infection)* and an international conference on Hospital Infection. Mortality, cost, and length of stay are significantly higher in patients with HAIs compared with patients without HAIs (Graves et al 2007; Glance et al 2013; Roberts et al 2010). The overall estimated yearly costs vary between 4.56 billion dollars in the United States to 1.09 billion pounds in the UK. In Italy, estimated costs are 2.5 to 5.0 billion euros per year, with the cost of a single case ranging from 9000 to 10,500 Euro (Agozzino et al 2008). Methicillin-resistant *Staphylococcus aureus* (MRSA) was the first multiple-resistant pathogen. The latest one is *Acinetobacter baumannii* (Acinetobacter B). Acinetobacter B infection has become so serious that in 2013 there was a conference dedicated to it in Cologne, Germany (www.acinetobacter2013.com).

Wound infections occur in 2% of all surgical procedures and account for 20% of HAI (de Lissovoy et al 2009). In a UK study, catheter-associated bacteremic urinary tract infections (UTIs) caused by HAI were significantly associated with 7-day mortality (Melzer & Welch 2013). The main pathogens involved were *Escherichia coli*, *Proteus mirabilis*, and *Pseudomonas aeruginosa* (in order of prevalence). Of these, over 25% were multiple-drug resistant. There were similar instances in France, where one third of all hospital patients contracted an HAI (pneumonia, bacteremia, or UTI). The main pathogens involved were *Aspergillus* spp. (59.2%) for pneumonia, coagulase-negative *Staphylococcus* (44.2%) for bacteremia and *Enterobacteria* (60%) for UTI (Huoi et al 2013). In the United States, such is the extent of hospital-acquired UTIs due to urinary catheters that, from 2008, some hospitals are being denied payment from health insurance companies (Meddings et al 2012). The incidence of HAI is compounded by patients who are admitted to hospital with community-acquired MRSA (Abdallah et al 2013).

For a list of the most common hospital-acquired pathogens and areas of the body, please see Table 7-2. The cause of infection can be poor hospital hygiene, infected visitors, and those carrying infection, or can occur as a result of self-infection. Sometimes infection can be due to the enforced relocation of a commensal. (A commensal is a bacterium that is symbiotic to the health of its host. However, when the commensal is transplanted to another part of the body, an infection ensues. A common example is *E. coli*. *E coli* is fine in the gut, but causes cystitis in the urinary tract.)

COMMON HOSPITAL-ACQUIRED INFECTION

Pseudomonas aeruginosa

P. aeruginosa has become common in hospitals as the cause of urinary, wound, and respiratory infections. Sometimes it is overlooked as a possible cause of bacteremia (Gellen-Dautremer et al 2011). A strictly aerobic, gram-negative bacillus, *P. aeruginosa* flourishes in water and aqueous solutions. The organism produces a pigment called pyocyanin, as well as fluorescein, and these compounds together create the characteristic blue-green, musty-smelling pus (Brooker 2008). *Pseudomonas* is now

TABLE 7-2 *Common Hospital-Acquired Infections and Area of the Body*

Site of HAI	Pathogen	Author
Blood	*Serratia marcescens*	Shime et al 2013
	Pseudomonas aeruginosa	Kuang et al 2013
	Acinetobacter baumannii	Rattanaumpawan et al 2013
	Citrobacter freundii	Deal et al 2009
	ESBL-producing *Enterobacter* spp.	Mezzatesta et al 2012
	MRSA	Ahmed et al 2013
Urinary tract	*Escherichia coli*	Melzer & Welch 2013
	Proteus mirabilis	Mishra et al 2013
	Pseudomonas aeruginosa	Neuner et al 2012
	Serratia marcescens	Shigemura et al 2009
	MRSA	Shigemura et al 2013
Lungs	*Klebsiella pneumoniae*	Uvizl et al 2011
	Pseudomonas aeruginosa	Junkins et al 2013
	Burkholderia cepacia complex	Lopes et al 2012
	Escherichia coli	Reissig et al 2013
	Acinetobacter baumannii	El-Saed et al 2013
	MRSA	Barbier et al 2013
Wounds	*Staphylococcus aureus*	Misteli et al 2011
	Escherichia coli	Ahmed-Bentley et al 2013
	MRSA	Elliott et al 2010
	Serratia marcescens	Posluszny et al 2011
	Pseudomonas aeruginosa	Pastar et al 2013

resistant to most antibiotics (Jwu-Ching et al 2012). Nearly 70% of people with cystic fibrosis are chronically infected with this bacterium. Mechanical ventilation and previous exposure to the antibiotics imipenem and meropenem are risk factors for multiple-drug-resistant *Pseudomonas* (MDRP) infection (Shu et al 2012). *Pseudomonas* also has the ability to create biofilm—this is when the bacteria ooze a sticky substance that allows them to adhere to smooth surfaces. Please see Table 7-3 for essential oils effective against *P. aeruginosa*.

Methicillin-Resistant *Staphylococcus aureus*

Staphylococceus aureus is a gram-positive spherical bacteria that groups together and, under the microscope, looks like bunches of grapes. The bacteria is yellow, hence its name, *aureus*—from the Latin '*aurum*' meaning golden. Methicillin-resistant *Staphylococcus aureus* (MRSA) is resistant to flucloxacillin and has been responsible for outbreaks of infection throughout the world (Tavares 2013; Nichol et al 2013; Rodrigues et al 2013). *Staphylococcus* wound infections tend to remain localized, possibly because of the production of coagulase that causes plasma to thicken (Brooker 2008). However, MRSA can infect any part of the body. For

TABLE 7-3 *Essential Oils Effective Against Pseudomonas in vitro*

Author	Year	Common Name	Botanical Name	Method	Results MIC
Opalchenova & Obreshkova	2003	Basil	*Ocimum basilicum*	Broth	0.0030% and 0.0007% (v/v)
Mahboubi et al	2006	Clove Lavender Geranium	*Eugenia caryophyllata* *Lavandula angustifolia* *Pelargonium graveolens*	Broth	32-64 µg/mL Ratio 3:1:1 showed strong synergy with gentamicin
Hosseini et al	2008	Cumin	*Cuminum cyminium*	Broth	0.015-0.25 mL
Owlia et al	2009	Zataria True myrtle River red gum	*Zataria multiflora* *Myrtus communis* *Eucalyptus camaldulensis*	Vapor	0.125 to 256 µg/mL
Tyagi & Malik	2010	Lemongrass Corn mint Peppermint Blue gum	*Cymbopogon citratus* *Mentha arvensis* *Mentha piperita* *Eucalyptus globulus*	Vapor	0.567 mg/mL 0.567 mg/mL 1.125. mg/mL 2.25 mg/mL
Bouhdid et al	2010	Cinnamon bark	*Cinnamomum verum*	Broth dilution	0.125% (v/v)
Kavanaugh & Ribbeck	2012	Cassia	*Cinnamomum aromaticum*	Broth	0.2% dilution prevented biofilming

example, MRSA UTIs can also lead to bacteremia (Shigemura 2013). MRSA pneumonia is common in ventilated (and non-ventilated) hospital patients (Barbier et al 2013). MRSA is also common in burns units (Rodrigues et al 2013). Patients admitted to the hospital for scheduled operations are routinely tested for MRSA and, where necessary, topical mupirocin is used to eliminate nasal or skin carriage. The spread of MRSA can be contained with scrupulous environmental cleaning, hand washing, and isolation (Brooker 2008; Hess et al 2013). Please see Table 7-4 for some of the essential oils that are effective against MRSA.

Vancomycin-Resistant *Escherichia coli*

Escherichia is a gram-negative bacterium, which under the microscope is shaped like a rod with a small tail. It is widely distributed in nature (Brooker 2008). *Escherichia coli (E. coli)* is part of the normal intestinal flora. Some strains are pathogenic and can cause gastroenteritis, UTI, meningitis, and wound infections. Some serotypes of *E. coli* can produce toxins that result in blood-stained diarrhea or hemolytic-uremic syndrome. Vancomycin-resistant *E. coli* (VRE) is one of the most common causes of infection in hospitals, accounting for up to 20% of all infections (Zhanel 2013). It is a frequent cause of UTIs (Tantry & Rahiman 2012; Mishra et al 2013) and of meningitis in children (Jiang et al 2013). Please see Table 7-5 for essential oils that are effective against *E. coli*.

Streptococcus

Streptococcus is a gram-positive coccus that, under the microscope, occurs in chains. There are various varieties—hemolytic and nonhemolytic—and some produce powerful toxins (Brooker 2008). Some species of *Streptococcus* are commensals and occur (without any ill effect) in the respiratory and intestinal tracts. However, some species are pathogenic and can cause serious illnesses. Necrotizing fasciitis (flesh-eating bacteria) is caused by *Streptococcus pyogenes* (Brooker 2008). It is a rare condition but the mortality rate is high. Eight percent of necrotizing soft tissue infections is attributable to *Streptococcal* infection and among these, 50% develop streptococcal toxic shock syndrome. The mortality rate for *streptococcal* toxic shock syndrome is approximately 32% (Lanitis et al 2012). Sepsis is now the leading direct cause of maternal death in the UK and *Streptococcus pyogenes* is the leading pathogen (Turner et al 2013). *Streptococcus pneumonia* caused an outbreak of severe chest infection in an assisted living facility of whom, 50% needed hospitalization (CDC 2013). *Streptococcus pneumoniae* is spread by droplet infection. It causes an estimated 175,000 hospitalizations each year and the fatality rate can be as high as 60% among the elderly (CDC 2013). Please see Table 7-6 for essential oils that are effective against *Streptococcus*.

Acinetobacter baumannii

Acinetobacter baumannii (A. baumannii) is a gram-negative, aerobic bacterium, which belongs to the family Neisseriaceae. Under the microscope, it looks halfway between a rod and a ball. *A. baumannii* is a relatively new pathogen and is

TABLE 7-4 *Essential Oils Effective Against MRSA in vitro and in vivo*

Author	Year	Common Name	Botanical Name	Method	Results MIC
Carson et al	2006	Tea tree	*Melaleuca alternifolia*	Broth dilution	0.25%
Chao et al	2008	Lemongrass Lemon myrtle Mountain savory Cinnamon Melissa	*Cymbopogon citratus* *Backhousia citriodora* *Satureja montana* *Cinnamomum zeylanicum* *Melissa officinalis*	Disk diffusion	Inhibition zones = 60 mm Lemongrass inhibited every strain of MRSA
Roller et al	2009	True lavender Spike lavender Spanish lavender Castillian lavender	*Lavandula angustifolia,* *Lavandula latifolia,* *Lavandula stoechas* *Lavandula luisieri**	Disc diffusion	Combined lavenders had best results
Doran et al	2009	Geranium Lemongrass	*Pelargonium graveolens* *Cymbopogon citratus*	Disc and vapor	Mixture was 89<70% effective
Tohidpour et al	2010	Common thyme Blue gum	*Thymus vulgaris* *Eucalyptus globulus*	Disk diffusion	18.5 µL/L 85.6 µL/L
Khanavi et al	2011	Kotschyam thyme	*Thymus kotschyanus*	Microdilution	Enhances effect of oxacillin and methicillin × 32
Nedorostova et al	2011	Horseradish Syrian marjoram Garlic Summer savory Winter savory Common thyme Breckland thyme	*Armoracia rusticana* *Origanum syriacum* *Allium sativum* *Satureja hortensis* *Satureja montana* *Thymus vulgaris* *Thymus serpyllum*	Vapor	8.3–17 µL/L 8.3–130 µL/L 8.3–530 µL/L 17–130 µL/L 33–260 µL/L 33–260 µL/L 33–530 µL/L
Warnke et al	2013	Lemongrass Eucalyptus Tea tree	*Cymbopogon citratus* *Eucalyptus globulus* *Melaleuca alternifolia*	Disc diffusion	20–29 mm 8–14 mm 9–15 mm Inhibition zones

**Lavandula luisieri* is a subspecies of *Lavandula stoechas* that is high in necrodane.

TABLE 7-5 *Essential Oils Effective Against E. coli in vitro*

Author	Year	Common Name	Botanical Name	Results
Duarte et al	2007	Palma rosa	*Cymbopogon martinii*	MIC 100-500 μg/mL
Si et al	2008	Oregano	*Oreganum vulgare*	MIC 0.5 μL/mL
Rath et al	2008	Jasmine	*Jasminum sambac*	MIC 100-500 μg/mL
Fisher et al	2009	Sweet orange Bergamot Lemon	*Citrus sinensis* *Citrus bergamia* *Citrus limon*	Orange and bergamot MIC = 0.25%-0.5% v/v
Mahboubi et al	2012	Iranian lemongrass	*Cymbopogon olivieri*	MIC of 4 μL/mL = 0.4%
Bachir & Benali	2012	Blue gum	*Eucalyptus globulus*	MIC = 0.1%
Tadtong et al	2012	Clary sage Lavender Ylang ylang	*Salvia sclarea* *Lavandula angustifolia* *Cananga odorata*	Used together 3:4:3 much better

TABLE 7-6 *Essential Oils Effective Against Streptococcus*

Author	Year	Common Name	Botanical Name	Results MIC
Shin & Kim	2005	Korean thyme	*Thymus magnus*	0.125 μL/mL
Cermelli et al	2008	Blue gum	*Eucalyptus globulus*	50 μL/mL
Singh et al	2011	Peppermint	*Mentha piperita*	0.5 μL/mL
Mahboubi et al	2012	Iranian Lemongrass	*Cymbopogon olivieri*	0.5 μL/mL
Saidi et al	2012	Black thyme	*Thymbra spicata*	3.12 μL/mL
Elaissi et al	2012	Peppermint box	*Eucalyptus odorata*	9.792 μL/mL

thought to have first appeared in military treatment facilities during the Iraq War (Scott et al 2007). *A. baumannii* is now common in Intensive Care Units globally and has rapidly become resistant to most antibiotics. *A. baumannii* can infiltrate open wounds, catheters, and ventilation tubes (Bassetti et al 2008). It causes fatal meningitis (Moon et al 2013) and pneumonia (Durante-Mangoni et al 2013). Please see Table 7-7 for essential oils that are effective against *A. baumannii*.

Klebsiella pneumoniae
Klebsiella is a gram-negative, anaerobic bacterium, which under the microscope is shaped like a rod. It belongs to the family Enterobacteriaceae and is a normal commensal living in the mouth and gut. However, when *Klebsiella* becomes transported

TABLE 7-7 *Essential Oils Effective Against Acinetobacter baumannii in vitro*

Author	Year	Common Name	Botanical Name	Result
Messager et al	2005	Teatree	*Melaleuca alternifolia*	>10(4)-fold reduction
Jazani et al	2009	Fennel	*Foeniculum vulgare*	3.9×10^{-3}
Lorenzi et al	2009	Everlasting	*Helicrysum italicum*	Enhances chloramphenicol × 8
Rosato et al	2010	Rosewood Geranium	*Aniba rosaeodora* *Pelargonium graveolens*	FIC index = 0.11
Lysakowska et al	2011	Thyme	*Thymus vulgaris*	0.25-1.0 µL/mL
Yang et al	2011	Palm ginger	*Zingiber corillinum*	MIC 1457.81 mg/L
Duarte et al	2012	Coriander	*Coriandrum sativum*	MIC between 1 and 4 µL/mL

FIC, Frational inhibitory index.

elsewhere it becomes pathogenic and is commonly associated with UTIs, wounds and respiratory infections (Brooker 2008). *Klebsiella pneumoniae* causes serious pneumonia, particularly in ventilated patients. *Klebsiella* is now resistant to many antibiotics including one of the latest antibiotics—carbapenem (Clock et al 2013; Alp et al 2013). Carbapenemase-resistant *Klebsiella pneumoniae* (CRKP) is very challenging to treat, especially in Intensive Care Units (Borer et al 2009; Ben-David et al 2010; Marchaim et al 2011; Llaca-Díaz et al 2012). Please see Table 7-8 for essential oils that are effective against *Klebsiella*.

Clostridum difficile

Clostridum is a large, gram-positive, spore-forming, anaerobic bacterium, which under the microscope is shaped like a rod (Brooker 2008). It occurs naturally in the intestinal tract, and also occurs in soil. *Clostridium botulinum* causes botulism. *Clostridium difficile* (*C. diff*) is a frequently occurring HAI and is the most common cause of nosocomial diarrhea (CDAD). One of the challenging aspects of treating CDAD is the recurrence that occurs in approximately 15 to 30% of patients after the first episode and up to 50 to 60% subsequently (Sears et al 2013). Treatment is with fidaxomicin, clindamycin, and vancomycin. The incidence and severity of *C. diff* have been increasing (Kee 2012). An antibacterial strain is now evident (Huang et al 2009; Shah et al 2010). Pretreating patients will probiotics can prevent infection with *C. diff* (Johnston et al 2012) but this is not standard practice in hospitals. This might be a preferable option to potential fecal microbiotica implantation, although the latter is 91% successful (Kelly 2012). Please see Table 7-9 for essential oils that are effective against *Clostridium*.

TABLE 7-8 *Essential Oils Effective Against Klebsiella pneumonia in vitro*

Author	Year	Common Name	Botanical Name	Result
Derakhshan et al	2010	Cumin	*Cuminum cyminum*	MIC 0.8-3.5 µg/mL
Orhan et al	2011	Fennel Peppermint Spearmint Basil Marjoram Turkish oregano Oregano Spanish savory	*Foeniculum vulgare* *Mentha piperita* *Mentha spicata* *Ocimum basilicum* *Origanum mar-* *jorana Origanum* *onites* *Origanum vulgare* *Satureja cuneifolia*	MIC 32 and 64 µg/mL for all the essential oils and against multiple resistant strains
Saidi et al	2012	Black thyme	*Thymbra spicata*	MIC = 3.12 µL/mL
Goncalves et al	2012	Cuban oregano	*Plectranthus amboinicus*	MIC = 0.09%
Warnke et al	2013	Tea tree Lemongrass Eucalyptus	*Melaleuca alternifolia* *Cymbopgon citratus* *Eucalyptus globulus*	Inhibition zones 11-14 2.5-4 3.5-5.5
Nadir et al	2013	Iranian sage	*Salvia santolinifolia*	22 mm; MIC 300 µg/mL

SEM, Scanning electrode microscopy.

TABLE 7-9 *Essential Oils Effective Against Clostridium difficile in vitro*

Author	Year	Common Name	Botanical Name	Result
Shahverdi et al	2007	Cinnamon	*Cinnamomum zeylanicum bark*	Enhanced clindamycin × 16
Doran et al	2008	Lemongrass Geranium	*Cymbopogon citratus* *Pelargonium graveolens*	MIC = 0.34 MIC = 2.4
Jeong et al	2009	Manuka	*Leptospermum scoparium*	MIC = 1.0

Multiple-Resistant *Serratia marcescens*

Serratia marcescens (S. marcescens) is a gram-negative bacillus that occurs naturally in soil and water and produces a red pigment at room temperature. It is associated with urinary and respiratory infections, endocarditis, osteomyelitis, septicemia, wound infections, eye infections, and meningitis. Transmission is by direct contact. Droplets of *S. marcescens* have been found growing on catheters, and in supposedly sterile solutions. Contaminated intravenous pain control fluids were the course of an outbreak of *S. marcescens* in a hospital in Taiwan (Chiang et al 2013). Most strains are resistant to several antibiotics. Between 1951 and 1952, the US Army conducted a study called Operation Sea-Spray to study wind-currents that might carry biological weapons. They filled balloons with *S. marcescens* and burst them over San Francisco. Shortly afterward, doctors noted a dramatic increase in pneumonia and UTIs (www.sunysccc.edu/academic/mst/microbes/23smarc.htm). *S. marcescens* in baby shampoo caused multiple infections in a neonatal ICU in Saudi Arabia (Lima et al., 2011; Madani et al 2011). Prefilled heparin and saline syringes infected with *S. marcescens* were the cause of bacteremia in a U.S. hospital (Chemaly et al 2011). *S. marcescens* was isolated persistently from the grating and drains of eight central sinks in an Australian ICU (Kotsanas 2013), and *S. marcescens* was found in the exit ports of oscillators in a Canadian pediatric ICU (Macdonald et al 2011). There is little research on the use of essential oils on *Serratia*.

Proteus mirabilis
Proteus is a gram-negative, anaerobic bacterium of the Enterobacteriaceae family (Brooker 2008). Under the microscope it is rod shaped, motile (can move due to its flagella) and has a characteristic "swarming" ability that allows it to migrate across catheter surfaces (Armbruster 2013). *Proteus mirabilis* and *Proteus vulgaris* cause UTIs (Melzer & Welch 2013), wound infections (Bessa et al 2013) and meningitis (Hammad et al 2011; Juyal et al 2013). Multiple-drug-resistant *Proteus mirabilis* has emerged, including resistance to nitrofurantoin and co-trimoxazole, the most preferred antibiotics for UTI (Mishra et al 2013). There is little research on the use of essential oils on *Proteus*.

Enterobacter
Enterobacter aerogenes and *Enterobacter cloacae* are gram-negative bacteria that belong to the family Enterobacteriaceae. They can be both aerobic and anaerobic. Under the microscope, Enterobacter is rod-shaped with rounded ends. *Enterobacter aerogenes* and *Enterobacter cloacae* cause wound (Múñez et al 2012), respiratory (Wang et al 2012), and urinary tract infections (Edlin 2013). A drug-resistant strain of *Enterobacter aerogenes* has emerged (Karlowsky et al 2013). *Enterobacter cloacae* can also cause ESBL-bacteremia (extended-spectrum β-lactamase producing bacteria) (Ahmed et al., 2009; Frakking et al 2013). There is little research on the use of essential oils on *Enterobacter*.

Citrobacter freundii
Citrobacter freundii is a gram-negative, aerobic bacterium that causes opportunistic infections of the respiratory system, urinary tract, the blood, and several other normally sterile sites in immune-compromised patients (Whalen et al 2007; Rosenberger et al 2011) . There is little research on the use of essential oils on *Citrobacter freundii*.

Burkholderia cepacia Complex (BCC) or Burkholderia cepacia

BCC or *Burkholderia cepacia* covers a group of gram-negative bacteria (Lipuma 2005) that can cause pneumonia in immune-compromised patients, especially those with cystic fibrosis. BCC infection can lead to a rapid decline in those with lung problems and strict isolation is necessary. BCC can also cause bacteremia (Rattanaumpawan et al 2013). There is little research on the use of essential oils on BCC.

Each of the bacteria outlined is becoming more common in hospitals, but there is a whole range of potential pathogenic organisms that surround us every day.

BACTERIAL CLASSIFICATION

Bacteria are classified according to their shape. The two main groups of bacteria are cocci (spherical-shaped) and bacilli (rod-shaped) (Brooker 2008). These two groups are then subdivided into gram-positive and gram-negative bacteria. (Gram was the microbiologist who devised the staining method.) Gram staining uses a mixture of violet dye and iodine to stain the magnesium ribonucleate found in some bacteria, deep purple. The purple stain cannot be washed out by alcohol. Bacteria that stain purple are gram-positive. Those that stain pink are gram-negative (Brooker 2008). *Mycobacterium* (the cause of TB and leprosy) is not revealed by the gram-stain method and instead is stained with an acid-fast method called the Ziehl-Nielsen method (Brooker 2008). A second subdivision of bacteria is between aerobic and anaerobic organisms.

Coccus Bacteria

The cocci bacteria include *Staphylococcus,* named for the Greek word *staphyl,* meaning grapes, because, seen under a microscope, all bacteria have this characteristic shape. *Staphylococcus* is the cause of many skin infections. *Streptococcus* often causes throat infections. Other members of the coccus family include *Pneumococcus,* which causes pneumonia, and *Neisseria,* which causes gonorrhea. *Streptococcus* can be further classified into A, B, or nonhemolytic types and aerobic or anaerobic types.

Bacillus Bacteria

The bacillus group are all rod-shaped and include Enterobacteriaceae such as *E. coli, E. faecalis,* and *Salmonella:* all cause diarrhea. It also includes *Proteus mirabilis* and *Bacillus anthracis* that cause proteus and anthrax, respectively. Other bacteria in the bacillus group include *Corynebacterium diphtheriae, Pseudomonas aeruginosa,* and *M. tuberculosis.* Anaerobic bacilli include *Clostridium tetani,* which causes tetanus, and *C. difficile,* which causes pseudomembranous colitis.

In addition to the two main groups, there is another group of organisms that are neither viruses nor bacteria, but something in between. This group includes *Chlamydia trachomatis* that causes genitourinary infections in 50 million women each year (Darville 2013).

BACTERIA AND ANTIBIOTICS

Bacteria are the oldest form of life on this planet (Buhner 2013). Their unique and extraordinary genetic abilities have enabled them to develop multiple mechanisms of resistance for each new antibiotic produced (Davies & Davies 2010). Global Industry Analysis, a market research company that publishes 1200 full-scale research reports each year, forecasts that the global antibiotics market will reach US$40.3 billion by 2015 (www.prweb.com). The focus will be on drugs with "improved effectiveness and reduced resistance."

Antibiotics work by inhibiting the growth of a microorganism or destroying it. They do this by:
  i) Stopping the synthesis of the bacteria's cell wall.
 ii) Preventing protein or nucleic acid production.
iii) Reducing the permeability of the cytoplasmic membrane.
These all prevent the bacteria from reproducing. Although most antibiotics today are synthetic, originally they were derived from natural substances. The most commonly used type is a broad-spectrum antibiotic that is nonselective. Broad-spectrum antibiotics do not always succeed in killing the bacterium causing the disease, and they destroy "friendly" gut bacteria. This can lead to an overgrowth of *Candida albicans.*

However, certain antibiotics do target gram-positive pathogens (such as *Staphylococcus* and *Streptococcus*) or gram-negative pathogens *(Clostridium difficile, Acetinobacter baumannii)*. But bacteria are very clever. They can destroy or degrade an antibiotic, even if it infiltrates the bacteria's membrane, by creating enzymes like extended-spectrum beta-lactamase (ESBL) or NDM-1 (New Delhi metallo-beta-lactamase) (Alp et al 2013; Mukherjee et al 2013). Bacteria can produce a new generation every 20 minutes, and they can share their resistance information with other forms of bacteria, regardless of if they are gram-positive or gram-negative, anaerobic or aerobic (Salyers et al 2007). Bacteria weave the new information into their DNA and this is then passed on to the next generation of bacteria.

Antibiotics are listed in the group of drugs most frequently associated with adverse reactions such as nausea and gastrointestinal problems, skin rashes, and headaches (Kronman et al., 2012). A search on PubMed using the words "antibiotics" and "side-effects" produced 92,952 hits. The use of antibiotics in childhood has been linked to inflammatory bowel disease (Kronman et al 2012). A Finnish population study of 3 million people showed that multiple use of antibiotics is associated with increased incidence of cancer in later life (Kilkkinen et al 2008). According to Buhner (2103), there are no new antibiotics in any stage of development after 2012, and there are no plans for any. Despite the $100 billion global profit of the top 12 pharmaceutical companies, there is no money in developing new antibiotics. There is more profit to be made in developing drugs for chronic conditions that will always be needed. Once an antibiotic has done its work, it does not to be used again until the next infection.

Resistance to Antibiotics

Most of the world's water supplies (industrialized countries) are contaminated with minute amounts of antibiotics. This means that bacteria have a constant source of antibiotics in the tiny amounts they can deal with, and they learn from it. And, of course, the place where most of the resistant bacteria can be found is in hospitals.

Although manmade antibiotics have become increasingly sophisticated in an attempt to compete with organisms that can mutate and initiate resistant colonies, this appears to be a losing battle. As early as 1942, Fleming (who discovered penicillin) told the medical profession that *Staphylococcus* could become resistant to penicillin. Today, 95% of *Staphylococcus* is resistant to penicillin. Bacteria have become resistant to antibiotics for various reasons:

1. Patients have not completed the prescribed course of antibiotics. This means the bacteria are not completely eradicated and they become immune to the next dose of that particular antibiotic.
2. Antibiotics have been prescribed for viral illness, e.g., the common cold.
3. Antibiotics have been used prophylactically.
4. During the past 40 years, antibiotics (penicillin and tetracycline) have been added to animal feed to increase growth as well as reduce possible infection from over-crowding, despite years of warning (Jukes 1973).
5. Antibiotics are used by the food industry to protect fruits and vegetables.
6. Antibiotics are used in the fish industry.
7. Overprescription of antibiotics has been widespread.

Many of the meats that we eat, such as chickens, turkeys, pigs, calves, beef cattle, and replacement dairy heifers, are given antibiotics to increase growth. In Canada, the approved antibiotics added to animal feed include chlortetracycline, virginiamycin, bacitracin, bambermycins, lincomycin, salinomycin, penicillin, monensin, tylosin, and lasalocid. The use of antibiotics in animal feed has lessened over the last 20 years in England, Scandinavia, The Netherlands, and most European countries. These countries agreed to ban the same antibiotics that were used in human medicine as growth stimulants for animals (Fisher 1994). The United States did not agree to the ban and 80% of the antibiotics currently sold in the United States are used in animal farming (Millet & Maertens 2011). In Africa, antibiotic residues in animal-derived foods have exceeded the WHO maximum residue levels. Tetracycline, the most commonly used antibiotic in Africa, was found in 41% animal-derived food (Darwish et al 2013).

ESSENTIAL OILS AS ANTIBACTERIAL AGENTS

It has been known for some time that all essential oils are antiseptic and some are effective against bacteria, fungi, and viruses (Belaiche 1979; Belaiche 1985; Belaiche 1985a; Benouda 1988; Benencia & Courreges 1999). Scientific research is certainly now giving credence to this historical knowledge. Nearly 20 years ago, Nelson (1997) found essential oils of peppermint, thyme, lavender, tea tree, and juniper were effective against MRSA in vitro. Warnke et al (2009) suggest that essential oils "represent a cheap and effective treatment option even for antibiotic resistant strains."

There is a long history of essential oils being used against pestilence. A large number of perfumers and glovemakers appeared to survive the Black Death in Europe. This could be because glovemakers were licensed to impregnate their wares with essential oils and because perfumes were made with real essential oils not synthetics. Deinenger (1995) cites Schweistheimer, who wrote that the English town of Bucklesbury was spared from the plague. At that time, Bucklesbury was the center of the lavender trade. Several lavenders are effective against MRSA (Roller & Buckle 2009). Nostradamus was supposed to have successfully treated the plague with pills of crushed roses placed under the tongues of plague victims. *Rosa damascena* has antiviral (HIV) properties (Mahmood 1996) and antibacterial properties (Mahboubi et al 2011) so perhaps Nostradamus was right to use rose.

RESEARCH ON THE ANTIBACTERIAL PROPERTIES OF ESSENTIAL OILS

To say there is a plethora of research on the antibacterial effects of essential oils is an understatement. There is certainly far too much to cover in this chapter, but what I hope to do is show a small selection of published studies. This increase in research is a huge change from when I wrote the second edition of this book, some 12 years ago. It is exciting to see how in vitro research is being followed by human tests and studies. For example, Casetti et al (2012) explored the effect of coriander essential oil on bacteria (*Streptococcus pyogenes* and MRSA) that cause skin infections. They found the minimum inhibitory concentration (MIC) required was 0.04% v/v and 0.25% v/v respectively. They followed this in vitro discovery with a 0.5% cream and a 1.0% lotion that they tried out on 40 health volunteers using a skin occlusion patch test. There was no skin irritation. This German study could lead the way to coriander treating skin complaints.

One of the most prolific researchers on the antimicrobial activity of tea tree (*Melaleuca alternifolia*) is Christine Carson, a microbiologist at the University of Western Australia in Perth (Carson et al 1993; Carson et al 1994; Carson et al 1995; Carson et al 1995a; Carson et al 1996; Carson et al 2001; Carson et al 2002; Carson et al 2007; Edmondson et al, Carson 2011). I had the great pleasure of meeting Dr. Carson again in Perth in 2013.

Edward-Jones et al (2004) tested patchouli, tea tree, geranium, and lavender essential oils, singly and combined, against three strains of MRSA in vitro. The most effective combinations were then tested using a "dressing model." This consisted of four layers of dressing. The first layer was either Jelonet or TelfaClear with or without Flamazine; the second layer was gauze, the third layer was Gamgee and the fourth layer was a crepe bandage. The "dressing model" was placed over three agar dishes (containing different strains of MRSA) and incubated for 24 hours at 37 °C. The combination of geranium and tea tree oil was most active against MRSA (Oxford strain). Geranium and citricidal (grapefruit seed extract) were most effective against MRSA (untypable).

Chin et al (2013) conducted an in vivo study based on Edward-Jones' in vitro study. Ten participants who had wounds infected with MRSA volunteered for the study. Four of the ten were used as matched subjects to compare standard treatment to treatment with tea tree. The differences were striking and hopefully will lead the way to a large randomized controlled trial soon.

Halcon et al (2010) developed a tea tree oil wound product and tested its feasibility on patients with chronic lower extremity wounds. Halcon had to complete the IND (Investigational New Drug) document for the FDA (Food and Drug Administration). This is not for the faint hearted as I found out when I was attending University of Pennyslvania! Fortunately, the FDA approved Halcon's IND and she was able to develop the product and test its feasibility. Her protocol included first washing the wound with sterile water to remove any debris, then applying the tea tree oil (or a placebo) to a clean gauze swab and place it directly on to the wound. Each subject was given 56 syringes containing 5 mL of a gel mixture and asked to keep the syringes in a refrigerator. The experimental (tea tree) group had 8% tea tree gel and the placebo had plain gel. Although recruitment was low, the study did demonstrate it was possible to make a product that was acceptable to the FDA and offer it to patients with positive results.

There have been several studies exploring the potential for using essential oils in a hand wash or gel (Caelli et al 2001; Messager et al 2005; Blackwood et al 2008; Rotter et al 2009; Blackwood et al 2013; Caelli et al 2001) found that a combination of 4% tea tree oil nasal ointment and a 5% body wash was more effective than the standard 2% mupirocin nasal ointment and triclosan body wash to eradicate MRSA. Messager et al (2005) found 5% tea tree oil in skin wash was more effective at reducing *E. coli* than a nonmedicated soft soap on 27 volunteers. In 2008, Blackwood et al published a research protocol for a multicentered phase 2/3 prospective open-label randomized, controlled clinical trial to compare 5% tea tree oil (TTO) with Johnsons' Baby Softwash (JBS) against MRSA. In 2013, they published the results of their randomized, controlled study. A total of 445 patients were randomized to the study. Of these, 39 developed new MRSA colonization: 22 were in the JBS group and 17 were in the TTO group. Unfortunately, their hypothesis—that TTO would produce a statistically significant lower incidence of MRSA—was not proven (P = 0.85). As a result, TTO could not be recommended above JBS. This was disappointing. However, the good outcome was that they showed clinically that TTO was as good as JBS. Perhaps further studies with more patients, or a higher percentage of TTO, will produce a statistically significant result. Or maybe TTO will always only be as good as JBS. Perhaps TTO needs to be mixed with another essential oil as combinations of essential oils have often been found to have a stronger antimicrobial activity than single essential oils. A combination of essential oils in a hand gel would also smell more pleasant than tea tree on its own.

However, some hospitals such as St. Clare's Hospital, Baraboo, WI, are using essential oils with good results and some physicians on staff recommend products containing essential oils (that have been developed in the hospital) to their patients for soft tissue infections. For example, an 8-month pregnant lady presented with CR-MRSA infection to the medial aspect of her thighs, bilaterally, secondary to contracting scabies. She was informed she would need a C-section. The patient received approval from her OB doctor to use an essential oil mixture (supplied by the hospital) on her thighs. Her MRSA cleared and she was able to have a vaginal delivery the following month. Another case was a 29-year-old female who had developed a soft tissue abscess to her left thigh. She was instructed on how to use the essential oil product supplied by the hospital pharmacy. The pain stopped within 3 days and the abscess cleared in 8 days (Rodriguez 2013).

Another hospital using essential oils for MRSA is Aurora Healthcare in Milwaukee, United States. The following case study shows how simple it is to add clinical aromatherapy to patient care. An elderly female living in a nursing home had been treated for MRSA for 9 months. She had infections in multiple locations including blood, urine, nares, and oropharynx. Her standard of care included several rounds of oral and topical antibiotics that were completed without eradication of the oropharynx. The patient had dementia so a mouthwash using swish and spit was not an option. One drop of tea tree was added to her toothpaste every day plus two drops of tea tree to her denture bath. After 1 week of treatment, her oropharynx cultured negative and the essential oil treatment was discontinued. Subsequent negative cultures were obtained the second and third week as well. This was an inexpensive treatment that was very successful (Ames 2013).

In an Iranian study, Mahboubi et al (2010) compared the use of an essential oil based antimicrobial hand gel with standard 0.1% triclosan hand gel on 63 healthy volunteers. The cream, marketed as Barij hand gel, contained blue gum (*Eucalyptus globulus*) at 0.05%, key lime (*Citrus aurantifolia*) at 0.3% and geranium (*Pelargonium gravelons*) at 0.1%. The volunteers were their own controls. The essential oil gel was rubbed onto one palm of the participants and the triclosan gel was rubbed on the other—both for 20 seconds. The results showed Barij gel was as effective as triclosan (P = 0.001) and certainly the smell would be nicer.

In Germany, an ointment containing essential oils of eucalyptus, pine needles, and menthol was found effective in adolescents (greater than 12 years old) with upper respiratory infections (Kamin et al 2007). This was a multicentered study where the data of 3060 patients was collected. Most patients were diagnosed with a cold, acute or chronic bronchitis, catarrh or hoarseness. The essential oil ointment was applied to the neck area and/or inhaled. The treatment was judged to be excellent (88%) by both physicians and patients.

The Christie Hospital, Manchester, UK, uses clinical aromatherapy—mainly to reduce the side effects of cancer treatment. However, Stringer (2010) writes about her use of essential oils for infection in a middle-aged obese woman with acute leukemia and diabetes. She had excoriated skin under both breasts, on both sides of her groin and underneath the abdominal apron. These areas were infected with *Candida, Pseudomonas*, and MRSA and exuded a distinct unpleasant odor that the patient found humiliating. An aqueous cream containing 3% lavender (*Lavandula angustifolia*), geranium (*Pelargonium graveolens*) and rosewood (*Aniba rosaeodora*) was applied daily. The amount of exudate decreased substantially in 1 week. The patient felt much happier as she was less sore and smelled much more pleasant. Despite starting chemotherapy, the sores continued to shrink and by the end of the chemotherapy, all excoriated areas had healed.

A study by Sherry et al (2001) indicates that essential oils can be effective when nothing else works. The authors reported on a chronic case of MRSA osteomyelitis. A 49-year-old man sustained an open fracture to his left tibia. He underwent numerous surgical treatments and IV antibiotics over a 15-month period to try to eradicate chronic osteomyelitis (MRSA). Amputation was being considered. In 2000, via a 3-cm percutaneous incision, the lower tibia was drilled and washed out with 4000 mL of saline. Then it was packed with calcium sulfate pellets impregnated with lemongrass, eucalyptus, tea tree, clove, and thyme essential oils in an ethanol base. A catheter was left in situ to allow delivery of further essential oils. One milliliter of antiseptic essential oil mixture was administrated daily. The dilution and ratio of the essential oils was not given. The wound healed and the culture was clear within 3 months. The symptoms resolved, and a plain X-ray examination showed resolution of the infective process with incorporation of the bone graft.

My students have had some impressive case-study results using essential oil compresses on wound infections and infected bedsores. Swabs to indicate infectious pathogens were taken, and the relevant essential oil selected. One particularly impressive case study was conducted by a nurse practitioner. A female patient had a chronically infected bedsore. This patient had been on systemic antibiotics without effect. A wound swab showed the infection had been caused by *Clostridium*. Searching through her notes, the nurse practitioner found a reference to a paper by Ross et al (1980). After she had discussed the safety and potential efficacy of sweet marjoram *(Origanum majorana)* with the patient's physician and had shown him the monograph, he gave his consent for her to use this essential oil. The treatment was discussed with the patient and consent obtained. A compress was applied directly to the infected site, using a 5% solution of sweet marjoram. The compress was reapplied three times a day. Within 24 hours there was a dramatic improvement, and within 5 days the wound was healed. In other case studies, essential oils with antibacterial properties have been selected without a swab being taken. Dilutions of up to 10% have been used with no negative effects. In most instances, the infection has healed very rapidly.

VIRUSES

A virus is different than any other pathogen because it is a coiled strand of nucleic acid protected by a protein coat that can only survive and reproduce inside a host cell (Brooker 2008). Viruses are smaller than bacteria and need electron microscopy to be seen. There are basically two types of virus: those that attack bacteria and those that attack the cells of other living organisms, such as animals and humans. The basic structure of a virus is illustrated in Fig. 7-1.

Viruses are classified as either DNA or RNA viruses and subdivided into single-strand and double-strand. A retrovirus contains an enzyme called reverse transcriptase that allows the RNA in the virus to be reverse-transcribed into DNA. Drugs such as zidovudine (AZT) and zalcitabine (HIVID) are designed to inhibit production of reverse transcriptase. Drug-resistant viruses are well documented (Romano et al 2012; Thai et al 2012; Newman et al 2013).

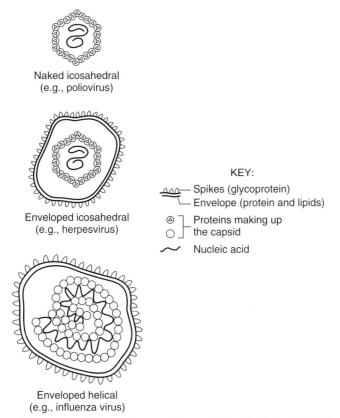

Naked icosahedral
(e.g., poliovirus)

Enveloped icosahedral
(e.g., herpesvirus)

KEY:

Spikes (glycoprotein)
Envelope (protein and lipids)
Proteins making up
the capsid
Nucleic acid

Enveloped helical
(e.g., influenza virus)

FIGURE 7-1 | Structure of viruses. (From Ackerman B, Dunk-Richards G. Microbiology: An Introduction for the Health Sciences. Australia: WB Saunders. 1991.)

In 2008, the Nobel Prize for Medicine/Physiology was divided between the discovery of the human papillomavirus (HPV) and its correlation with cervical cancer in women, and the discovery of the human immunodeficiency virus (HIV) (Rogowska-Szadkowska 2008).

Viruses such as the common cold, influenza, warts, mumps, measles, chickenpox, polio, and glandular fever (Epstein-Barr) are well known; less common are viruses that cause rabies and Lassa fever. Although herpes has been around supposedly since Roman time, HSV1 and HSV2 have become much more prevalent in the last 10 years. Of the common viruses, only smallpox has been eradicated through immunization. A compulsory immunization program in the West has controlled mumps and measles. However, concern over the safety of the MMR vaccine led to an outbreak of measles in Wales during 2013.

Synthetic virucides are difficult to manufacture, and most have moderate to severe side effects (Stasi et al 2013; Fortana 2012; Gallant 2012). Virucides work in one of three ways: through immunologic control, through stimulation of the

TABLE 7-10 *Databases Searched Using Virus Name AND "Essential Oil"*

Virus	PubMed	ScienceDirect	Quintessential
Herpes	42	704	20
Influenza	23	680	6
Warts	5	313	2

natural resistance mechanism of the host, or through chemotherapy. One of the most successful, AZT (azidothymidine), stops the phosphate linkage from being formed—thus the virus cannot manufacture DNA. However, many viruses are now resistant to AZT (Praparattanapan et al 2012).

Current antivirals include acyclovir (Zovirax), famcyclovir (Famvir), Vidara-bine (Vira-A), and rimantadine (Flumadine). Ribavirin, a broad-spectrum anti-viral, has been approved for the treatment of infections with respiratory syncytial virus, HCV and Lassa virus (Debing et al 2013). Retinazole inhibits *Ebola* (Kesel et al 2013). However, there are no drugs available for many other viruses that cause life-threatening infections.

Highly active antiretroviral therapy (HAART) has increased survival time in AIDS patients to more than 10 years (Husstedt et al 2009). HAART has also low-ered the incidence of various opportunistic diseases in HIV-positive women, and decreased the incidence of mother to child infection (Linguissi et al 2012). However, its impact on cervical squamous intraepithelial lesions (SILs) is unclear (Heard et al 2006). HAART drugs have potent side effects on the central and peripheral nervous system and muscles. These side effects make it difficult for patients to completely adhere to the treatment regimen (Husstedt et al 2009).

ANTIVIRAL PROPERTIES OF ESSENTIAL OILS

For the number of articles found on viruses and essential oils in different databases, please see Table 7-10. A list of published research on essential oils and HSV1 and HSV2 is given in Table 7-11. The antiviral effects of essential oils (and their com-ponents) have been evaluated over the last 10 years against diseases such as SARS, influenza, Dengue fever, West Nile fever and yellow fever and the in vitro research is very encouraging (Reichling et al 2009). Many of the studies carried out since 2005 are listed in Table 7-12. Essential oils appeared to have a direct effect on the mechanism of a virus, either by interfering with the virus envelope or by affect-ing the virus's ability to enter the host cell. However, unlike acyclovir, they do not prevent viral replication (Reichling 2010). Star anise essential oil (and all isolated compounds) deactivated free virus particles (Astani et al 2011). Oregano and clove appeared to disrupt the virus envelope (Siddiqui et al 1996).

Over 40 years ago, Kucera and Herrmann (1967) explored the antiviral effects of the aqueous extract of *Melissa officinalis* against influenza, mumps, and influ-enza and found it had an antiviral effect on mumps but had no effect on influenza.

TABLE 7-11 *Antiviral Essential Oils Against HSV1 and HSV2*

Author	Year	Essential oil	Botanical Name	Effective Against
Allahverdiyev	2004	Melissa	*Melissa officinalis*	HSV2; similar to acyclovir
Reichling et al	2005	Manuka	*Leptospermum scoparium*	HSV1 and 2
Tragoolpua & Jatisatienr	2007	Clove	*Eugenia caryophyllus bud*	HSV1 and 2
Saddi et al	2007	Great mugwort	*Artemisia arborescens*	HSV1
Schnitzler et al	2007	Hyssop Sandalwood Thyme Ginger	*Hyssopus officinalis* *Santalum album* *Thymus vulgaris* *Zingiber officinalis*	Drug-resistant HSV1 and 2
Koch et al	2008	Star anise Dwarf pine German chamomile	*Illicium verum* *Pinus mugo* *Matricaria recutita*	Drug-resistant HSV1
Koch et al	2008a	Lemon	*Citrus limon*	HSV1 and 2
Schnitzler et al	2008	Melissa	*Melissa officinalis*	HSV1 and 2
Garozzo et al	2011	Tea tree Blue gum	*Melaleuca alternifolia* *Eucalyptus globulus*	HSV1 and 2
Astani et al	2011	Star anise	*Illicium verum*	HSV1
Astani et al	2012	Melissa	*Melissa officinalis*	HSV1 and 2

TABLE 7-12 *Antiviral Essential Oils*

Author	Year	Essential oil	Botanical Name	Virus
Loizzo et al	2008	Bay laurel	*Laurus nobilis*	SARS
Wu et al	2010	On Guard™ Orange Clove Cinnamon Eucalyptus Rosemary	*Citrus sinensis* *Eugenia caryophyllus* *Cinnamomum* *Eucalyptus globulus* *Rosmarinus officianlis*	Influenza
Ocazionez et al	2010	Lemon verbena Bushy lippia	*Lippia citriadora* *Lippia alba*	Dengue fever
Gorozzo et al	2011	Tea tree	*Melaleuca alternifolia*	Influenza
Vourlioti-Arapi et al	2012	Syrian juniper	*Juniperus drupacea*	West Nile fever
Gómez et al	2013	Lemon verbena Bushy lippia	*Lippia citriadora* *Lippia alba*	Yellow fever

More recently, *Melissa officinalis* was found to be effective against HSV1 and HSV2 (Schnitzler et al 2008; Cermelli et al 2008).

Lemon gum *(Eucalyptus citriadora)* was found to be an effective antiviral by Mendes et al (1990). *Eucalyptus globulus* (blue gum) was found to be an effective antiviral (Schnitzler et al 2001). This may be of particular interest to patients with HIV/AIDS as *Eucalyptus globulus* is also effective against MRTB (multiple-drug-resistant tuberculosis) that is common in AIDS patients (Sadlon & Lamson 2010). I am a little surprised there is no research on *Ravansara aromatica, Ravansara anisata* (sometimes called *Ravintsara*) or *Eucalyptus smithii* as these are all excellent antiviral agents—especially against HSV1 and HSV2.

Duke (1985) wrote that cinnamon *(Cinnamomum verum)* and clove *(Syzygium aromaticum)* had antiviral properties. Current research shows he is correct (Ovadia et al 2009; Yeh et al 2013; Elizaquível et al 2013). Cinnamon produces two essential oils: one from the leaf and one from the bark. The leaf essential oil contains less than 7% cinnamic aldehyde (a known skin irritant) but the essential oil obtained from the bark contains up to 90% cinnamic aldehyde (Lovell 1993). The latter is therefore contraindicated for topical applications, as even at such low dilutions as 0.01%, reactions have been found in patch testing (Mathias 1980). A physician reported that cinnamon oil caused a 10×12 cm^2 second degree burn on the thigh of an 11-year-old boy that came to the University of Mexico pediatric clinic (Sparks 1985).

FUNGAL INFECTIONS

A fungus is a primitive organism classified as neither a plant nor an animal. Only a few fungi are pathogenic to man, and most cause superficial, mild lesions (MacSween & Whaley 1992). Fungi are divided into three categories: superficial, subcutaneous, and systemic. All can be environmental in origin. Fungal infections are caused by airborne allergens, elaborating toxins, or by direct infection. With an airborne allergen (such as tinea, or ringworm) the spores, or hyphae, of the fungus infiltrate the outer layers of the skin and cause destruction of the epidermis. With mycetoma, a localized infection occurs that may slowly spread, although with *candidiasis* and *cryptococcosis* the infection can become systemic.

Opportunistic yeast infections, such as *candidiasis, cryptococcosis, trichosporonosis,* and *geotrichosis,* are diseases caused by fungi that normally are saprophytic and do not cause disease in humans or animals (Vázquez-González et al 2013). However, morbidity and mortality remain high for patients with invasive fungal infections (IFIs) such as invasive *candidiasis* (IC), invasive *aspergillosis* (IA), *cryptococcal* meningitis despite an increasing number of antifungals and other treatments (Perfect 2013).

Cryptococcosis

Cryptococcosis is a yeast infection that is spread by bird droppings and begins as a sporadic disease manifesting with lung infestation. From the lungs, yeast cells migrate to the central nervous system (CNS). Technically there is a blood-brain barrier (BBB) but this barrier is not 100% leakproof and under certain conditions, such as

TABLE 7-13 *Essential Oils Effective Against Cryptococcus spp.*

Author	Year	Common Name	Botanical Name	MIC
Lemos et al	2005	Clove basil	*Ocimum gratissimum*	62.5 µL/mL
Angiolella et at	2010	Apple mint	*Mentha sauveolens*	0.03%
Vale-Silva et al	2010	Portuguese thyme	*Thymus × viciosoi*	0.04-0.64 µL/mL
Zuzarte et al	2011	White lavender	*Lavandula viridis*	0.32-0.64 µL/mL
Pinto et al	2013	Ferulago	*Ferulago capillaris*	0.08-5.0 µL/mL

immune deficiency, the BBB is compromised and CNS infection can occur. Meningoencephalitis is the most common form of *cryptococcosis*, followed by pulmonary infection (Tseng et al 2013). Standard treatment is intravenous Liposomal amphotericin B (AmBisome)—a lipid-associated formulation of amphotericin B or micafungin (Moen et al 2009). Fluconazole and intraconazole are also used and they are less expensive. Some essential oils such as *Artemisia dracunculus* (tarragon) are effective against *Cryptococcus* (Lopes-Lutz et al 2008). However, the majority of effective essential oils appear to be less well known. I have included a small selection in Table 7-13.

ASPERGILLOSIS

Spores of this *Aspergillosis* are present in the atmosphere, and many species are infectious to man. The most common is *Aspergillus fumigatus*. Although the effect of this fungus is not as rapid as that of *Cryptococcus,* the resulting bronchial asthma can be debilitating. The fungus may colonize a bronchial cavity and can result in necrotizing pneumonia. This tends to occur only in immunocompromised patients. Invasive *aspergillosis* (IA) is a major cause of mortality in patients with hematologic malignancies (Morrissey et al 2011) and morbidity and mortality are increasing (Maschmeyer 2007). Aspergillus is becoming resistant to standard treatment with azole-based drugs such as voriconazole (Badali et al 2013; van der Linden 2013).

Khan and Ahmad (2011) tested essential oils for their ability to enhance the effect of fluconazole against *Aspergillus*. They found that essential oils containing cinnamaldehyde reduced the MIC of fluconazole by 8-fold. A further study by Khan and Ahmad found (2011a) found palma rosa *(Cymbopogon martini)* and lemongrass *(Cymbopogon citratus)* also had promising activity against *Aspergillus*. Other essential oils such as *Juniperus communis* (juniper) and *Lavandula luisieri* have also been found effective against *Aspergillus* (Cabral et al 2012; Zuzarte et al 2012).

CANDIDA ALBICANS

Candida is normally present in the mouth, intestinal tract, vagina, and on moist skin and does not pose a problem. However, in certain circumstances, the fungus begins a mucocutaneous, or systemic, invasion. The mucosal infection occurs when an alteration in the pH of the body tissue produces an alkaline medium that allows the yeast fungus to proliferate. From the mucosa, *Candida* can invade surrounding surfaces such as nail beds, producing chronic granulomatous inflammation of the underlying tissue. It can also spread throughout the body, invading the heart valves, lungs, liver, and kidneys with multiple, small abscesses. Thus, *Candida* can cause severe mucosal and life-threatening invasive infections, especially in immunocompromised hosts (Smeekens et al 2013) although this is mainly with *Candida glabrata*. Critically ill patients in the intensive care unit (ICU) are at increased risk of encountering bloodstream infections (BSIs) with *Candida* (Chahoud et al 2013). The symptoms of candidal mucosal infestation are severe itching, with creamy, curd-like deposits. *Candida* is a common infection in diabetes, pregnancy, during antibiotic therapy, and following radiation and chemotherapy (Brooker 2008). A more in depth review of essential oils for *Candida* and table of essential oils that are effective against *Candida* can be found in the chapter on women's health.

EVOLUTIONARY PHARMACOLOGY

Clearly, further research is needed. I hope this chapter will encourage a paradigm shift in pharmaceutical research. The pharmaceutical industry has invested billions in creating antibiotics, antivirals, and antifungals. Now they are faced with increasing evidence that these medicines are no longer working because the pathogens have become resistant. But could it be possible that these medicines, that used to save lives, no longer work just because they are fixed entities?

Let me elucidate: when pharmaceutical companies find a novel substance that works, they reduce it down to the main active ingredient. Then they extract it, synthesize it and a new drug is born. The drug is always exactly the same. Every ampicillin is identical, no matter where you buy it. Every fluconozole is identical. So, a pathogen can mutate fairly quickly and simply. This is the same with the standardized essential oils (SEOs) that are used by the pharmaceutical industry. For example SO 856:2006 specifies certain characteristics for peppermint essential oil *(Mentha piperita)*.

But this does not happen in nature. In nature, nonstandardized essential oils, (NSEOs) are not identical. Their exact chemical makeup depends on geography and harvest: that is, where the plant grows (altitude, temperature, rainfall) and the process of distillation (length, temperature). These subtle changes in the chemistry of an NSEO mean that each batch of essential oil is slightly different—but within certain general parameters. Also, the chemical makeup of an NSEO has synergy—the whole exerts more than the sum of all the parts.

Research has already shown that the components in some essential oils enhance drug permeation and drug potency (Choi & Shin 2007; Krishnaiah et al 2008; Rosata 2010; Duarte et al 2012). Mostly, these are standardized components, or (SEOs). Therefore, over a short period of time, the pathogen will mutate to accommodate them. But, what if a whole NSEO was added to a conventional antibiotic?

What if the essential oil was changed daily or weekly? Or if a mixture of essential oils was used? The subtle changes and synergy of an NSEO might prove more difficult for a pathogen to accommodate. I first postulated this idea at the Gattefosse Foundation (Buckle 2010).

If the pharmaceutical industry tried this new different way of thinking—away from a fixed, reductionist paradigm, perhaps they might discover that NSEO or mixtures of NSEOs could "recharge" an antibiotic and make it work again. What about other medicines? It is worth trying. If my hypothesis is right, this idea of Evolutionary Pharmacology could be generalized to a whole range of different medicines. Perhaps evolutionary pharmacologic medicines (EPM) could be the future.

REFERENCES

Abdallah S, Al-Asfoor K, Salama M, Al-Awadi B. 2013. Prospective Analysis Methicillin-resistant Staphylococcus aureus and its Risk Factors. *J Glob Infect Dis*. 5(1):19–25.

Agozzino E, Di Palma MA, Gimigliano A, Piro A. 2008. Economic impact of healthcare-associated infections. *Ig Sanita Pubbl*. 64(5):655–70.

Ahmed S, Daef E, Badary M, Mahmoud M, Abd-Elsayed A. 2009. Nosocomial blood stream infection in intensive care units at Assiut University Hospitals (Upper Egypt) with special reference to extended spectrum beta-lactamase producing organisms. *BMC Res Notes*. 6(2):76.

Ahmed-Bentley J, Chandran A, Joffe A, French D, Peirano G, Pitout J. 2013. Gram-negative bacteria that produce carbapenemases causing death attributed to recent foreign hospitalization. *Antimicrob Agents Chemother*. Apr 22. [Epub ahead of print] PMID: 23612195. Accessed 29 April 2013.

Allahverdiyev A, Duran N, Ozguven M, Koltas S. 2004. Antiviral activity of the volatile oils of Melissa officinalis L. against Herpes simplex virus type-2. *Phytomedicine*. 11(7-8):657–661.

Alp E, Perçin D, Colakoğlu S, Durmaz S, Kürkcü C et al. 2013. Molecular characterization of carbapenem-resistant Klebsiella pneumoniae in a tertiary university hospital in Turkey. *J Hosp Infect*. 2013 Apr 26. doi:pii: S0195–6701(13)00111-4. Accessed 29 April 2013.

Ames D. 2013. Personal communication.

Angiolella L, Vavala E, Sivric S, Diodata D, Ragno R. 2010. In vitro activity of Mentha suaveolens essential oil against Cryptococcus neoformans and dermatophytes. *Int J of Essential Oil Therapeutics*. 4(1-2): 35–36.

Arnold C. 2012. West Nile Virus Bites Back. *The Lancet Neurology*. 11(12): 1023–1024.

Armbruster C, Hodges S, Mobley H. 2013. Initiation of swarming motility by Proteus mirabilis occurs in response to specific cues present in urine and requires excess L-glutamine. *J Bacteriol*. 195(6):1305–19.

Astani A, Reichling J, Schnitzler P. 2011. Screening for antiviral activities of isolated compounds from essential oils. *Evid Based Complement Alternat Med*. 2011:253643. Accessed May 8, 2013.

Astani A, Reichling J, Schnitzler P. 2012. Melissa officinalis extract inhibits attachment of herpes simplex virus in vitro. *Chemotherapy*. 58(1):70–7.

Bachir R, Benali M. 2012. Antibacterial activity of the essential oils from the leaves of Eucalyptus globulus against Escherichia coli and Staphylococcus aureus. *Asian Pac J Trop Biomed*. 2(9):739–42.

Badali H, Vaezi A, Haghani I, Yazdanparast SA, Hedayati M et al. 2013. Environmental study of azole-resistant Aspergillus fumigatus with TR34 /L98H mutations in the cyp51A gene in Iran. Mycoses. May 14. doi: 10.1111/myc.12089. Accessed May 15, 2013.

Badiou-Bénéteau A, Carvalho S, Brunet J, Carvalho G, Buleté. A 2012. Development of biomarkers of exposure to xenobiotics in the honey bee *Apis mellifera*: Application to the systemic insecticide thiamethoxam. *Ecotoxicology and Environmental Safety*. 82(1):22–31.

Barbier F, Andremont A, Wolff M, Bouadma L. 2013. Hospital-acquired pneumonia and ventilator-associated pneumonia: recent advances in epidemiology and management. *Curr Opin Pulm Med*. 19(3):216–28.

Başer K, Kurkcuoğlu M, Askun T, Tumen G. 2009. Anti-tuberculosis activity of Daucus littoralis Sibth. et Sm. (Apiaceae) from Turkey. *J Essential Oil Res.* 21(6): 572–575

Bassetti M, Repetto E, Righi E, Boni S, Diverio M et al. 2008. Colistin and rifampicin in the treatment of multidrug-resistant Acinetobacter baumannii infections. *J Antimicrob Chemother.* 61(2):417–20.

Belaiche P. 1979. Traite de phytotherapie et d'aromatherapie, Tome 1: L'aromatogramme. Paris: Maloine.

Belaiche P. 1985. Treatment of vaginal infections of *Candida albicans* with essential oils of *Melaleuca alternifolia*. Phytotherapy. 15:13–14.

Belaiche P. 1985a. Treatment of skin infections with essential oils *of Melaleuca alternifolia. Phytotherapy.* 15:15–17.

Ben-David D, Maor Y, Keller N, Regev-Yochay G, Tal I et al. 2010. Potential role of active surveillance in the control of a hospital-wide outbreak of carbapenem-resistant Klebsiella pneumoniae infection. *Infect Control Hosp Epidemiol.* 31(6):620–6.

Benencia F, Courreges M. 1999. Antiviral activity of sandalwood oil against herpes simplex viruses 1 and 2. *Phytomedicine.* 6(2): 119–123.

Benouda A, Hassar M Benjilali B. 1988. In vitro antibacterial properties of essential oils tested against hospital pathogenic bacteria. *Fitoterapia.* 59(2): 115–119.

Bessa L, Fazii P, Di Giulio M, Cellini L. 2013. Bacterial isolates from infected wounds and their antibiotic susceptibility pattern: some remarks about wound infection. *Int Wound J.* Feb 24. doi: 10.1111/iwj.12049. [Epub ahead of print]. Accessed May 1, 2013.

Blackwood B, Thompson G, McMullan R, Stevenson M, Riley T et al. 2008. Tea tree oil (5%) body wash versus standard care (Johnson's Baby Softwash) to prevent colonization with methicillin-resistant Staphylococcus aureus in critically ill adults: a randomized controlled trial. *J Antimicrob Chemother.* 68(5):1193–9.

Blackwood B, Thompson G, Mcgullan R, Stevenson M, Riley T et al. 2013. Tea tree oil (5%) body wash versus standard care (Johnson's Baby Softwash) to prevent colonization with methicillin-resistant Staphylococcus aureus in critically ill adults: a randomized controlled trial. *J Antimicrob Chemo.* 68(5):1193–9.

Borer A, Saidel-Odes L, Riesenberg K, Eskira S, Peled N et al. 2009. Attributable mortality rate for carbapenem-resistant Klebsiella pneumoniae bacteremia. *Infect Control Hosp Epidemiol.* 30(10):972–6.

Bouhdid S, Abrini J, Zhiri A, Espuny M J, Manresa A. 2010. Functional and ultrastructural changes in Pseudomonas aeruginosa and Staphylococcus aureus cells induced by Cinnamomum verum essential oil. *Journal of Applied Microbiology.* 109(4): 1139–1149.

Brooker C. 2008. *Medical Dictionary.* Churchill Livingstone. London.

Buckle J. 2010. Aromatherapy: is there role for essential oils in current and future healthcare? Bulletin Technique Gattefosse. Foundation Gattefosse, France. 103. 95–101.

Bueno J, Escobar P, Martínez J, Leal S, Stashenko E. 2011. Composition of three essential oils, and their mammalian cell toxicity and antimycobacterial activity against drug resistant-tuberculosis and non-tuberculous Mycobacteria strains. *Natural Product Communications.* 6(11): 1743–1748.

Buhner S, 2013. *Herbal Antibiotics: Natural Alternative to Treating Resistant Bacteria.* 2nd edition. Storey Publishing, North Adam, MA.

Cabral C, Francisco V, Cavaleiro C, Gonçalves M, Cruz M et al. 2012. Essential oil of Juniperus communis subsp. alpina (Suter) needles: chemical composition, antifungal activity and cytotoxicity. *Phytother Res.* 26(9):1352–7.

Caelli M, Porteous J, Carson C et al. 2001. Tea tree oil as an alternative topical decolonization for methicillin-resistant Staphylococcus aureus. *Journal of Hospital Infection.* 46(3) 236–237.

Carson C, Riley T. 1993. Antimicrobial activity of the essential oil of *Melaleuca alternifolia. Lett Appl Microbiol.* 16:49–55.

Carson C, Riley T. 1994. Susceptibility of *Propionibacterium acnes* to the essential oil of *Melaleuca alternifolia. Lett Appl Microbiol.* 19:24–25.

Carson C, Cookson B, Farrelly B, Riley T. 1995. Susceptibility of methicillin-resistant *Staphylococcus aureus* to the essential oil of *Melaleuca alternifolia Antimicrob Chemother.* 35:421–4.

Carson C, Hammer K, Riley T. 1995. Broth micro-dilution method for determining the susceptibility of *Escherichia coli and Staphylococcus aureus* to the essential oil of *Melaleuca alternifolia* (tea tree oil). *Microbios*. 82:181–185.

Carson C, Hammer K, Riley T. 1996. In-vitro activity of the essential oil of *Melaleuca alternifolia* against *Streptococcus* spp. *J Antimicrob Chemother*. 37:1177–1178.

Carson C, Dry A, Smith A, Riley T. 2001. *Melaleuca alternifolia* (tea tree) oil gel (6%) for the treatment of recurrent herpes labialis *Antimicrob Chemother*. 48:450–451.

Carson C, Mee B, Riley T. 2002. Mechanism of action of *Melaleuca alternifolia* (tea tree) oil on *Staphylococcus aureus* determined by time-kill, lysis, leakage, and salt tolerance assays and electron microscopy. *Antimicrob Agents Chemother*. 48:1914-1920.

Carson C, Hammer K, Riley T. 2006. *Melaleuca alternifolia* (Tea Tree) Oil: a Review of Antimicrobial and Other Medicinal Properties. *Clin Microbiol Reviews*.19(1): 50–62.

Casetti F, Bartelke S, Biehler K, Augustin M, Schempp C, Frank U. 2012. Antimicrobial activity against bacteria with dermatological relevance and skin tolerance of the essential oil from Corandrum sativum L fruits. *Phytotherapy Research*. 26(3):420–4.

DVD. Centers for Disease Control and Prevention. 2013. Notes from the field: outbreak of severe respiratory illness in an assisted-living facility – Colorado. *Morb Mortal Wkly Rep*. 62:230–1.

Cermelli C, Fabio A, Fabio G, Quaglio P. 2008. Effect of Eucalyptus essential oil on Respiratory Bacteria and Viruses. *Current Microbiology*. 56(1): 89–92.

Chao S, Young G, Oberg C, Nakaoka K. 2008. Inhibition of methicillin-resistant Staphylococcus aureus (MRSA) by essential oils. *Flavour and Fragrance Journal*. 23(6):444–449.

Chahoud J, Kanafani Z, Kanj S. 2013. Management of candidaemia and invasive candidiasis in critically ill patients. *Int J Antimicrob Agents*. May 8. doi:pii: S0924–8579(13)00134-9. Accessed May 15, 2013.

Chemaly RF, Rathod DB, Sikka MK, Hayden MK, Hutchins M et al 2011. Serratia marcescens bacteremia because of contaminated prefilled heparin and saline syringes: a multi-state report. *Am J Infect Control*. 39(6):521–4.

Chiang P, Wu T, Kuo A, Huang Y, Chung T et al 2013. Outbreak of Serratia marcescens postsurgical bloodstream infection due to contaminated intravenous pain control fluids. *Int J Infect Dis*. Apr 1. doi:pii: S1201–9712(13)00102-1. Accessed April 28, 2013.

Chien H, Chen C, Chen Y, Chang P, Tsai T, Chen C. 2013. The Use of Chitosan to Enhance Photodynamic Inactivation against Candida albicans and Its Drug-Resistant Clinical Isolates. *Int J Mol Sci*. 14(4): 7445–56.

Chin K, Cordell B. 2013. The effect of Teatree oil (Melaleuca alternifolia) on wound healing using a dressing model. *J Alternative & Complementary Medicine*. In press.

Choi S, Shin S. 2007. Activity of essential oil from Mentha piperita against some antibiotic-resistant Streptococcus pneumoniae strains and its combination effects with antibiotics. *Natural Product Sciences*. 13(2): 164–168.

Chomvarin C, Jumroenjit W, Wongboot W, Kanoktippornchai B, Chaimanee P et al. 2012. Molecular analysis and antimicrobial resistance of Vibrio cholerae O1 in northeastern Thailand. *Southeast Asian J Trop Med Public Health*. 43(6):1437–46.

Clock S, Tabibi S, Alba L, Kubin C, Whittier S, Saiman L. 2013. In vitro activity of doripenem alone and in multi-agent combinations against extensively drug-resistant Acinetobacter baumannii and Klebsiella pneumoniae. *Diagn Microbiol Infect Dis*. 2013 Apr 16. doi:pii: S0732–8893(13)00147-8. Accessed April/29, 2013.

Crandall P, Ricke S, O'Bryan C, Parrish N. 2012. In vitro effects of citrus oils against Mycobacterium tuberculosis and non-tuberculous Mycobacteria of clinical importance. *J Environ Sci Health B*. 47(7):736–41

Darville T. 2013. Recognition and treatment of chlamydial infections from birth to adolescence. *Adv Exp Med Biol*. 764:109–22.

Darwish WS, Eldaly EA, El-Abbasy MT, Ikenaka Y, Nakayama S, Ishizuka M. 2013. Antibiotic residues in food: the African scenario. *Jpn J Vet Res*. 61 (Suppl):S13–22.

Davies J, Davies D. 2010. Origins and Evolution of Antibiotic Resistance. *Microbiol Rev*. 74 (3): 417–433.

de Lissovoy G, Fraeman K, Hutchins V, Murphy D, Song D, Vaughn B. 2009. Surgical site infection: incidence and impact on hospital utilization and treatment costs. *Am J Infect Control*. 37(5):387–97.

Deal E, Micek S, Reichley R, Ritchie D. 2009. Effects of an alternative cefepime dosing strategy in pulmonary and bloodstream infections caused by Enterobacter spp, Citrobacter freundii, and Pseudomonas aeruginosa: a single-center, open-label, prospective, observational study. *Clin Ther*. 31(2):299–310.

Debing Y, Jochmans D, Neyts J. 2013. Intervention strategies for emerging viruses: use of antivirals. *Curr Opin Virology*. 3(2): 217–24.

Deinenger E. 1995. The spectrum of activity of plant drugs containing essential oils. In Conference Proceedings, Holistic Aromatherapy. San Francisco: Pacific Institute of Aromatherapy, 15–43.

Derakhshan S, Sattari M, Bigdeli M. 2010. Effect of cumin (Cuminum cyminum) seed essential oil on biofilm formation and plasmid Integrity of Klebsiella pneumoniae. *Pharmacogn Mag*. 6(21):57–61.

Doran A, Morden W, Dunn K, Edwards-Jones V. 2009. Vapour-phase activities of essential oils against antibiotic sensitive and resistant bacteria including MRSA. *Letters in Applied Microbiology*. 48(4):387–392.

Duarte M, Leme, Delarmelina E, Soares A, Figueira G, Sartoratto A. 2007. Activity of essential oils from Brazilian medicinal plants on Escherichia coli. *Journal of Ethnopharmacology*. 111(2):197–201.

Duarte A, Ferriera S, Silva F, Dominigues F. 2012. Synergistic activity of coriander oil and conventional antibiotics against *Acinetobacter baumannii*. *Phytomedicine*. 19(3-4):236–238.

Duke J. 1985. *Handbook of Medicinal Herbs*. Boca Raton, FL: CRC Press.

Durante-Mangoni E, Signoriello G, Andini R, Mattei A, De Cristoforo M et al 2013. Colistin and Rifampicin compared with Colistin alone for the treatment of serious infections due to extensively drug-resistant Acinetobacter baumannii. A multicentre, randomised, clinical trial. *Clin Infect Dis*. 2013 Apr 24. [Epub ahead of print]. Accessed 28 April 2013.

Edlin R, Shapiro D, Hersh A, Copp H.2013. Antibiotic Resistance Patterns in Outpatient Pediatric Urinary Tract Infections. *J Urol*. Jan 28. doi:pii: S0022–5347(13)00105-5. Accessed May 1, 2013.

Edmondson M, Newell N, Carville K, Smith J, Riley T, Carson C. 2011. Uncontrolled, open-label, pilot study of tea tree (Melaleuca alternifolia) oil solution in the decolonisation of methicillin-resistant Staphylococcus aureus positive wounds and its influence on wound healing. *Int Wound J*. 8(4):375–84.

Edwards-Jones V, Buck R, Shawcross S, Dawson M, Dunn K. 2004. The effect of essential oils on methicillin-resistant Staphylococcus aureus using a dressing model. *Burns*. 30(8):772–7.

Elizaquível P, Azizkhani M, Aznar R, Sánchez G. 2013. The effect of essential oils on norovirus surrogates. *Food Control*. 32(1): 275–278.

Elliott R, Weatherly H, Hawkins N, Cranny G, Chambers D, Myers L et al. 2010. An economic model for the prevention of MRSA infections after surgery: non-glycopeptide or glycopeptide antibiotic prophylaxis? *Eur J Health Econ*. 11(1):57–66.

El-Saed A, Balkhy H, Al-Dorzi H, Khan R, Rishu A, Arabi Y. 2013. Acinetobacter is the most common pathogen associated with late-onset and recurrent ventilator-associated pneumonia in an adult intensive care unit in Saudi Arabia. *Int J Infect Dis*. Mar 18. doi:pii: S1201–9712(13)00084-2. Accessed 29 April 2013.

El Abed, S Houari, A Latrache, H Remmal, A. Koraichi, S. 2011. In vitro activity of four common essential oil components against biofilm-producing Pseudomonas aeruginosa. *Research Journal of Microbiology*. 6(4):394–401.

Elaissi A, Rouis Z, Salem NA, Mabrouk S, ben Salem Y et al. 2012. Chemical composition of 8 *eucalyptus* species' essential oils and the evaluation of their antibacterial, antifungal and antiviral activities. *BMC Complement Altern Med*. doi: 10.1186/1472-6882-12-81. Accessed 16 May 2013.

Ena J, Dick R, Wenzel R. 1993. The epidemiology of intravenous vancomycin usage in a university hospital: A ten-year study. *Journal of the American Medical Association*. 269(5) 598–602.

Fisher J. 1994. *The Plague Makers*. New York: Simon & Schuster.

Fisher K, Phillips C. 2009. In vitro inhibition of vancomycin-susceptible and vancomycin-resistant Enterococcus faecium and E faecalis in the presence of citrus essential oils. *Br J Biomedical Science*. 66(4):180–5.

Fontana R. 2012. Side effects of long-term oral antiviral therapy for hepatitis B. *Hepatology*. 49(5 Suppl):S185–95.

Frakking F, Rottier W, Dorigo-Zetsma J, van Hattem J, van Hees B et al. 2013. Appropriateness of empirical treatment and outcome in bacteremia caused by extended-spectrum β-lactamase producing bacteria. *Antimicrob Agents Chemother*. Apr 22. [Epub ahead of print]. Accessed May 1, 2013.

Gallant J. 2012. Antiretroviral therapy in resource-limited settings: is there still a role for stavudine? *Antivir Ther*. 17(8):1507–9.

Garozzo A, Timpanaro R, Bisignano B, Furneri P, Bisignano G et al. 2009. In vitro antiviral activity of Melaleuca alternifolia essential oil. *Lett Appl Microbiol*. 49(6):806–8.

Garozzo A, Timpanaro R, Stivala A, Bisignano G, Castro A. 2011. Activity of Melaleuca alternifolia (tea tree) oil on Influenza virus A/PR/8: study on the mechanism of action. *Antiviral Res*. 89(1):83–8

Gellen-Dautremer J, Bert F, Panhard X, Fantin B, Lefort A. 2011. Physicians fail to consider *Pseudomonas aeruginosa* as a potential pathogen in medicine patients with bacteremia *Journal of Infection*. 63(1): 99–101.

Glance L, Stone P, Mukamel D, Dick A. 2013. Increases in mortality, length of stay, and cost associated with hospital-acquired infections in trauma patients *Arch Surg*. 146(7):794–801.

Gómez L, Stashenko E, Ocazionez R. 2013. Comparative study on in vitro activities of citral, limonene and essential oils from Lippia citriodora and L. alba on yellow fever virus. *Nat Prod Commun*. 8(2):249–52.

Goncalves T, Braga M, de Oliveira F, Santiago G, Carvalho C et al. 2012. Effect of subinihibitory and inhibitory concentrations of Plectranthus amboinicus (Lour.) Spreng essential oil on Klebsiella pneumoniae. *Phytomedicine*. 19(11):962–968.

Govindarajan M, Sivakumar R, Rajeswari M, Yogalakshmi K. 2012 Chemical composition and larvicidal activity of essential oil from Mentha spicata (Linn.) against three mosquito species. *Parasitol Res*.110(5):2023-32.

Graves N, Weinhold D, Tong E, Birrell F, Doidge S et al. 2007. Effect of healthcare-acquired infection on length of hospital stay and cost. *Infect Control Hosp Epidemiol*. 28(3):280–92.

Greenwood B, Fidock D, Kyle D. 2008. Malaria: Progress, perils and prospects for eradication. *J Clin Invest*. 118.

Gupta R, Alkhateeb F, Latif D, Farley K. 2013. Parental attitudes affecting compliance with the recommendation for two doses of 2009 pandemic influenza A (H1N1) vaccine in children less than 10 years of age in West Virginia. *W V Med J*. 109(2):10–4.

Halcon L, Swiontkowski M, Tsukayama D, Thiel T, Lillehei A. 2010. Tea tree oil (Melaleuca alternifolia) to treat wounds with Staphylococcus aureus: product development, clinical protocol and feasibility. *Int J Clin Aromatherapy*. 7(1): 3–10.

Hammad O, Hifnawy T, Omran D, Zaki S, Daraz A. 2011. Gram-negative bacillary meningitis in Egypt. *J Egypt Public Health Assoc*. 86(1-2):16–20.

Harijanto P. 2010. Malaria treatment by using artemisinin in Indonesia. *Acta Med Indones*. 42(1):51–6.

Heard I, Potard V, Costagliola D. 2006. Limited impact of immunosuppression and HAART on the incidence of cervical squamous intraepithelial lesions in HIV-positive women. *Antivir Ther*. 11(8):1091–6.

Hess A, Shardell M, Johnson J, Thom K, Roghmann M, et al. 2013. A randomized controlled trial of enhanced cleaning to reduce contamination of healthcare worker gowns and gloves with multidrug-resistant bacteria. *Infect Control Hosp Epidemiol*. 34(5):487–93.

Huoi C, Vanhems P, Nicolle M, Michallet M, Bénet T. 2013. Incidence of hospital-acquired pneumonia, bacteraemia and urinary tract infections in patients with haematological malignancies, 2004-2010: a surveillance-based study. *PLoS One*. 2013;8(3):e58121. doi: 10.1371/journal.pone.0058121. Accessed 29 April 2013.

Hosseini Jazani N, Zartoshti M, Shahabi S. 2008. Antibacterial effects of Iranian Cuminum cyminum essential oil on burn isolates of Pseudomonas aeruginosa. *International Journal of Pharmacology*. 4(2): 157–159.

Huang H, Weintraub A, Fang H, Nord CE. 2009. Antimicrobial resistance in Clostridium difficile. *Int J Antimicrob Agents*. 34(6):516–22.

Husstedt IW, Reichelt D, Neuen-Jakob E, Hahn K, Kästner F et al. 2009. Highly active antiretroviral therapy of neuro-AIDS. Side effects on the nervous system and interactions. *Nervenarzt.* 80(10):1133–4, 1136–8, 1140–2.

Jazani N, Zartoshti M, Babazadeh H, Ali-Daiee N, Zarrin S, Hosseini S. 2009. Antibacterial effects of Iranian fennel essential oil on isolates of Acinetobacter baumannii. *Pakistan Journal of Biological Sciences.* 12(9):738–741.

Jeong E, Ju-Hyun J, Hyung-Wook K, Min-Gi K, Hoi-Seon L. 2009. Antimicrobial activity of Leptospermum and its derivatives against human intestinal flora. *Food Chemistry.* 115(4): 1401–1404

Jiang H, Kui L, Huang H, Su M, Wen B. 2013. Frequency distribution and antibiotic resistance of pathogens from the cerebrospinal fluid of 116 children with bacterial meningitis. *Zhongguo Dang Dai Er Ke Za Zhi.* 15(4):264–7.

Johnston B, Ma S, Goldenberg J, Thorlund K, Vandvik P et al. 2012 Probiotics for the prevention of Clostridium difficile-associated diarrhea: a systematic review and meta-analysis. *Ann Intern Med.* 157(12):878–88.

Jukes T. 1973. Public health significance of feeding low levels of antibiotics to animals. *Advances in Applied Microbiology.* 16:1–29.

Junkins R, Macneil A, Wu Z, McCormick C, Lin T. 2013. Regulator of Calcineurin 1 Suppresses Inflammation during Respiratory Tract Infections. *J Immunol.* Apr 15. [Epub ahead of print] PMID: 23589609. Accessed 29 April 2013.

Juyal D, Rathaur VK, Sharma N. 2013. Neonatal meningoventriculitis due to proteus mirabilis - a case report. *J Clin Diagn Res.* 7(2):369–70.

Jwu-Ching S, Ju-Hsin C, Leung-Kei S, An-Jing K, Shu-Huan H et al. 2012. Interplay between mutational and horizontally acquired resistance mechanisms and its association with carbapenem resistance amongst extensively drug-resistant Pseudomonas aeruginosa (XDR-PA). *Int J Antimicrob Agents.* 39(3):217–22.

Kamin W, Kieser M. 2007. Pinimenthol ointment in patients suffering from upper respiratory tract infections - a post-marketing observational study. *Phytomedicine.* 14(12):787–91.

Kandel N, Shrestha J, Upadhyay B, Shrestha A, Shakya G. 2012. Pandemic (H1N1) 2009 Cases in Nepal. *J Nepal Med Assoc.* 52(188):201–4.

Karlowsky J, Adam H, Desjardins M, Lagacé-Wiens P, Hoban D et al. 2013. Changes in fluoroquinolone resistance over 5 years (CANWARD 2007-11) in bacterial pathogens isolated in Canadian hospitals. *J Antimicrob Chemother.* 68. Suppl 1:i39–i46.

Kavanaugh N, Ribbeck K. 2012. Selected Antimicrobial Essential Oils Eradicate Pseudomonas spp. and Staphylococcus aureus Biofilms. *Applied & Environmental Microbiology.* 78(11):4057–4061.

Kee V. 2012. Clostridium difficile infection in older adults: a review and update on its management. *Am J Geriatr Pharmacother.* 10(1):14-24.

Kelly CR, de Leon L, Jasutkar N. 2012. Fecal microbiota transplantation for relapsing Clostridium difficile infection in 26 patients: methodology and results. *J Clin Gastroenterol.* 46(2):145–9.

Kesel A, Huang Z, Murray M, Prichard M, Caboni L et al 2013. Retinazone inhibits certain blood-borne human viruses including Ebola virus Zaire. *Antivir Chem Chemother.* May 2. doi: 10.3851/IMP2568. Accessed May 6, 2013.

Khan and Ahmad. (2011). Antifungal activity of essential oils and their synergy with fluconazole against drug-resistant strains of Aspergillus fumigatus and Trichophyton rubrum. *Appl Microbiol Biotechnol.* 90(3):1083–94.

Khan and Ahmad (2011a). In vitro antifungal, anti-elastase and anti-keratinase activity of essential oils of Cinnamomum-, Syzygium- and Cymbopogon-species against Aspergillus fumigatus and Trichophyton rubrum. *Phytomedicine.* 19(1):48–55.

Kilkkinen A, Rissanen H, Klaukka T, Pukkala E, Heliövaara M. 2008. Antibiotic use predicts and increase risk of cancer. *International Journal of Cancer.* 123(9):2152–2155.

Khanavi M, Farahanikia, B, Rafiee F, Dalili D, Safaripour E, Samadi N. 2011. Reversal of resistance in MRSA strains by Thymus kotschyanus essential oil. *Journal of Essential Oil Bearing Plants.* 14(6):684–692.

Koch C, Reichling J, Kehm R, Sharaf M, Zentgraf M et al. 2008. Efficacy of anise oil, dwarf-pine oil and chamomile oil against thymidine-kinase-positive and thymidine-kinase-negative herpesviruses. *Journal of Pharmacy and Pharmacology.* 60(11):1545–1550.

Koch C, Reichling J, Schnitler P. 2008a. Essential oils inhibit the replication of herpes simples cirus (HSV-1) and type 2 (HSV-2). In *Botanical Medicine in Clinical Practice*. Ed Watson R and Preddy V. pages 192-197. CAB International.

Kotsanas D, Wijesooriya WR, Korman TM, Gillespie EE, Wright L. 2013. "Down the drain": carbapenem-resistant bacteria in intensive care unit patients and handwashing sinks. *Med J Aust*. 198(5):267–9.

Krawczyk A, Arndt M, Grosse-Hovest L, Weichert W, Giebel B et al. 2013. Overcoming drug-resistant herpes simplex virus (HSV) infection by a humanized antibody. *Proc Natl Acad Sci USA*. 10(17):6760–5.

Krishnaiah YS, Al-Saidan SM. 2008. Limonene enhances the in vitro and in vivo permeation of trimetazidine across a membrane-controlled transdermal therapeutic system. *Curr Drug Deliv*. 5(1):70-6.

Kronman M, Zaoutis T, Haynes K, Feng R, Coffin S. 2012. Antibiotic exposure and IBD development among children: a population-based cohort study. *Pediatrics*. 130(4)e794–803.

Kuang L, Jiang Y, Hu Z, Mu L, Su M, Zhou W. 2013. Species and drug resistance of pathogens in blood cultures from the pediatric hematology ward. *Zhongguo Dang Dai Er Ke Za Zhi*. 15(4):259–63.

Kucera L, Herrmann E. 1967. Antiviral substances in plants of the mint family (Labiatae). 1. Tannin of *Melissa officinalis*. Proceedings of the Society for Experimental Biology and Medicine. 124:865, 874.

Lanitis S, Khan M, Sgourakis G, Kontovounisios C, Papaconstandinou T, Karaliotas C. 2012. Severe monobacterial necrotizing soft tissue infection by group A Streptococcus: A surgical emergency. *Asian Pac J Trop Biomed*. 2(3):250–2.

Lapidus N, de Lamballerie X, Salez N, Setbon M, Delabre R et al. 2013. Factors Associated with Post-Seasonal Serological Titer and Risk Factors for Infection with the Pandemic A/H1N1 Virus in the French General Population. *PLoS One*. 8(4):e60127.

Lemos J, Passos X, Fernandes F, Paula J, Ferri P et al 2005. Antifungal activity from Ocimum gratissimum L. towards Cryptococcus neoformans. *Mem Inst Oswaldo Cruz*.100(1):55–8

Lima K, Carvalho R, Carneiro I, Lima J, Sousa Cde O, et al 2011. Serratia marcescens-contaminated baby shampoo caused an outbreak among newborns at King Abdulaziz University Hospital, Jeddah, Saudi Arabia. *Pediatr Crit Care Med*. 12(6):e282–6.

Linguissi L, Bisseye C, Sagna T, Nagalo B, Ouermi D et al. 2012. Efficiency of HAART in the prevention of mother to children HIV-1 transmission at Saint Camille medical centre in Burkina Faso, West Africa. *Asian Pac J Trop Med*. 5(12):991–4.

Lipuma J. 2005. Update on the Burkholderia cepacia complex. *Curr Opin Pulm Med*. 11(6): 528–33.

Llaca-Díaz J, Mendoza-Olazarán S, Camacho-Ortiz A, Flores S, Garza-González E. 2012. One-Year Surveillance of ESKAPE Pathogens in an Intensive Care Unit of Monterrey, Mexico. *Chemotherapy*. 58(6):475–81.

Loizzo M, Saab A, Tundis R. 2008. Phytochemical analysis and in vitro antiviral activities of the essential oils of seven Lebanon species. *Chem Biodivers*. 5:461–70.

Lopes A, Mafort T, de Sá Ferreira A, Santos de Castro M, Cássia de Firmida M, de Andrade Marques E. 2012. Is the type of chronic pulmonary infection a determinant of lung function outcomes in adult patients with cystic fibrosis? *Monaldi Arch Chest Dis*. 77(3-4):122–8.

Lopes-Lutz D, Alviano D, Alviano C, Kolodziejczyk P. 2008. Screening of chemical composition, antimicrobial and antioxidant activities of *Artemisia* essential oils. *Phytochemistry*, 69(8):1732–1738.

Lorenzi V, Muselli A, Bernardini AF, Berti L, Pagès J et al 2009. Geraniol restores antibiotic activities against multidrug-resistant isolates from gram-negative species. *Antimicrob Agents Chemother*. 53(5):2209–11.

Lovell C. 1993. *Plants and the Skin*. Oxford, UK: Blackwell Scientific Publications.

Lysakowska M, Denys A, Sienkiewicz M. 2011. The activity of thyme essential oil against Acinetobacter spp. *Central European Journal of Biology*. 6(3):405–413.

Macdonald T, Langley J, Mailman T, Allain K, Nelson G et al 2011. Serratia marcescens outbreak in a neonatal intensive care unit related to the exit port of an oscillator. *Pediatr Crit Care Med*. 12(6):e282–6.

Machan T, Korth J, Liawruangrath B, Liawruangrath S, Pyne S G. 2006. Composition and antituberculosis activity of the volatile oil of Heliotropium indicum Linn. growing in Phitsanulok, Thailand. *Flavour and Fragrance Journal*. 21(2): 265–267.

MacSween R, Whaley M. 1992. Eds. Muir's Book of Pathology. 13th ed. London. Edward Arnold.

Madani T, Alsaedi S, James L, Eldeek B, Jiman-Fatani A et al. 2011. Serratia marcescens-contaminated baby shampoo causing an outbreak among newborns at King Abdulaziz University Hospital, Jeddah, Saudi Arabia. *J Hospi Infect.* 78(1): 16–9.

Mahboubi M, Shahcheraghi F, Deizabadi M. 2006. Bactericidal effects of essential oils from clove, lavender and geranium on multi-drug resistant isolates of Pseudomonas aeruginosa. *Iranian Journal of Biotechnology.* 4(2):137–40.

Mahboubi M, Kazempour N. 2012. Biochemical Activities of Iranian Cymbopogon olivieri (Boiss) Bor. Essential Oil. *Indian J Pharm Sci.* 74(4):356–60.

Mahboubi M, Kazempour N, Akbari H. 2010. Evaluation of the antimicrobial activity of natural hand rub get (Barij antimicrobial gel) in comparison to chemical hand rub gel including 0.1% triclosan under in vitro and in vivo conditions. *Int J Clinical Aromatherapy.* 7(1):18–2.

Mahboubi M, Kazempour N, Khamechian T, Fallah M, Memar Kermani M. 2011. Chemical composition and antimicrobial activity of Rosa damascena essential oil. *Journal of Biologically Active Products from Nature.* 1(1):19–26.

Mahmood N, Pacente S, Pizza C, Burke A, Khan A, Hav A. 1996. The anti-HIV activity and mechanisms of action of pure compounds isolated from Rosa damascena. *Biochem Biophys Res Commun.* 229(1):73–9.

Mansour S, Foda M, Aly A. 2012. Mosquitocidal activity of two *Bacillus* bacterial endotoxins combined with plant oils and conventional insecticides. *Industrial Crops and Products.* 35(1):44–52.

Marchaim D, Chopra T, Pogue JM, Perez F, Hujer AM et al. 2011. Outbreak of colistin-resistant, carbapenem-resistant Klebsiella pneumoniae in metropolitan Detroit, Michigan. *Antimicrob Agents Chemother.* 55(2):593–9.

Maschmeyer G, Haas A, Cornely OA. 2007. Invasive aspergillosis: epidemiology, diagnosis and management in immunocompromised patients. *Drugs.* 67(11):1567–601.

Mathias C. 1980. Contact urticaria from cinnamic aldehyde. Archives of Dermatology. 116(1) 74–76.

Meddings J, Reichert H, Rogers M, Saint S, Stephansky J, McMahon L. 2012. Effect of nonpayment for hospital-acquired, catheter-associated urinary tract infection: a statewide analysis. *Ann Intern Med.* 157(5):305–12.

Melzer M, Welch C. 2013. Outcomes in UK patients with hospital-acquired bacteraemia and the risk of catheter-associated urinary tract infections. *Postgrad Med J.* Mar 21. [Epub ahead of print] PMID: 23520064. Accessed April 29, 2013.

Mendes N, Araujo N, De Souza C et al. 1990. Molluscicidal and carcaricidal activity of different species of *Eucalyptus. Revista Societe Brasilia Medicinale Tropicale.* 23(4) 197–199.

Messager S, Hammer K, Carson C, Riley T. 2005 Effectiveness of hand-cleansing formulations containing tea tree oil assessed ex vivo on human skin and in vivo with volunteers using European standard EN 1499. *Journal of Hospital Infection.* 59(3):220–8

Mezzatesta M, Gona F, Stefani S. 2012. Enterobacter cloacae complex: clinical impact and emerging antibiotic resistance. *Future Microbiol.* 7(7):887–902.

Mishra M, Debata N, Padhy R, Rosenthal V. 2013. Surveillance of multidrug resistant uropathogenic bacteria in hospitalized patients in India. *Asian Pac J Trop Biomed.* 3(4):315–324.

Millet S, Maertens L. 2011. The European ban on antibiotic growth promoters in animal feed: from challenges to opportunities. *Vet J.* 187(2):143–4.

Misteli H, Widmer A, Rosenthal R, Oertli D, Marti W, Weber W. 2011. Spectrum of pathogens in surgical site infections at a Swiss university hospital. *Swiss Med Wkly.* :w13146. Epub 2011 Jan 20. Accessed April 29, 2013.

Moen M, Lysend-Williamson K, Scott L. 2009. Liposomal amphotericin B: a review of its use as empirical therapy in febrile neutropenia and in the treatment of invasive fungal infections. *Drugs.* 69(3): 361–92.

Moon C, Kwak YG, Kim BN, Kim ES, Lee CS. 2013. Implications of postneurosurgical meningitis caused by carbapenem-resistant Acinetobacter baumannii. *J Infect Chemother.* Apr 26. [Epub ahead of print] Accessed 29 April 2013.

Morrissey C, Chen S, Sorrell T, Bradstock K, Szer J et al. 2011. Design issues in a randomized controlled trial of a pre-emptive versus empiric antifungal strategy for invasive aspergillosis in patients with high-risk hematologic malignancies. *Leuk Lymphoma.* 52(2):179–93.

Mukherjee M, Basu S, Mukherjee S, Majumder M. 2013. Multidrug-Resistance and Extended Spectrum Beta-Lactamase Production in Uropathogenic E. Coli which were Isolated from Hospitalized Patients in Kolkata, India. *J Clin Diagn Res*. 7(3):449–53.

Múñez E, Ramos A, Alvarez de Espejo T, Vaqué J, Sánchez-Payá J et al 2012. Aetiology of surgical infections in patients undergoing craniotomy. *Neurocirugia (Astur)*. 23(2):54–9.

Nadir M, Rasheed M, Sherwani S, Kazmi S, Ahmad V. 2013. Chemical and antimicrobial studies on the essential oil from Salvia santolinifolia Boiss. *Pak J Pharm Sci*. 26(1): 39–52.

Ndiaye M, Tine R, Faye B, Ndiaye J, Lo A et al. 2013. Selection of Antimalarial Drug Resistance after Intermittent Preventive Treatment of Infants and Children (IPTi/c) in Senegal. *Am J Trop Med Hyg*. [Epub ahead of print]PMID: 23589534. Accessed April 28, 2013.

Nedorostove L, Kloucek P, Urbanova K, Kokoska L, Smid J, et al. 2011. Antibacterial effect of essential oil vapours against different strains of Staphylococcus aureus, including MRSA. *Flavour and Fragrance Journal*. 26(6):403–407.

Nelson R. 1997. In vitro activities of five plant essential oils against methicillin-resistant *Staphylococcus aureus* and vancomycin-resistant *Entericoccus faecium*. *Journal of Antimicrobial Chemotherapy*. 40(2) 305–306.

Neuner E, Sekeres J, Hall G, van Duin D. 2012. Experience with fosfomycin for treatment of urinary tract infections due to multidrug-resistant organisms. *Antimicrob Agents Chemother*. 56(11):5744–8.

Newman RM, Kuntzen T, Weiner B, Berical A, Charlebois P et al. 2012. Whole Genome Pyrosequencing of Rare Hepatitis C Virus Genotypes Enhances Subtype Classification and Identification of Naturally Occurring Drug Resistance Variants. *J Infect Dis*. 2012 Dec 13; Accessed May 7 2013.

Nichol K, Adam H, Roscoe D, Golding G, Lagacé-Wiens P et al. 2013. Changing epidemiology of methicillin-resistant Staphylococcus aureus in Canada..*J Antimicrob Chemother*. 68 Suppl 1:i47–i55.

Ocazionez R, Meneses R, Torres F, Stashenko E. 2010. Virucidal activity of Colombian Lippia essential oils on dengue virus replication in vitro. *Mem Inst Oswaldo Cruz*. 105(3):304–9.

Oliveira Carvalho V, Okay T, Melhem M, Walderez Szeszs M, Del Negro G. 2013. The new mutation L321F in Candida albicans ERG11 gene may be associated with fluconazole resistance. *Rev Iberoam Micol*. Feb 9. doi:pii: S1130–1406(13)00013-2. 10.1016/j.riam.2013.01.001. [Epub ahead of print]

Opalchenova G, Obreshkova D. 2003. Comparative studies on the activity of basil—an essential oil from Ocimum basilicum L. -against multidrug resistant clinical isolates of the genera Staphylococcus, Enterococcus and Pseudomonas by using different test methods. *Journal of Microbiological Methods*. 54(1): 105–110.

Orhan I, Ozcelik B, Kan Y, Kartal M. 2011. Inhibitory effects of various essential oils and individual components against extended-spectrum beta-lactamase (ESBL) produced by Klebsiella pneumoniae and their chemical compositions. *J Food Science*. 76(8):M538–46.

Ovadia M, Kalily I, Berstein E. 2009. Cinnamon Fraction Neutralizes Avian Influenza H5N1 Both In Vitro and In Vivo. Antiviral Research 82(2): A35.

Owlia P, Saderi H, Rasooli I, Sefidkon F. 2009. Antimicrobial characteristics of some herbal oils on Pseudomonas aeruginosa with special reference to their chemical compositions. *Iranian Journal of Pharmaceutical Research*. 8(2):107–114.

Pastar I, Nusbaum A, Gil J, Patel S, Chen J. 2013. Interactions of methicillin resistant Staphylococcus aureus USA300 and Pseudomonas aeruginosa in polymicrobial wound infection. *PLoS One*. 8(2):e56846. doi: 10.1371/.

Pinto E, Hrimpeng K, Lopes G, Vaz S, Gonçalves M et al 2013. Antifungal activity of Ferulago capillaris essential oil against Candida, Cryptococcus, Aspergillus and dermatophyte species. Eur *J Clin Microbiol Infect Dis*. 2013 Apr 26. [Epub ahead of print]. Accessed May 15, 2013.

Praparattanapan J, Kotarathitithum W, Chaiwarith R, Nuntachit N, Sirisanthana T, Supparatpinyo K. 2012. Resistance-associated mutations after initial antiretroviral treatment failure in a large cohort of patients infected with HIV-1 subtype CRF01_AE. *Curr HIV Res*. 10(8):647–52.

Perfect JR. 2013. Fungal diagnosis: how do we do it and can we do better? *Curr Med Res Opin*. 29(4):3–11.

Posluszny J Jr, Conrad P, Halerz M, Shankar R, Gamelli R. 2011. Surgical burn wound infections and their clinical implications. *J Burn Care Res*. 32(2):324–33.

Rath C, Devi S, Dash S, Mishra R. 2008. Antibacterial potential assessment of jasmine essential oil against E. coli. *Journal of Ethnopharmacology.* 70(2): 197–201.

Rattanaumpawan P, Ussavasodhi P, Kiratisin P, Aswapokee N. 2013. Epidemiology of bacteremia caused by uncommon non-fermentative gram-negative bacteria. *BMC Infect Dis.* 13(1):167.

Reichling J J, Koch C, Stahl-Biskup E, Sojka C, Schnitzler P. 2005. Virucidal activity of a beta-triketone-rich essential oil of Leptospermum scoparium (manuka oil) against HSV-1 and HSV-2 in cell culture. *Planta Med.* 71(12):1123–7.

Reichling J, Schnitzler P, Suschke U, Saller R. 2009. Essential oils of aromatic plants with antibacterial, antifungal, antiviral and cytotoxic properties—an overview. *Forsch Komplementmed.* 16: 79–90.

Reichling J. 2010. Antiviral effects of essential oils used traditionally in aromatherapy. *Int J Clinical Aromatherapy.* 7(1):29–35.

Reissig A, Mempel C, Schumacher U, Copetti R, Gross F, Aliberti S. 2013. Microbiological Diagnosis and Antibiotic Therapy in Patients with Community-Acquired Pneumonia and Acute COPD Exacerbation in Daily Clinical Practice: Comparison to Current Guidelines. *Lung.* Apr 6. [Epub ahead of print] PMID: 23564195. Accessed April 29, 2013.

Roberts R, Scott R 2nd, Hota B, Kampe L, Abbasi F et al. 2010. Costs attributable to healthcare-acquired infection in hospitalized adults and a comparison of economic methods. *Med Care.* 48(11):1026–35.

Rodrigues D. 2013. Personal communication.

Rodrigues M, Fortaleza C, Riboli D, Rocha R, Rocha C, Cunha. M. 2013. Molecular epidemiology of methicillin-resistant Staphylococcus aureus in a burn unit from Brazil. *Burns.* S0305-4179(13) 00047–8.

Rogowska-Szadkowska D. 2008. 2008 Nobel Prize for Medicine or Physiology for discovery of HPV and HIV viruses – short history of discovery of HIV. *HIV & AIDS Review.* 7(4):5–9.

Roller S, Ernest N, Buckle J. 2009. The antimicrobial activity of high-necrodane and other lavender oils on methicillin-sensitive and -resistant Staphylococcus aureus (MSSA and MRSA). *Journal of Alternative and Complementary Medicine.* 15(3):275–279.

Romano K, Ali A, Aydin C, Soumana D, Ozen A et al. 2012. The molecular basis of drug resistance against hepatitis C virus NS3/4A protease inhibitors. *PLoS Pathog.* 8(7):e1002832. Accessed May 7, 2013.

Rosato A, Piarulli M, Corbo F, Muraglia M, Carone A et al. 2010. In vitro synergistic antibacterial action of certain combinations of gentamicin and essential oils. *Curr Med Chem.* 17(28):3289–95.

Rosenberger L, Hranjec T, Politano A, Swenson B, Metzger R et al 2011. Effective cohorting and "superisolation" in a single intensive care unit in response to an outbreak of diverse multi-drug-resistant organisms. *Surg Infect (Larchmt).* 12(5):345–50.

Ross S, El-Keltawi N, Megella, S. 1980. Antimicrobial activity of some Egyptian aromatic plants. *Fitoterapia.* 51(4) 201–205.

Rotter M, Sattar S, Dharan S, Allegranzi B, Mathai E, Pittet D. 2009. Methods to evaluate the microbicidal activities of hand-rub and hand-wash agents. *J Hosp Infect.* 73(3):191–9.

Saddi M, Senna A, Cottiglia F, Chisu L, Casu L et al. 2007. Antiherpevirus activity of Artemisia arborescens essential oil and inhibition of lateral diffusion in Vero cells. *Ann Clin Microbiol Antimicrob.* 6:1–10.

Saidi M, Ghafourian S, Zarin-Abaadi M, Movahedi K, Sadeghifard N. 2012. In vitro antimicrobial and antioxidant activity of black thyme (Thymbra spicata L.) essential oils. *Roum Arch Microbiol Immunol.* 71(2):61–9.

Sadlon A, Lamson D. 2010. Immune-modifying and antimicrobial effects of Eucalyptus oil and simple inhalation devices. *Altern Med Rev.* 15(1):33–47.

Salyers A, Moon K, David Schlessinger D. 2007. The Human Intestinal Tract- a hotbed of resistant gene transfer? Part 11. *Clinical Microbiology Newsletter.* 29(4): 25–30.

Schnitzler P, Koch C, Reichling J. 2007. Susceptibility of drug-resistant clinical Herpes simplex virus type 1 strains to essential oils of ginger, thyme, hyssop, and sandalwood. *Antimicrobial Agents and Chemotherapy.* 51(5):1859–1862.

Schnitzler P, Schön K, Reichling J. 2001. Antiviral activity of Australian tea tree oil and eucalyptus oil against herpes simplex virus in cell culture. *Pharmazie.* 56(4): 343–7.

Schnitzler P, Schuhmacher A, Astani A, Reichling J. 2008. Melissa officinalis oil affects infectivity of enveloped herpesviruses. *Phytomedicine.* 15(9):734–40.

Scott P, Deye G, Srinivasan A, Murray C, Moran K et al. 2007. US Military Health Care System Associated with Military Operations in Iraq. *Clinical Infectious Diseases.* 44:1577–84.

Sears P, Ichikawa Y, Ruiz N, Gorbach S. 2013. Advances in the treatment of Clostridium difficile with fidaxomicin: a narrow spectrum antibiotic. *Ann N Y Acad Sci.* May 14. doi: 10.1111/nyas. Accessed May 20, 2013.

Shah D, Dang M, Hasbun R, Koo H, Jiang Z et al. 2010. Clostridium difficile infection: update on emerging antibiotic treatment options and antibiotic resistance. *Expert Rev Anti Infect Ther.* 8(5):555–64.

Shahverdi A R, Monsef-Esfahani H R, Tavasoli F, Zaheri A, Mirjani R. 2007. Trans-cinnamaldehyde from cinnamomum zeylanicum bark essential oil reduces the clindamycin resistance of Clostridium difficile in vitro. *Journal of Food Science.* 72(1):S055–S058.

Sherry E, Boeck H, Warnke P. 2001. Percutaneous treatment of chronic MRSA osteomyelitis with a novel plant-derived antiseptic. BioMed Central Surgery. www.biomedcentral.com.

Sherry E, Reynolds M, Sivananthan S, Mainawalala S, Warnke P. 2004. Inhalational phytochemicals as possible treatment for pulmonary tuberculosis: two case reports. *American Journal of Infection Control.* 32(6): 369–370.

Shigemura K, Arakawa S, Tanaka K, Fujisawa M. 2009. Clinical investigation of isolated bacteria from urinary tracts of hospitalized patients and their susceptibilities to antibiotics. *J Infect Chemother.* 15(1):18–22.

Shigemura K, Tanaka K, Osawa K, Arakawa S, Miyake H, Fujisawa M. 2013. Clinical factors associated with shock in bacteremic UTI. *Int Urol Nephrol.* Apr 25. Accessed April 28, 2013.

Shin S, Kim J. 2005. In vitro inhibitory activities of essential oils from two Korean thymus species against antibiotic-resistant pathogens. *Arch Pharm Res.* 28(8):897–901.

Shime N, Kosaka T, Fujita N. 2013. De-escalation of antimicrobial therapy for bacteraemia due to difficult-to-treat Gram-negative bacilli. *Infection.* 41(1):203–10.

Shu J, Su L, Chia J, Huang S, Kao Y et al. 2012. Identification of a hidden outbreak due to the spread of a VIM-3-producing, extensive drug-resistant Pseudomonas aeruginosa (XDRPA) clone at a regional hospital in Taiwan. *Epidemiol Infect.* 9:1–4.

Si H, Hu J, Liu Z, Zeng L. 2008. Antibacterial effect of oregano essential oil alone and in combination with antibiotics against extended-spectrum β-lactamase-producing Escherichia coli. *FEMS immunology and medical microbiology.* 53(2): 190–4.

Siddiqui Y, Ettayebi M, Haddad A, Al-Ahdal M. 1996. Effect of essential oils on enveloped viruses: antiviral activity of oregano and clove oils on herpes simplex virus type 1 and Newcastle disease virus. *Med Sci Res.* 24: 185–186.

Singh R, Shushni M, Belkheir A. 2011. Antibacterial and antioxidant activities of *Mentha piperita. Arabian Journal of Chemistry.* http://dx.doi.org/10.1016/j.arabjc.2011.01.019, Accessed May 16, 2013.

Smeekens S, van de Veerdonk F, Kullberg B, Netea M. 2013. Genetic susceptibility to Candida infections. *EMBO Mol Med.* 2013 Apr 30. doi: 10.1002/emmm.201201678. Accessed May 15, 2013.

Sparks T. 1985. Cinnamon oil burns. *Western Journal of Medicine.* 142(6): 835.

Stasi C, Rosselli M, Zignego AL, Laffi G, Milani S. 2013. Serotonin and its implication in the side-effects of interferon-based treatment of patients with chronic viral hepatitis: Pharmacological interventions. *Hepatol Res.* Mar 25. doi: 10.1111/hepr.12116. Accessed May 7, 2013.

Stringer J. 2010. Infection in the clinical environment: challenges and benefits of using essential oils – a therapist's perspective. *Int J of Clinical Aromatherapy.* 7(1): 11–17.

Tadtong S, Suppawat S, Tintawee A, Saramas P, Jareonvong S, Hongratanaworakit T. 2012. Antimicrobial activity of blended essential oil preparation. *Nat Prod Commun.* 7(10):1401–4.

Tantry B, Rahiman S. 2012. Antibacterial resistance and trend of urinary tract pathogens to commonly used antibiotics in Kashmir Valley. *West Indian Med J.* 61(7):703–7.

Tavares A, Miragaia M, Rolo J, Coelho C, de Lencastre H. 2013. High prevalence of hospital-associated methicillin-resistant Staphylococcus aureus in the community in Portugal: evidence for the blurring of community-hospital boundaries. *Eur J Clin Microbiol Infect Dis.* 2013 Apr 21. Apr 21. [Epub ahead of print]. Accessed. 29 April 2013.

Thai H, Campo D, Lara J, Dimitrova Z, Ramachandran S et al. 2012. Convergence and coevolution of hepatitis B virus drug resistance. *Nat Commun.* Apr 17; 3:789. Epub 2012 Apr 17. Accessed 7 May 2013.

Tohidpour A, Sattari M, Omidbaigi R, Yadegar A, Nazemi J. 2010. Antibacterial effect of essential oils from two medicinal plants against Methicillin-resistant Staphylococcus aureus (MRSA). *Phytomedicine.* 17(2):142–145.

Tragoolpua Y, Jatisatienr A. 2007. Anti-herpes simplex virus activities of Eugenia caryophyllus (Spreng.) Bullock & S. G. Harrison and essential oil, eugenol. *Phytotherapy Research.* 21(12):1153–1158.

Tsai A, Dueger E, Macalino G, Montano S, Tilley D et al. 2013. The U.S. military's Neisseria gonorrhoeae resistance surveillance initiatives in selected populations of five countries. *MSMR.* 20(2):25–7.

Tseng H, Liu C, Ho M, Lu P, Lo H et al 2013. Microbiological, epidemiological, and clinical characteristics and outcomes of patients with cryptococcosis in Taiwan, 1997-2010. *PLoS One.* 17;8(4):e61921.

Turner C, Dryden M, Holden M, Davies F, Lawrenson R, et al 2013. Lethal Streptococcus pyogenes postpartum sepsis: Molecular analysis of an outbreak. *J Clin Microbiol.* Apr 24. [Epub ahead of print]. Accessed 28 April, 2013.

Tyagi A, Malik A. 2010. Antimicrobial action of essential oil vapours and negative air ions against Pseudomonas fluorescens. *Int J Food Microbiology.* 143(3):205–210.

Uvizl R, Hanulik V, Husickova V, Sedlakova M, Adamus M, Kolar M. 2011. Hospital-acquired pneumonia in ICU patients. *Biomed Pap Med Fac Univ Palacky Olomouc Czech Repub.* 155(4):373–8.

Vale-Silva LA, Gonçalves MJ, Cavaleiro C, Salgueiro L, Pinto E. 2010. Antifungal activity of the essential oil of Thymus x viciosoi against Candida, Cryptococcus, Aspergillus and dermatophyte species. *Planta Med.* 76(9):882–8.

van der Linden J, Camps S, Kampinga G, Arends J, Debets-Ossenkopp Y et al 2013. Aspergillosis due to Voriconazole Highly-resistant Aspergillus fumigatus and Recovery of Genetically Related Resistant Isolates from Domestic Homes. *Clin Infect Dis.* May 10. Accessed May 15, 2013.

Vázquez-González D, Perusquía-Ortiz AM, Hundeiker M, Bonifaz A. 2013.Opportunistic yeast infections: candidiasis, cryptococcosis, trichosporonosis and geotrichosis. *J Dtsch Dermatol Ges.* 11(5):381–94.

Vourlioti-Arapi F, Michaelakis A, Evergetis E, Koliopoulos G, Haroutounian SA. 2012. Essential oils of indigenous in Greece six Juniperus taxa: chemical composition and larvicidal activity against the West Nile virus vector Culex pipiens. *Parasitol Res.* 110(5):1829–39.

Wang H, Shi H, Zhou W, Hu Z, Mu L et al. 2012. Common pathogens and clinical characteristics of neonatal pneumonia. *Int J Infect Dis.* Mar 18. S1201–9712(13)00084-2. Accessed 1 May, 2013.

Warnke P, Becker S, Podschun R, Sivananthan S, Springer I et al. 2009. The battle against multi-resistant strains: renaissance of antimicrobial essential oils as a promising force to fight hospital-acquired infections. *J of Cranio-Maxillo-Facial Surgery.* 37(7):392–7.

Warnke P, Lott A, Sherry E, Podschun R. 2013. The ongoing battle against multi-resistant strains: *In-vitro* inhibition of hospital-acquired MRSA, VRE, *Pseudomonas*, ESBL *E. coli* and *Klebsiella* species in the presence of plant-derived antiseptic oils. *J Cranio-Maxillofacial Surgery.* 41(4):321–236.

Waturangi D, Wennars M, Suhartono M, Wijaya Y. 2013. Edible ice in Jakarta, Indonesia, is contaminated with multidrug-resistant Vibrio cholerae with virulence potential. *J Med Microbiol.* 62(Pt 3):352–9.

Whalen J, Mully T, English J 3rd. 2007. Spontaneous Citrobacter freundii infection in an immunocompetent patient. *Archives Dermatology.* 143(1):124–5.

Wu S, Patel K, Booth L, Metcalf J, Lin H, Wu W. 2010. Protective essential oil attenuates influenza virus infection: an in vitro study in MDCK cells. *BMC Complement Altern Med.* 10:69. doi: 10.1186/1472-6882-10-69.

Yang C, Zhou LL, Wang HY, Huang SN, Liu Q et al. 2011. The inhibitory effect of Zingiber corallinum Hance essential oil on drug-resistant bacteria and evaluation of its acute toxicity. *Med Sci Monit.* 17(5):BR139–46.

Yeh C, Chang, J, Wang K, Shieh D, Chiang L. 2013. Water extract of *Cinnamomum cassia* Blume inhibited human respiratory syncytial virus by preventing viral attachment, internalization, and syncytium formation. *Journal of Ethnopharmacology.* 147(2):321–326.

Zhanel GG, Adam HJ, Baxter MR, Fuller J, Nichol KA. 2013. Antimicrobial susceptibility of 22746 pathogens from Canadian hospitals: results of the CANWARD 2007-11 study. *J Antimicrob Chemother.* 68 Suppl 1:i7–i22.

Zeller H, Marrama L, Sudre B, Van Bortel W, Warns-Petit E. 2013. Mosquito-borne disease surveillance by the European Centre for Disease Prevention and Control. *Clin Microbiol Infect.* Apr 22. doi: 10.1111/1469-0691.12230. Accessed April 28, 2013.

Zuzarte M, Gonçalves MJ, Cavaleiro C, Canhoto J, Vale-Silva L et al. 2011. Chemical composition and antifungal activity of the essential oils of Lavandula viridis L'Her. *J Med Microbiol.* 60(Pt 5):612–8.

Zuzarte M, Gonçalves MJ, Cruz MT, Cavaleiro C, Canhoto J et al. 2012. Lavandula luisieri essential oil as a source of antifungal drugs. *Food Chem.* 135(3):1505–10.

Chapter 8

Insomnia

"Each night, when I go to sleep, I die. And the next morning, when I wake up, I am reborn."

Mahatma Gandhi

CHAPTER ASSETS

OVERVIEW

Today's society is fast-moving and thousands of people travel daily, often across time zones. Regularity and sleep patterns are constantly disturbed as new sounds and unfamiliar surroundings compound the sense of timelessness caused by continuous movement. Sleep has become a commodity to be bought and sold. Approximately 30% of the general population has insomnia (Jahangir et al 2008). It is estimated that 40% of all insomnia patients have a coexisting psychiatric condition (Ancoli-Israel 2006). Insomnia and depression share a common pathologic process. This makes people susceptible to both conditions—specifically, abnormal regulation of corticotropin-releasing factor (CRF). Arroll et al (2012) found 50% insomnia participants (n = 388) had depression. Insomnia impairs cognitive and physical functioning and insomniacs are more prone to accidents. Insomnia affects job performance and results in time off work. Insomnia affects quality of life. Women are 1.4 times more likely to have insomnia than men with elderly females the most at risk (Jahangir et al 2008).

Patients in the hospital are separated from everything that enables them to feel relaxed. They are in a strange bed, with strange smells, strange noises, and a strange routine. Unsurprisingly, many patients feel apprehensive and are unable to sleep. Even frequently hospitalized patients find sleep difficult (Boonstra et al 2011;

Haynes et al 2011; Isaia et al 2011). Good sleep hygiene, for example, going to bed when sleepy and not napping during the day, can alleviate symptoms in 30% of insomniacs (Falloon et al 2011) and, in some studies, is as effective as sleeping pills. However, good sleep hygiene may be difficult in a hospital environment. Cognitive behavioral therapy (CBT) has been successful for insomnia (Morgenthaler et al 2006). However, CBT is not available in hospitals; therefore, night sedation may be the only choice for hospital patients.

Sleep

Sleep is defined by Brooker (2008) as a "naturally altered state of consciousness occurring in humans in a 24 hour biological rhythm." Sleep occurs in two forms: rapid eye movement (REM), when dreaming occurs, and non-rapid eye movement (NREM). Both types are important. REM sleep occurs three to four times each night and lasts from 5 minutes to over 1 hour (Hsieh et al., 2012). During this time, the brain waves are fast, low voltage and both heart rate and respiration are irregular. During NREM, brain waves are slow, high voltage and both heart rate and blood pressure are low and regular. Humans have a 24-hour circadian rhythm that is controlled by a central circadian pacemaker located in the suprachiasmatic nucleus (SCN) of the hypothalamus (Dijk et al 2012). Twelve percent of insomniacs have delayed sleep circadian rhythm disorder (Falloon et al 2011). Hospitalized patients sometimes require high-dose opioids. This produces a complete lack of REM sleep (Gay 2010). Patients who require mechanical ventilation also lack a normal circadian rhythm. Sleep is controlled by melatonin—a signaling hormone secreted by the pineal gland. Melatonin is also synthesized in various other organs and tissues in the body (Hardeland 2012).

Insomnia

Insomnia is either primary, with no underlying cause, or secondary, with an underlying condition (Falloon et al 2011). According to the American Sleep Disorders Association (2005), insomnia is repeated difficulty in falling asleep, staying asleep, or poor quality of sleep for at least 1 month. Roth (2007) states this difficulty is "present despite adequate opportunity and circumstance to sleep. The impairment in sleep is associated with daytime impairment or distress. Sleep difficulty occurs at least 3 times per week and has been a problem for at least 1 month." All the above types of insomnia may occur in hospital patients, where strange noises and smells permeate dreams or prevent sleep from occurring.

Night Sedation

Several websites, including The Mayo Clinic, suggest there are two types of night sedation: sedatives (anxiolytics) and sedative/hypnotics. Thorpy and Roth (2013) suggest dividing sedative/hypnotics that induce and/or maintain sleep into the following categories (Tables 8-1 and 8-2).
1. Benzodiazepine receptor agonists (BZDs). These can be short, medium, or long acting and are for short-term use—up to 1 month. Examples are estazolam (ProSom), flurazepam (Dalmane), quazepam (Dormalin), temazepam (Restoril),

TABLE 8-1 *Some Short-Acting Drugs That Initiate Sleep*

Name	Type	Precautions	Side Effects
Zopiclone (Lunesta)	Z	Drug/alcohol abuse Depression Respiratory problems	Heavy meals may slow absorption Sudden withdrawal may lead to unpleasant symptoms
Ramelteon (Rozerem)	M	Pregnancy, breast-feeding Liver, kidney, or respiratory disease Depression or sleep apnea	May interact with alcohol Heavy meals may slow absorption
Triazolam (Halcion)	B	Pregnancy, breast-feeding Depression, respiratory conditions History of drug abuse	Interacts with grapefruit juice, alcohol, and some medications Drug must be halted gradually Seldom prescribed because of habit-forming property
Zaleplon (Sonata)	Z	Pregnancy, breast-feeding Liver, kidney, or respiratory disease Depression	May interact with other medications Heavy meals may slow absorption Fast and short acting Can be habit-forming
Zolpidem (Ambien, Edluar)	Z	Liver, kidney, or respiratory disease Depression	May become less effective over time Sleep effects such as sleep-driving and sleep-eating may occur

Information has been gleaned from individual drug websites and The Mayo Clinic website (2012).
B = Benzodiazepine; M = melatonin receptor agonist; Z = nonbenzodiazepine (Z medicine).

triazolam (Halcion), diazepam (Valium), lorazepam (Ativan), and nitrazepam (Mogadon).

2. Nonbenzodiazepines (Z medicines). Examples are zolpidem, zaleplon, and zopiclone. These act via γ-aminobutyric acid (GABA)ergic neurotransmission. It is important to have at least 7 hours sleep after taking Z medicines (NHS Choices 2013).

3. Histamine-1 receptor antagonists. Examples are doxepin and diphenhydramine.

4. Melatonin receptor agonists. Ramelteon (Rozerem) is approved for sleep-onset insomnia in the United States and Japan, but not yet in Europe (Takeda 2011). Circadin is the brand name for melatonin in the UK (NHS Choices 2013). Melatonin plus light box therapy can also be useful for circadian rhythm sleep disorder (Murakami et al 2012). Melatonin is available online as a food supplement.

5. Circadian regulators. These drugs reset the circadian clock in the SCN of the hypothalamus. Agomelatine (Valdoxan, Melitor, Thymanax) is a melatonergic antidepressant that appears to also have positive effects on insomnia (O'Neill et al 2013).

TABLE 8-2 *Some Drugs That Prolong Sleep*

Name	Type	Precautions	Pointers
Estazolam (ProSom)	B	Pregnancy, breast-feeding Elderly patient	May interact with many medications Can be habit-forming Falls in the elderly

Eszopiclone (Lunesta)	Z	Depression, lung disease
		Alcohol abuse
		Metabolic disorders
			Heavy meals may slow
			  absorption
			Sudden withdrawal may lead
			  to unpleasant symptoms

Temazepam (Restoril)	B	Pregnancy, breast-feeding
		Kidney or liver problems
		Depression, substance
		  abuse
		Lung disease
			May interact with many
			  medications
			May react with alcohol
			Can be habit-forming

Zolpidem (Ambien CR)	Z	Pregnancy, breast-feeding Kidney or liver problems Depression	Extended-release formula

Information has been gleaned from research (Jacob et al., 2012; Majdan et al., 2012), individual drug websites and The Mayo Clinic website (2012).
B = Benzodiazepine; Z = nonbenzodiazepine (Z medicine).

AROMATHERAPY FOR INSOMNIA

Background

Nearly 30 years ago, the headline "Lavender Beats Benzodiazepines" (Tisserand 1988) introduced the idea that aromatherapy could be useful for insomnia. Tisserand outlined the use of essential oils of lavender, marjoram, geranium, mandarin, and cardamom as sleep aids in a hospital. Aromatherapy can be beneficial to relax patients, thus enabling them to sleep or to restore a normal sleep pattern.

Helen Passant, possibly the most holistic nurse after Florence Nightingale, introduced aromatherapy into the Churchill Hospital in Oxford, England, in the 1980s, when she was in charge of a ward for the elderly. Remarkably, Passant reduced her original drug bill by one third by gradually replacing analgesia and night sedation with essential oils. She found her patients seemed to "get off to sleep just as easily, if not better, with oils of lavender or marjoram, either vaporized or applied by massage" (Tisserand 1988). Around the same time, another hospital in Oxford, The Radcliffe Infirmary, introduced aromatherapy into the Beeson Ward. Patients were given the option of aromatherapy instead of night sedation or analgesics. Nearly all of the patients chose aromatherapy (Tisserand 1988).

In a survey of six countries (Canada, Germany, Japan, Mexico, UK, and the United States), 84% of UK residents could recall "the distinct smell of how their bedroom smelled" (National Sleep Foundation 2013, http://www.sleepfoundation.org). More than 50% of residents of all other countries in the survey (except Japan) could also remember. According to this study, 50% of residents of five countries (except Germany) liked the smell of lavender or jasmine in their bedroom. Seventy percent of residents of five countries (except Japan) said the smell of antiseptic detracted them from sleep. This is not surprising because aromas have an affect even when we are sleeping (Arzi et al 2010). If we can make a hospital bed smell more like the patient's bed at home, there is increased chance they will be able to sleep.

PUBLISHED AROMATHERAPY STUDIES

The following selection has been chosen to give a broad overview of some of the aromatherapy studies that have been published on insomnia. It is not intended to be a systematic review. New additions to this third edition include studies from 2000 onwards. I have selected studies from as many countries as possible, using a range of databases (Pubmed, Science Direct, Royal College of Nursing, Quintessential.co.uk, and Herbalgram), and I have chosen essential oils that are readily available and safe to use on hospital patients. It is difficult to conceal aroma, and lavender is well recognized and associated with relaxation. However, the studies outlined below will hopefully give some credence to a nurse or physician's wish to try aromatherapy for their patient's insomnia.

LAVENDER

Background

True lavender *(Lavandula angustifolia)* has a long history of use in aromatherapy to promote sleep and relaxation and to relieve anxiety. In Bulgaria, Atanassova-Shopova et al (1973) found that linalol and terpineol were the active components of lavender and they had a depressing effect on the central nervous system (CNS). Oral doses of linalool were found to be hypnotic and anticonvulsant in mice in a study by Elisabetsky et al (1995a). Elisabetsky et al (1995b) also established that linalol inhibited glutamate binding in rat cortex in a way similar to phenobarbital. The glutamate binding involved all receptor subtypes investigated. A Japanese study (Yamada et al 1994) concurred that inhaled lavender had anticonvulsant effects in mice. Linalool, one of the main components of lavender, was found to induce sleep in mice in a later study by de Moura Lincke et al (2009).

In France, Guillemain et al (1989) agreed that oral doses of lavender (diluted 1:60 in olive oil) had marked sedative effects on mice and enhanced barbiturate sleep time. In Germany, Buchbauer et al (1991) in Germany discovered that lavender had a sedative effect when inhaled by mice. Interestingly, the more agitated the animal was (as a result of injecting caffeine), the stronger the sedative effect of the lavender. Jager et al (1992a) established that lavender diluted in peanut oil was absorbed through the skin.

Henry et al (1994) carried out a 7-week study on human subjects at Newholme Hospital in Bakewell, England. Lavender was diffused at night in a ward of patients with dementia. Diffused lavender had a statistically significant sedative effect. Hudson (1996) also found lavender was effective for elderly patients in a long-term unit. Eight of the nine patients in the study had improved sleep at night and improved alertness during the day. Lavender straw (the byproduct of distillation) was itself found to reduce the stress of pigs in transit in a study by Bradshaw et al (1998).

Recent Studies

Recent published studies include an American one by Goel et al (2005) who found that inhaled lavender increased the percentage of deep or slow-wave sleep (SWS) in 31 men and women in a sleep laboratory. Goel describes aromatherapy as an "anecdotal method for modifying sleep and mood." At the end of the study, Goel concludes "lavender serves as a mild sedative and has practical applications as a novel, nonphotic method for promoting deep sleep in young men and women and for producing gender-dependent sleep effects." His study showed a difference between the effect of lavender on sleep patterns in men and women. A 12-week controlled trial in Taiwan monitored the effect of lavender on heart rate variation (HRV) in 67 women with insomnia (Chien et al 2012). Outcomes measured included the Chinese version of the Pittsburgh Sleep Quality Index (PSQI). The experimental group received lavender inhalation twice a week for 12 weeks. The control group received a health education program on sleep. Women receiving aromatherapy experienced a significant improvement in sleep quality after intervention (P = 0.001). A Korean study (Lee & Lee 2006) explored the effects of inhaled lavender on 42 women college students with insomnia. The 4-week protocol comprised 1 week baseline, 1 week lavender, 1 week washout, and 1 week lavender. The length of time taken to fall asleep plus quality of sleep and satisfaction of sleep all improved by 60% (P = 0.0001).

A British study in 2005 led by Lewith, a physician, explored the effects of lavender using a diffuser. The 4-week protocol was similar to the Korean study with a baseline, lavender week, washout week, and second lavender week. Ten volunteers with insomnia rated PSQI as well as other questionnaires rating treatment credibility and attitudes to complementary alternative medicine (CAM). The lavender group had a 2.5 point reduction in the PSQI scale (P = 0.07). Women and younger volunteers improved the most.

An Iranian study (Moeini et al 2010) explored the use of lavender for insomnia in patients with ischemic heart disease in a hospital coronary care unit (CCU). Sixty-four patients took part in the controlled study that lasted three nights. Each time, aromatherapy was diffused for 9 hours. The sleep quality of the lavender group was better than that of the control group (P = 0.001).

Expectancy may play a role in aromatherapy and a double-blind, placebo-controlled trial study by Howard & Hughes (2008) concluded "previous associations of lavender aroma with assisted relaxation may have been influenced by expectancy biases." Because of this, a Moroccan team led by Alnamer (2012) explored the sedative and hypnotic effects of methanolic and aqueous extracts of lavender on mice (who could not be accused of being biased by expectancy) using diazepam as the control. They found that "extracts of *Lavandula officinalis* have potent sedative and hypnotic activities." However, a systematic review of all complementary therapies

TABLE 8-3 *Published Studies on Insomnia and Essential Oils*

Author	Year	Number	Essential Oil	Method	Result
Lewith et al	2005	10	Lavender	Inhaled	+ve
Goel et al	2005	31	Lavender	Inhaled	+ve
Lee & Lee	2006	42	Lavender	Inhaled	+ve
Fewell et al	2007	36	Sweet orange	Topical	−ve
Howard & Hughes	2008	96	Lavender	Inhaled	−ve
Komori et al	2006	29	Mixture*	Inhaled	+ve
Jahangir et al	2008	36	Rose	Oral	+ve
Hongratanawor-akit	2009	40	Rose	Topical	+ve
Arzi et al	2010	36	Lavender, vetivert	Inhaled	Affected respiration during sleep
Moeini et al	2010	64	Lavender	Inhaled	+ve
Chien et al	2012	67	Lavender	Inhaled	+ve
Alnamer	2012	Mice	Lavender	Inhaled	+ve
Johannessen	2013	24	Lavender	Inhaled	+ve

*A mixture of sandalwood (35%), juniper berry (12%), rose (8%), and orris (6%).

used in insomnia concluded that aromatherapy was poorly represented (Sarris & Byrne 2011). Table 8-3 shows that there are surprisingly few studies on aromatherapy and insomnia and most involve lavender. This is disappointing because aromatherapy is a very simple complementary therapy to try.

Despite this lack of evidence, essential oils are being used for insomnia. A recent Norwegian survey of 12 nurses working in four different establishments found that lavender *(Lavandula augustifolia)* essential oil had been diffused nightly and this had reduced insomnia in all four residential homes for dementia patients (Johannessen 2013). In the UK, a 28-month audit of aromatherapy at the Royal Marsden Hospital, London showed that aromasticks (containing either lavender plus petitgrain or lavender plus mandarin) were offered to cancer patients with insomnia (Dyer et al 2013).

RJ Buckle students have conducted 21 pilot studies on insomnia (Table 8-4). Seven of these studies used lavender. The patient populations included children, adults, night nurses, and children with autism. Methodology was varied and used topical application, inhalers, and diffusers. Blyth (2011) explored the effect of aromatherapy on the sleep patterns of children with autism. Parents applied 2% *Lavandula angustifolia* cream to the forearms of their children just before bedtime (n =10). The parents documented the hours of sleep and the waking episodes for a 3-week period. The first week was baseline, followed by the lavender week, then washout. The length of time the children slept did not change. However, 8 of the 10 children had a dramatic reduction in the number of times they awoke and needed

TABLE 8-4 *Studies Carried out by RJ Buckle Students*

Name	Year	State	N	Adults/Children	Essential Oil
Davis	1997	NM	11	Adults	Lavender
Weihbrecht	1999	PA	9	Adults	Lavender
Knuteson	2000	IN	8	Children	Mandarin
Hull	2000	WA	12	Adults	Ravensara
King	2001	IN	10	Adults	Sweet marjoram and Roman chamomile
Cashman	2002	PA	10	Adults	Clary sage and sweet marjoram
Tisdale	2002	PA	10	Night nurses	Ravensara
Knowles	2002	WA	20	Adults	Lavender
Dupos	2002	PA	12	Adults	Lavender and Roman chamomile
Vought	2003	MN	10	Adults	Lavender and sweet marjoram
Tomanino	2005	MN	9	Adults	Lavender and sweet marjoram
Schauer	2006	MN	10	Children	Lavender
Esch	2006	WI	10	Adults	Lavender
Hebert	2006	MN	10	Adults	Sweet marjoram and Roman chamomile
Luedtke	2006	MN	10	Night nurses	Roman chamomile
Anderson	2007	CT	10	Adults	Sweet marjoram
Dolcimascola	2007	PA	10	Night nurses	Lavender
Nickman	2007	NE	10	Adults	Ravensara
Fandrich	2007	WI	9	Children	Mandarin
Blyth	2011	WI	10	Autistic children	Lavender
Goodwin	2011	MA	13	Adults	Lavender and clary sage

attention during the lavender week. As every mother will tell you, that is important! The effect could be attributed to the rubbing, the gentle evaporation of lavender that was inhaled by the child while he/she was asleep, or the combination of the two.

NEROLI

Jager et al (1992b) found that neroli (*Citrus aurantium var. amara* [flos]) had a sedative effect on mice. In this study, the sedative effects were observed during the first 30 minutes of exposure to the aroma. More recent studies have focused on gerbils inhaling neroli (Chen et al 2008). In this study, neroli showed a measurable anxiolytic effect with Xanax as the control. Xanax is a benzodiazepine that is sometimes used to treat insomnia. Neroli is often suggested for anxiety. However, as one of the most expensive essential oils, this could be why there is so little published research.

PASSIONFLOWER AND LIME BLOSSOM

Buchbauer et al (1992) found that essential oils of passionflower *(Passiflora incarnata)* and lime blossom *(Tilia cordata)* had sedative effects. Lime blossom and its major component, benzyl alcohol, decreased the motility of animals in both normal and induced-agitation states. Interestingly, passionflower and its main components, maltol and 2-phenylethanol, only reduced motility when the animals were in an agitated state. A recent review of herbal preparations used for anxiety, depression, and insomnia in humans (Sarris et al 2011) found that although human studies indicated that passionflower had a measurable anxiolytic effect, more studies were required. Passionflower appears to work by modulating the GABA system (Appel et al 2011). In these studies, passionflower was taken internally.

BLACK CUMIN

Khanna et al (1993) found that black cumin *(Nigella sativa)* essential oil had a sedative effect more powerful than the drug chlorpromazine (Largactil) and was also an analgesic. The study suggested that black cumin contained an opioid-like component. More recent studies on animals have concentrated on anxiolytic effects (Gilhotra & Dhingra 2011) and anticonvulsant effects (Hosseinzadeh & Parvardeh 2004) in mice. It would be interesting to study inhaled black cumin on human insomnia. Because black cumin has a strong, pungent aroma, it would probably need to be "softened" with another calming aroma such as lavender, clary sage, or Roman chamomile.

ROMAN CHAMOMILE

Surprisingly, there are few published studies on Roman chamomile *(Chamaemelum nobile)* for insomnia; those that are in the literature focus on chamomile extract. It is well known that chamomile tea has a sedative effect (Gould et al 1973). RJ Buckle students have conducted five pilot studies on insomnia using Roman chamomile on its own or in a mixture. However, the studies have been inconclusive, either because the participants did not keep to the research protocol or because the effects, although positive, were very small. Roman chamomile may be a useful essential oil to add to a mixture for insomnia, but I am not convinced that it is effective enough on its own. It certainly has a more pleasing aroma than German chamomile *(Matricaria recutita)*.

RAVENSARA

This is an interesting choice and not one that would immediately come to mind. Nevertheless, three RJ Buckle students carried out studies on insomnia using ravensara. Nickman (2007) explored the effects of inhaled *Ravensara aromatica* for three nights (n = 10). Participants inhaled three drops of ravensara on a cotton ball and then placed the cotton ball by their pillow. Each night they replaced the old cotton ball with a new cotton ball with three drops of ravensara. In the aromatherapy group, three participants slept better, one experienced reduced snoring, and one noticed some sinus clearing. In the control group, two participants said the placebo had no effect, two participants had congested sinuses and did not sleep, but one participant said they had the best sleep ever! Ravensara would not be my first choice for insomnia. However, it would be an excellent addition to a mixture if the person had a cold or sinus problems.

ROSE

Most people enjoy the smell of roses. Rose is perhaps the most recognized and popular aroma in the world. Despite essential oil of rose being expensive, the cost may be justified where chronic insomnia is concerned. Both Macht and Ting (1921) and Rovesti and Columbo (1973) demonstrated that rose *(Rosa damascena)* essential oil has sedative effects. The sedative effects were replicated in a later study by Hongratanaworakit (2009). This study found that rose oil caused "significant decreases of breathing rate and systolic blood pressure that indicate a decrease of autonomic arousal." Jahangir et al (2008) compared the effect of steam-distilled rose petals (Ruh gulaab), rose distillate, or diluted rose distillate when given orally (three times daily) to 36 people with insomnia. The distilled rose petals had the greatest effect on insomnia with 66.6% (eight people) claiming total relief from insomnia. An added bonus was that rose had a positive effect on constipation.

In my experience, as well as that of my students and patients, rose is a strong contender to use for anxiety and for insomnia. Rose is in my own personal sleep potion when I travel and it certainly works for me.

MIXTURES

Komori et al (2006) explored the effect of a mixture of inhaled essential oils on 29 primary insomniacs with benzodiazepine dependency. The mixture was sandalwood (35%), juniper berry (12%), rose (8%), and orris (6%). Twenty-six participants were able to reduce their drug dose and 12 participants were able to come off the sleeping pill completely. Seong et al (2013) used a mixture of ylang ylang *(Cananga odorata)*, sweet marjoram *(Origanum majoranum)*, lavender *(Lavandula angustifolia)*, and neroli *(Citrus aurantium* var *amara* [flos]) in this randomized, controlled 2-week study. Participants were newly enlisted soldiers (undergoing training before placement) who were diagnosed with essential hypertension. Soldiers in the experimental group used aroma stones at night and wore aroma necklaces during the day. Results showed a significant reduction in blood pressure and pulse. It would be interesting to repeat this study and look at levels of insomnia.

It would be simple to design an insomnia study using personal patches or personal packets (please see the chapter on application methods) for patients in hospital. These modern methods of application would give constant delivery, or ready availability to the patient and not affect other people in the room (unlike a diffuser). It would be useful if such studies could include a baseline week, an intervention week, and a washout week. The oils I suggest could include some of the following: lavender, ylang ylang, mandarin, neroli, rose, clary sage, Roman chamomile, and sweet marjoram. The mixture I use when I can't sleep contains rose, lavender, mandarin, and frankincense.

REFERENCES

Alnamer R, Alaoui K, Bouidida H, Benjouad A, Cherrah Y. 2012. Sedative and hypnotic activities of the methanolic and aqueous extracts of *Lavandula officinalis* from Morocco. *Adv Pharmacol Sci.* Epub 2011 Nov 20.

American Sleep Disorders Association. 2005. *International Classification of Sleep Disorders. 2nd Edition: Diagnostic and Coding Manual.*

Ancoli-Israel S. 2006. The impact and prevalence of chronic insomnia and other sleep disturbances associated with chronic illness. *Am J Managed Care.* 12(8):S221–9.

Anderson S. 2007. Sweet marjoram for insomnia. Unpublished dissertation for RJ Buckle Associates.

Appel K, Rose T, Fiebich B, Kammler T, Hoffman C, Weiss G. 2011. Modulation of the γ-aminobutric acid (GABA) system by *Passiflora incarnata*. *Phytother Res.* 25(6):838–43.

Arroll B, Fernando A, Falloon K, Goodyear-Smith F, Samaranayake C et al. 2012. Prevalence of causes of insomnia in primary care: a cross-sectional study. *Br J Gen Pract.* 62(595):e99–e103.

Arzi A, Sela L, Green A, Givaty G, Dagan Y, Sobel N. 2010. The influence of odorants on respiration in sleep. *Chemical Senses.* 35(1):31–40.

Atanassova-Shopova S, Roussinov K, Boycheva I. 1973. On certain central neurotropic effects of lavender essential oils. II. Communications: studies on the effects of linalol and of terpineol. *Bull Instit Physiol.* 55:149–56.

Blyth. 2011. Effect of lavender on the sleep of autistic children. Unpublished RJBA dissertation.

Bradshaw R, Marchant J, Meredith M et al. 1998. Effects of lavender straw on stress and travel sickness in pigs. *J Alternative Complement Med.* 4(3):271–5.

Boonstra L, Harden K, Jarvis S, Palmer S, Kavanaugh-Carveth P, Barnett J, Friese C. 2011. Sleep disturbance in hospitalized recipients of stem cell transplantation. *Clin J Oncol Nurs.* 15(3):271–6.

Brooker C. 2008. *Medical Dictionary.* 16th Edition. Churchill Livingstone. London. p 444.

Buchbauer G, Jirovetz L, Jager W. 1991. Aromatherapy: evidence for sedative effects of the essential oil of lavender after inhalation. *Zeitschrift fur Naturforschung.* 46(11-12):1067–72.

Buchbauer G, Jirovetz L, Jager W. 1992. Kurzmitteilungen: passiflora and lime-blossoms—motility effects after inhalation of the essential oils and of some of the main constituents in animal experiments. *Archiv der Pharmazie (Weinheim).* 325(4):247–8.

Cashman 2002. Clary sage for insomnia. Unpublished dissertation for RJ Buckle Associates.

Chen Y, Cheng F, Shih Y, Chang T, Wang M, Lan S. 2008. Inhalation of neroli essential oil and its anxiolytic effects. *J Complement Integrative Med.* 5(1). doi:10.2202/1553-3840.1143. Accessed October 29, 2012.

Chien L, Cheng S, Liu C. 2012. The effect of lavender aromatherapy on autonomic nervous system in midlife women with insomnia. *Evid Based Complement Alternat Med.* doi:10.1155/2012/740813. Accessed October 26, 2012.

Davis M. 1997. Lavender for insomnia. Unpublished dissertation for RJ Buckle Associates.

de Moura Lincke V, da Silva A, Figueiro M, Piato A, Herrmann A et al. 2009. Inhaled linalool-induced sedation in mice. *Phytomedicine.* 16:303–7.

Dijk D, Duffy J, Silva E, Shanahan T, Boivin D, Czeisler C. 2012. Amplitude reduction and phase sifts of melatonin, cortisol and other circadian rhythms after a gradual advance of sleep and light exposure in humans. *PLoS One.* 7(2):e30037. doi:10.1371/journal.pone.0030037. Accessed October 27, 2012.

Docimascola L. 2007. Lavender for insomnia. Unpublished dissertation for RJ Buckle Associates.

Dupois G. 2002. Roman chamomile and lavender for insomnia. Unpublished dissertation for RJ Buckle Associates.

Dyer J, Cleary L, Ragsdale-Lowe M, McNeill S, Osland C. 2013. The use of aromastix at a cancer centre: a retrospective audit. *Complement Ther Clin Practice.* http://www.sciencedirect.com/science/article/pii/S1744388113000947. Accessed November 28, 2012.

Elisabetsky E, de Souza G, Dos Santos M et al. 1995a. Sedative properties of linalool. *Fitoterapia.* 66(5):407–15.

Elisabetsky E, Marschner J, Souza D. 1995b. Effects of linalool on glutamatergic system in the rat cerebral cortex. *Neurochem Res.* 20(4):461–5.

Esch K. 2006. Lavender for insomnia. Unpublished dissertation for RJ Buckle Associates.

Falloon K, Arool B, Raina Elley C, Fernando A. 2011. The assessment and management of insomnia in primary care. *BMJ.* doi:10.1136/bmj.2009.d2899.

Fandrich M. 2007. Mandarin for insomnia in children. Unpublished dissertation for RJ Buckle Associates.

Fewell F, McVicar R, Gransby P, Morgan P. 2007. Blood concentration and uptake of D-limonene during aromatherapy massage with sweet orange oil. A pilot study. *Intern J Essential Oil Ther.* 1:97–102.

Gay P. 2010. Sleep and sleep-disordered breathing in the hospitalized patient. *Respir Care.* 55(9):1240–54.

Gilhotra N, Dhingra D. 2011. Thymoquinone produced antianxiety-like effects in mice through modulation of GABA and NO levels. *Pharmacol Rep.* 63(3):660–9.

Goel N, Kim H, Lao R. 2005. An olfactory stimulus modifies night time sleep in young men and women. *Chronobiol Int.* 22(5):889–904.

Goodwin G. 2011. Lavender and clary sage for insomnia in menopausal women. Unpublished dissertation for RJ Buckle Associates.

Gould L, Reddy C, Gomprecht R. 1973. Cardiac effects of chamomile tea. *J Clin Pharmacol.* 13(11):475–9.

Guillemain J, Rousseau A, Delaveau P. 1989. Effects neurodepresseurs de l'huile essentielle de *Lavandula angustifolia*. Annales Pharmaceutiques Francaises. 47(6):337–43.

Hardeland R. 2012. Neurobiology, pathophysiology, and treatment of melatonin deficiency and dysfunction. *ScientificWorldJournal.* 640389. doi:10.1100/2012/640389.

Haynes PL, Parthasarathy S, Kersh B, Bootzin RR. 2011. Examination of insomnia and insomnia treatments in psychiatric inpatients. *Int J Ment Health Nurs.* 20(2):130–6.

Hebert R. 2006. Sweet marjoram and Roman chamomile for insomnia. Unpublished dissertation for RJ Buckle Associates.

Henry J, Rusius C, Davies M et al. 1994. Lavender for night sedation of people with dementia. *Int J Aromather.* 6(2):28–30.

Hongratanaworakit T. 2009. Relaxing effect of rose oil on humans. *Nat Prod Commun.* 4: 291–6.

Hosseinzadeh H, Parvardeh S. 2004. Anticonvulsant effects of thymoquinone, the major constituent of *Nigella sativa* seeds, in mice. *Phytomedicine.* 11(1):56–64.

Howard S, Hughes M. 2008. Expectancies, not aroma, explain impact of lavender aromatherapy on psychophysiological indices of relaxation in young healthy women. *Br J Health Psychol.* 13(Pt 4):603–17.

Hsieh K, Nguyen D, Siegel J, Lai Y. 2012. New pathways and data on REM sleep behaviour disorder in a rat model. *Sleep Med.* Oct 8. pii: S1389–9457(12)00318-8. doi:10.1016/j.sleep.2012.08.008. [Epub ahead of print].

Hudson R. 1996. The value of lavender for rest and activity in the elderly patient. *Complement Ther Med.* 4(1):52–7.

Hull S. 2000. Ravensara for insomnia. Unpublished dissertation for RJ Buckle Associates.

Isaia G, Corsinovi L, Bo M, Santos-Pereira P, Michelis G, Aimonino N, Zanocchi M. 2011. Insomnia among hospitalized elderly patients: prevalence, clinical characteristics and factors. *Arch Gerontol Geriatr.* 52(2):133–7.

Jager W, Buchbauer G, Jirovetz L et al. 1992a. Percutaneous absorption of lavender oil from a massage oil. *J Soc Cosmetic Chemists.* 43(1):49–54.

Jager W, Buchbauer G, Jirovetz L. 1992b. Evidence of the sedative effect of neroli oil, citronella and phenylethyl acetate on mice. *J Essential Oil Res.* 4(4):387–394.

Jacob T, Michels G, Silayeva L, Haydon J, Succol F, Moss S. 2012. Benzodiazepine treatment induces subtype-specific changes in GABAA receptor trafficking and decreases synaptic inhibition. *Proc Natl Acad Sci USA.* Oct 22. [Epub ahead of print].

Jahangir U, Urooj A, Shah A, Ishaaq M, Habib A. 2008. A comparative clinical trial of rose petal (Gul gulaab), rose hydrosol diluted (Arq gulaab) and rose hydrosol (Ruh gulaab) in insomnia. *Internet J Neurol.* 11(2). http://ispub.com/IJN/11/2/11966. Accessed December 18, 2013.

Johannessen B. 2013. Nurses experience of aromatherapy use with dementia patients experiencing disturbed sleep patterns. An action research project. *Comp Ther Clinical Practice.* 19(4):2009–13.

King P. 2001. Roman chamomile and sweet marjoram for insomnia. Unpublished dissertation for RJ Buckle Associates.

Khanna T, Zaidi F, Dandiya P. 1993. CNS and analgesic studies on *Nigella sativa. Fitoterapia.* 64(5):407–10.

Knowles S. 2002. Lavender for insomnia. Unpublished dissertation for RJ Buckle Associates.

Knuteson 2000. Mandarin and insomnia in children. Unpublished dissertation for RJ Buckle Associates.

Komori T, Matsumoto T, Yamamoto M, Motomura E, Shiroyama T, Okazaki Y. 2006. Application of fragrance in discontinuing the long-term use of hypnotic benzodiazepines. *Intern J Aroma.* 16(1):3–7.

Lee I, Lee G. 2006. Effects of lavender aromatherapy on insomnia and depression in women college students. *Taehan Kanho Hakhoe Chi.* 36(1):136–43.

Lewith G, Godfrey A, Prescott P. 2005. A single-blinded, randomized pilot study evaluating the aroma of *Lavandula angustifolia* as a treatment for mild insomnia. *J Altern Complement Med.* 11(4):631–7.

Luedtk L. 2006. Roman chamomile for insomnia. Unpublished dissertation for RJ Buckle Associates.

Macht D, Ting G. 1921. Experimental enquiry into the sedative of some aromatic drugs and fumes. *J Pharmacol Exp Ther.* 18(5):361–72.

Majdan M, Mauritz W, Brazinova A, Wilbacher I, Rusnak M, Leirgeb J. 2012. Barbiturates use and its effects in patients with severe TBI in five European Counties. *J Neurotrauma.* Sep 5. http://www.ncbi.nlm.nih.gov/pubmed/22950895. [Epub ahead of print]. Accessed October 29, 2012.

Mayo Clinic. 2012. http://www.mayoclinic.com/health/sleeping-pills/SL00010. Accessed July 2014.

Moeini M, Khadibi M, Bekhadi R, Mahmoudian S, Nazari F. 2010. Effect of aromatherapy on the quality of sleep in ischemic heart disease patients hospitalized in intensive care units of heart hospitals of the Isfahan University of Medical Sciences. *Iran J Nurs Midwifery Res.* 15(4):234–9.

Morgenthaler T, Kramer M, Alessi C, Friedman L, Boehlecke B et al. 2006. Practice parameters for the psychological and behavioral treatment of insomnia: an update. An American Academy of Sleep Medicine report. *Sleep.* 29(11):1415–9.

Murakami J, Imai M, Yamada N. 2012. Diagnosis and treatment in circadian rhythm sleep disorders. *Nihon Rinsho.* 70(7):1155–60.

National Sleep Foundation. 2013. Orexin receptor antagonists: a new class of sleeping pill. http://www.sleepfoundation.org. Accessed December 18, 2013.

NHS Choices. 2013. Melatonin. http://www.nhs.uk/medicine-guides/pages/MedicineOverview.aspx?condition=Insomnia&medicine=Melatonin&preparationMelatonin%202mg%20modified-release%20tablets. Accessed January 4, 2013.

Nickman K. 2007. *Ravensara aromatica* for insomnia. Unpublished RJBA dissertation.

O'Neill B, Gardani M, Findlay G, Whyte T, Cullen T. 2013. Challenging behaviour and sleep cycle disorder following brain injury: a preliminary response to agomelatine treatment. *Brain Inj.* [Epub ahead of print]. Accessed January 4, 2013.

Roth T. 2007. Insomnia: definition, prevalence, etiology, and consequences. *J Clin Sleep Med.* 3(5 Suppl):S7–S10.

Rovesti P, Columbo E. 1973. Aromatherapy and aerosols. *Soap Perfumery Cosmetics.* 46:475–7.

Schauer B. 2006. Does mandarin improve infant sleep? Unpublished dissertation for RJ Buckle Associates.

Sarris J, Byrne G. 2011. Systematic review of insomnia and complementary medicine. *Sleep Med Rev.* 15(2):99–106.

Sarris J, Panossian A, Schweitzer I, Stough C, Schloley A. 2011. Herbal medicine for repression, anxiety and insomnia: a review of psychopharmacology and clinical evidence. *Eur Neuropyschopharmacol.* 21(12):841–60.

Seong K, Hong J-H, Hur M-J, Lee M. 2013. Two week aroma inhalation effects on blood pressure in young men with essential hypertension. *Eur J Integr Med.* 5(3):254–60.

Takeda. 2011. Takeda discontinues development of Ramelteon in Europe for the treatment of insomnia. http://www.takeda.com/news/2011/20111007_3902.html. Accessed July 2014.

Thorpy M, Roth T. 2013. Towards a classification of medications for sleep and circadian rhythym disorders. Nat Sci Sleep. 5:143–5. doi:10.2147/NSS.S55679. eCollection 2013.

Tisdale 2002. Ravensara for insomnia. Unpublished dissertation for RJ Buckle Associates.

Tisserand R. 1988. Lavender beats benzodiazepines. *Int J Aromather.* 1(1):1–2.

Tomaino J. 2005. Sweet marjoram for insomnia. Unpublished dissertation for RJ Buckle Associates.

Vought T. 2003. Lavender and sweet marjoram for insomnia. Unpublished dissertation for RJ Buckle Associates.

Weihbrecht L. 1999. Lavender for insomnia. Unpublished dissertation for RJ Buckle Associates.

Yamada K, Mimaki Y, Sashida Y et al. 1994. Anticonvulsant effects of inhaling lavender oil vapor. *Biol Pharma Bull.* 17(2):359–60.

Chapter 9

Nausea and Vomiting

"Sweetest things turn sourest by their deeds: Lilies that fester smell far worse than weeds."

William Shakespeare (1564-1616), Sonnet XCIV

CHAPTER ASSETS

This chapter will discuss some of the published research on nausea and is divided into different essential oils for easy reading. It also includes some unpublished studies carried out by my students. A table of relevant research is provided in each section.

Nausea can have many causes, but the two main ones in a clinical setting are chemo-induced and postoperative nausea. Nausea and vomiting are symptoms experienced by 50% of patients receiving chemotherapy and radiotherapy (Lua & Zakaria 2012). Postoperative nausea and vomiting (PONV) continue to be a major cause of patient dissatisfaction affecting up to 60% of patients (Reagan et al 2009). Between 20% and 60% of patients who receive morphine become nauseated (de Pradier 2006).

Although nausea does not always lead to actual vomiting, the causes of nausea and vomiting are similar. Nausea is activated by the chemoreceptor trigger zone (CTZ) and has five different receptors that may activate it. Nausea and vomiting can have numerous causes (Box 9-1).

CONVENTIONAL APPROACHES TO TREATING VOMITING

The choice of antiemetic drug prescribed is determined by the cause of the nausea (Clare et al 2011). There are seven basic categories of antiemetic agents used in

BOX 9-1 *Some Causes of Nausea and Vomiting*

Gastrointestinal Causes
Stomach or intestinal irritation, gastroenteritis
Any type of abdominal surgery, but in particular gall bladder and gynecologic
    surgeries
Obstruction
Hypertrophic pyloric stenosis

Central Nervous System Causes
Loss of sense of balance resulting from middle or inner ear trauma, labyrinthitis
Sensory responses in the brain activated by smell, sight, or emotion
Increased pressure in the brain (caused by tumors, hemorrhage, meningitis)
Head injury
Migraine
Psychiatric disorder/anxiety
Chemoreceptor trigger areas that respond either to natural chemicals produced by the
    body (e.g., kidney and pancreas) or to motion sickness

Metabolic Causes
Pregnancy
Uremia
Alcohol
Diabetes with gastroparesis
Pain

Drugs
Prescription: narcotics/opiates (McNatty 2008)
Recreational (Hill & Thomas 2011)
Anesthetic inhalational volatile gases

conventional medicine: antihistamines, anticholinergics, corticosteroids, cannabinoids, benzodiazepines, dopamine antagonists, and serotonin antagonists.

Antihistamines (dramamine, diphenhydramine, hydroxyzine) affect the organ
of balance as well as the vomiting center of the brain. These drugs also have an effect
on the CTZ, and they block the histamine and dopamine receptors. In addition,
they inhibit acetylcholine. Antihistamines work by reducing the sensitivity of the
vomiting center to input from the inner ear, although they do not directly affect
the inner ear.

Because the vomiting center of the brain is stimulated by the neurotransmitter
acetylcholine, one of the most direct ways of inhibiting vomiting is to use anticholinergic drugs (atropine, scopolamine, hyoscyamine). Transdermal scopolamine
provides up to 72 hours of antiemetic treatment and is mainly used for the treatment of motion sickness. However, long-term use of anticholinergic drugs can
cause side effects such as poor digestion, dry mouth, blurred vision, and constipation. Corticosteroids (dexamethasone, prednisone) can help to reduce nausea

associated with chemotherapy but can cause side effects such as mania, insomnia, gastric irritation, and avascular necrosis (AVN). Cannabinoids (dronabinol) have been used to treat nausea and vomiting in patients with end-stage illness, but they have limited effectiveness as a result of irregular absorption rates. Cannabinoids often take several days to weeks to reach therapeutic blood levels and have the side effect of uncomfortable dizziness or euphoria. Benzodiazepines such as lorazepam have been used to treat nausea. These drugs often cause dry mouth and drowsiness.

The neurochemical that stimulates the CTZ is dopamine. Dopamine antagonists (e.g., prochlorperazine, chlorpromazine, haloperidol, metoclopramide, and droperidol) work by blocking dopamine-mediated transmission, thereby relieving nausea. Dopamine antagonists have common side effects of extrapyramidal symptoms, which limit their use.

Serotonin agonists (5-HT$_3$) such as granisetron, azesetron, and odansetron (Zofran) are safe and effective in controlling nausea (Endo et al 2012) and are frequently considered first-line antiemetic agents. These medications have fewer side effects compared to other classes of antiemetics; however, these drugs are often prohibitively expensive (Ishimuru 2008).

Because the etiology of nausea and vomiting is multifactorial, using several different medications makes the most sense. Numerous studies have shown that combination therapy using different categories of antiemetic medications works better than single-agent antiemetic treatment.

Nonpharmacologic Techniques

Nontraditional techniques used for treatment of nausea and vomiting include methods such as acupuncture, acupressure, electroacupuncture, and hypnosis.

AROMATHERAPY FOR NAUSEA

Although conventional approaches are often very effective in managing nausea and vomiting, some patients are intolerant of drug side effects or unable to afford them. Aromatherapy can be tried before conventional medicine and used alongside it (Buckle 2007). The main method of use is direct inhalation to the patient via: (1) aromasticks; (2) aromapatches; (3) aromapackets; and (4) aroma nasal clips. For more information on these methods, please see the section of applications in Chapter 2.

There are several published reviews on aromatherapy for nausea (Ernst & Pittler 2000; Kitzler & Nolan 2009; Hines et al 2012; Lua & Zakaria 2012). These reviews will be discussed in relation to the relevant essential oil.

Peppermint

Peppermint *(Mentha piperita)* has been a classic choice for the treatment of nausea for hundreds of years. Used primarily to treat nausea, rather than actual vomiting, peppermint essential oil is effective both in vitro and in vivo. Peppermint also has recognized antispasmodic effects and relieves colonic spasm within 30 seconds (Leicester & Hunt 1982). It also reduced postoperative colic and nausea following colostomies (McKenzie & Gallacher 1989; Asao et al 2001). Both Valnet (1990) and Franchomme and Penoel (1980), pioneers of clinical aromatherapy, state that peppermint is an antiemetic. Grigoleit and Grigoleit (2005) reviewed nine clinical trials on the use of peppermint essential oil given orally for gastrointestinal disorders. In most of the studies, there was a substantial soothing effect on the gut with a single dose (0.1 to 0.24 mL per participant).

A recent review of the scientific evidence by Lua & Zakaria (2012) found that the existing evidence for inhaling essential oil of peppermint as an antiemetic was "encouraging, but not yet compelling." They searched CINAHL (Cumulative Index to Nursing and Allied Health Literature), Pubmed, EBSCO Host, and Science Direct and found five articles that met their criteria with 328 patients. The results suggested that inhaled peppermint or ginger reduced the incidence and severity of both nausea and vomiting and decreased the need for conventional medication. It is worth noting that databases such as Chemical Abstracts, AGRICOLA, EMBASE, and specialist journals such as *Flavor & Fragrance Journal*, *Journal of Essential Oils Research*, and the *International Journal of Clinical Aromatherapy* were not searched; information from these sources might have added more weight to the conclusion.

One of the earliest promising studies on postoperative nausea using peppermint was by Tate (1997). This was a controlled study on 18 patients following major gynecologic surgery. Group 1 received no treatment, group 2 received peppermint essence, and group 3 received peppermint essential oil. Participants in group 3 were asked to inhale directly from the bottle when they were nauseated. Measurement was made on a five-point scale ranging from 0 (no nausea) to 4 (about to vomit). The amount of antiemetic drug (metoclopramide [Maxolon], prochlorperazine [Stemetil], and ondansetron [Zofran]) used was measured. Participants in the experimental group needed 50% fewer antiemetics. The Kruskal–Wallis test was used to establish significance, $P = 0.0487$. The cost per treatment was approximately US 75 cents (UK 48 pence).

Stringer & Donald (2011) found that aromasticks containing peppermint and lemon were effective to reduce nausea in patients at the Christie Hospital, Manchester, UK, using a retrospective service evaluation. Patients referred to the complementary therapy service were offered an aromastick to help with anxiety, nausea, or sleep; 160 patients accepted the offer. Patient details were taken. One week later participants were followed up by a different person who documented how often the aromastick was used and the perceived benefits. Forty-seven percent of nauseous patients said the aromastick had settled their nausea.

One of the "noncompelling" clinical trials mentioned by Lua and Zakaria (2012) was a study on the effect of inhaled peppermint on 33 postoperative patients in Connecticut conducted by Anderson and Gross (2004). Participants discovered that inhaling peppermint essential oil from a gauze swab reduced their nausea ($P = 0.005$); however, so did taking deep breaths. A second "noncompelling" study was by Ferruggiari et al (2012). Their results were also disappointing; however, the authors state that "most participants received intraoperative antiemetics and did not report nausea postoperatively." Then, in a Cochrane review, Hines et al (2012) dismissed the use of inhaled peppermint as an effective antiemetic.

However, a very positive study by Hunt et al (2012) from the Department of Anesthesia at Carolinas Medical Center, Charlotte, North Carolina, was published almost at the same time as the Cochrane review. This study did not use peppermint on its own but a mixture that contained peppermint. This study will be discussed further under the section on essential oil mixture.

RJ Buckle students have conducted six pilot studies on inhaled peppermint for nausea for their certification (Table 9-1). For published studies on nausea, please see Tables 9-2, 9-3, 9-4, and 9-5.

One of the first RJ Buckle studies was carried out at the oncology center of St. Luke's Hospital in New Bedford, Massachusetts (Figuenick 1998). Ten chemotherapy patients inhaled peppermint and found it effective in reducing their nausea and were able to reduce their use of medication (Zofran and Compazine). Zofran is very expensive, and Compazine causes sedation. In fact, peppermint proved so effective that those in the control group demanded the peppermint, and the control part of the

TABLE 9-1 *Nausea Studies Carried out by RJ Buckle Students*

Name	Year	State	N	Type of Nausea	Essential Oil
Beagham	2002	MI	15	Postoperative	Peppermint
Figuenick	1998	MA	8	Chemo-induced	Peppermint
Chalifour	2005	MA	9	Opiate detox	Peppermint
Piotroswki	2005	WI	17	General nausea	Peppermint
Irby	2006	MN	8	Chemo-induced	Peppermint
Lowdermilk	2007	WI	10	Chemo-induced	Peppermint
Geiger	2005	AZ	92	Postoperative	Ginger
Karas-Irwin	2006	NJ	9	Postoperative (adult)	Ginger
Nord	2006	MN	99	Postoperative (pediatric)	Ginger and lavender
Annis	2011	MN	13	Motion sickness (sea)	Ginger, lavender, and fennel
Evenson	2000	AZ	10	Postoperative	Lavandin

TABLE 9-2 *Published Research on Nausea and Peppermint*

Author	Year	N	Nausea	Essential Oil	Result
Tate	1997	18	Postoperative	Peppermint	+ve
Anderson & Gross	2004	33	Postoperative	Peppermint	−ve
Stringer & Donald	2011	123	Chemo-induced	Peppermint/lemon	+ve
Ferruggiari et al	2012	70	Postoperative	Peppermint	−ve
Hines et al	2012	402	Postoperative	Peppermint	−ve

study collapsed. Of the patients in this study, 84% stated that essential oil of peppermint relieved their nausea, and 71% found that it enhanced their standard antiemetic medication. One patient found that it enhanced his appetite. Inhaled peppermint is now routinely offered in many chemotherapy units in the United States and in the UK.

Chalifour (2005) conducted a pilot study using peppermint to ease nausea in patients detoxing from opiate and crack addiction at the Cooley-Dickenson Hospital, Northampton, Massachusetts. Peppermint was inhaled 30 minutes before meals. Subjects rated their nausea using a Clinical Institute Withdrawal Assessment (CIWA) form. This scale was used before meals (breakfast and lunch). There appeared to be a 100% reduction in nausea.

Piotroswki (2005) offered an aromastick containing peppermint to 17 hospital patients with nausea in Madison, Wisconsin. Nausea was rated pre- and posttest with the Edmonton Symptom Assessment System numerical scale. The results were statistically significant using a paired t test (P = 0.0002). Irby (2006) recruited participants from a Woman's Cancer Resource Center in St. Paul, Minnesota. All participants (8) were taking antinausea medication (Compazine or Zofran). Seven participants had marked relief from inhaling peppermint that lasted from 30 minutes to several hours. Lowdermilk (2007) offered her participants a choice of either peppermint or ginger for their chemo-induced nausea. All participants (10) were taking conventional antiemetic drugs but were having breakthroughs. All preferred peppermint to ginger, and all found it helpful.

SPEARMINT

Spearmint has an antiemetic effect and may be effective for longer periods than peppermint because it works on different areas of the brain to peppermint (Lawrence 2001). Tayarani-Najaran et al (2013) conducted a randomized, placebo-controlled, double-blind study comparing spearmint *(Mentha spicata)* and peppermint *(Mentha piperita)* against placebo and control. Two drops of spearmint essential oil and two drops of peppermint essential oil were added to sugar and given in capsules. The first treatment was given 30 minutes before the patients received their chemotherapy treatment, then 4 hours later, and the last dose was given after a further 4 hours at home. There was a significant reduction in the "number of emetic events" in the first 24 hours after chemotherapy for both spearmint and peppermint essential oil (P < 0.05). There was no difference between the antiemetic effects of peppermint and spearmint. The cost of conventional drugs was also reduced when an essential oil was used. Reagan et al (2009) and Hunt et al (2012) both used spearmint in the mixtures of essential oils they used in their studies. Please see the section on mixtures.

GINGER

Ginger *(Zingiber officinale)* was introduced in Europe during the middle ages. The essential oil, which does not smell anything like the dried root or candied ginger, contains zingiberene. Ginger is an effective remedy for nausea and is particularly suitable for pregnancy. Vutyavanich et al (1997) studied 70 expectant mothers over a period of 5 months in a double-blind, placebo-controlled trial. They found that baseline nausea and vomiting decreased significantly in the group using ginger. Ginger had no adverse effects on the mothers' pregnancy outcomes.

Published Reviews on Ginger

Ernst and Pittler (2000) conducted a systematic review of randomized trials on the use of ginger for nausea caused by seasickness, morning sickness, and chemotherapy-induced nausea. Although their findings were inconclusive, they conclude "the studies collectively favored ginger over placebo." Chaiyakunapruk et al (2006) conducted a meta-analysis of ginger studies for the treatment of postoperative nausea and vomiting and his conclusion was "a fixed dose of at least 1 g of ginger is more effective than placebo for the prevention of postoperative nausea and vomiting and postoperative vomiting." In 2005, a review by Borrelli et al found that "ginger may be an effective treatment for nausea and vomiting in pregnancy." Boone and Shields (2005) conducted a review of studies using ginger (orally) for pregnancy-related nausea. The conclusion was that ginger was a "low-risk, cost effective and efficacious treatment for nausea in pregnancy." However, a Cochrane review (Matthews et al 2010) found "the use of ginger products may be helpful to women, but evidence of effectiveness was limited and not consistent."

Published Studies on Ginger

In 2004, Tad Gieger, MD, completed his study on the use of inhaled ginger essential oil on 92 patients with PONV for RJ Buckle certification (Table 9-1). As an anesthesiologist, he had a personal interest in PONV. Patients were randomly allocated to the ginger group or a control group. In the ginger group, patients received 5% ginger administered nasocutaneously before surgery and applied immediately postoperatively (so the effect would be primarily inhalation). The control group received standard medical treatment. The results showed that in the ginger group only 7/43 patients had PONV nausea, and in the control group 24/49 had PONV. He published his study in 2005.

Panahi et al (2012) used ginger to reduce chemo-induced nausea in a study of 100 female patients with advanced breast cancer in the oncology unit of Baqiyatallah Hospital, Tehran, Iran. In this case, ginger root was taken orally in capsules 30 minutes before chemotherapy. It appeared to cause a significant reduction in nausea. Ginger essential oil would be a logical follow on from Panahi's study. The chemistry of ginger essential oil supports this because many of the antiemetic components in the whole herb are also found in the essential oil (Hertz 2009).

In the study by Hunt et al (2012) participants were randomly allocated to one of four groups. Group 1 received ginger essential oil on its own. Group 2 received a mixture of ginger, spearmint, peppermint, and cardamom. Group 3 received isopropyl alcohol as the placebo. Group 4 received saline as the control. Hospital patients (n = 303) were randomly allocated to one of the four arms. Patients with a nausea level of 1 to 3 on a verbal descriptive scale (0-3) received a 2 × 2 gauze pad. The gauze pad contained one cubic centimeter that had been saturated with the randomly chosen aromatherapy agent (ginger, aromatherapy mixture, placebo or control) and were told to inhale deeply three times. Nausea (0-3) was measured again 5 minutes later. Ginger produced a statistically significant reduction in nausea ($P = 0.002$), but not in the placebo control group ($P = 0.76$). The essential oil mixture produced a greater effect ($P = 0.001$) than ginger on its own. The number of antiemetic medications requested after aromatherapy was significantly reduced for both the ginger and the aromatherapy mixture versus placebo ($P = 0.002$ and $P < 0.001$, respectively).

RJ Buckle students have conducted two pilot studies on inhaled ginger for nausea for their certification (Table 9-1). Tad Geiger's study (2005) has already been discussed in this section. The second study was by Karas-Irwin (2006). This was a feasibility study conducted at Valley Hospital, Ridgewood, New Jersey, to test the number of patients affected by PONV and was to be followed by a randomized controlled trial to test the effectiveness of inhaled ginger essential oil as an antiemetic. All patients who agreed to take part and who experienced nausea were offered ginger aromasticks for nausea within 24 hours of orthopedic surgery. The aromasticks were so effective that the study was stopped and patients are now regularly offered ginger essential oil in an aromastick to inhale (Mazzer 2013). See Table 9-3 for published studies on ginger and nausea.

LAVENDER

There are no studies in the literature using lavender essential oil on its own as an antiemetic, but several studies have used lavender in a mixture. Lavender was used with ginger in a mixture by Nord and Belew (2006), and in an RJ Buckle (RJBA) student study lavender was mixed with fennel and ginger (Annis 2011). These will be covered in the section on mixtures below.

Everson, another RJBA student, carried out a small project with lavandin (*Lavandula intermedia* CT Super) to treat postoperative nausea (2000). She became intrigued with the antiemetic properties of lavender while undergoing chemotherapy herself. During the 26 weeks Everson received chemotherapy, she never

TABLE 9-3 *Published Research on Nausea and Ginger*

Author	Year	N	Nausea	Essential Oil	Result
Pongrojpaw & Chiamchanya	2003	80	Postoperative	Ginger	+ve
Eberhart et al	2003	180	Postoperative	Ginger	−ve
Morin et al	2004	538	Postoperative	Review: ginger	−ve
Smith et al	2004	291	Pregnancy	Ginger	+ve
Geiger	2005	92	Postoperative	Ginger	+ve
Borrelli et al	2005	675	Pregnancy	Ginger	+ve
Boone & Shields	2005	915	Pregnancy	Review: ginger	+ve
Zick et al	2009	162	Postoperative	Ginger	−ve
Ensiyeh & Sakineh	2009	70	Pregnancy	Ginger	+ve
Panahi et al	2005	100	Chemo-induced	Ginger	+ve

vomited and only used six of the prescribed antiemetic pills. All of the women in her cancer support group were nauseated, and all used most of their antiemetic pills. Ten patients were included in the exploratory postoperative study, which was not randomized or controlled. Consent was given by the hospital and each patient signed an informed consent. After inhaling lavender, only two patients required an antiemetic postoperatively—a much lower than usual incidence. Although no conclusions can be reached from this study, this chemotype of lavandin might be worth trying in a mixture with spearmint, peppermint, cardamom, and ginger.

CARDAMOM

Cardamom *(Elettaria cardamomum)* is listed in the *Indian Materia Medica* as relieving vomiting and nausea (Nadkarni 1992); it is one of the oldest essential oils known (Arctander 1994). Cardamom contains 50% α-terpinyl acetate and 1,8-cineole, with small amounts of borneol, α-terpineol, and limonene. Borneol was shown to be an effective antagonist of acetylcholine in a study by Cabo et al (1986), and perhaps this compound imbues cardamom with its antiemetic property. A study in rats by Jamal et al (2006) showed that cardamom has antiemetic properties. However, there are no studies using cardamom (as a single essential oil) on humans for nausea in the published literature. However, cardamom has been used as part of an aromatherapy mixture in two clinical trials. The first mixture was with ginger, spearmint, and peppermint (Hunt et al 2012). The results of this study supported the investigators' hypothesis that "aromatherapy would be effective as a treatment for PON." The other study was by de Pradier (2006). This study used a mixture of cardamom, ginger, and tarragon applied to the necks of 73 patients. Seventy-five percent reported a reduction in nausea. It would be worth exploring the effect of cardamom singly for human nausea.

CITRUS PEEL OILS

In a study by Ndao et al (2012), 37 pediatric patients undergoing stem cell infusion were offered bergamot to inhale before therapy. Bergamot did not appear to reduce either anxiety or nausea. However, in a study by Potter et al (2011) in Portland, Oregon, sweet orange appeared to significantly reduce nausea in 72 patients (P = 0.032). In this study, orange was either inhaled or eaten in slices. This is not as strange as it seems; Sicilian mothers offer their children slices of orange when their children become seasick. Price and Price (2012) cite lemon as being effective against nausea. However, I could find nothing to substantiate this in the published literature. Just because there is nothing yet in the published literature does not mean they are not effective clinically, so lemon essential oil would be interesting to try either singly or in a mixture. For published studies on citrus and nausea, please see Table 9-4.

ANISEED, CARAWAY, CLOVE, AND FENNEL

Aniseed *(Anethum graveolens)*, caraway *(Carvum carvi)*, fennel *(Foeniculum vulgare)*, and clove (Eugenia caryophyllata) are listed in *Potter's New Cyclopaedia of Botanical Drugs and Preparations* as carminatives (Wren 1988). Although these are not antiemetic, they may make an antinausea mixture more robust.

TABLE 9-4 *Published Research on Nausea and Citrus Oils*

Author	Year	N	Nausea	Essential Oil	Result
Stringer & Donald	2011	123	Chemo-induced	Peppermint/lemon	+ve
Potter et al	2011	60	Stem cell	Orange*	+ve
Ndao et al	2012	37	Stem cell	Bergamot	ve

*Orange slices eaten and/or sweet orange essential oil inhaled.

Carum copticum (related to caraway and with a similar kind of smell) was found to reduce contraction activity in rat's ileum (Hejazian et al 2009). *Carum copticum* has a long history of use in Iran for intestinal complaints going back as far as Avicenna (Avesina 1985). This might be another essential oil to add to an antiemetic mixture.

MIXTURES

Reagan et al (2009) used a mixture containing ginger, peppermint, spearmint, and lavender delivered in an aromastick on 98 patients in the postanesthesia care unit (PACU) following total join replacement at Gaston Memorial Hospital, North Carolina. Fifty percent of patients experienced nausea. Thirty-nine percent of patients used the aromastick and it reduced their nausea.

Hunt et al (2012), who conducted a study on 303 patients (see the Ginger section), found that the aromatherapy mixture (ginger, spearmint, peppermint, and cardamom) produced a greater reduction in nausea than ginger on its own. The study concludes "aromatherapy is promising as an inexpensive, noninvasive treatment for PON."

RJBA STUDIES

Two RJBA students (Nord and Annis) conducted pilot studies using mixtures for nausea for their certification. Nord (2006) used a lavender/ginger mixture on 99 pediatric patients. The lavender/ginger mixture or placebo (jojoba) was applied to pulse points before surgery and covered with a Band-Aid. One drop was also placed on a cotton ball that was then attached to the patient's hospital gown for future inhalation. The mixture was reapplied 3 hours later when necessary. The outcome measure was a standard pediatric tool: face, legs, activity, cry, and consolation (the FLACC scale). The hospital statistician reviewed the data and the results were significant ($P = 0.04$). For published studies on nausea and mixtures of essential oils, please see Table 9-5.

Annis (2011) explored the antiemetic effects of fennel and ginger on motion sickness (seasickness). Originally, 24 people had been approached, but only 13 were recruited. However, five of the dissenting people then wanted to join the study when they saw the positive effects of inhaling the mixture on reducing seasickness. All 18 who took part and inhaled the fennel and ginger mixture had a reduction in nausea. This was an interesting informal study on a group of people during a whale-watching boat trip.

TABLE 9-5 *Published Research on Nausea and Mixtures of Essential Oils*

Author	Year	N	Nausea	Essential Oil	Result
Gilligan	2005	25	Hospice	Mixture*	+ve
de Pradier	2006	73	Postoperative	Ginger, cardamom, tarragon	+ve
Stringer & Donald	2011	123	Chemo-induced	Peppermint/lemon	+ve
Hunt et al	2012	303	Postoperative	Ginger/peppermint Spearmint/cardamom	+ve

*Mixture = *Pimpinella anisum, Foeniculum vulgare* var. *dulce, Anthemis nobilis*, and *Mentha* × *piperita*.

IMPORTANCE OF INDIVIDUAL PREFERENCE IN CHOICE OF ESSENTIAL OIL

Because there are several essential oils with antiemetic effects, it is a good idea to ask patients which essential oils they prefer because this is more likely to produce a positive effect. This highlights the importance of learned memory and of involving patients in choosing their oils. The method of application is usually inhalation—aromasticks, patches, or packets. However, a gentle abdominal rub can be very beneficial to a child or anxious patient who is sick with worry rather than nauseated for physical reasons.

REFERENCES

Anderson L, Gross J. 2004. Aromatherapy with peppermint, isopropyl alcohol or placebo is equally effective in relieving postoperative nausea. *J Perianesth Nurs.* 19(1):29–35

Annis M. 2011. Inhaled ginger for seasickness during boat trip to watch whales. Unpublished dissertation for RJBA certification.

Arctander S. 1994. *Perfume and Flavor Materials of Natural Origin.* Carol Stream, IL: Allured Publishing.

Asao T, Mochiki E, Suzuki H et al. 2001. An easy method for the intraluminal administration of peppermint oil before colonoscopy and its effectiveness in reducing colonic spasm. *Gastrointest Endosc.* 53:172–7.

Avesina A. 1985. *Law in Medicine.* Soroush Press, Tehran, 2:187.

Beagham C. 2002. *Peppermint for postoperative nausea.* Unpublished dissertation for RJ Buckle Associates.

Boone S, Shields K. 2005. Treatment of pregnancy-related nausea and vomiting with ginger. *Ann Pharmacother.* 39:1710–3.

Borrelli F, Capasso R, Aviello G, Pittler M, Izzo A. 2005. Effectiveness and safety of ginger in the treatment of pregnancy-induced nausea and vomiting. *Obstet Gynecol.* 105(4):849–56.

Buckle J. 2007. Should nursing take aromatherapy more seriously? *J Advanced Nurs.* 16:116–20.

Cabo J, Crespo M, Jimenez J, Navarro C. 1986. The spasmolytic activity of various aromatic plants from the province of Granada. The activity of the major components of their essential oils. *Plantes Medicinales et Phytotherapy.* 20(5):213–218

Chaiyakunapruk N, Kitakannakom N, Nathisuwan S, Leeprakobboon K, Leelasettagool C. 2006. The efficacy of ginger for the prevention of postoperative nausea and vomiting: a meta-analysis. *Am J Obstet Gynecol.* 194(1):95–9.

Chalifour M. 2005. Peppermint as anti-emetic in Opiate detox. Unpublished dissertation for RJBA certification.

Clare P, Miller J, Nikolova T, Tickoo R. 2011. Treating nausea and vomiting in palliative care: a review. *Clin Interv Aging*. 6:243–59.

de Pradier. 2006. A trial of a mixture of three essential oils in the treatment of postoperative nausea and vomiting. *Int J Aromather*. 16(1):15–20.

Eberhart LH, Mayer R, Betz O, Tsolakidis S, Hilpert W et al. 2003. Ginger does not prevent post-operative nausea and vomiting after laparoscopic surgery. *Anesth Analg*. 96(4):995–8.

Endo J, Iihara H, Yamada M, Yanase K, Kamiya F, Ito F, Funaguchi N, Ohno Y, Minatoguchi S, Itoh Y. 2012. A randomized, controlled non-inferiority study comparing the antiemetic effect of intravenous granisetron and oral azesetron based on estimated 5-HT3 receptor occupancy. *Anticancer Res*. 32(9):3939–47.

Ensiyeh J, Sakineh M. 2009. Comparing ginger and vitamin B6 for the treatment of nausea and vomiting in pregnancy: a randomised controlled trial. *Midwifery*. 25(6):649–53.

Ernst E, Pittler M. 2000. Efficacy of ginger for nausea and vomiting: a systematic review of randomized clinical trials. *Br J Anaesth*. 84(3):367–71.

Evenson C. 2000. *Lavandula intermedia* (DT Super) as a post-operative anti-emetic. Unpublished dissertation. RJ Buckle Associates LLC.

Ferruggiari L, Ragione B, Rich E, Lock K. 2012. The effect of aromatherapy on postoperative nausea in women undergoing surgical procedures. *J Perianesth Nurse*. 27(4):246–51.

Figuenick R. 1998. Essential oil of peppermint: a 3-part audit on nausea. Unpublished dissertation. RJ Buckle Associates LLC.

Franchomme P, Penoel D. 1980. *L'aromatherapie Exactement*. Jollois, Limoge, France.

Geiger J. 2005. The essential oil of ginger, *Zingiber officinale*, and anaesthesia. *Int J Aromather*. 15:7–14.

Gilligan N. 2005. The palliation of nausea in hospice and palliative care patients with essential oils of Pimpinella anisum (aniseed), Foeniculum vul-gar var (sweet fennel), Anthemis nobilis (Roman Chamomile) and Mentha x piperita (peppermint). *The International Journal of Aromatherapy*. 15: 163-167.

Grigoleit HG, Grigoleit P. 2005. Gastrointestinal clinical pharmacology of peppermint oil. *Phytomed*. 12:607–11.

Hejazian S, Dashti M, Mahdavi S, Qureshi M. 2009. The effect of Carum copticun on acetylcholine induced contraction in isolated rat's ileum. *J Acupunct Meridian Stud*. 2(1): 75–78.

Hertz R. 2009. Aromatherapy facts and fictions: a scientific analysis of olfactory effects on mood, physiology and behaviour. *Int J Neurosc*. 119:263–90.

Hill S, Thomas S. 2011. Clinical toxicology of recreational drugs. *Clin Toxicol (Phila)*. 49(8):705–19.

Hines S, Steels E, Change A, Gibbons K. 2012. Aromatherapy for treatment of postoperative nausea and vomiting. *Cochrane Database Syst Rev*. 18(4):CD007598.

Hunt R, Dienemann J, Norton J, Hartley W et al. 2012. Aromatherapy as treatment for postoperative nausea: a randomized trial. *Anesth Anal*. [Epub ahead of print].

Irby S. 2006. Inhaled peppermint for relief of chemo induced nausea. Unpublished dissertation for RJBA.

Ishimuru H, Takayama S, Shiokawa M, Inoue T. 2008. Cost-effectiveness analysis of 5-HT3 receptor antagonist drugs in cancer chemotherapy. *Gan To Kagaku Ryoho*. 35(4):619–23.

Jamal A, Jarved K, Aslam M, Jafri M. 2006. Gastroprotective effect of cardamom, *Elettaria cardamomum* Maton fruits in rats. *J Ethnopharmacol*. 103(2):149–53.

Karas-Irwin B. 2006. A feasibility study on inhaled ginger for post operative nausea. Unpublished dissertation for RJBA certification.

Kitzler R, Nolan S. 2009. The role of aromatherapy in postoperative nausea and vomiting. *Onc Nurs Forum*. 36: 47.

Leicester R, Hunt R. 1982. Peppermint oil to reduce colonic spasm during endoscopy. *Lancet*. 2(8305):989–90.

Lawrence B. 2001. Personal communication, September 2001.

Lowdermilk G. 2007. Peppermint and ginger for chemo-induced nausea. Unpublished dissertation for RJBA.

Lua P, Zakaria N. 2012. A brief review of current scientific evidence involving aromatherapy use for nausea and vomiting. *J Alt Comp Med*. 18(6):534–40.

McKenzie J, Gallacher M. 1989. A sweet-smelling success: use of peppermint oil in helping patients accept their colostomies. *Nursing Times.* 85(27):48–9.

Matthews A, Dowswell T, Haas D, Doyle M, O'Mathuna D. 2010. Interventions for nausea and vomiting in early pregnancy. *Cochrane Database Syst Review.* 8(9):CD007575. doi: 10.1002/14651858. CD007575.pub2.

Mazzer M. 2013. Holistic Nursing Department, Valley Hospital, Ridgewood, NJ. Personal communication.

McNatty D. 2008. Side effect solutions: helping patients avoid drug-induced nausea. *Pharmacy Times.* http:// www.pharmacytimes.com/publications/issue/2008/2008-08/2008-08-8642. Accessed October 20, 2012.

Morin A, Betz O, Kranke P, Geldner G, Wulf H, Eberhart L. 2004. Is ginger a relevant antiemetic for post-operative nausea and vomiting? *Anasthesiol Intensivmed Notfallmed Schmerzther.* 39(5):281-5.

Nadkarni K. 1992. *Indian Materia Medica,* Vol. 1. Prakashan, India: Bombay Popular.

Ndao D, Ladas E, Cheng B, Sands S et al. 2012. Inhalation aromatherapy in children and adolescents undergoing stem cell infusion: results of a placebo-controlled double-blind trial. *Psychooncology.* 21(3):247–54.

Nord D, 2006. *Ginger and Lavender for post operative nausea in children.* Unpublished dissertation for RJ Buckle Associates.

Panahi Y, Saadat A, Sahebkar A et al. 2012. Effect of ginger on acute and delayed chemotherapy-induced nausea and vomiting: a pilot, randomized, open-label clinical trial. *Integr Cancer Ther.* [Epub ahead of print.]

Piotroswki A. 2005. *Peppermint to relieve nausea in hospitalized patients.* Unpublished dissertation. RJ Buckle Associates LLC.

Pongrojpar D, Chiamchanya C. 2003. The efficacy of ginger in preventing post-operative nausea and vomiting after outpatient gynecological laparoscopy. *J Med Assoc Thai.* 86(3):244–50.

Potter P, Eisenberg S, Cain K, Berry D. 2011. Orange interventions for symptoms associated with dimethyl sylfoxide during stem cell reinfusions: a feasibility study. *Cancer Nurs.* 34(5):361–8.

Price S, Price L. 2012. *Aromatherapy for Health Professionals.* Churchill Livingstone.

Reagan S, Kind L, Clements F. 2009. *Quease Ease Aromatherapy for Treatment of PONV.* American Association of Critical Care Nurses.

Smith C, Crowther C, Willson K, Hotham N, McMillian V. 2004. A randomized controlled trial of ginger to treat nausea and vomiting in pregnancy. *Obstet Gynecol.* 103(4):639–45.

Stringer J, Donald G. 2011 Aromasticks in cancer care: an innovation not to be sniffed at. *Complement Ther Clin Pract.* 17:116–21.

Tate S. 1997. Peppermint oil: a treatment for postoperative nausea. *J Adv Nurs.* 26(3):543–9.

Tayarani-Najaran Z, Talasaz-Firoozi E, Nasiri R, Jalai N, Hassanzadeh M. 2013. Ecancermedicalscience. 2013:7.290. Accessed May 29, 2013.

Valnet J. 1990. *The Practice of Aromatherapy.* Saffron Walden, UK: CW Daniels.

Vutyavanich T, Kraisarin T, Ruangsri R. 1997. Ginger for nausea and vomiting in pregnancy: randomized, double-masked, placebo controlled trial. *Obstet Gynecol.* 97(4):577–82.

Wren R. 1988. *Potter's New Cyclopaedia of Botanical Drugs and Preparations.* London: Churchill Livingstone.

Zick SM, Ruffin MT, Lee J, Normolle DP, Siden R. 2009. Phase II trial of encapsulated ginger as a treatment for chemotherapy-induced nausea and vomiting. *Support Care Cancer.* 17(5):563–72.

Chapter 10

Pain and Inflammation

"I've learned that people will forget what you said, people will forget what you did, but people will never forget how you made them feel."

Maya Angelou

CHAPTER ASSETS

PAIN

Pain is an unpleasant sensation experienced when nociceptors are stimulated (Brooker 2008). Although there are physical dimensions that reflect a commonality of pain in humans, the experience of pain is unique to the individual (Fields 1997) and pain relief is influenced by individual perceptions and experience (Shi et al 2010). People who live with pain on a daily basis have, what is to them, a clear way of describing what they feel. If the pain changes, they know it. However, describing pain to someone who does not experience that pain can be problematic. Descriptions of pain vary greatly. Apart from the site of the pain (for example, abdominal), one of the most important aspects to consider is the onset of pain. The onset clarifies which kind of pain is involved: acute or chronic.

Aromatherapy may be useful with some of the problems associated with acute pain, for example, prolonged length of healing and increased length of stay in acute care facilities. However, this chapter will concentrate on aromatherapy for chronic pain because it appears to be more beneficial for chronic pain according to the research.

Chronic pain is a global issue. According to the Institute of Medicine (IOM) report (2011), chronic pain affects about 100 million Americans, and associated medical charges and lost productivity cost around $635 billion annually. This is a low estimate because it excludes children, those in the armed services, residents of nursing homes or those in long-term care facilities. Under the *Patient Protection and Affordable Care Act (2012)* in the United States, there are 16 recommendations for action and these include "reducing barriers to pain control." In the UK, the *UK Pain Proposal Report* (2011) found that 45% of the estimated 7.8 million people living with chronic pain did not have access to adequate management for their pain. In Australia, according to ABC national radio (2011), one in five Australians has chronic pain, costing the government an estimated $34.4 billion per year. Canadians are also struggling with the management of chronic pain and have estimated costs of over $6 billion per year (Schopflocher & Taenmzer 2011). Chronic pain has also become a major issue in Japan (Yamamoto et al 2010).

Pain is one of the most commonly addressed symptoms in a clinical setting, and of all the symptoms we experience in hospitals, it is the one we fear the most. Because pain is such a complex subject, specific types of pain such as arthritis, childbirth, menstrual pain, and neuralgic pain will be discussed in the chapters on care of the elderly, OB/GYN, and neurology, respectively. This chapter will examine the use of aromatherapy for alleviating various kinds of chronic pain. It discusses animal and human research regarding the use of whole essential oils and individual components within essential oils.

PHYSIOLOGY OF PAIN

Pain is an experience that affects us on many different levels: emotional, sensory, motivational, and cognitive (Mersky 1986). Pain is a complex neurophysiologic phenomenon (Alavi et al 1997) that can be described as somatic, neuropathic, or visceral. Somatic pain is well localized, persistent, and is often described as sharp or stabbing. Neuropathic pain is usually described as burning, numbing, or shooting and originates from compression or stimulation of a nerve. Visceral pain tends to be poorly localized, dull, and aching and involves an AC fiber ratio of 1:10 in visceral afferents. In normal adults, the ability to detect pain is completely removed when A and C axons are blocked (Fields 1997). When pain triggers the nociceptors (pain receptors), it is translated or transduced into electrical activity. The electrical impulse is then transmitted to the spinal cord via the dorsal root and relayed to the thalamus in the brain via the afferent pathways.

Pain is often divided into acute and chronic. Acute pain is short lasting and has a well-defined pattern of onset. Chronic pain persists beyond the expected period of healing (Casey 2002) and is associated with a degenerative or chronic pathologic process such as arthritis. However, sometimes the cause of pain is elusive, for example, in fibromyalgia and complex regional pain syndrome.

The thalamus is involved in pain perception and interpretation (Alavi et al 1997) and is part of the limbic system that analyzes smell; therefore, there is an implicit suggestion that smell may affect the perception of pain. Primary nociceptors activate spinal pain-transmission cells through two neurotransmitters, glutamate (an amine) and substance P (a peptide), which are present in C fibers (Fields 1997). Greer (1995) noted substance P immunoreactive processes throughout the laminae of the olfactory bulb. Substance P is released from peripheral sensory neurons in inflammatory and neuropathic pain (Teodoro et al 2012). A variety of chemical agents can activate the primary afferent nociceptors. These include serotonin and potassium. If the tissue is damaged or inflamed, the sensitivity of the nociceptors is heightened. The whole process results in a subjective, sensory, and emotional experience of pain.

Visceral pain is usually blocked by substances similar to opioids that are naturally produced (Sofaer & Foord 1993). The body can produce enkephalin, an opioid-like peptide that occurs in three forms: beta-endorphin, the met- and leu-enkephalins, and the dynorphins. These peptides work as neurotransmitters and neuromodulators at three major classes of receptors, mu, delta, and kappa, to produce analgesia (Holden et al 2005).

Etiology of Pain

There are many possible causes of pain: a simple headache can have a dozen predisposing factors including low blood sugar, sinusitis, stress, alcohol, hormonal imbalance, or a brain tumor. Pain is a complex issue because it is so intensely personal and closely linked to feelings and expectations (Atlas & Wager 2012). Pain may affect psychosocial issues, such as decreased social interactions, decreased work productivity, financial problems, impaired relationships, etc. Some people lose their faith. Some feel vulnerable and feel a sense of hopelessness. Goleman (1996) writes in his book *Emotional Intelligence* that humanity is most evident in our feelings and "emotional intervention should be a standard part of medical care" (p 165). Anxiety and tension are thought to heighten pain, whereas pleasure and relaxation may decrease pain. Most people find it difficult to relax when they are in pain and difficult to alter their own perception of pain unaided.

Orthodox Approaches to Pain

Over a decade ago, the Joint Commission on Accreditation of Healthcare Organizations (JCAHO), an organization that accredits the majority of the medical facilities in the United States, developed a new mandatory standard for the assessment and treatment of pain (Berry & Dahl 2000). They mandated that pain assessment should be the "5th vital sign." It was the first time JCAHO (now known as The Joint Commission) or any other accrediting body had issued standards focusing on pain awareness and management. Institutions had to work out how they were going to meet the new standards and what they needed to do to deal effectively with a patient in pain. As part of these standards, medical institutions are required to inform patients of their right to appropriate pain assessment and treatment. The assessment includes documenting the level and characteristics of each person's pain using a numeric scale of 0-10 or pictures of expressive faces (http://www.jointcommission.org/). No patient should score his or her pain above a four. Institutions are required to develop protocols for pain management and to educate their staff on pain management.

Analgesics are among the most widely used medications in the United States (Sinclair 2012) and probably worldwide. Analgesics are divided into opioids (narcotics) and nonopioids. The use of opioids is strictly regulated. Originally, narcotics were opioid derivatives and came from the plant *Papaver somniferum.* Recent advances in pharmacology have resulted in the development of several synthetic analgesics that work on the opioid receptors in the brain.

Narcotic/Opioid Drugs

Morphine, diamorphine, dihydrocodeine, hydrocodone, and fentanyl are examples of opioid drugs. Derived from the opium poppy, morphine and its derivatives work by binding to opioid receptors in the central nervous system (CNS) to reduce pain. Newer synthetic opioid drugs, for example, tramadol and hydrocodone, may have additional effects on serotonin and norepinephrine levels. Opioid drugs may reduce the ability to concentrate as well as reduce pain. The respiratory and cough centers are also depressed by morphine, as is the neurotransmitter acetylcholine. Codeine, a common but milder narcotic, is also derived from the opium poppy (Martin 1994). Codeine is used to suppress dry coughs as well as for the relief of general pain. Opioids are potentially addictive. Although previously it was thought that narcotics were less likely to be addictive for someone experiencing chronic pain (Carter 1996), some people dispute this (Juurlink & Dhalia 2012). Major side effects of opioids are constipation, nausea, and dry mouth. Adding other analgesics, such as paracetamol, nonsteroidal antiinflammatory drugs (NSAIDs), or cyclooxygenase-2 (COX-2) inhibitors to patient-controlled analgesia (PCA) reduced the amount of morphine the patient used significantly (McDaid et al 2011). Continued use may lead to tolerance, dependence, or addiction.

Common Nonopioid/Nonnarcotic Drugs

Major drugs in this category are aspirin, acetaminophen (paracetamol), anticonvulsants, antidepressants, and nonsteroidal/steroidal antiinflammatory drugs (Sullivan & Robinson 2006). Aspirin (acetylsalicylic acid) has antiinflammatory as well as analgesic effects. Originally aspirin was derived from salacin, a glycoside found in the bark of the willow tree (*Salix* alba). Aspirin blocks prostaglandin synthesis in both the CNS and the peripheral nervous system. Acetaminophen (called Tylenol in the United States and panadol or paracetamol in the UK) is a painkiller that has no antiinflammatory effects (Brooker 2008). One of the main drawbacks to paracetamol is its toxicity at relatively low doses: 10 to 15 g can cause liver damage (Brooker 2008).

ANTIINFLAMMATORY DRUGS

Antiinflammatory drugs are also used for both acute and chronic pain. Despite being very useful, they can have adverse side effects. Antiinflammatory drugs are divided into two main categories: nonsteroidal (NSAIDs) and steroidal.

NSAIDs

Aspirin is the most common NSAID and has a long history of use. Yin et al (1998) found that aspirin inhibited transcription factors that coded the production of prostaglandin synthase enzymes. Lyss et al (1997) discovered that helenalin, a lactone found in *Arnica*, inhibited the same transcription factor, but in a different way. However, blocking prostaglandin synthesis can give rise to specific side effects. All NSAIDs, including aspirin-based antiinflammatories, can increase gastric bleeding in patients with gastric ulcers. This results from the inhibition of prostaglandin E2 (PGE2) that suppresses gastric acid secretion. NSAIDs can also prolong bleeding as they inhibit production of thromboxane (Ward 1993). They can also upset the fluid balance and affect renal blood flow. They can cause bronchospasm and nasal polyposis in susceptible individuals, and they can delay the onset of labor as they can reduce the contractile effects of prostaglandins on the uterine muscles (Kvam 1994). Indomethacin is often used when salicylates are not tolerated. However, in arthritic patients, indomethacin can lead to a high incidence of CNS effects if the dose is high.

Steroid-Based Antiinflammatory Drugs

Despite being superior to NSAIDs (and affecting the inflammatory process at each level), steroidal antiinflammatory drugs have many side effects. These include hyperglycemia leading to diabetes, myopathy, increased intraocular pressure with the potential for glaucoma, electrolyte imbalance leading to hypertension, thinning of the skin with an increased tendency for poor healing and skin breakdown, hirsutism, insomnia, depression, and psychosis (Craig 1994). These drugs are usually avoided in long-term treatment. However, steroidal antiinflammatory drugs have provided relief for chronic inflammation and will continue to be used until other drugs with fewer side effects are found. Infliximab, which belongs to a relatively new class of monoclonal antibody, is used as an antiinflammatory in the treatment of autoimmune diseases. For neuropathic pain, gabapentin and pregabalin are the drugs of choice.

LIMITATIONS OF ORTHODOX TREATMENTS

Despite advances in pain medication, many patients suffer chronic (and sometimes severe) pain over their lifetime. In some cases, this is despite the advent of PCA. Knowledge and attitude toward pain and pain management continue to be the most prominent barriers for effectively treating pain (Jablonski & Duke 2012). Controversies surrounding new analgesic drugs also exist. Oxycontin, a drug as potent as morphine, was heavily marketed to physicians but later found to be highly addictive (Meier & Petersen 2001).

CHRONIC PAIN SYNDROME

In 2011, an average of 31% of Americans reported having a neck or back condition, 26% had a knee or leg condition, and 18% had another condition causing recurring pain. The Gallup Poll found similar rates each year since tracking began in 2008. In all, 47% of Americans reported having a least one of the three types of chronic pain measured in the survey, including 7% who reported all three types (The Gallup Poll 2011). For essential oils that can be useful for chronic pain, please see Table 10-1.

TABLE 10-1 *Essential Oils Suitable for Chronic Pain*

Common Name	Botanical Name	Application
Black pepper	*Piper nigrum*	Topical
Clove bud[*][†]	*Syzygium aromaticum*	Topical
Frankincense	*Boswellia carteri*	Inhaled, topical
Ginger	*Zingiber officinale*	Topical, oral in capsules
Juniper	*Juniperus communis*	Topical
Lavender (spike)	*Lavandula latifolia*	Topical
Lavender (true)	*Lavandula angustifolia*	Inhaled, topical, oral capsules
Lemongrass	*Cymbopogon citrates*	Inhaled, topical
Marjoram (sweet)	*Origanum majorana*	Inhaled, topical
Myrrh	*Commiphora molmol*	Topical
Peppermint	*Mentha piperita*	Topical, oral capsules
Rose	*Rosa damascene*	Topical
Rosemary[‡]	*Rosmarinus officinalis*	Inhaled, topical
Verbena	*Aloysia triphylla*	Inhaled, topical
Ylang ylang	*Cananga odorata*	Inhaled

[*]Clove bud is safer than clove leaf. Phenols can be harsh on the skin.
[†]Best to avoid regular use of clove with patients on anticoagulant therapy.
[‡]Rosemary is a stimulant: best to avoid regular use in hypertension or epilepsy.

As well as chronic pain, there is chronic pain syndrome (CPS). CPS has been described as a complex dysfunction and is extremely difficult to treat successfully. Allopathic medicine treats CPS with a mixture of opioid and nonopioid drugs backed with tricyclic or valium-type drugs that are not antidepressants, although they are used for that purpose in this instance.

How patients could have rapid access to pain control was investigated in a recent study from Germany (Erlenwein et al 2012). This study found that standardizing postoperative pain management so nursing stuff could administer pain medication (within well-defined margins) reduced the dependence on the ward doctor and meant patients received analgesics much more quickly in the hospital setting.

Jablonski and Duke (2012) suggest that effective pain management should include alternative and complementary therapies. Gatlin and Schulmeister (2007) suggest that we should stop overlooking simple, noninvasive, nonpharmacologic measures shown to be effective in pain management.

AROMATHERAPY FOR PAIN

Touch, relaxation, and pleasure each play an important part in how individuals perceive the world around them and how they feel about themselves. This includes the perception of pain (Beck & Beck 1987). Aromatherapy works on the sensory system and enhances the parasympathetic response, which is closely linked with endorphins (Weil 1996). Inhaling sweet aromas has been found to increase pain tolerance (Prescott & Wilkie 2007). The intensity and depth of pain is influenced by external factors such as previous experience, attitude, and culture. Pain can be "put on hold" by strong emotions such as anger, fear, or elation. Conversely, fear can make pain feel worse. Pain is a warning system. By deadening it, the warning system is dulled. A headache pill does not make the cause of the headache go away; it just allows the person to carry on functioning.

Aromatherapy can be helpful in alleviating chronic pain (Buckle 1999). Essential oils have pharmacologically active components and some enhance the absorption and potency of orthodox pain medicines (Buckle 2010). For example, cardamom enhances absorption of indomethacin, an antiinflammatory drug (Huang et al 1999). Many components in essential oils are analgesic, so it is hardly surprising that aromatherapy is now part of many pain management programs in the United States, UK, Australia, Canada, and elsewhere.

As well as having analgesic properties (De Sousa 2011), the actual application of diluted essential oils in a massage, or the 'M' Technique®, can be very relaxing. The odor of most essential oils is pleasurable. Thus, aromatherapy enhances the parasympathetic response, encouraging relaxation at a deep level. Relaxation has been shown to alter perceptions of pain and allow a patient to "let go," often for the first time. The analgesic effects of aromatherapy can be traced to several factors, depending on whether the essential oils are used topically on the area of pain, inhaled to reduce the sensation of pain, or taken orally.

Inhalation

The two factors that contribute to the benefits associated with inhalation of essential oils for pain are as follows:

(1) A complex mixture of volatile chemicals reaches the "pleasure memory sites" within the brain. These include the nucleus accumbens and ventral pallidum in the subcortical region and the orbitofrontal cortex and anterior cingulated cortex in the cortical region.

(2) Certain analgesic components within the essential oil (that may or may not be known) affect the neurotransmitters dopamine, serotonin, and noradrenaline at receptor sites in the brain. For example, bergamot essential oil can affect the synaptic plasticity of neurotransmitters (Bagetta et al 2010). However, most essential oils are thought to merely affect the perception of pain (Gedney et al 2004).

Whatever the mechanism, inhaled essential oils appear to impact the perception of pain.

Topical Use

The factors associated with topical use of essential oils for pain are as follows:

(1) Certain components within essential oils are warming, for example, 1,8-cineole in eucalyptus (Liapi et al 2007). Some components are cooling, for example, menthol in peppermint (Kraemer et al 2005).

(2) Some components (such as esters) have antispasmodic action, for example, linalyl acetate in lavender (Koto et al 2006).

(3) Some components have an antiinflammatory action, such as the sesquiterpene chamazulene in German chamomile (Ramadan et al 2006).
(4) Certain components have a topical analgesic effect, for example, citronellal in lemongrass (Quintans-Junior et al 2011). Lavender and its two main components, linalyl acetate and linalool, also showed local anesthetic activity in a study by Ghelardini et al (1999).
(5) The interaction of touch with sensory fibers in the skin affects the transmission of referred pain (Schmelz 2011).
(6) There is a positive rubefacient effect of a warm bath or friction on the skin.

Oral Use

Although this may not be within the remit of some health professionals, research shows that certain components within essential oils have analgesic effect when taken orally. An example of this is gingerdione from ginger (Lee et al 2012). Whole essential oils can also have analgesic effects on specific areas when taken orally. For example, peppermint taken in enteric-coated capsules was found to be helpful in relieving the colonic spasm that follows colonoscopy (Shavakhi et al 2012). Peppermint oil capsules, such as Colpermin, are available from many health food stores and the internet and can be useful for irritable bowel syndrome (IBS). Anecdotal evidence suggests that *Lavandula angustifolia* (three drops in 15 mL of warm water) in a gargle and swallow is also good for relieving a sore throat. For more on the oral use of essential oils, please see Chapter 7.

Two thousand years ago, man used the plants *Salix* (willow) and *Populus* (poplar) to alleviate pain (Lewis & Elvin-Lewis 1977). Gattefosse, the grandfather of clinical aromatherapy (1937), wrote "almost all essential oils have analgesic properties."

Animal Studies

A literature search of the databases listed in the appendix found published research on essential oils with analgesic effects (on animals) for basil, bergamot, eucalyptus, frankincense, ginger, lavender, lemon, myrrh, patchouli, peppermint, rose, rosemary, and thyme. This does not mean that other essential oils do not have analgesic effects, just that they are not published as yet. The methods used on the animals were as follows:

Intraperitoneal (i.p.)	Into the abdominal cavity
Subcutaneous (s.c.)	Under the skin
Oral (p.o.)	Oral
Intraplantarly (i.pl.)	Between the paws
Intracerebroventricularly (i.c.v.)	Into the brain
Intrathecal (i.t.)	Into the spinal cord
Intragastrically (i.g.)	Into the stomach via nasogastric tube

Here are a few of the studies to give you an idea of what they involved. Brazilian basil *(Ocimum selloi)* was found to have analgesic properties in mice at 2, 20, and 200 mg/kg orally (Franca et al 2008). This basil contains up to 55.3% methylchavicol (estragole). In a later study, *Ocimum basilicum* (the basil more often used in aromatherapy) demonstrated peripheral and central analgesic effects related to the inhibition of pain mediators (such as prostaglandins and prostacyclins) as well as interaction with opioid receptors (Vanancio et al 2011). Another species of basil *(Ocimum gratissiumum)* had analgesic effects in mice: the active components were eugenol and myrcene (Paula-Friere et al 2012).

Rosemary had analgesic properties in rats when the rats' paws were subjected to acetic acid or hot plates (Takaki et al 2008; Martinez et al 2009). Frankincense and myrrh were found to be effective analgesic and antiinflammatory agents (both separately and combined) when used in rats that had paw pain induced by formalin and carrageenan (Su et al 2012).

Perez-Raya et al (1990) found that *Mentha rotundifolia* and *Mentha longifolia* (both types of peppermint) had analgesic properties in mice and rats. Peana et al (1999) found that essential oil of clary sage *(Salvia sclarea)* had antiinflammatory and analgesic action at a local level. An extract of myrrh *(Commiphora molmol)* had a strong local anesthetic effect in a study by Dolara et al (2000). The anesthetic action blocked the sodium current of excitable mammalian membranes. The local anesthetic activity on nerve cells was measured by incubating hippocampal brain slices, freshly dissected with a tissue chopper, from the brain of one of the experimental male rats. The slices were stimulated with a positive electrical current applied through electrodes.

Lavandula angustifolia had a local anesthetic effect in rabbits (Ghelardini et al 1999). Most animal research tends to inject the essential oil into the animal's peritoneal cavity, into its brain, or between the animal's paws. In some studies, the essential oil is administered via nasogastric tube. Other studies, such as the one by Maruyama et al (2005) using geranium, explore the topical analgesic effects of essential oils.

The analgesic effects of lemongrass in mice were explored by Viana et al (2000). They concluded that the essential oil worked at both central and peripheral levels when given by p.o. and i.p. routes. For animal studies, please see Table 10-2.

Human Studies

One of the earliest studies showing the analgesic effect of essential oils in humans was conducted by Woolfson and Hewitt (1992). They found a 50% pain reduction in patients in a critical care unit. Thirty-six patients were randomly allocated into three groups of 12: group A received massage plus lavender, group B received massage without lavender, and group C was the control group who received no treatment and were left to rest "curtained off" from the remainder of the unit. Treatment consisted of 20 minutes of foot massage twice a week for 5 weeks. This was an interesting study because some of the patients were artificially ventilated, so the effects of the essential oil could have come from inhalation or topical absorption. The largest difference between the groups was in heart rate. Ninety percent of Group A had a reduction of 11 to 15 beats per minute, whereas only 58% of Group B had a reduction, which was consistently less. Only 41% of the control group showed any reduction. The study provided no formal statistics or analysis.

Wilkinson (1995) investigated the effects of 1% Roman chamomile *(Chamomelum nobile)* in a massage on 51 patients with cancer in a randomized study. The participants ranged in age from 26 to 84 years. Ninety-four percent of the participants were female, and 6% were male. Forty-one percent had been referred for pain

TABLE 10-2 *Essential Oils and Animal Studies*

Essential Oil	Year	Author	Animal	Results
Basil	2008	Franca et al	Mice	+ve
	2011	Vanancio et al	Mice	+ve
	2012	Paula-Friere et al	Mice	+ve
Bergamot	2010	Sakurada et al	Mice	+ve
Eucalyptus	2003	Silva et al	Mice	+ve
Frankincense	2012	Su et al	Rats	+ve
Geranium	2005	Maruyama et al	Mice	+ve
Ginger	2009	Khushtar et al	Rats	+ve
Lavender	2003	Hajhashemi et al	Mice	+ve
Lavandin (Grosso)	2004	Barocelli et al	Rats	+ve
Lemon	2011	Campelo et al	Mice	+ve
Lemongrass	2000	Viana et al	Mice	+ve
Myrrh	2012	Su et al	Rats	+ve
Patchouli (extract)	2011	Tsung-Chun et al	Mice	+ve
Peppermint	2012	Taher	Mice	+ve
Rose otto	2010	Hajhashemi	Rats	+ve
Rosemary	2008	Takaki et al	Rats	+ve
	2009	Martinez et al	Rats	+ve
Thyme	2009	Taherian	Mice	+ve

+ve = positive result; *–ve* = negative result.

control. During the study, 45% of the participants were receiving morphine, with the remainder on weak opioids, nonopioids, or nothing. Seventy-six percent of the participants had metastases. Mann–Whitney U tests on all independent variables revealed no significant differences between conditions in the pretest scores for the Rotterdam Symptom Checklist on physical or psychological symptoms, activities, and the top 10 symptoms. The data were analyzed using the Statistical Package for the Social Sciences (Nie et al 1975) and nonparametric tests were employed for all statistical analyses. State Trait Anxiety Inventory (STAI) scores fell by an average of 16 points in the aromatherapy massage group but only 10 points in the plain massage or standard group ($P = 0.005$), and pain was reduced statistically ($P = 0.003$). One patient is quoted as saying "I know now, almost definitely, that it (aromatherapy) has helped me in my quest for pain relief. I have told Dr. R at the pain clinic how pain free I was while having regular (aromatherapy) treatment" (Wilkinson 1995).

Since the last edition of this book, there have been many published studies evaluating the effect of essential oils on human pain, as Table 10-3 indicates. RJ Buckle students have conducted many more studies on the use of aromatherapy on pain for their certification. These studies are mainly nonpublished (as yet) and are listed in Table 10-4. Studies have been on inhaled, topically applied (mainly as massage) and oral use of essential oils, and nearly all have shown positive results.

TABLE 10-3 *Essential Oils for Pain Relief in Human Studies*

Essential Oil	Year	Author	Type of Pain	Application	N	Result
Lavender	2004	Gedney et al	Induced pain	Inhaled	26	+ve
	2006	Kim et al	Postoperative pain	Inhaled	50	−ve
	2006	Yip & Tse	Neck pain	Acupressure	32	+ve
	2007	Kim et al	Postoperative pain	Inhaled	54	+ve
	2012	Sheikhan et al	Episiotomy	Topical	60	+ve
	2011	Hadi & Hanid	After cesarean	Inhaled	200	+ve
	2011	Kim et al	Needle insertion	Inhaled	30	+ve
	2011	Grunebaum et al	Botox inject	Inhaled	30	−ve
	2012	Sasannejad et al	Migraine	Inhaled	47	+ve
Mixture 1	2005	Kim et al	Arthritis	Topical	40	+ve
Mixture 2	2006	Han et al	Menstrual	Topical	67	+ve
Mixture 3	2012	Hur et al	Menstrual	Topical	23	+ve
Mixture 4	2012	Ou et al	Menstrual	Topical	48	+ve
Peppermint	2002	Davies et al	Postherpetic neuralgia	Topical	1	+ve
	2004	Raudenbush et al	GI	Inhaled	158	+ve
	2008	Khvorova & Neill	GI	Oral	R	+ve
	2008	Ford et al	IBS	Oral	R	+ve
	2010	Merat et al	Colonoscopy	Oral	90	+ve
	2012	Shavakhi et al	GI	Oral	32	+ve
	2012	Mann et al	GI	Oral	1634	+ve
Eucalyptus	2011	Smith D, Jacobson 2011 et al	Arthritis	Topical	43	+ve
Ginger	2005	Calvert	Labor	Bath	22	+ve
	2008	Leach & Kumar	Arthritis	Oral	R	+ve
	2008	Yip et al	Arthritis	Topical	59	+ve
Jasmine	2004	Raudenbush	Cold pressor	Inhaled	158	+ve
Tea tree	2012	Joksimovic et al	Hemorrhoids	Topical	36	+ve
Chamomile	2008	Pazandeh et al	Episiotomy	Topical	88	−ve
Bergamot	2008	Chang	Hospice	Topical	58	+ve
	2012	Ndao	Stem cell	Inhaled	37	−ve
Rose	2012	Ayan et al	Renal colic	Inhaled	80	+ve

GI = Gastrointestinal; *IBS* = irritable bowel syndrome; *N* = number in trial; *R* = review; *+ve* = positive result; *−ve* = negative/no result.

Mixture 1 = lavender, marjoram, eucalyptus, rosemary, and peppermint blended in proportions of 2:1:2:1:1.

Mixture 2 = two drops of lavender *(Lavandula officinalis)*, one drop of clary sage *(Salvia sclarea)*, and one drop of rose *(Rosa centifolia)* in 5 mL of almond oil.

Mixture 3 = clary sage, marjoram, cinnamon, ginger, and geranium in a ratio of 1:1:0.5:1.5:1.5 diluted in almond oil to 5%.

Mixture 4 = lavender *(Lavandula officinalis)*, clary sage *(Salvia sclarea)*, and marjoram *(Origanum majorana)* in a 2:1:1 ratio was diluted in unscented cream at 3% concentration.

TABLE 10-4 *Studies Carried out on Pain by RJ Buckle Students*

Name	Year	State	N	Type of Pain	Essential Oil
Costa	1997	MA	10	Back	Lavender
Solis	2000	AZ	6	Back	Sweet marjoram/black pepper
White	2002	PA	12	Neck pain	Peppermint
Hein	2002	AZ	10	Neck pain	Rosemary
Walters	2004	TX	10	Neck/shoulder	Eucalyptus/black pepper
Carpenter	2007	TX	10	Neck/shoulder	Roman chamomile/ marjoram/lavender
Kirkman	2008	TX	10	Neck/shoulder	Lavender/sweet marjoram/black pepper
Newell	2011	MS	10	Shoulder	Ginger
Herring	2006	MN	18	Fibromyalgia	Peppermint
Gilmore	2006	NJ	18	Chronic pain	Sweet marjoram/ lavender
Haynes	2007	PA	22	Chronic pain	Peppermint/basil/ lavender/Roman chamomile
Trull	2007	TX	18	Acute postoperative pain	Mandarin/sandalwood
Harper	2010	NY	12	Recent injury	Black pepper
Lippert	1997	KS	6	Arthritis	Mixture
Kinzelmann	1997	KS	6	Arthritis	*Eucalyptus citriadora*/ ginger
Peters	2002	PA	8	Arthritis	German chamomile/ ginger
Berguetski	2002	MN	8	Arthritis	German chamomile/ ginger
Tait	2002	OH	8	Arthritis	*Eucalyptus globulus*
Dullaghan	2002	NY	9	Arthritis	Black pepper
Cote	2002	WA	11	Arthritis	Black pepper
Beasley	2003	IN	10	Arthritis	German chamomile/ frankincense
Prommel	2003	NY	8	Arthritis	Black pepper/sweet marjoram
Gutierrez	2004	AZ	14	Arthritis	*Helicrysum*
Wiest	2005	MN	12	Arthritis	Black pepper
Pemberton	2007	TX	10	Arthritis	*Eucalyptus globulus*/ lavender

TABLE 10-4 *Studies Carried out on Pain by RJ Buckle Students—cont'd*

Name	Year	State	N	Type of Pain	Essential Oil
Bozarth	2009	TX	11	Arthritis	Black pepper/marjoram/ German chamomile
Gagnon	2010	MA	8	Arthritis	Peppermint/lemongrass
Estabrook	2012	NE	11	Arthritis	Lavender/frankincense
Flick	2008	TX	9	Raynaud's syndrome	Black pepper
Bonavia	2007	WI	11	Muscle pain	Sweet marjoram
Decker	2007	MA	8	Muscle pain	Roman chamomile
Hjersted-Smith	2008	TX	10	Muscle pain	Sweet marjoram
Colby	2009	MN	10	Muscle pain	Sweet marjoram
McCleod	2012	MN	12	Muscle ache after sport	Peppermint/sweet marjoram
Cavallo	2004	AZ	27	Dysmenorrhea	Clary sage
Rodriquez	2005	WI	14	Dysmenorrhea	Clary sage
Reimer	2005	WI	12	Dysmenorrhea	Clary sage
Nichols	2006	NC	7	Dysmenorrhea	Lavender/clary sage/ petitgrain
Clark	2007	NE	10	Dysmenorrhea	Mixture
Tibjas	2008	TX	11	Dysmenorrhea	Clary sage/geranium
Pray	2000	AZ	8	Headache	Peppermint/Roman chamomile
North-Doty	2008	WI	10	Headache	Peppermint
Arends	2012	SD	14	Headache	Lavender/frankincense
Adams	2000	AZ	23	Labor	Lavender
Swingle	2001	NY	25	Labor	Clary sage/frankincense
Marino	2004	AZ	11	Labor	Lavender
Bowles	2004	AZ	9	Labor	Lavender

Inhaled

Lavender, given via oxygen mask in a postanesthesia care unit, reduced opioid requirements of morbidly obese patients undergoing laparoscopic adjustable gastric banding in a Korean study (Kim et al 2007). Lavender, given in a face mask, was also effective in another randomized, controlled study by Kim et al (2011). In this study, healthy volunteers rated stress and pain during needle insertion. The results showed that the pain intensity of needle insertion was significantly decreased after aromatherapy compared with the control (P < 0.001).

However, inhaled lavender was not effective in two other studies on pain. Inhaled lavender did not reduce pain during elective cosmetic facial injections of

Botox (12 U) (Grunebaum et al 2011). Inhaled lavender did not reduce the pain scores of postsurgical patients (underdoing a breast biopsy) or the amount of narcotics required (Kim et al 2006), but it did produce a higher satisfaction with pain control. Similarly, inhaled oils of mandarin and sandalwood did not reduce acute postoperative pain (Trull 2007).

Ayan et al (2012) explored the use of inhaled rose oil on a group of 80 patients with renal colic. Half of the group received conventional analgesic (diclofenac sodium, 75 mg intramuscularly, i.m.) plus a placebo smell of saline. The other group received the same i.m. injection plus inhaled rose essential oil. Pain was measured using a visual analogue scale (VAS) where the worst pain was given a score of 10 and no pain was 0. Inhaling the rose impacted the perception of pain after 10 and 30 minutes. At 30 minutes, the difference in the two groups was 3.75 ± 2.08 for the diclofenac plus placebo group, versus 1.08 ± 1.07 for the diclofenac plus rose group.

Perhaps inhaled aroma has more to do with the perception of pain, rather than the actual pain itself. Gedney et al (2004) explored the effect of inhaled lavender and rosemary on acute pain. In this study, volunteers experiencing contact heat, pressure, and ischemic pain rated inhaled lavender and rosemary. They found the pain "unpleasantness" was reduced with lavender, and less so with rosemary. This idea that inhaled aroma could affect perception of pain was explored by Martin (2006) who used a pleasant aroma (lemon) versus an unpleasant aroma (machine oil) on a group of 60 healthy volunteers who had induced pain (cold pressor test). Pain was measured at 5, 10, and 15 minutes. In this study, both lemon and machine oil groups reported significantly greater pain than those in the control group at 5 minutes. However, at 15 minutes, individuals exposed to the unpleasant odor experienced greater pain than the other group.

Topical

Lavender in a bath reduced perineal discomfort following episiotomy in an Iranian study (Sheikhan et al 2012). However, a similar study (also from Iran) found that "essence of chamomile" in a bath following episiotomy did not reduce perineal discomfort (Pazandeh et al 2008).

Massage using essential oils is a popular way to reduce the perception of chronic pain. These studies are often completed in hospices (Soden et al 2004; Chang 2008). Some aromatherapy massage studies have targeted dysmenorrhea (Han et al 2006; Ou et al 2012) or muscular pain (Kraft & Uehleke 2005). Other studies have explored the effect of using different percentages of essential oils topically. For example, a study by Pittler & Ernst (2003) used 100%, 50%, and 10% geranium essential oil versus a placebo of mineral oil or capsaicin 0.025% on postherpetic neuralgia. Pain reduction was dose dependent ($P \leq 5.003$). A placebo-controlled study of a mixture of topically applied essential oils on 153 patients with fibromyalgia (Ko et al 2007) found improvement in the following measurement outcomes: VAS night pain rating ($P = 0.018$), Jamar grip strength ($P < 0.001$), number of trigeminal evoked potentials (TePs; $P < 0.001$), average TeP pain threshold ($P < 0.001$), and Lanier scale (P = 0.001). The mixture contained camphor, eucalyptus, peppermint, rosemary, lemon, and orange in aloe vera.

Gobel et al (1991) studied the effect of peppermint applied topically for headaches. Pain was induced in healthy humans using pressure, thermal, and ischemic stimuli. The intensity of the pain, neurophysiology, performance-related activity, and mood states were monitored. Peppermint diluted in ethanol and applied topically produced a significant analgesic effect. Krall and Krause (1993) conducted an open, randomized study of 100 patients to evaluate the effects of a topically applied gel containing peppermint oil (30%) on periarticular pain. Effects of the peppermint gel were measured in acute (n = 49) and subacute (n = 51) conditions compared to the standard treatment of 10% hydroxyethyl salicylate gel. Different aspects of pain (intensity on pressure and spontaneous and movement-induced pain) were examined using a VAS (ranging from 0 = no symptom to 100 = severe symptom) for a period of 20 days. No statistical details were given. In 78% of cases both the physician and the patient considered the results with the mint therapy to be highly effective as opposed to 50% and 34%, respectively, with the standard gel. There were 10 instances of side effects from the hydroxyethyl salicylate gel (three of erythema and seven of itching) and only one (smell of peppermint in the nose) from the mint oil. At the end of the study, 19% of the mint oil patients were still suffering from pain compared to 36% of the aspirin gel group. The results of this comparative study were dependent on the severity of the symptoms.

Ginger *(Zingiber officinale)* can have an analgesic and deeply warming action, but the topical analgesic gingerol (a phenol) only occurs in the CO_2 extract, not in the essential oil (Wren 1988). Any phenol-rich essential oil needs to be used with care in topical applications. Rose (1992) suggests that benzoin, camphor, clove, coriander, ginger, hops, lemongrass, marjoram, black pepper, pine, savory, and ylang ylang have analgesic properties. Other aromatherapy educators suggest that additional essential oils—such as basil, bay laurel, cajuput, cinnamon leaf, eucalyptus, geranium, juniper berry, nutmeg, sweet fennel, sweet marjoram, peppermint, rosemary CT 1,8-cineole, camphor, spearmint, tarragon, thyme CT thymol, wintergreen, and yarrow—have analgesic properties (e.g., Rhind 2012).

Oral

Peppermint was found to reduce gastric pain in several studies (Merat et al 2010; Shavakhi et al 2012). Merat's study was a randomized, double-blind, placebo-controlled study on 90 outpatients with IBS. Participants took one capsule of enteric-coated, delayed-release peppermint oil (Colpermin) or placebo three times a day for 8 weeks. At the end of the 8 weeks, 14 participants were free from abdominal pain in the Colpermin group compared to only six in the control group (P < 0.001). The severity of abdominal pain was also reduced significantly in the Colpermin group compared to controls. Shavakhi et al (2012) explored the effect of peppermint given orally before colonoscopy. Sixty-five adult patients undergoing colonoscopy were randomized to receive either peppermint oil (Colpermin; n = 33) or placebo capsules (n = 32) as premedication, 4 hours before colonoscopy. Oral peppermint oil reduced the pain in patients during and following colonoscopy.

There have been other studies on the oral use of aromatic herbs, such as ginger and fennel, but they have tended to be on the dried herb rather than the essential oil. For example, Modaress and Asadipour (2006) explored the effect of orally ingested fennel on dysmenorrhea and Rahnama et al (2012) explored the effect of orally ingested ginger, also for dysmenorrhea. Perhaps more studies on the oral use of essential oils will follow.

RESEARCH ON ISOLATED ANALGESIC COMPONENTS OF ESSENTIAL OILS

Whole essential oils are not patentable. However, isolated components from essential oils can be synthesized and added together to form a new patentable product. So, it is hardly surprising there is a lot of research on the isolated components of essential oils. Much of it is conducted by the pharmaceutical industry. Many essential oils contain components that have been shown to have analgesic (antinociceptive) effects in rats and mice (Santos et al 2005). Of these, perhaps the most well-known component is (-)linalool, found in large amounts in essential oils like lavender and clary sage. This linalool acts on several receptors, namely opioids, adenosine A1 and A2, and cholinergic M2, and it produces changes in potassium (K^+) channels (Peana et al 2006).

Lorenzetti et al (1991) found that myrcene had a direct analgesic effect on rats. Myrcene is a terpene found in up to 20% in some distillations of West Indian lemongrass *(Cymbopogon citratus)*—usually those that have aged (Clarke 2012). The analgesic effect lasted 3 hours and was similar to that of peripheral-acting opioids, but did not affect the CNS, which was remarkable because the essential oil was administered orally. The analgesic effects did not lead to tolerance within a period of 5 days (which would have occurred with a narcotic). This is interesting because Seth et al (1976) had previously investigated the effect of lemongrass on pain and found it enhanced the effect of morphine in rats. However, Seth also investigated *Cymbopogon nardus* (East Indian lemongrass) and found it to be less effective as an analgesic. *Cymbopogon nardus* contains considerably less myrcene than *Cymbopogon citratus* (Boelens 1994). Lorenzetti et al (1991) conclude their paper with the suggestion that terpenes should be investigated with the "possibility of developing a new class of analgesic with myrcene as the prototype." Myrcene is found (although in small amounts) in several essential oils such as rosemary, frankincense, juniper, rose, ginger, and verbena (Sheppard-Hangar 1995), all of which have traditional analgesic qualities. Surprisingly, there is little recent published research on myrcene. However, a paper by Gbenou et al (2012) compared *Eucalyptus citriadora* and *Cymbopogon citratus* in formol-induced edema and acetic acid-induced abdominal cramps in Wistar rats. In this study, geranial (an aldehyde that makes up to 93% of *Eucalyptus citriadora*) appeared to have more analgesic effect than the myrcene in *Cymbopogon citratus*.

Nepetalactone, a lactone found in *Nepeta caesarea* (catnip), was found to have analgesic properties in a controlled, comparative study with morphine on mice and was hailed the "new opioid" (Aydin et al 1998). The essential oil was given by i.p. injection. The lactone appeared to affect mechanical, not thermal, algesic receptors, which "suggests specificity for specific opioid receptor subtypes excluding mu-opioid receptors." Because the lactone is the main component of *Nepeta caesarea* (92% to 95%), it was thought to have specific, opioid-receptor-subtype agonistic activity. The essential oil also had marked sedative effects. Aydin et al (1996) had previously studied *Origanum onites* and found that it also had analgesic activity. Since then, nepatalactone does not appear to have received further interest.

de Sousa's excellent review (2011) summarizes the results of studies on 43 components of essential oils found to have analgesic properties: 62.8% were monoterpenes, 18.6% were sesquiterpenes, and 18.6% were other constituents. Her paper shows the potential of essential oils and/or their components to work either on their own or to enhance analgesic drugs. Table 10-5 shows a small sample of studies from her review, exploring specific analgesic components found within essential oils. I have listed the most common essential oil within which the component is found. For a more comprehensive overview, please read de Sousa's review.

Several over-the-counter (OTC) medicines include analgesic components found in essential oils, for example, Rowatinex®, which is used to relieve urinary pain and spasm associated with kidney stones (Bak et al 2007). Rowatinex contains pinene (α + β) 31 mg, camphene 15 mg, cineole B.P.C. 1973 (British Pharmaceutical Codex) 3 mg, fenchone 4 mg, borneol 10 mg, anethol U.S.P. 4 mg (United States

TABLE 10-5 *Analgesic Components Within Essential Oils*

Component	Functional Group	Essential Oil	Author	Year
(−)-Carvone	Ketone	Spearmint	Gonçalves et al	2008
β-Caryophyllene	Terpene	Black pepper	Gertsch et al	2008
Citronellal	Aldehyde	Lemongrass	Quintans et al	2011
		Lemongrass	Melo et al	2010
1,8-Cineole	Oxide	*Eucalyptus*	Liapi et al	2007
Eugenol	Phenol	Clove	Yano et al	2008
Fenchone	Ketone	Fennel	Him et al	2008
Geranial	Aldehyde	*Eucalyptus citriadora*	Gbenou et al	2012
(−)-Linalool	Alcohol	Lavender	Peana	2004
(+)-Limonene	Terpene	Lemon	Amaral et al	2007
Menthol	Alcohol	Peppermint	Kraemer et al	2005
β-Myrcene	Terpene	Basil	Paul-Friere et al	2012
		Rosemary	Martinez et al	2009
α-Pinene	Terpene	Fennel	Him et al	2008
Thymol	Phenol	Thyme	Mikaili et al	2010
α-Terpineol	Alcohol	Tea tree	Quintans-Júnior	2011

Pharmacopeia), and olive oil 33 mg. Radian-B linament, Radian massage cream, Deep Heat linament, Counterpain Balm, Tiger Balm, and Neotica Balm linament all contain menthol and methyl salicylate. Counterpain, Tiger Balm, and Neotica also contain eugenol (Harris 2004).

ANTISPASMODIC ESSENTIAL OILS FOR PAIN

Spasm may be the cause or the result of pain (Fahn 2007). Spasm and cramp are involuntary contractions, usually of the muscles, and are an attempt by the body to protect itself. Spasms can affect both skeletal and smooth muscle. Several essential oils have specific antispasmodic effects that can be useful when applied topically or taken internally. Anecdotally, the greater the number of different esters in an essential oil, the greater the antispasmodic effect (although there is no research to substantiate this yet). Roman chamomile has more esters than any other essential oil and has a history of use as an analgesic (Wren 1988). Lis-Balchin (1997) found that clary sage, dill, fennel, frankincense, lavender, Roman chamomile, and sage reduced the "twitch response to nerve stimulation, in isolated rat tissue."

Bowel spasm can be a cause of intense intestinal pain. One of the earliest human studies on intestinal pain was the use of enteric-coated peppermint oil capsules for IBS (Kline et al 2001). Fifty children took part in the controlled, multicentered study. The gelatin capsules did not release the oil until they were in the small intestine (an environment of pH 6.8 or higher). Between one capsule (187 mg) and two capsules were given three times a day. During the study, eight children withdrew for various reasons. However, 76% of the peppermint group had a significant reduction in symptoms compared to the placebo group (43%). No side effects were reported and there was no change in stool consistency. A more recent randomized, double-blind, placebo-controlled study (Merat et al 2010) found that enteric-coated, delayed-release peppermint oil (Colpermin) taken three times daily for 8 weeks significantly reduced the severity of abdominal pain ($P < 0.001$).

INFLAMMATION

Sometimes pain is caused by inflammation. Inflammation is a nonspecific local defense mechanism initiated by tissue injury (Brooker 2008). Derived from the Latin *infiammare*, meaning "to burn," the function of inflammation is to restore the body to normal functioning as quickly as possible. The symptoms of inflammation are redness, swelling, heat, and pain—sometimes called rubor, tumor, calor, and dolor (Mills 1991)—with concomitant loss of function (Craig & Stitzel 1994). During the inflammatory process, chemical mediators are released such as histamine, kinin, interleukins, and prostaglandins. Histamine is an amine that causes capillary dilation and increased vessel permeability. Kinin is a protein that causes vasodilation and smooth muscle contraction. Prostaglandins (PGE1, PGE2, and PGE3) are a group of lipids that modulate the action of several hormones that cause inflammation and blood clotting (Brooker 2008).

Antiinflammatory Essential Oils

Some essential oils have strong antiinflammatory effects on the dermis and epidermis (Bowles 2000). There has been considerable research on the antiinflammatory components of essential oils and some on the whole essential oil.

Antiinflammatory Components

1,8-Cineole was found to reduce colon inflammation in rats when it significantly reduced myeloperoxidase activity and caused repletion of glutathione (Santos 2004). Eugenol reduced the tongue edema that was induced in mice (Dip et al 2004). Chainy et al (2000) explored the mechanism that gives anethole (found in large amounts in anise, camphor, and fennel) its antiinflammatory effect. His research found that anethole acts on IκBα kinase. It also blocked nuclear factor (NF)-κB activation and suppressed tumor necrosis factor (TNF)-induced activation of the transcription factor AP-l, c-jun N-terminal kinase (JNK), and mitogen-activated protein kinase (MAPK). Finally, anethole cancelled TNF-induced apoptosis (as measured by both caspase activation and cell viability). In other words, anethole has a very good antiinflammatory effect.

COX-2 is an enzyme that plays a key role in inflammation, and COX-2 inhibitors (e.g., Celebrex) are a group of drugs that are commonly used for arthritis. Carvacrol suppressed lipopolysaccharide-induced COX-2 mRNA and protein expression in human macrophage-like U937 cells, suggesting that carvacrol regulates COX-2 expression through its agonistic effect on peroxisome proliferator-activated receptor-gamma (PPARγ; Hotta et al 2010). Juhás et al (2008) showed that borneol significantly suppressed proinflammatory cytokine mRNA expression in mice. There are other antiinflammatory components, but these are some of the main ones.

Antiinflammatory Essential Oils

Rossi et al (1988) investigated Roman chamomile *(Anthemis nobilis)* in a comparative, controlled study on rats with carrageenan-induced edema. The control was indomethacin. Three essential oils of chamomile were used. White-headed, double-flowered chamomile flowers showed a greater antiinflammatory action than the yellow-flowered variety. Nevertheless, all three essential oils of Roman chamomile produced significant antiinflammatory effects. In this study the chamomile was given subcutaneously. Jakovlev et al (1979) demonstrated the antiinflammatory effect of German chamomile and suggested that the antiphlogistic effects could be attributed to bisabolol and bisabolol oxides. Tubaro et al (1984) found when German chamomile *(Matricaria recutita)* was applied topically to mouse ears (with hydrocortisone as the control) the chamomile showed an antiinflammatory action, although the effect was only half as strong as that of the steroid. There do not appear to be any more recent studies on either Roman or German chamomile for antiinflammatory conditions.

Nutmeg *(Myristica fragrans)* may have been the inspiration for Nostradamus' prophecies, but it also has antiinflammatory activities. Benet et al (1988) attributed the antiinflammatory action of nutmeg to eugenol. They found the greatest effect was observed after 4 hours and was comparable to the effects of phenylbutazone and indomethacin. However, nutmeg did not ameliorate painful diabetic neuropathy (PDN) in a study by Motilal and Maharaj (2013) carried out in Trinidad. In this randomized, double-blind, placebo-controlled study, 74 patients were randomly allocated to receive topical nutmeg extracts (NEMM; mace oil [2%], nutmeg oil [14%], methyl salicylate [6%], menthol [6%], and coconut oil) or placebo (MM; methyl salicylate [6%], menthol [6%], coconut oil, and alcohol). Although there were significant reductions in pain, there were no statistically significant differences between both groups after 4 weeks.

Wagner et al (1986) screened various essential oils traditionally used for their antiinflammatory action. They found that eugenol, eugenyl acetate, thymol, capsaicin, curcumin, and carvacrol were present in most of the essential oils screened, and the antiphlogistic effects were closely linked to the vascular reaction of early inflammation. In herbal medicine, this is called the counterirritant effect. Clove and cinnamon had the strongest effect, Dwarf pine (*Pinus mugo* var. *pumilo*) and eucalyptus *(Eucalyptus globulus)* had a mild effect, and *Chamomelum nobile* had a weak antiinflammatory effect.

Where there is topical inflammation, essential oils should be applied topically. Essential oils are absorbed into and through the skin (Hongratanaworakit & Buchbauer, 2007; Buckle 2010). This was once disputed, but components in essential oils are currently used to enhance drug delivery both topical and oral (Aggarwal & Dhawan 2012). For example, cardamom enhances absorption of indomethacin, an antiinflammatory drug (Huang et al 1999).

Sometimes, in cases of arthritic pain, heat can help. If this is the case, essential oils that have rubefacient effects, such as *Piper nigrum* (black pepper), *Syzygium aromaticum* (clove), or *Zingiber officinale* (ginger), can be useful. These can be added to an essential oil high in a component with analgesic and/or antiinflammatory action. Sometimes cooling will help relieve the pain. In this case, *Mentha piperita* (peppermint) can be added to the mix. Kraemer et al (2005) found that adding menthol to a cetylated fatty acid opical cream improved functional performance in people with arthritis. These topically applied creams became popular in early 2000 when researchers concluded that they could be an alternative to nonsteroidal antiinflammatory drugs for the treatment of osteoarthritis (Hesslink et al 2002).

It is important to allow patients to smell the mixture before it is applied; they will have to live with it, after all! Be gentle and slow. Allowing someone to touch a painful area takes courage, and that courage needs to be rewarded with respect. All the essential oils mentioned are safe to use for the relief of pain. Although a 5% solution is usually adequate, much higher concentrations can be used (20% to 40%). In some circumstances, and depending on the essential oils selected, 100% solutions can be used. Lavender and tea tree are good examples of safe oils that can be used at full strength. Do not use phenol-rich essential oils undiluted on the skin. Please see the section on safety and contraindications.

Woelk and Schläfke (2010) demonstrated in their 6-week study that the oral use of silexan (lavender oil in a capsule) was as effective as lorazepam (and as safe) in adults with anxiety. With the arrival of OTC oral capsules containing essential oils for anxiety, it will not be long before an essential oil/s or essential oil component/s are marketed in capsule form for analgesia. Aromatherapy has moved a long way in the last 10 years.

CONCLUSIONS

There is no suggestion that essential oils should replace conventional analgesia. However, topical, inhaled, and (in some instances) oral applications of essential oils do have analgesic effects, and some appear to enhance orthodox analgesia. The positive effect of essential oils could be through the placebo response, the effect of touch and smell on the parasympathetic nervous system, or because components in essential oils have analgesic, antiinflammatory, and/or antispasmodic activity.

REFERENCES

Adams A. 2000. Lavender to reduce pain in labor. Unpublished dissertation for RJ Buckle Associates.

Aggarwal G, Dhawan S, HariKumar S. 2012. Natural oils as skin permeation enhancers for transdermal delivery of olanzapine: in vitro and in vivo evaluation. *Curr Drug Deliv* 9(2):172–81.

Alavi A, LaRiccia P, Sadek A et al. 1997. Neuroimaging of acupuncture in patients with chronic pain. *J Alternat Complement Med.* 3(Suppl 1):S47–S53.

Amaral J, Silva M, Neto M, Neto P, Moura B et al. 2007. Antinociceptive effect of the monoterpene R-(+)-limonene in mice. *Biol. Pharm. Bull.* 30:1217–1220.

Arends R. 2012. Lavender and frankincense for tension headaches. Unpublished dissertation for RJ Buckle Associates.

Atlas L, Wager T. 2012. How expectations shape pain. *Neurosci Lett.* 520(2):140–8.

Ayan M, Ufuk T, Erkan S, Suren, Gurbuzler L, Koyuncu F. 2012. Investigating the effect of aromatherapy in patients with renal colic. *J Alternat Complement Med.* 1–5.

Aydin S, Beis R, Ozturk Y et al. 1998. Nepetalactone: a new opioid analgesic from *Nepeta casesarea* Boiss. *J Pharm Pharmacol.* 50(7):813–817.

Aydin S, Ozturk Y, Beis R et al. 1996. Investigation of *Origanum onites, Sideritis congesta* and *Saturega cuneifolia* essential oils for analgesic activity. *Phytother Res* 10:342–344.

Bagetta G, Morrone L, Rombola L, Amantea D, Russo R et al. 2010. Neuropharmacology of the essential oil of bergamot. *Fitoterapia.* 81(6):453–61.

Bak C, Yoon W, Chung H. 2007. Effects of an α-blocker and terpene mixture for pain control and spontaneous expulsion of ureter stone. *Korean J Urol.* 48:517–521.

Barocelli E, Calcina F, Chiavarini M, Impicciatore M, Bruni R et al. 2004. Antinociceptive and gastroprotective effects of inhaled and orally administered *Lavandula hybrida* Reverchon "Grosso" essential oil. *J Ethnopharmacol.* 89(1):67–71.

Beasley A. 2003. German chamomile and frankincense for arthritic pain. Unpublished dissertation for RJ Buckle Associates.

Beck D, Beck J. 1987. *The Pleasure Connection: How Endorphins Affect our Health and Happiness.* Anaheim, CA: Synthesis Press.

Benett A, Stamford F, Tavares I. 1988. The biological activity of eugenol, a major constituent of nutmeg: studies on prostaglandins, the intestine and other tissues. *Phytother Res.* 2(3):125–129.

Berry P, Dahl J. 2000. The new JCAHO pain standards: implications for pain management nurses. *Pain Mngt Nurs.* 1(1):3–12.

Boelens M. 1994. Sensory and chemical evaluation of tropical grass oils. *Perfumer & Flavorist.* 19:29–45.

Bonavia H. 2007. Sweet marjoram for muscle pain. Unpublished dissertation for RJ Buckle Associates.

Bowles J. 2000. *The Basic Chemistry of Aromatherapeutic Essential Oils.* Sydney, Australia: Pirie Publishing.

Bowles V. 2004. Lavender to reduce pain in labor. Unpublished dissertation for RJ Buckle Associates.

Bozarth C. 2009. Black pepper, German chamomile and sweet marjoram for arthritis pain. Unpublished dissertation for RJ Buckle Associates.

Brooker C. 2008. *Medical Dictionary.* 16th Edition. Churchill Livingstone.

Buckle J. 2010. Aromatherapy: is there a role for essential oils in current and future healthcare? *Bulletin Technique 2010. Gattefosse Foundation Symposium.* St Remy de Provence, France.

Calvert I. 2005. Ginger: an essential oil for shortening labour? *Pract Midwife.* 8(1):30–4.

Campelo L, de Almeida A, de Freitas R, Cerqueira G et al. 2011. Antioxidant and antinociceptive effects of *Citrus limon* essential oil in mice. *J Biomed Biotechnol.* 2011:678673. [Epub 2011 May 31].

Carpenter K. 2007. Topically applied Roman chamomile, lavender and sweet marjoram for neck and shoulder pain. Unpublished dissertation for RJ Buckle Associates.

Carter R. 1996. Give a drug a bad name. *New Scientist.* 150(2024):27–29.

Casey M. 2002. Aromatherapy: pain management. *Aromather Today.* 21:26–29.

Cavallo D. 2004. Clary sage for dysmenorrhea. Unpublished dissertation for RJ Buckle Associates.

Chainy G, Manna S, Chaturvedi M, Aggarwal B. 2000. Anethole blocks both early and late cellular responses transduced by tumor necrosis factor: effect on NF-κB, AP-1, JNK, MAPKK and apoptosis. *Oncogene.* 19:2943–2950.

Chang S. 2008. Effects of aroma hand massage on pain, state anxiety and depression in hospice patients with terminal cancer. *Taehan Kanho Hakhoe Chi.* 38(4):492–502.

Clarke M. 2012. Verbal communication. Nature's Gift Essential Oils. www.naturesgift.com.

Clark M. 2007. Geranium, Roman chamomile, clary sage and fennel mixture topically applied for dysmenorrhea. Unpublished dissertation for RJ Buckle Associates.

Colby BJ. 2009. Sweet marjoram for muscle pain. Unpublished dissertation for RJ Buckle Associates.

Costa D. 1997. Topically applied lavender for back pain. Unpublished dissertation for RJ Buckle Associates.

Cote S. 2002. Black pepper for arthritic pain. Unpublished dissertation for RJ Buckle Associates.

Craig C. 1994. Introduction to CNS pharmacology. In Craig C, Stitzel R (eds). *Modern Pharmocology.* 4th edition. Boston. Little, Brown & Co. pages 477–485.

Davies S, Harding L, Baranowski A. 2002. A novel treatment of postherpetic neuralgia using peppermint oil. *Clin J Pain.* 18(5):297–301.

Decker R. 2007. Roman chamomile baths for muscle pain. Unpublished dissertation for RJ Buckle Associates.

de Sousa D. 2011. Analgesic-like activity of essential oil components. *Molecules.* 16(3):2233–2252.

Dip E, Pereira N, Fernandes P. 2004. Ability of eugenol to reduce tongue edema induced by *Dieffenbachia picta* Schott in mice. Toxicon. 43(6):729–735.

Dolara P, Corte B, Ghelardini C et al. 2000. Local anesthetic, antibacterial and antifungal properties of sesquiterpenes from myrrh. *Planta Medica.* 66(4):356–358.

Dullaghan C. 2002. Black pepper for arthritis pain. Unpublished dissertation for RJ Buckle Associates.

Erlenwein J, Studer D, Lange J, Bauer M et al. 2012. Process optimization by central control of acute pain therapy: implementation of standardized treatment concepts and central pain management in hospitals. *Anaesthetist.* http://www.ncbi.nlm.nih.gov/pubmed/23135771. Accessed November 9, 2012. [Epub ahead of print].

Estabrook S. 2012. Lavender and frankincense for arthritic pain. Unpublished dissertation for RJ Buckle Associates.

Fahn. 2007. *DANA Guide to Brain Health.* Dana Press.

Fields H. 1997. Pain: anatomy and physiology. *J Alternat Complement Med.* 3(Suppl 1):S41–S46.

Flick M. 2008. Black pepper for Raynaud's syndrome. Unpublished dissertation for RJ Buckle Associates.

Ford A, Talley N, Spiegal B, Foxx-Orenstein A, Schiller L et al. 2008. Effect of fibre, antispasmodics, and peppermint oil in the treatment of irritable bowel syndrome: systematic review and meta-analysis. *BMJ.* Nov 13;337:a2313. doi:10.1136/bmj.a2313.

Franca C, Menezes F, Costa L, Alves P et al. 2008. Analgesic and antidiarrheal properties of *Occimum selloi* essential oil in mice. *Fitoterapia.* 79(7-8):569–73.

Gagnon M. 2010. Peppermint and lemongrass for arthritic pain. Unpublished dissertation for RJ Buckle Associates.

Gallup Poll. 2011. http://www.gallup.com/poll/154169/chronic-pain-rates-shoot-until-americans-reach-late-50s.aspx. Accessed March 13, 2013.

Gatlin C, Schulmeister L. 2007. When medication is not enough: nonpharmacological management of pain. *Clin J Oncol Nurs.* 11(5):699–704.

Gbenou J, Ahounou J, Akakpo H, Laleye A, Yayi E et al. 2012. Phytochemical composition of *Cymbopogon citratus* and *Eucalyptus citriodora* essential oils and their anti-inflammatory and analgesic properties on Wistar rats. *Mol Bio Rep.* Oct 14. Accessed October 29, 2012. [Epub ahead of print].

Gedney J, Glover T, Fillingim R. 2004. Sensory and affective pain discrimination after inhalation of essential oils. *Psychosom Med.* 66(4):599–606.

Gertsch J, Leonti J, Raduner M, Racz S, Chen I et al. 2008. β-Caryophyllene is a dietary cannabinoid. *Proc Natl Acad Sci.* 105(26):9099–9104.

Ghelardini C, Galeotti N, Salvatore G et al. 1999. Local anesthetic activity of essential oil of *Lavandula angustifolia*. *Planta Medica.* 65(8):700–703.

Gilmore K. 2006. Sweet marjoram and lavender for chronic pain. Unpublished dissertation for RJ Buckle Associates.

Gobel H, Schmidt G, Soyka, D. 1991. Effect of peppermint and eucalyptus oil preparations on neurophysiological and experimental algesimetric headache parameters. *Cephalalgia.* 14:228–234.

Goleman D. 1996. *Emotional Intelligence.* New York: Bantam.

Gonçalves J, Oliveira C, Benedito F, de Sousa R, de Almemeida D et al. 2008. Antinociceptive activity of (-)-carvone: evidence of association with decreased peripheral nerve excitability. *Biol Pharm Bull.* 31(5):1017–20.

Greer C. 1995. Anatomical organization of the human olfactory system. In Gilbert A (ed.), *Compendium of Olfactory Research.* 1982-1994, 3–7.

Grunebaum L, Murdock J, Castanedo-Tardan M, Baumann L. 2011. Effects of lavender olfactory input on cosmetic procedures. *J Cosmetic Dermatol.* 10:89–93.

Gutierrez C. 2004. Helicrysum italicum for arthritic pain. Unpublished dissertation for RJ Buckle Associates.

Hadi N, Hanid A. 2011. Lavender essence for post-cesarean pain. *Pakistan J Biol Sci.* 14(11):664–667.

Hajhashemi V, Ghannadi A, Sharif B. 2003. Anti-inflammatory and analgesic properties of the leaf extracts and essential oil of *Lavandula angustifolia* Mill. *J Ethnopharmacol.* 89(1):67–71.

Hajhashemi V, Ghannadi A, Hajiloo M. 2010. Analgesic and anti-inflammatory effects of *Rosa damascena* hydroalcoholic extract and its essential oil in animal models. *Iranian J Pharm Res.* 9(2):163–8.

Han S, Hur M, Buckle J, Choi J, Lee M. 2006. Effect of aromatherapy on symptoms of dysmenorrheal in college students: a randomized, controlled clinical trial. *J Alternat Complement Med.* 12(6):535–541.

Harper L. 2007. Black pepper for recent injury pain. Unpublished dissertation for RJ Buckle Associates.

Harris B. 2004. The role of menthol, methyl salicylate and eugenol in pain relief. *Int J Clin Aromather.* 1(1):16–23.

Haynes O. 2007. Peppermint, Roman chamomile, basil and lavender for chronic pain. Unpublished dissertation for RJ Buckle Associates.

Hein J. 2002. Topically applied rosemary for neck pain. Unpublished dissertation for RJ Buckle Associates.

Herring D. 2006. Peppermint for fibromyalgia. Unpublished dissertation for RJ Buckle Associates.

Hesslink R, Armstrong S, Nagendran M, Streevatsan S, Barathur R. 2002. Cetylated fatty acids improve knee function in patients with osteoarthritis. *J Rheumatol.* 29(8):1708–12.

Him A, Ozbek H, Turel I, Oner A. 2008. Antinociceptive activity of a-pinene and fenchone. *Pharmacol Online* 3:363–9.

Hjersted-Smith C. 2008. Sweet marjoram for muscle pain. Unpublished dissertation for RJ Buckle Associates.

Holden J, Jeong Y, Forrest J. 2005. The endogenous opioid system and clinical pain management. *AACN Clin Issues.* 6(3):291–301.

Hotta M, MNakata R, Katsukawa M, Hori K, Takahashi S, Inoue H. 2010. Carvacrol, a component of thyme oil, activates PPARα and γ and suppresses COX-2 expression. *J Lipid Res.* 51:132–139.

Hongratanaworakit T, Buchbauer G. 2007. Autonomic and emotional responses after transdermal absorption of sweet orange oil in humans: placebo controlled trial. *Int J Essential Oil Ther.* 1(1):29–34.

Huang Y, Fang J, Hung C, Wu P, Tsai H. 1999. Cyclic monoterpene extract from cardamom oil as a skin permeation enhancer for indomethacin: in vitro and in vivo studies, *Biol Pharm Bull.* 22:642–646.

Hur M, Lee M, Seong K, Lee. 2012. Aromatherapy massage on the abdomen for alleviating menstrual pain in high school girls: a preliminary controlled clinical study. *Evidence-Based Complement Alternat Med.* 187163.

Jablonski K, Duke G. 2012. Pain management in persons who are terminally ill in rural acute care: barriers and facilitators. *J Hospice Palliative Nurs.* 14(8):533–540.

Jakovlev V, Isaac O, Thiemer K et al. 1979. Pharmacological investigations with compounds of chamomile. II. New investigations on the antiphlogistic effects of a bisabolol and bisabolol oxide. *Planta Medica.* 35:125–140.

Joksimovic N, Spasovski G, Joksimovic V, Andreevski V, Zuccari C, Omini C. 2012. Efficacy and tolerability of hyaluronic acid, tea tree oil and methyl-sulfonyl-methane in a new gel medical device for treatment of haemorrhoids in a double-blind, placebo-controlled clinical trial. *Updates Surg.* 64(3):195–201.

Juurlink D, Dhalia I. 2012. Dependence and addiction during chronic opioid therapy. *J Med Toxicol.* http://www.ncbi.nlm.nih.gov/pubmed/23073725. [Epub ahead of print].

Juhás Š, Čikoš S, Czikková S, Veselá J, Il'ková G. 2008. Effects of borneol and thymoquinone on TNBS-induced colitis in mice. *Folia Biologica (Praha).* 54:1–7.

Kirkman J. 2008. Topically applied lavender, sweet marjoram and black pepper for neck and shoulder pain. Unpublished dissertation for RJ Buckle Associates.

Khushtar M, Kumar V, Javed K, Bhandari U. 2009. Protective effect of ginger oil on aspirin and pyloris ligation-induced gastric ulcer model in rats. *Indian J Pharm Sci.* 71(5):554–8.

Khvorova Y, Neill J. 2008. A review of the effect of peppermint oil in various gastrointestinal conditions. *J Gastroenterol Nurses College of Australia.* 18(3):6–15.

Kim M, Nam E, Paik S. 2005. The effects of aromatherapy on pain, depression, and life satisfaction of arthritis patients. *Taehan Kanho Hakhoe Chi.* 35(1):186–94.

Kim J, Ren C, Fielding G, Pitti A, Kasumi T et al. 2007. Treatment with lavender aromatherapy in the post-anesthesia care unit reduces opioid requirements of morbidly obese patients undergoing laparoscopic adjustable gastric banding. *Obes Surg.* 17(7):920–5.

Kim J, Wadja M, Cuff G, Serota D et al. 2006. Evaluation of aromatherapy in treating postoperative pain: pilot study. *Pain Practice.* 6(4):273–277.

Kim S, Kim H, Yeo J, Hong S, Lee J, Jeon Y. 2011. The effect of lavender oil on stress, bispectral index values, and needle insertion pain in volunteers. *J Alternat Complement Med.* 17(9):823–6.

Kinzelmann A. 1997. Eucalyptus citriadora and ginger topically applied for arthritic pain. Unpublished dissertation for RJ Buckle Associates.

Kline R, Kline J, Di Palma J et al. 2001. Enteric coated pH dependent peppermint oil capsules for the treatment of irritable bowel syndrome in children. *J. Pediatr.* 138(1):125–128.

Ko G, Hum A, Traitses G, Berbrayer D. 2007. Effects of topical 024 essential oils on patients with fibromyalgia syndrome: a randomized, placebo controlled pilot study. *J. Musculoskeletal Pain.* 15(1):11–19.

Koto R, Imamura M, Watanabe C, Obayashi S, Shiraishi M, Sasaki Y. 2006. Linalyl acetate as a major ingredient of lavender essential oil relaxes the rabbit vascular smooth muscle through dephosphorylation of myosin light chain. *J Cardiovasc Pharmacol.* 48:850–856.

Kraemer W, Ratamess N, Anderson J, Volek J et al. 2005. A cetylated fatty acid topical cream with menthol reduces the pain and improves functional performance in individuals with arthritis. *J Strength Condition Res.* 19(2):475–480.

Kraft K, Uehleke B. 2005. Muscular pain reduction after standardized training by external essential oils. *Focus Alternat Complement Ther.* 11(2):136–7.

Krall B, Krause W. 1993. Efficacy and tolerance of *Mentha arvensis aethoeroleum.* Paper presented July 21–24 at 24th International Symposium on Essential Oils. Berlin, Germany.

Kvam D. 1994. Anti-inflammatory and anti-rheumatic drugs. In Craig C, Stitzel R (eds.), *Modern Pharmacology*, 4th ed. Boston: Little, Brown & Co., pp 485–500.

Lee H, Parl S, Lee M, Kim H, Ryu S et al. 2012. 1-Dehydro-(10)-gingerdione from ginger inhibits IKKβ activity for NF-Kβ activiation and suppresses NF-Kβ-regulated expression of inflammatory genes. *Br J Pharmacol.* 167(1):128–40.

Leach M, Kumar S. 2008. The clinical effectiveness of ginger (*Zingiber officinale*) in adults with osteoarthritis. *Int J Evid Based Healthc.* 6(3):311–20.

Lewis W, Elvin-Lewis M. 1977. *Medical Botany*. New York: Wiley Interscience.

Liapi C, Anifandis G, Chinou I, Kourounakis A et al. 2007. Antinociceptive properties of 1,8 cineole and beta-pinene, from the essential oil of *Eucalyptus camuldulensis* leaves, in rodents. *Planta Medica.* 73(12):1247–54.

Lippert C. 1997. Topically applied mixture of essential oils for arthritis. Unpublished dissertation for RJ Buckle Associates.

Lis-Balchin M. 1997. A preliminary study of the effect of essential oils on skeletal and smooth muscle in vitro. *J Ethnopharmacol.* 58(3):183–187.

Lorenzetti B, Souza G, Sarti S et al. 1991. Myrcene mimics the peripheral analgesic activity of lemongrass tea. *J Ethnopharmacol.* 34(1):43–48.

Lyss G, Schmidt T, Merfort I et al. 1997. Helenalin, an anti-inflammatory sesquiterpene lactone from arnica, selectively inhibits transcription factor NF-kappaB. *Biol Chem.* 378(9):951–961.

Mann N, Sandhu K. 2012. Peppermint oil in irritable bowel syndrome: systematic evaluation of 1634 cases with meta-analysis. *Int Med J.* 19(1):5–6.

Marino D. 2004. Lavender to reduce pain in labor. Unpublished dissertation for RJ Buckle Associates.

Martin B. 1994. Opioid and nonopioid analgesics. In Craig C, Stitzel R (eds.), *Modern Pharmacology*, 4th ed. Boston: Little, Brown & Co., 431–450.

Martin G. 2006. The effect of exposure to odor on the perception of pain. *Psychosomatic Med.* 68:613–616.

Martinez A, Gonzales-Trujano M, Pellicer F, Lopen-Munoz F Navarrete A. 2009. Antinociceptive effect and GC/MS analysis of *Rosmarinus officinalis* essential oil from its aerial parts. *Planta Medica.* 75(5):508–11.

Maruyama N, Sekimoto Y, Ishibashi H, Inouye S, Oshima. 2005. Suppression of neutrophil accumulation in mice by cutaneous application of geranium essential oil. *J Inflammation.* 2:1–11.

McDaid C, Maund E, Rice S, Wright K, Jenkins B. 2011. Paracetamol and selective and non-selective non-steroidal anti-inflammatory drugs for the reduction in morphine-related side-effects after major surgery: a systematic review. *Br J Anaesth.* 106(3):292–297.

Meier B, Petersen M. 2001. Sales of painkiller grew rapidly but success brought a high cost. *New York Times.* CL(51,683) A15.

Melo M, Sena L, Barreto F, Bonjardim L, Almeida J, et al. 2010. Antinociceptive effect of citronellal in mice. *Pharm. Biol.* 248:411–416.

Merat S, KhaliliS, Mostajabi P, Ghorbani A, Ansari R, Malekzadeh R. 2010. The effect of enteric-coated, delayed-release peppermint oil on irritable bowel syndrome. *Digest Dis Sci.* 55(5):1385–90.

Mersky Y. 1986. Classification of chronic pain. Descriptions of chronic pain syndromes and definitions of pain terms. Prepared by the International Association for the Study of Pain, Subcommittee on Taxonomy. *Pain Suppl.* 3:S1–S226.

Mikaili P, Nezhady M, Shayegh J, Asghari M. 2010. Study of antinociceptive of *Thymus vulgaris* and *Foeniculum vulgare* essential oil in mouse. *Int. J Acad Res.* 2:374–376.

Mills S. 1991. *Out of the Earth.* London: Viking Arkana.

Modaress N, Asadipour M. 2006. Comparison of the effectiveness of fennel and mefenamic acid on pain intensity in dysmenorrhoea. *Eastern Med Health J.* 12(3-4):423–7.

Motilal S, Maharaj R. (2013). Nutmeg extracts for painful diabetic neuropathy: a randomized, double-blind, controlled study. *J Altern Complement Med.* 19(4):347–52.

Newell S. 2011. Ginger for shoulder pain. Unpublished dissertation for RJ Buckle Associates.

Ndao D, Ladas E, Cheng B, Sands S, Snyder K et al. 2012. Inhalation aromatherapy in children and adolescents undergoing stem-cell infusion: results of a placebo-controlled, double-blind trial. *Psychooncology.* 21(3):247–54.

Nichols A. 2006. Clary sage, lavender and petitgrain for dysmenorrhea. Unpublished dissertation for RJ Buckle Associates.

Nie N, Hull C, Jenkins J et al. 1975. *Statistical Package for the Social Sciences*. New York. McGraw-Hill.

North-Doty A. 2008. 2% Peppermint topically applied for headaches. Unpublished dissertation for RJ Buckle Associates.

IOM Report. 2011. http://www.iom.edu/~/media/Files/Report%20Files/2011/Relieving-Pain-in-America-A-Blueprint-for-Transforming-Prevention-Care-Education-Research/Pain%20Research%202011%20Report%20Brief.pdf.

Ou M, Hsu T, Lai A, Lin Y, Lin C. 2012. Pain relief assessment by aromatic essential oil massage on outpatients with primary dysmenorrheal: a randomized, double-blind clinical trial. *J Obstet Gynaecol Res*. 38(5):817–22.

Paula-Freire L, Andersen M, Molska G, Köhn D, Carlini E. 2012. Evaluation of the antinociceptive activity of *Ocimum gratissimum* L. (Lamiaceae) essential oil and its isolated active principles in mice. *Phytother Res*. Oct 10. doi:10.1002/ptr.4845. [Epub ahead of print].

Pazandeh F, Savadzadeh S, Mojab F, Majd A. 2008. Effects of chamomile essence aromatherapy on episiotomy pain of primiparous women. *Iranian J Nurs Midwifery*. 18(62): 1.

Peana A, Moretti M, Juliano C. 1999. Chemical composition and antimicrobial action of the essential oils of *Salvia desoleana* and *Salvia sclarea*. *Planta Medica*. 65(8):752–754.

Peana A. 2004. Effects of (-)-linalool in the acute hyperalgesia induced by carrageenan, L-glutamate and prostaglandin E2. *Eur J Pharmacol*. 497(3):279–284.

Peana A, Marzocco S, Popolo A, Pinto A. 2006. (-)-Linalool inhibits in vitro NO formation: probable involvement in the antinociceptive activity of this monoterpene compound. *Life Sci*. 78: 719–723.

Pemberton E. 2007. Eucalyptus globulus and lavender for arthritic pain. Unpublished dissertation for RJ Buckle Associates.

Perez-Raya M, Utrilla M, Navarro M et al. 1990. CNS activity of *Mentha rotundifolia* and *Mentha longifolia* essential oil in mice and rats. *Phytother Res*. 4:232–234.

Peters D. 2002. German chamomile and ginger topically applied for arthritic pain. Unpublished dissertation for RJ Buckle Associates.

Pittler M, Ernst E. 2003. Temporary relief of postherpetci neuralgia pain with topical geranium oil. *Am J Med*. 115:586–587.

Pray C. 2000. Peppermint and Roman chamomile for headaches. Unpublished dissertation for RJ Buckle Associates.

Prescott J, Wilkie J. 2007. Pain tolerance selectively increased by a sweet-smelling odor. *Psychol Sci*. 18(4):308–11.

Prommel D. 2003. Black pepper and sweet marjoram for arthritic pain. Unpublished dissertation for RJ Buckle Associates.

Quintans-Junior L, da Rocha R, Caregnato F, Joreira J et al. 2011. Antinociceptive action and redox properties of citronellal, an essential oil present in lemongrass. *J Medicinal Food*. 14(6):630–9.

Quintans-Júnior L, Oliveira L, Santana M, Santana M, Guimarães M. 2011. α-Terpineol reduces nociceptive behavior in mice. *Pharmaceutical Biology*. 49(6):583–6.

Rahnama P, Montazeri A, Huseini H, Kianbakht S, Naseri M. 2012. Effect of Zingiber officinale R. rhizomes (ginger) on pain relief in primary dysmenorrhea: a placebo randomized trial. *BMC Complement Altern Med*. 2:92. doi:10.1186/1472-6882-12-92.

Ramadan M, Goeters S, Watzer B, Krause E, Lohmann K. 2006. Chamazulene carboxylic acid and matricin: a natural profen and its natural prodrug, identified through similarity to synthetic drug substances. *J Natural Products*. 69:1041–1045.

Raudenbush B, Koon J, Meyer B, Corley N, Flower N. 2004. Effects of odorant administration on pain and psychophysiological measures in humans. *North Am J Psychol*. 6(3):361–370.

Reimer J. 2005. Clary sage for dysmenorrhea. Unpublished dissertation for RJ Buckle Associates.

Rhind J P. 2012. *Essential Oils*. 2nd edition. Singing Dragon. London.

Rodriquez D. 2005. Clary sage for dysmenorrhea. Unpublished dissertation for RJ Buckle Associates.

Rose J. 1992. *The Aromatherapy Book*. San Francisco: North Atlantic Books.

Rossi T, Melegari M, Bianchi A et al. 1988. Sedative, anti-inflammatory and antidiuretic effects induced in rats by essential oils of varieties of *Anthemis nobilis:* a comparative study. *Pharmacol Res Commun.* 20(Suppl.):71–74.

Sakurada T, Mizogushi H, Kuwahata H, Katsuyama S et al. 2010. Intraplantar injection of bergamot essential oil induces peripheral antinociception mediated by opioid mechanism. *Pharmacol Biochem Behav.* 97(3):436–43.

Sasannejad P, Saeedi M, Shoeibi A, Gorji A, Abassi M, Foroughipour M. 2012. Lavender essential oil in the treatment of migraine headache: a placebo-controlled clinical trial. *Eur Neurol* 67(5):288–91.

Santos F, Jeferson F, Santos C, Silveira E, Rao V. 2005. Antinociceptive effect of leaf essential oil from *Croton sonderianus* in mice. *Life Sci.* 77:2953–2963.

Santos F. 2004. 1,8-Cineole (eucalyptol), a monoterpene oxide attenuates the colonic damage in rats on acute TNBS-colitis. *Food Chem Toxicol.* 42(4):579–584.

Schmelz M. 2011. Neuronal sensitivity of the skin. *Eur J Dermatol.* 21(Suppl. 2):43–7.

Schopflocher D, Taenmzer P. 2011. The prevalence of pain in Canada. *Pain Res Manag.* 16(6):445–50.

Seth G, Kokate C, Varma K. 1976. The effect of essential oil of *Cymbopogon citratus* on central nervous system. *Indian J Exp Biol.* 14(3):370–371.

Shavakhi A, Ardestani S, Taki M, Goli M, Keshteli A. 2012. Premedication with peppermint oil capsules in colonoscopy: a double blind placebo-controlled randomized trial study. *Acta Gastronenterol Belg.* 75(3):349–53.

Sheikhan F, Jahdi F, Khoei E, Shamsalizadeh N, Sheikhan M. 2012. Episiotomy pain relief: use of lavender oil essence in primiparous Iranian women. *Complement Ther Clin Practice.* 18(1):66–70.

Sheppard-Hangar S. 1995. *Aromatherapy Practitioner Reference Manual*, Vol. II. Tampa, FL: Atlantic School of Aromatherapy.

Shi Q, Cleeland C, Klepstad P, Miaskowski C, Pedersen N. 2010. Biological pathways and genetic variables involved in pain. *Qual. Life Res.* 19:1407–1417.

Silva J, Abebe W, Sousa S., Duarte V, Machado M. 2003. Analgesic and anti-inflammatory effects of essential oils of eucalyptus. *J Ethnopharmacol.* 89:277–283.

Sinclair M. 2012. Environmental costs of pain management: pharmaceuticals vs physical therapies. *Integrat Med.* 11(5):38.

Smith D, Jacobson B. 2011. Effect of a blend of comfrey root extract (*Symphytum officinale* L.) and tannic acid creams in the treatment of osteoarthritis of the knee: randomized, placebo-controlled, double-blind, multiclinical trials. *J Chiropract Med.* 10(3):147–56.

Sofaer B, Foord J. 1993. Care of the person in pain. In Hinchcliff S, Norman S, Schrober J (eds.), *Nursing Practice and Health Care.* London: Edward Arnold, pp 374–401.

Soden K, Vincent K, Craske S, Lucas C, Ashley S. 2004. A randomized controlled study of aromatherapy massage in a hospice setting. *Palliative Med.* 18:87–92.

Solits 2000. Sweet marjoram and black pepper for back pain. Unpublished dissertation for RJ Buckle Associates.

Su S, Hua Y, Wang Y, Gu W, Zhoi W, Duan J et al. 2012. Evaluation of the anti-inflammatory and analgesic properties of individual and combined extracts from *Commiphora myrrha* and *Boswellia caterii.* *J Ethnopharmacol.* 139(2):649–56.

Sullivan M, Robinson J. 2006. Antidepressant and anticonvulsant medication for chronic pain. *Phys Med Rehab Clin North Am.* 17, 381–400.

Swingle J. 2001. Clary sage and frankincense for labor pain. Unpublished dissertation for RJ Buckle Associates.

Taher Y. 2012. Antinociceptive activity of *Mentha piperita* leaf aqueous extract in mice. *Libyan J Med.* 2012;7. doi:10.3402/ljm.v7i0.16205. [Epub 2012 Mar 27].

Taherian A, Babaei M, Vafaei A, Jarrahi M, Jadidi M, et al. 2009. Antinociceptive effects of hydroalcoholic extract of *Thymus vulgaris.* *Pak J Pharm Sci.* 22(1):83–9.

Tait J. 2002. Eucalyptus globulus for arthritis. Unpublished dissertation for RJ Buckle Associates.

Takaki I, Bersani-Amado L, Vendruscolo A, Sartoretto S, Diniz S, Bersani-Amado C, Cuman R. 2008. Anti-inflammatory & antinoceptive effects of Rosmarinus officinalis essential oil in experimental animal models. *J Medicinal Food.* 11(4): 741–6.

Teodoro F, Tronco Júnior M, Zampronio A, Martini A et al. 2012. Peripheral substance P and neurokinin-1 receptors have a role in inflammatory and neuropathic orofacial pain models. *Neuropeptides.* Nov 21. doi:pii.S0143–4179(12)00110-2. 10.1016/j.npep.2012.10.005. [Epub ahead of print].

Tibjlas T. 2008. Clary sage and geranium for dysmennorhea. Unpublished dissertation for RJ Buckle Associates.

Trull K. 2007. Aromatherapy for pain following elective cardiac surgery. Unpublished dissertation for RJ Buckle Associates.

Tsung-Chun L, Jung-Chun L, Tai-Hung H, Ying Chih L et al. 2011. Analgesic and anti-inflammatory activities of methanol extract from *Pogostemon cablis. Evid Based Complement Alternat Med.* doi:10.1093/ecam/nep183.

Tubaro A, Zillia, C, Redaeli C, et al. 1984. Evaluation of anti-inflammatory activity of chamomile extract topical application. *Planta Medica.* 50(4):359–360.

UK Pain Proposal Report 2011. Accessed March 13, 2013. www.arthritiscare.org.uk

Vanancio A, Onofre A, Lira A, Alves P, Blank A et al. 2011. Chemcial composition, acute toxicity and antinociceptive activity of the essential oil of a plant breeding cultivar of basil (*Ocimum basilicum*). *Planta Med.* 77(8):825–9.

Viana G, Vale T, Pinho R, Matos F. 2000. Antinociceptive effect of the essential oil from *Cymbopon citratus* in mice. *J Ethnopharmacol.* 70:323–327.

Wagner H, Wierer M, Bauer R. 1986. In vitro inhibition of prostaglandin biosynthesis by essential oils and phenolic compounds. *Planta Medica.* 52(3):184–187.

Walters B. 2004. Topically applied eucalyptus and black pepper for neck and shoulder pain. Unpublished dissertation for RJ Buckle Associates.

Ward K. 1993. Care of the person with an infection. In Hinchcliff S, Norman S, Schrober J (eds.), *Nursing Practice and Health Care.* London: Edward Arnold, pp 402–434.

Weil A. 1996. *Spontaneous Healing.* New York: Fawcett.

White L. 2002. Peppermint topically applied for neck pain. Unpublished dissertation for RJ Buckle Associates.

Wiest C. 2005. Black pepper for arthritic pain. Unpublished dissertation for RJ Buckle Associates.

Wilkinson S. 1995. Aromatherapy and massage in palliative care. *Int J Palliative Nurs.* 1(1):21–30.

Woelk H, Schläfke S. 2010. A multi-center, double-blind, randomized study of the lavender oil preparation Silexan in comparison to Lorazepam for generalized anxiety disorder. *Phytomedicine.* 17(2):94–99.

Woolfson A, Hewitt D. 1992. Intensive aromacare. *Int J Aromather.* 4(2):12–14.

Wren R. 1988. *Potter's New Cyclopaedia of Botanical Drugs and Preparations.* London: Churchill Livingstone.

Yamamoto K, Kanbara K, Matsuura H, Ban I, Mizuno Y et al. 2010. Psychological characteristics of Japanese patients with chronic pain assessed with the Rorschach test. *Biopsychosocial Med.* http://www.bpsmedicine.com/content/4/1/20. Accessed November 18, 2012.

Yano S, Suzuki Y, Yuzurihara M, Kase Y, Takeda S. 2008. Antinociceptive effect of methyleugenol on formalin-induced hyperalgesia in mice. *Eur J Pharmacol.* 553(103):99–103.

Yin M, Yamamoto Y, Gaynor R. 1998. The anti-inflammatory agent aspirin and salicylate inhibit the activity of I(kappa) Bkinase-beta. *Nature.* 396(6706):77–80.

Yip Y, Tam A. 2008. An experimental study on the effectiveness of massage with aromatic ginger and orange essential oil for moderate-to-severe knee pain among the elderly in Hong Kong. *Complement Ther Med.* 16(3):131–8.

Yip Y, Tse S. 2006. An experimental study on the effectiveness of acupressure with aromatic lavender essential oil for sub-acute, non-specific neck pain in Hong Kong. *Complement Ther Clin Pract.* 12(1):18–26.

Chapter 11

Stress and Well-Being

"It's not stress that kills us, it is our reaction to stress."

Hans Seyle

CHAPTER ASSETS

STRESS

Most people experience some stress during their life. It is how we cope with stress that determines if it will affect our health. When we talk about stress, we often assume mental or emotional stress. But physical stress also exists. Running a marathon, changing shift work, intense manual labor, prolonged heat or cold, chronic pain, malnutrition, and prolonged lack of a vital mineral or vitamin are all examples of physical stressors. Stress fractures can be caused by overuse—when muscles become fatigued and are unable to absorb added shock (Brooker 2008). This description helps clarify emotional and mental stress. Simply put, if we continue to overdo it, we will reach a point when we cannot cope with or adapt to the stress, and our body and mind begin to breakdown. Stress-related disorders have a great impact on healthcare systems (Kormos & Gaszner 2013).

DEFINITION OF STRESS

Hans Selye, an Austrian–Canadian endocrinologist who worked at McGill University, Canada, conceived the idea of stress in 1935. He was carrying out research on rats and found that rats injected with various hormonal extracts developed enlarged adrenal glands, shrunken lymphatic glands, and bleeding gastrointestinal ulcers. He named this phenomenon "the stress syndrome" (Anthony & Thibodeau 1983).

Rahe (1975), a psychiatrist at the University of Washington School of Medicine, found that the more stress a person experienced, the more likely he or she was to fall ill. He interviewed more than 5000 people and devised what was to become a classic, systematized method for correlating the events in people's lives with their illnesses (Pelletier 1992). Until that time it had been assumed that only adverse stress would have a significant effect. However, the survey showed that **any** change in the normal pattern of life, even good stress, produced symptoms. Stress can be divided into that which is necessary for survival (acute) and that which will eventually lead to breakdown (chronic). Acute stress is processed by the sympathetic adrenal–medullary (SAM) system. Chronic stress is processed via the hypothalamic–pituitary adrenocortical (HPA) axis (Scott et al 2012).

The alarm response (acute stress) can be life-saving. Physiologic changes (produced by receptors in the brain) increase heartbeat and respiration. Unnecessary metabolism is curbed, while blood and oxygen are swiftly redirected to the vital centers of the body (brain and heart). When the danger is over, the body quickly returns to its original state. Clammy hands and feet become warm and dry again. Respiration and pulse slowly return to normal and digestion recommences. However, if stress continues (chronic stress), the person will not be able to overcome stress responses, and will eventually become exhausted through loss of energy (Yoshiyama 2014). This can lead to physical, mental, and emotional problems, and ultimately breakdown.

STRESSORS

A major conference held in Arizona in the 1980s brought together leading psychologists, immunologists, and physicians to discuss stress and try to define it. After heated debate, it was agreed there was no absolute definition of stress but that "things" outside people caused stress. These "things" were labeled *stressors*. People react and adapt to stressors differently. Some people are able to cope; others cannot. Stressors have measurable psychological and physiologic effects and psychological stress can lower immunity. Perhaps the most common symptom that stands for anxiety or stress is a dry mouth. In China, individuals suspected of lying were forced to chew rice powder and then spit it out (Yount 2007, p 88) because it was believed the stress of lying would render a person incapable of salivation. In fact, salivary cortisol is a biomarker for stress (Ng et al 2004). The brain has a remarkable ability to change our body's normal functions in response to stressful experiences (McEwen et al 2012). The mind–body connection is very strong (Littrell 2008).

Stressors can be divided into four categories: physical, physiologic, psychological, and sociocultural (Brooker 2008). Our responses to stress are governed by the hypothalamus, which is part of the limbic system. Odor has a direct pathway to the limbic system, in particular to the amygdala, so it makes sense that aromatherapy can reduce stress. Toda and Morimoto (2008) found that lavender reduced stress using saliva tests.

CHRONIC STRESS

In chronic stress, the "arousal state" of a person is never completely switched off and cortisol levels remain above average. This shows up in the saliva

(Van Holland et al 2012), hair (Wosu et al 2013), urine, and blood (Sauvé 2007). Over time, small but damaging physiologic changes occur. Increase in blood sugar induced by chronic stress has been linked to type 2 diabetes (Lukaschek 2013). Chronic stress also affects hormonal balance (Scott et al 2012), digestion (Blanchard 2008), and immune function (Bellingrath et al 2010). Chronic stress also changes cognitive ability: reducing flexibility to rigid habit action (Ohira 2011).

Chronic stress accounts for 80% of all healthcare problems in the United States (Lee 2010). This situation is similar in many other countries such as the UK (Chandola et al 2006), Germany (Backé et al 2012), and Finland (Heikkilä et al 2013). Despite this, the workforce is still encouraged to push itself to the limit and being "stressed" or a "workaholic" is often the acceptable face of modern life. However, if stress remains relentless, breakdown is inevitable.

MEASURABLE PHYSICAL RESPONSES TO CHRONIC STRESS

Stress increases:
(1) Adrenaline/noradrenaline in the blood and urine;
(2) Rate and force of the heartbeat;
(3) Blood adrenocorticoids;
(4) Lactate in the blood;
(5) Urinary adrenocorticoids;
(6) Systolic blood pressure;
(7) Dilation of the pupils.
Stress decreases the number of white blood cells (eosinophils and lymphocytes).

An increase in eosinophils and lymphocytes leads to immunosuppression and decreased resistance to infection. An increase in aldosterone, thyroxine, and glucagon increases the level of blood glucocorticoids. An increase in cortisol levels affects carbohydrate, lipid, and protein metabolism. This can lead to muscle wasting, thinning of the skin, and a reduced immune response (Garg et al 2001). It also raises blood cholesterol levels and reduces vitamin D and calcium absorption, resulting in osteoporosis.

For 50 common symptoms of stress, please see the American Institute of Stress (AIS; 2013).

STRESS AND PATIENTS

Arguably, one of the most stressful situations in anyone's life is to be institutionalized. To many people a hospital can seem like a prison where patients lose their sense of control, their identity, and feel helpless and anonymous. This feeling of anonymity is compounded by Western medicine, which treats the medical condition rather than the patient. Patients may have chronic stress (from being ill) or acute stress (from being in the hospital). The more seriously ill the patient, the more severe the loss of control and the resulting stress. Compounding this sense of loss is the feeling of invasion: of privacy, personal space, and the body itself. A patient in a hospital could experience all four stressors (physical, physiologic, psychological, and sociocultural).

A patient's stress levels will directly impact the rate of his or her recovery (Gouin & Kiecolt-Glazer 2011; Marshall 2011). Stress can also affect patient survival. A Swiss study of 504 patients (Nickel et al 2013) found that stress biomarker levels were significantly greater in nonsurvivors than survivors (P < 0.0001).

Although anxiety is a symptom of stress, it is often used as a synonym for stress. Frazier et al (2002) found that reliance on the top recognized stress indicators—patients' verbalization of anxiety, agitation, increased blood pressure, increased heart rate, and restlessness—produced an inaccurate and incomplete stress evaluation. The GAD-7 scale (generalized anxiety disorder) is a self-assessment that contains seven questions relevant to patient stress (Spitzer et al 2006). The Patient Health Questionnaires PHQ-9 and PHQ-15 have 9 and 15 questions, respectively, that measure and monitor depression, anxiety, and somatization (where a patient experiences psychological distress in the form of physical symptoms). Chronic stress often accompanies chronic illness and is associated with depression, reduced mental acuity, and increased sensitivity to pain (Bergmann et al 2013).

Because patient stress has such serious consequences, procedures are needed to reduce it whenever possible. Acute patient stress can occur immediately before an invasive procedure, such as magnetic resonance imaging (MRI) or cardiac catheterization, or following surgery. Chronic stress can occur in hospitalized patients who have no control over their own environment or uncertain prospects for their lives.

Aromatherapy for Patient Stress

Aromatherapy is a simple, safe, cost-effective method that can reduce both acute and chronic stress. Inhaling a relaxing essential oil before a procedure can help a patient with acute stress. Examples of this are the aromasticks used in a British hospital for cancer patients prior to radiotherapy (Stringer & Donald 2011), the ambient odor used both in India (Bhargava et al 2009) and in Austria (Lehrner et al 2005) before dental surgery, and the inhalation given to U.S. patients prior to colonoscopy (Muzzarelli et al 2006). The chronic stress of lengthy treatments, such as renal hemodialysis, can be soothed with aromatherapy massage (Heath & Lewis 2008). In this study, as well as reducing stress in 21 patients, aromatherapy reduced blood pooling and outbreaks of pustules in one patient with chronic renal asteatotic eczema. The mixture used on the legs was *Helichrysum italicum*, *Juniperus communis*, and *Lavandula angustifolia*.

Familiar smells associated with happy memories can help reestablish feelings of happiness. To be happy is to be unstressed. Certain essential oils have their own relaxing properties. Essential oils such as lavender, lavandin, mandarin, rose, bergamot, and frankincense have all shown their potential to reduce stress (Field et al 2005; Chang 2008; Thomas 2011; Holm & Fitzmaurice 2008; Bhargava et al 2009; Conrad & Adams 2012).

Each hospital department carries its own particular brand of stress and fear. One of the most common, but least life-threatening, stresses in oncology is a woman's fear of losing her hair. The simple act of a gentle head massage with a diluted essential oil such as lavender *(Lavandula angustifolia)* can do a tremendous amount to "touch the spot" and help reassure the patient that their hair *will* grow back. In a randomized, controlled study, hair loss as a result of alopecia responded well to topically applied essential oils (Hay et al 1998). It is a shame this study has not been repeated.

Essential oil of lavandin *(Lavandula × hybrida)* reduced the stress of patients waiting for an operation (Braden et al 2009). One hundred and fifty adult patients were randomly allocated to either control (standard care), experimental (standard care plus essential oil lavandin), or sham (standard care plus jojoba oil) groups. One drop of lavender essential oil was applied to a cotton ball. The patient was asked to sniff the cotton ball prior to the nurse taping the cotton ball to the patient's hospital gown, near the chest area. Visual analog scale (VAS) scores were used to assess anxiety. Muzzarelli et al (2006) used lavender in their study of 118 patients awaiting either colonoscopy or esophagogastroduodenoscopy. The "state" part of the State Trait Anxiety Inventory (STAI) was used to measure patients' anxiety levels before and after breathing in lavender. Although the patients said the smell of lavender was pleasant, it did not reduce their anxiety. In both these studies on preoperative anxiety, the gas chromatography/mass spectrometry (GC/MS) charts were not given. This makes it impossible to know the chemical profile of the lavender that was used. For a selection of published studies on aromatherapy and stress, please see Table 11-1.

This is really important to know! I remember my own randomized, controlled study about 20 years ago (Buckle 1993), when I compared lavandin *(Lavandula x intermedia)* with lavender *(Lavandula angustifolia)*. No one was more surprised than me when the results found that lavandin was more effective at reducing post-cardiotomy stress in an intensive care unit (ICU) than lavender! However, chemical analysis showed that the lavandin used was chemotype (CT) super. This has almost twice as many esters (calming and soothing) as the *Lavandula angustifolia* used. Therefore, it really is vital to know the chemistry, particularly for lavender because there are so many varieties, and some lavenders such as *latifolia* can be stimulating. Please see the chemistry section for more information.

Lehrner et al (2000) explored the effect of two essential oils: sweet orange *(Citrus sinensis)* or lavender *(Lavandula angustifolia)* on patients waiting for a dental procedure. The study had four groups: (1) sweet orange; (2) lavender; (3) music; and (4) no music. Statistical analyses revealed that compared to the control condition both ambient odors of orange and lavender reduced anxiety and improved mood in patients waiting for dental treatment. Tukey–Kramer multiple comparisons showed a statistical difference between the control group and the orange group ($P = 0.049$) and between the control group and the lavender group ($P = 0.039$). There was no statistically significant difference between the control group and the music group ($P = 0.371$).

Kritsidima et al (2010) explored the effect of diffused lavender in a cluster randomized-controlled trial of 340 patients awaiting dental surgery. Analyses of variance (ANOVAs) showed that although both groups had similar levels of generalized dental anxiety, the lavender group reported significantly lower current anxiety ($P < 0.001$) than the control group. Doshi (2012), an RJBA student, explored the effect of aromatherapy (bergamot and frankincense) on 24 women who were about

TABLE 11-1 *Selection of Published Studies on Aromatherapy and Anxiety*

Author	Year	Essential Oils	Common Names	Method	Number of Participants
Bhargava et al	2009	*Lavandula angustifolia*	Lavender	Inhaled	140
		Citrus sinensis	Sweet orange		
Braden et al	2009	*Lavandula x intermedia*	Lavandin	Inhaled	150
Chang	2008	*Citrus bergamia*	Bergamot	Hand massage	58
		Lavandula angustifolia	Lavender		
		Boswellia carteri	Frankincense		
Conrad & Adams	2012	*Rosa damascena*	Rose	Hand 'M' Technique vs. inhalation	28
		Lavandula angustifolia	Lavender		
Holm & Fitzmaurice	2008	*Citrus aurantium* var *amara* [flos]	Neroli	Inhaled	1104
Kasper et al	2010	Silexan	Lavender	Oral	221
Kritsidima et al	2010	*Lavandula angustifolia*	Lavender	Inhaled	340
Lee et al	2011	Various	Various	Various	16 (review and RCT)
Lehrner et al	2005	*Lavandula angustifolia*	Lavender	Inhaled	200
		Citrus sinensis	Sweet orange		
McCaffrey et al	2009	*Lavandula angustifolia*	Lavender Rosemary	Inhaled	40
Muzzarelli et al	2006	*Lavandula angustifolia*	Lavender	Inhaled	118

RCT = Randomized, controlled trial.

to undergo breast needle biopsy at a hospital in New Jersey, United States. The women were randomly allocated to one of four groups: (1) inhaling essential oils (on a patch on the hospital gown); (2) receiving the hand 'M' Technique®; (3) receiving the hand 'M' Technique plus aromatherapy; and (4) the control group. The group who received both the hand 'M' Technique plus aromatherapy had the greatest reduction in stress. The intervention was only given for 10 minutes.

Graham et al (2003) found that essential oils of lavender, bergamot, and cedarwood reduced the stress of patients during radiotherapy. Lavender and Japanese cedarwood (Hiba oil, botanical name *Thujopsis dolabrata*) both reduced anxiety in 14 female patients who were receiving regular hemodialysis (Itai et al 2000). The outcome measure was the Hamilton rating scale for anxiety (HAMA). Markish, an RJBA student and dialysis nurse, conducted a study (2011) on 16 patients undergoing hemodialysis 3 times a week for 4 hours in a busy teaching hospital in Texas. She used a combination of angelica root *(Angelica archangelica)*, bergamot *(Citrus bergamia)*, and lavender *(Lavandula angustifolia)* on a cotton ball placed in the patient pillowcase close to the nose. The outcome measure was the VAS. Patients were receiving pro re nata (prn) morphine, valium, and Benadryl. The essential oil mix showed a positive difference—reduction in anxiety in the patients and reduction in prn medicines needed.

STRESS AND HOSPITAL STAFF

Stress in hospitals is not confined to patients. Nursing staff are under tremendous stress; their numbers have been cut even though their workload has remained just as heavy, and morale is very low. Nursing stress is a global issue (Gandi et al 2011; Toh et al 2012; Chacón 2013; Wang et al 2013). A recent UK survey of 1865 healthworkers found nurses were more stressed than combat troops (Calkin 2013) with nurses frequently having a stress score of 43.35 on the internationally recognized Impact of Event Scale (a score above 44 is categorized as severe and may reduce the individual's ability to function). Physicians are also feeling stressed, even in countries where the health system is perceived to be less stressful. A German study (Bauer & Groneberg 2013) found a high prevalence (55.5%) of distress among physicians in hospitals and even more with female doctors (59.7%). A Norwegian study found high levels of stress and deteriorating mental health among medical students (Gramstad et al 2013). A French study found a high proportion of burnout among doctors and nurses working in the ICU and anesthesia (Mon et al 2013). Health professionals find it hard to look after themselves.

Aromatherapy for Hospital Staff

Health professionals experience many emotional and disturbing scenes. Often there is no way of ameliorating emotions until the next break and frequently there are no breaks. The pressure can be eased if aromatherapy is used. Mandarin *(Citrus reticulata)*, lavender *(Lavandula angustifolia)*, or chamomile *(Chamaemelum nobile)* inhaled in an aromasticks can have a calming effect very quickly. Peppermint *(Mentha piperita)*, black pepper *(Piper nigrum)*, or rosemary *(Rosmarinus officinalis)* can revive and stimulate, making night shifts more tolerable. Nurses, physicians, physical therapists, and others represent a large reservoir of professionals who touch other people throughout life—from pediatrics to the care of the elderly. This is procedural touch: necessary for the medical or nursing intervention and not intended to relax or calm the patient. However, a 5-minute hand 'M' Technique with bergamot *(Citrus bergamot)* can provide rapid, therapeutic help for a colleague following a traumatic experience. If this is not possible, just inhaling angelica or rose can be useful. Touch and smell may be as old as the hills, but they can be deeply comforting.

RJBA students have carried out numerous studies on stress in hospital staff. Please see a selection from 2004 in Table 11-2.

Pemberton (2007) conducted a study on 14 ICU nurses to test if a 5% mixture of lavender and clary sage (self-applied to the inner aspect of the arms) reduced work-induced stress more than a placebo (carrier oil only). The study lasted 2 weeks. Each nurse was asked to evaluate his or her own stress using a VAS (0-10) 3 hours into a 12-hour shift. Then they applied Application 1 oil for the first three shifts and Application 2 oil for the next three shifts. The results found that the nurses' stress decreased 50% more for Application 2 oil. Application 2 was the aromatherapy mixture. The study was published a few years later in *Holistic Nursing Practice* (Pemberton & Turpin 2008).

Moonan (2012), another RJBA student, explored the effects of lavender and Roman chamomile on the stress levels of the leadership and administrative group for surgical programs and the pediatric transplant center at a large pediatric hospital in Massachusetts, United States. Participants were randomly allocated to one of two groups. Intervention was five drops each of chamomile *(Chamaemelum nobile)* and lavender *(Lavandula angustifolia)* in 20 mL of jojoba oil to be applied by a roller ball when the participant felt stressed. The control group received a roller ball with rose water only. The study took 3 weeks: baseline, intervention, washout. The perceived stress score (PSS) was measured for each week and compared (n = 10). Participants had greater reduction with the essential oil roller ball than with just rose water.

Yusui (2006), another RJBA student, explored the effect of inhaling peppermint and bergamot in aromasticks on oncology night nurses. They measured stress at the beginning, the midpoint, and at the end of their 12-hour shift using the PSS and the VAS. The control group received an inhaler with jojoba vegetable oil that has a slight smell but no essential oils. Both groups had some stress reduction, possibly as a result of breathing deeply. However, stress reduction in the aromatherapy group was 34% and in the control group only 12%.

STRESS AND HOSPITAL VISITORS

Visiting a sick relative in the hospital is stressful. What to say? What to do? Where to sit? Frequently, the patient has insufficient energy to carry on a conversation and the silences become longer and longer. The sicker the patient, the more stressed the visitors (Auerbach et al 2005) and the less likely they are to touch their relative. Families often do not know what to do and can feel marginalized by hospital staff (Molter 2007). The stress of families can communicate itself to the patient, increasing the patient's sense of helplessness. However, relatives and visitors want to be able to help their loved one (Eldridge 2004). When you are a patient, the small things in life become very important. These include fresh air, natural light, living plants, kind touch, and pleasant smells. Few of these occur in a hospital. Perhaps this is what Florence Nightingale meant when she is purported to have said the

TABLE 11-2 *RJBA Student Studies on Nurse Stress*

Name	Year	State	Essential Oils	Participants	Method	Number
Tiller	2006	AZ	Lavender	Child abuse hotline	Inhaled	12
Yusui	2006	NY	Peppermint, bergamot	Night nurses	Aromastick	10
Pemberton	2007	TX	Lavender, clary sage	ICU nurses	Topical	14
Meyer	2007	NE	Mandarin, geranium	Nurses	Hand 'M' Technique	18
Lucier	2010	MA	Lavender, bergamot, ylang ylang	Behavioral health nurses	Aromastick	30
Scheller	2010	MN	Lavender, clary sage	Community hospital nurses	Hand 'M' Technique	14
Doshi	2012	NJ	Bergamot, frankincense	Patients pre-breast biopsy	Inhaled and 'M' Technique	24
Finneron	2011	MA	Lavender, clary sage	Clinical nurse managers	Roller ball	9
Markish	2011	TX	Lavender, bergamot, angelica	Hemodialysis patients	Cotton ball	16
Moonan	2012	MA	Lavender/Roman chamomile	Surgical pediatric transplant staff	Roller ball	10
Palmer	2010	MA	Lavender, bergamot	Outpatient clinic staff	Aromastick	10
Pritchard	2012	TX	Bergamot	Relatives and patients	'M' Technique	30
Romanello	2012	CT	Lavender; Geranium, bergamot, black pepper	Operating room staff	Aromastick	14
St. Michel	2011	MN	Lavandin	Nurse leadership	Rollerball	13

ICU = Intensive care unit.

"least fortunate were those who found themselves nearest to a hospital." Hospital visitors can do quite a lot to help alleviate their relatives' stress as well as their own stress.

Aromatherapy for Stressed Visitors
Chang (2008) found that aromatherapy hand massage eased anxiety, pain, and depression in patients. Learning a simple hand massage or 'M' Technique and using gentle essential oils can empower a visitor (even a child) and make the patient feel special. No words are necessary; touch and smell can say it all. Aromatherapy costs little in terms of money, time, or energy, but it communicates a great deal. Many relatives are keen to learn something that can help their loved one (Eldridge 2004).

In a ground-breaking study in Texas (2012), Pritchard, an RJBA student who works as a nurse in a trauma ICU, explored the effect of relatives using aromatherapy to help their loved ones. In this controlled study, Pritchard recruited relatives of 30 trauma patients in two separate groups of 15. The Hospital Anxiety and Depression Scale (HADS tool) was administered on the first day to 15 relatives. Following this, the 15 relatives were asked to visit their loved one twice a day for three consecutive days (Days 2, 3, and 4). They were asked to behave as usual and this included touching and talking to the patient. The HADS tool was readministered to the participant after the Day 4 visit. During the following week, no recruitment took place. During the third week, a further 15 relatives were recruited. These relatives were taught the hand 'M' Technique and were given a bottle of 5% bergamot to use with the M. All relatives were patch-tested before taking part in the study. These relatives performed the 'M' Technique plus bergamot on their loved one twice a day for approximately 5 minutes per session for a total of 3 days (Days 2, 3, and 4). The HADS tool was given to the participant again after the final 'M' Technique on Day 4. There was a statistically significant reduction in the anxiety and depression levels of relatives in the aromatherapy plus 'M' Technique group. This is the only study I am aware of where relatives have been taught a simple aromatherapy technique by members of the hospital staff. The study is certainly worth repeating on relatives of different types of patients and perhaps measuring patient stress and anxiety levels as well as relative stress and anxiety. This simple study has huge implications for hospitals—to make them more hospitable for visitors as well as patients and staff. Holism can occur simply in the interaction of all people concerned with a patient's care (Yoshiyama 2014).

Burnout
If chronic stress continues unabated, it is possible to reach burnout. Maslach and Leiter (2008) define burnout as "a prolonged response to chronic emotional and interpersonal stressors." They found that people who reach burnout had increased cynicism and inefficacy. Varney, an RJBA student, explored the effect of a mixture of inhaled essential oils on mental exhaustion and moderate burnout in a randomized, controlled, double-blind study (2010). What makes her study unusual was that she chose ordinary people suffering from burnout, not healthcare professionals

or those in accepted high-stress jobs. Their burnout resulted from juggling child-care or care of an elderly relative with a full-time job or academic study. Fourteen participants were randomly allocated to receive an aromastick containing (1) basil, peppermint, and helichrysum or (2) rose water (control). During this 3-week study, participants rated their symptoms on a VAS (0-10). The results found that inhaling the mixture of peppermint, basil, and helichrysum essential oils several times a day reduced the symptoms of burnout more than placebo. The study was published in the *Journal of Alternative and Complementary Medicine* (Varney & Buckle 2012).

POSTTRAUMATIC STRESS DISORDER

In 1980, the American Psychiatric Association (APA) added posttraumatic stress disorder (PTSD) to the third edition of its *Diagnostic and Statistical Manual of Mental Disorders (DSM-III)* nosologic classification scheme. Army personnel who have been trained to handle chronic stress sometimes can suffer from PTSD when the situation is over and it is safe for them to "let go." The memory of certain smells can be associated with highly emotional experiences. Because the olfactory cortex and amygdala are involved in fear responsivity and survival, aromas can induce trauma symptoms in anyone with PTSD (Vasterling et al 2000). In a randomized, controlled study (Vermetten et al 2007) using positron emission tomography (PET) brain scanning, the aromas of vanilla and diesel were tested on eight veterans with PTSD and eight without PTSD against a control of plain air. The smell of diesel produced the signs of stress only in the veterans with PTSD, not the veterans without PTSD who rated it as only slightly less agreeable to vanilla. It is not just combat troops with PTSD who are affected more severely by aromas. This is the case for others such as refugees where aromas have triggered panic attacks (Hinton et al 2004). It appears that those with PTSD are hypersensitive to stimuli and this includes aromas. Interestingly, an Australian study (Dileo et al 2008) found that people with PTSD exhibited significant olfactory identification deficits (OIDs) compared to controls, even though their cognitive measures were not compromised. Therefore, it is important when using aromatherapy with anyone with PTSD to use essential oils that will trigger good memories rather than traumatic ones. This is a fascinating area for future study.

PTSD and Aromatherapy

Is it possible to reprogram the brain using aromas so that traumas can be overcome? According to Abramovitch and Lichtenberg (2009), this may be so. They found that needle phobia, panic disorder, and combat-induced PTSD all responded to olfactory conditioning under hypnosis. This article covers three case studies. The first one, a 42-year-old male with needle fear who needed urgent dental surgery, was successfully programmed using red mandarin under hypnosis not to fear needles and dental surgery. The second case was a 37-year-old male with panic attacks and agoraphobia who was taking venlafaxine 225 mg, alprazolam 2 mg, and risperidone 2 mg daily. After 3 months of olfactory conditioning with basil, he was able to go without drugs. At his 1-year follow-up, he was smelling basil only once or

TABLE 11-3 *Published Studies on Posttraumatic Stress Disorder (PTSD) and Aroma*

Author	Year	Type	Number of Participants
Abramovitz & Lichtenberg	2009	Hypnotherapy	3
Dileo et al	2008	War veterans	31
Hinton et al	2004	Cambodian refugees	100
Vasterling et al	2000	War veterans	68
Vermetten et al	2007	War veterans	16

twice a month and no longer suffered from panic attacks or agoraphobia. The third case was a 51-year-old recently retired veteran who had full PTSD with secondary depression, anxiety attacks, severe insomnia, and suicidal thoughts. Everyone else in his armored carrier had been killed except him when it went over a mine. His daily drug regimen included olanzapine 10 mg (antipsychotic), escitalopram 30 mg (antidepressant), and clonazepam (mild tranquilizer). He also selected basil out of several other aromas. After six sessions of olfactory conditioning with the hypnotherapist, his well-being had greatly improved. A year later this improvement had been maintained. He was well enough to try and patch up his broken marriage. The authors comment that they have had good results with essential oils in their hypnotherapeutic conditioning and have started formal research. For a list of published studies on aromatherapy and PTSD, please see Table 11-3.

REFERENCES

Abramovitz E, Lichtenberg P. 2009. Hypnotherapeutic olfactory conditioning (HOC): case studies of needle phobia, panic disorder, and combat-induced PTSD. *Int J Clin Exp Hypnosis.* 57(2):184–197.
American Institute of Stress (AIS). 2013. http://www.stress.org/stress-effects. Accessed November 28, 2013.
Anthony G, Thibodeau G. 1983. *Textbook of Anatomy and Physiology.* London: CV Mosby.
Auerbach S, Kiesler D, Wartella J, Rausch S, Ward K, Ivatury R. 2005. Optimism, satisfaction with needs met, interpersonal perceptions of the healthcare team, and emotional distress in patients' family members during critical care hospitalization. *Am J Crit Care.* 14(3):202–10.
Backé E, Seidler A, Latza U, Rossnagel K, Schumann B. 2012. The role of psychosocial stress at work for the development of cardiovascular diseases: a systematic review. *Int Arch Occup Environ Health.* 85(1):67–79.
Bauer J, Groneberg D. 2013. Distress among physicians in hospitals – an investigation in Baden-Württemberg, Germany. *Dtsch Med Wochenschr.* 138(47):2401–6.
Bellingrath S, Rohleder N, Kudielka B. 2010. Healthy working school teachers with high effort-reward imbalance and over commitment show increased pro-inflammatory immune activity and a dampened inert immune defence. *Brain Behav Immun.* 24(8):1332–1339.
Bergmann N, Ballegaard S, Holmager P, Kristiansen J, Gyntelberg F et al. 2013. Pressure pain sensitivity: a new method of stress measurement in patients with ischemic heart disease. *Scand J Clin Lab Invest.* 73(5):373–9.
Bhargava R, Dileep C, Jyothi C, Jayaprakash K. 2009. The effect of ambient odours and ambient music on the anxiety of patients in a dental setting. *Int J Clin Aroma.* 6(2):3–8.

Blanchard E, Lackner J, Jaccard J, Rowell D, Carosella A et al. 2008. The role of stress in symptom exacerbation among IBS patients. *J Psychosomatic Research*. 64(2):119–12.

Braden R, Reichow S, Halm M. 2009. The use of essential oil of lavandin to reduce preoperative anxiety in surgical patients. *J Perianesth Nurs*. 24(6):348–355.

Brooker C. 2008. *Medical Dictionary*. 16th edition. Churchill Livingstone. London.

Buckle J. 1993. Aromatherapy. *Nursing Times*. 89(20):32–5.

Calkin S. 2013. Nurses More Stressed than Combat Troops. *Nursing Times*. http://www.nursingtimes.net/nursing-practice/clinical-zones/management/nurses-more-stressed-than-combat-troops/5053522.article. Accessed November 26, 2013.

Chacón M. 2013. Burnout among Cuban nurses: out of the shadows. *MEDICC Rev*. 15(4):60.

Chandola T, Brunner E, Marmot M. 2006. Chronic stress at work and the metabolic syndrome: prospective study. *BMJ*. 332(7540):521–525.

Chang S. 2008. Effects of aroma hand massage on pain, state anxiety and depression in hospice patients with terminal cancer. *Taehan Kanho Hakhoe Chi*. 38(4):492–502.

Conrad P, Adams C. 2012. The effect of clinical aromatherapy for anxiety and depression in the high risk postpartum woman – a pilot study. *Comp Ther Clin Practice*. 19(3):164–168.

Dileo J, Brewer W, Hopwood M, Anderson V, Creamer M. 2008. Olfactory identification dysfunction, aggression and impulsivity in war veterans with post-traumatic stress disorder. *Psychol Med*. 38(4):523–531.

Doshi M. 2012. Effects of *Citrus bergamia* and *Boswellia carterii* on women undergoing stereotactic breast biopsy. RJBA unpublished dissertation.

Eldridge D. 2004. Helping at the bedside: spouses' preferences for helping critically ill patients. *Res Nurse Health*. 27(5):307–321.

Field T, Diego M, Hernandez Reil M, Cisneros W, Feijo J et al. 2005. Lavender fragrance cleansing gel effects on relaxation. *Int J Neurosci*. 115(2):207–222.

Finneron K. 2011. The effect of essential oils on work-related stress for nurse clinical risk managers. Unpublished RJBA dissertation.

Frazier S, Moser D, Riegel B et al. 2002. Critical care nurses' assessment of patients' anxiety: reliance on physiological and behavioral parameters. *Am J Critical Care*. 11(1):57–64.

Gandi J, Wai P, Karick H, Dagona Z. 2011. The role of stress and level of burnout in job performance among nurses. *Ment Health Fam Med*. 8(3):181–94.

Garg A, Chren M, Sands L et al. 2001. Psychological stress perturbs epidermal permeability barrier homeostasis. *Arch Dermatol*. 137(1):53–59.

Gouin J-P, Kiecolt-Glazer J. 2011. The impact of psychological stress on wound healing. Methods and mechanisms. *Immunol Allergy Clin North Am*. 31(1):81–93.

Graham P, Browne L, Cox H, Graham J. 2003. Inhalation aromatherapy during radiotherapy: results of a placebo-controlled double-blind randomized trial. *J Clin Oncol*. 21(12):2372–2376.

Gramstad T, Gjestad R, Haver B. 2013. Personality traits predict job stress, depression and anxiety among junior physicians. *BMC Med Educ*. 13(1):15.

Hay L, Jamieson M, Ormerod D. 1998. Randomized trial of aromatherapy: successful treatment for alopecia areata. *Arch Dermatol* 134(11):1349–1352.

Heath J, Lewis W. 2008. Complementary therapy practice aids stress reduction in patients receiving renal haemodialysis. *Int J Clin Aromather*. 5(1):19–25.

Heikkilä K, Nyberg S, Theorell T, Fransson EI, Alfredsson L et al. 2013. Work stress and risk of cancer: meta-analysis of 5700 incident cancer events in 116,000 European men and women. *BMJ*. 346:f165.

Hinton D, Pich V, Chhean D, Pollark M, Barlow D. 2004. Olfactory-triggered panic attacks among Cambodian refugees attending a psychiatric clinic. *General Hospital Psychiatry*. 26(5):390–397.

Holm L, Fitzmaurice L. 2008. Emergency department waiting room stress: can music or aromatherapy improve anxiety scores? *Pediatr Emerg Care*. 24(12):836–838.

Itai T, Amayasu H, Kuribayashi M, Kawamura N, Okada M, Momose A et al. 2000. Psychological effects of aromatherapy on chronic hemodialysis patients. *Psych Clin Neurosci*. 54(4):393–397.

Kasper S, Gastpar M, Muller W, Volz H, Moller H, Dienel A, Schlafke S. 2010. Silexan, an orally administered lavandula oil preparation, is effective in the treatment of subsyndromal anxiety disorder. A randomized, double-blind, placebo controlled trial. *Int Clin Psychopharmacol.* 15(5):277–287.

Kormos V, Gaszner B. 2013. Role of neuropeptides in anxiety, stress, and depression: from animals to humans. *Neuropeptides.* 47(6):401–19.

Kritsidima M, Newton T, Asimakopoulou K. 2010. The effects of lavender scent on dental patient anxiety levels: a cluster randomised-controlled trial. *Commun Dentist Oral Epidemiol.* 38(1):83–87.

Lee Y, Wu Y, Tsang H, Leung A, Cheung M. 2011. A systematic review on the anxiolytic effects of aromatherapy in people with anxiety symptoms. *J Alt Comp Med.* 17(2):101–108.

Lee R. 2010. The new pandemic: superstress? *Explore: Journal of Science & Healing.* 6(1):7–10.

Lehrner J, Eckersberger C, Walla P et al. 2000. Ambient odor of orange in a dental office reduces anxiety and improves mood in female patients. *Physiol Behav.* 71(1-2):83–86.

Lehrner J, Marwinski G, Lehr S, Johren P, Deecke L. 2005. Ambient odors of orange and lavender reduce anxiety and improve mood in a dental office. *Physiol Behav.* 86(1-2):92–95.

Littrell. 2008. The body–mind connection: not just a theory anymore. *Soc Works Health Care.* 46(4):17–37.

Lucier J. 2010. The effect of essential oils on work-related stress in behavioral health nurses. Published RJBA dissertation.

Lukaschek K, Baumert J, Kruse J, Thwing Emeny R, Lacruz M et al. 2013. Relationship between post-traumatic stress disorder and type 2 diabetes in a population-based, cross-sectional study with 2,970 participants. *J Psychosom Res.* 74(4):340–345.

Markish M. 2011. The effect of essential oils on hemodialysis patients. Unpublished RJBA dissertation.

Marshall G Jr. 2011. The adverse effects of psychological stress on immunoregulatory balance: applications to human inflammatory disease. *Immunol Allergy Clin North Am.* 31(1):133-40.

Maslach C, Leiter MP. 2008. Early predictors of job burnout and engagement. *J Appl Psychol.* 93(3):498–512.

McEwen B, Eiland L, Hunter R, Miller M. 2012. Stress and anxiety: structural plasticity and epigenetic regulation as a consequence of stress. *Neuropharmacology.* 62(1):3–12.

McCaffrey R, Thomas D, Kinzelman A. 2009. The effects of lavender and rosemary essential oils on test-taking anxiety among graduate nursing students. *Holistic Nursing Practice.* 13(2):88–93.

Meyer P. 2007. Effects of *Citrus reticulata* (mandarin) and *Pelargonium graveolens* (geranium) on the stress levels of nurses and nursing assistants working on an adult oncology unit. Unpublished RJBA dissertation.

Molter N. 2007. *Creating Healing Environments,* 2nd edition. Jones and Bartlett Publishers, MA: Sudbury.

Mon G, Libert N, Journois D. 2013. Burnout-associated factors in anesthesia and intensive care medicine. 2009 Survey of the French Society of Anesthesiology and Intensive Care. *Ann Fr Anesth Reanim.* 32(3):175–88.

Moonan M. 2012. The effects of lavender and Roman chamomile on stress levels in surgical and transplant leadership and administrative staff at a children's hospital. Unpublished RJBA dissertation.

Muzzarelli L, Force M, Sebold M. 2006. Aromatherapy and reducing preprocedural anxiety: a controlled prospective study. *Gastroenterol Nursing.* 29(6):466–471.

Ng V, Koh D, Mok B et al. 2004. Stressful life events of dental students and salivary immunoglobulin A. *Int J Immunopathol Pharmacol.* 17(2):49–56.

Nickel C, Messmer A, Geigy N, Misch F, Mueller B et al. 2013. Stress markers predict mortality in patients with nonspecific complaints presenting to the emergency department and may be a useful risk stratification tool to support disposition planning. *Acad Emerg Med.* 20(7):670–9.

Ohira H, Matsunaga M, Kimura K, Murakami H, Osumi T et al. 2011. Chronic stress modulates neural and cardiovascular responses during reversal learning. *Neuroscience.* 193(13):193–204.

Palmer D. 2010. Does inhaling essential oils reduce the perceived stress levels of employees in an outpatient multispecialty physician office? Unpublished RJBA dissertation.

Pelletier K. 1992. Mind–body health: research, clinical and policy implications. *Am J Health Promotion.* 6(5):345–348.

Pemberton E. 2007. The effect of essential oils on work-related stress on nurses in intensive care. Unpublished RJBA dissertation.

Pemberton E, Turpin P. 2008. The effect of essential oils on work-related stress in intensive care unit nurses. *Holist Nurse Practice*. 22(2):97–102.

Pritchard C. 2012. Aromatherapy intervention to reduce the anxiety and depression levels of family members and friends of patients with traumatic injury. Unpublished RJBA dissertation.

Rahe R. 1975. Epidemiological studies of life change and illness. *Int J Psych Med*. 6(2):133–146.

Romanello V. 2012. Aromatherapy on the work-related stress of operating room staff. Unpublished RJBA dissertation.

Sauvé B, Koren G, Walsh, G, Tokmakejian S, Van Uum S. 2007. Measurement of cortisol in human hair as a biomarker of systemic exposure. *Clin Invest Med*. 30(5):E183–E191.

Scheller M. 2010. Effects of *Salvia sclarea* (clary sage) and *Lavandula angustifolia* (lavender) on stress levels of nurses and nursing assistants in a rural community hospital in Minnesota. Unpublished RJBA dissertation.

Scott K, Tamashiro K, Sakai R. 2012. Chronic social stress: effect of neuroendocrine function. *Handbook Neuroendocrinol*. 521–534.

Spitzer R, Kroenke K, Williams J, Lowe B. 2006. A brief measure for assessing generalized anxiety disorder: the GAD-7. *Arch Internal Med*. 166(10):1092–7.

St. Michel J. 2011. Effect of lavandin on nurse manager stress. Unpublished RJBA dissertation.

Stringer J, Donald G. 2011. Aromasticks in Cancer Care: an innovation not to be sniffed at. *Comp Ther Cl Practice*. 17(2):116–121.

Tiller L. 2006. Effect of lavender on the stress of a Child Abuse Hotline in AZ. Unpublished RJBA dissertation.

Thomas J. 2011. Immunity over inability: the spontaneous regression of cancer. *J Nat Sci Biol Med*. 2(1):43–49.

Toda M, Morimoto K. 2008. Effect of lavender aroma on salivary endocrinological stress markers. *Arch Oral Biol*. 51(10):964–968.

Toh S, Ang E, Devi M. 2012. Systematic review on the relationship between the nursing shortage and job satisfaction, stress and burnout levels among nurses in oncology/haematology settings. *Int J Evid Based Healthc*. 10(2):126–41.

Van Holland B, Frings-Dresen, Sluiter M. 2012. Measuring short-term and long-term physiological stress effects by cortisol reactivity in saliva and hair. *Int Arch Occup Environ Health*. 85(8):849–852.

Varney E, Buckle J. 2012. Effects of inhaled essential oils on mental exhaustion and moderate burnout: a pilot study. *J Alt Comp Med*. 18(12):69–71.

Vasterling J, Brailey K, Sutker P. 2000. Olfactory identification in combat-related posttraumatic stress disorder. *J Traumatic Stress*. 13(2):241–253.

Vermetten E, Schmahl C. Southwick S, Bremner J. 2007. Positron tomographic emission study of olfactory induced emotional recall in veterans with and without combat-related stress disorder. *Psychopharmacol Bull*. 40(1):8–30.

Wang S, Liu Y, Wang L. Nurse burnout. 2013. Personal and environmental factors as predictors. *Int J Nurs Pract*. doi:10.1111/ijn.12216. Accessed November 26, 2013.

Wosu A, Valdimarsdóttir U, Shields A, Williams D, Williams M. 2013. Correlates of cortisol in human hair: implication for epidemiologic studies of health effects of chronic stress. *Ann Epidemiol*. (23)12:797–811.

Yount. 2007. *Forensic Science: from Fibers to Fingerprints*. Chelsea House Publishing. New York, USA. p 88.

Yoshiyama K. 2014. Personal communication.

Yusui T. 2006. Essential oil on work-related stress among oncology nurses working the night shift. Unpublished RJBA dissertation.

Section III

AROMATHERAPY IN CLINICAL SPECIALTIES

Section III covers a selection of clinical specialties (arranged in alphabetical order). Each chapter focuses on a handful of specific problems within each specialty and explores how aromatherapy might help alleviate those problems. As in Sections I and II, each chapter has been peer reviewed by an expert in that field and is backed up with published research, clinical experience, case studies, and small pilot studies. The aim in writing this section is to spotlight the clinical potential of aromatherapy within specific departments. Obviously there will be some overlap among chapters, and the reader is advised to refer to the general index at the back of the book to find other areas where the symptom has been discussed.

Finally, in the words of Abraham Lincoln "Character is like a tree and reputation like a shadow. The shadow is what we think of it; the tree is the real thing." I am trying to present the real thing—the *clinical* use of aromatherapy.

Chapter 12

Care of the Elderly

"Growing old is like being increasingly penalized for a crime you have not committed."

Temporary Kings, by Anthony Powell (1973)

CHAPTER ASSETS

TABLE 12-1 | *A Selection of Recently Published Studies on Dementia, 243*

TABLE 12-2 | *Dementia Studies by RJBA Students, 245*

TABLE 12-3 | *Selection of Some Recent Published Studies on Aromatherapy of Arthritis, 248*

BOX 12-1 | *Essential Oils for Dementia in Alphabetical Order, 246*

THE ELDERLY

The world population is growing older. People are living longer and surviving diseases that would previously have been fatal. This longevity produces an increasing burden on healthcare services (Grover & Niecko-Najjum 2013). By 2022, there will be an estimated 18 million cancer survivors in the United States alone (Mitka 2013). In the UK, the aging population has produced major issues for healthcare provision and planning (Caley & Sidhu 2011). In Japan, a single payment system has allowed total healthcare spending to be controlled despite Japan's growing elderly population (Ikegama & Anderson 2012). In The Netherlands, the estimated cost of healthcare, as a percentage of the Gross Domestic Product (GDP), will rise from 13% in 2011 (€90 billion) up to 31% in 2040 (Eddes 2013).

Exercise, both mental and physical, plus good nutrition and a sense of contentment are important in successful aging (Ayers & Verghese 2013; Webster & Ma 2013; Wijsman et al 2013). It also helps to have good genes as a recent Canadian genome study showed (Omoumi et al 2013). According to one survey, Japan has the oldest population with approximately 25% of the population over 65 years of age (Chartsbin 2011). However, the oldest woman, Jeanne Calment, who was French, died aged 121 years. It is a sad part of Western culture that age is not revered, and those who could impart so much information and life experience to

240

younger members of society are frequently isolated in residential homes. This is not to denigrate such institutions, but to question why "civilized" society does not want to look after its elderly. Perhaps the world has become so busy that there is no time to just "be" with those whose sense of time has gone.

AROMATHERAPY AND THE ELDERLY

I remember seeing Helen Passant speak about using aromatherapy and touch in her geriatric ward at a nursing conference in England during the 1980s; later I read her article (Passant 1990). Her talk made a major impression on me and I decided that integrating aromatherapy and gentle touch (the 'M' Technique®) into nursing care would become my life's work. I wanted to change the face of nursing—to put the caring back into it. Helen talked about how lavender seemed to open the box of memories in her patients and how they became alive again. More recently, Verboomen (2005), an RJBA student, conducted a fascinating study on the memories elicited in 10 elderly people (aged 76 to 90 years) using five essential oils (bergamot, sweet marjoram, ylang ylang, myrrh, and angelica). Despite growing up in the same area and having similar life experiences, the aromas produced different thoughts. Interestingly, ylang ylang was the most liked aroma.

Aromatherapy in the care of the elderly has grown exponentially in the last 20 years. An example is an Australian study (Bowles et al 2005) on the use of aromatherapy in 28 separate residential geriatric care facilities. They found aromatherapy was used extensively to manage symptoms of dementia and age-related physical discomfort. Fifty-nine percent of residents were receiving aromatherapy regularly and 47% received daily treatments. The most commonly used essential oils were lavender *(Lavandula angustifolia)*, tea tree *(Melaleuca alternifolia)*, geranium *(Pelargonium graveolens)*, eucalyptus *(Eucalyptus globulus)*, and bergamot *(Citrus bergamia)*. Most facilities used aromatic foot-baths or hand, foot, limb, and neck-and-shoulders massage with essential oils. Fifteen facilities used commercial blends.

Nishimura (2004) discusses the use of aromatherapy (hand and foot massage with essential oils) in a nursing home for the elderly in Tokyo, Japan. The 800-bed facility was established about 30 years ago and has a long waiting list. Its motto is "the hospital to which you want to admit your aging mother for the best care." A team of aromatherapists (supplied by TEN Aroma Association) has offered treatments to its elderly residents (average age 90 years) twice a week for the past 10 years and the program is now well integrated into the facility. Staff state that the residents really enjoy the treatments and it makes a substantial impact on their quality of life. This gives the team of aromatherapists very high job satisfaction.

A Japanese study (Satou et al 2013) found that a 5-minute aromatherapy massage using 2% geranium *(Pelagonium graveolens)* and peppermint *(Mentha piperita)* in jojoba oil twice a week reduced psychological stress among 11 elderly patients in long-term hospitalization. A clear reduction was observed in the 12-question General Health Questionnaire ($P < 0.05$). A Norwegian study (Johannessen 2013) found that diffusing lavender *(Lavandula angustifolia)* at night reduced sleep disturbance in the elderly. A Korean study found a thrice weekly 20-minute aromatherapy massage with lavender, chamomile, rosemary, and lemon increased the self-esteem of elderly women (Rho et al 2006).

In France, aromatherapy is included in the care of elderly residents at a retirement home for people with handicaps and special needs in the Lorraine region (Barat-Dupont 2008). Essential oils were first introduced via cleaning materials in 2004. Integration then progressed through room disinfection to patient massage with essential oils. All essential oils are dispensed on prescription and those providing treatment have trained for 2 years. At the time of writing, all residents' rooms are equipped with a diffuser and essential oils are diffused at regular times in the dining area. In addition, essential oils such as Ravansara (*Commiphora camphora* CT 1,8-cineole) and *Eucalyptus radiata* are used to protect residents from respiratory complaints during autumn and winter.

Dementia and Alzheimer's Disease

Dementia is an irreversible brain disease that causes progressive memory disturbance and personality disintegration (Brooker 2008). One of the most common causes of dementia in the elderly is Alzheimer's disease. This is when plaques containing abnormal protein appear in the cortex, leading to brain atrophy and the presence of the characteristic neurofibrillary "tangles." In this chapter, aromatherapy in dementia and Alzheimer's disease will be discussed together, although it is possible for dementia to occur without Alzheimer's disease. See Table 12-1 for a list of recently published studies on dementia.

Cases of mild cognitive impairment, dementia, and Alzheimer's disease are increasing (Brodaty et al 2013). According to a UK study, one in 14 people over 65 years of age and one in six people over 80 years of age have some form of dementia (Alzheimers Society UK 2012). The Alzheimers Society of the United States claims that 8 million Americans have Alzheimer's disease (Alzheimers Society USA 2013). Conventional treatment is with drugs such as donepezil (Kim et al 2013). Olfactory dysfunction is thought to be a marker for detecting early Alzheimer's disease (Burns 2000; Jimbo et al 2011; Naudin et al 2013). This may be because individuals who are positive for the apolipoprotein E (ApoE) ε4 allele are at higher risk for developing Alzheimer's and the ε4 allele is linked to olfactory decline (Green et al 2013). However, smell and touch are powerful messengers and can sometimes penetrate the fog of dementia in a way words do not (MacMohan & Kermode 1998; Smith et al 2002; Staal et al 2007).

Ho (1996) described the sensory-stimulation groups developed at Burton Hospital in Dudley, England. Odors were matched with colors, such as lavender with shades of mauve and purple. Music associated with the aroma was played, such as the nursery rhyme "Lavender Blue Dilly Dilly," and patients had access to herbs and photographs connected to the aroma. Frequently, patients with dementia were able to make the correct connections. More recently, Snoezelen (a Dutch concept that was initiated in the 1970s as a leisure activity for severely disabled people) has been expanded for use with dementia patients (Berg et al 2010). Snoezelen rooms give the user a combined experience of vision, touch, sounds, and aromas (Lofan & Gold 2009).

TABLE 12-1 *A Selection of Recently Published Studies on Dementia*

Author	Year	Essential Oil	Common Name	Number of Participants
Bowles et al	2002	Various*	Various	56
Bowles et al	2005	Various†	Various	1032
Lin et al	2007	*Lavandula angustifolia*	Lavender lotion	70
Fujii et al	2008	*Lavandula angustifolia*	Lavender, two drops on the collar	14
Bowles	2009	Various‡	Various	98
Jimbo et al	2009	*Lavandula angustifolia* *Rosmarinus officinalis* *Citrus sinensis*	Lemon and rosemary, am Lavender and orange, pm Diffused	28
Burns et al	2011	*Melissa officinalis*	Melissa, topical	114
Fung et al	2012	Review	Various	11 trials
Fu et al	2013	*Lavandula angustifolia*	Lavender spray	67
Kimura & Takamatsu	2013	*Lavandula angustifolia*	Lavender	?
Johannessen	2013	*Lavandula angustifolia*	Lavender, diffused	24

*Lavender *(Lavandula angustifolia)*, sweet marjoram *(Origanum majorana)*, patchouli *(Pogostemon cablin)*, and vetiver *(Vetiveria zizanioides)*.
†Lavender *(Lavandula angustifolia)*, tea tree *(Melaleuca alternifolia)*, geranium *(Pelargonium graveolens)*, eucalyptus *(Eucalyptus globulus)*, and bergamot *(Citrus bergamia)*.
‡Eucalyptus *(Eucalyptus globulus)*, cypress *(Cupressus serpervirens)*, Persian lime *(Citrus latifolia)*, mandarin *(Citrus reticulata)*, lemongrass *(Cymbopogon citratus)*, and ginger *(Zingiber officinale)*.

Ballard et al (2002) conducted one of the earliest randomized controlled trials (RCTs) on 72 patients with severe dementia. In this British study, 10% melissa *(Melissa officinalis)* in a lotion was applied to each participant's face and arms twice a day. The control group received sunflower oil. Results showed a highly significant reduction in agitation using the Cohen–Mansfield Agitation Inventory (CMAI) score for the aromatherapy group compared to the placebo group (35% and 11%, respectively). An RCT by Lin et al (2007) found inhaled lavender *(Lavandula angustifolia)* was effective in alleviating agitated behaviors in Chinese patients with dementia in Hong Kong.

Snow et al (2004) suggest that the effects of essential oils are greatly enhanced (and actually may not be effective) without touch or massage. In their 10-week study of seven nursing home residents with advanced dementia, split-middle analyses conducted separately for each patient revealed no treatment effects specific to inhaled lavender without touch. However, a Japanese RCT on 28 patients with dementia (Fujii et al 2008) found that inhaled lavender **did** have a measurable effect on symptoms of dementia. The aromatherapy group received two drops of lavender on their collar three times daily. Outcome measures included the Neuropsychiatric Inventory (NPI), Mini-Mental State Examination (MMSE), and Barthel Index tests. There was significant improvement in the NPI score in the lavender group but not in the control group.

In a second Japanese study without touch, Jimbo et al (2009) explored the effect of diffusing rosemary and lemon essential oils in the morning and diffusing lavender and orange essential oils in the evening. The study involved 28 elderly people with dementia and 17 had Alzheimer's disease. The study lasted for 84 days. The study started with 28 days control, followed by 28 days aromatherapy, and then a further 28 days of washout. Outcome measures included the Japanese version of the Gottfries, Brane, Steen scale (GBSS-J), Functional Assessment Staging of Alzheimer's disease (FAST), a revised version of Hasegawa's Dementia Scale (HDS-R), and the Touch Panel-type Dementia Assessment Scale (DTAS). All patients showed significant improvement in personal orientation related to cognitive function on both the GBSS-J and TDAS after the aromatherapy intervention.

A Chinese systematic review (Fung et al 2012) of 11 RCTs shortlisted from electronic databases between 1995 and 2011 found that aromatherapy had reduced the behavioral and psychological symptoms of dementia (BPSD), improved cognitive functions, increased quality of life, and enhanced independence in activities of daily living. The authors concluded that aromatherapy was a safe and effective complementary therapy to use in dementia.

In an Australian study, Fu et al (2013) conducted an RCT (n = 67) to examine the reduction of agitation in dementia. One group received 3% lavender *(Lavandula angustifolia)*, sprayed directly on to the skin of the lower neck and upper chest, and a 2.5-minute hand massage twice a day for 6 weeks. The second group just received the lavender spray, and the control group received a water mist spray. The results did not show any significant reduction in agitation for either aromatherapy group. The authors comment that spraying the aromatherapy mist on the chest (rather than inhaling it directly or massaging it into the skin) may have contributed to the lack of effect. The hand massage was also a little short. The hand 'M' Technique is usually given for 5 minutes, so it would be interesting to repeat this study using a longer hand massage or the 'M' Technique.

Taking care of patients with Alzheimer's disease can be challenging. In cases where patients will not remain stationary, walking alongside them while simultaneously conducting a gentle hand 'M' Technique (with or without essential oils) can lead to positive changes in the patient, such as renewed eye contact and speech coherence. Several RJBA students have conducted studies on patients with dementia (Table 12-2). Quate (2002) used the 'M' Technique plus a 2% mixture of four essential oils: lavender *(Lavandula angustifolia)*, mandarin *(Citrus sinensis)*, bergamot *(Citrus bergamia)*, and petitgrain *(Citrus aurantium* var. *amara* fol). Her study was carried out at a residential hospital for dementia patients in Ohio, United States, and involved eight residents. Outcome measures included the Dementia Care Mapping (DCM) tool that was used regularly every 3 months. Results were compared with previous months and years. Aromatherapy plus the 'M' Technique had an increased positive effect on 87% of residents.

TABLE 12-2 *Dementia Studies by RJBA Students*

Name	Year	State	Essential Oil	Common Name	Method	Number of Participants
Quate	2002	MI	*Citrus bergamia*	Mixture*	Topical	6
Smith	1999	MA	*Lavandula angustifolia*	Lavender	Diffused	17
			Origanum marjorana	Sweet marjoram		
Brook	2003	NY	*Boswellia carterii*	Frankincense	Topical	6
Trumbull	2003	MA	*Lavandula angustifolia*	Lavender	Ribbon*	6
Curran	2003	MA	*Lavandula angustifolia*	Lavender	Diffused	10
Denert	2005	MA	*Citrus bergamia*	Bergamot	Inhaled	10

*Lavender *(Lavandula angustifolia)*, mandarin *(Citrus sinensis)*, bergamot *(Citrus bergamia)*, and petit-grain *(Citrus aurantium* var. *amara fol)*.

Room diffusers, nebulizers, and personal patches can be used in situations where patients are confined to bed or who dislike any form of touch. Curran (2003), another RJBA student, diffused lavender *(Lavandula angustifolia)* at sunset in the main common room of a large residential long-term facility for dementia in Massachusetts, United States. Ambulatory patients frequently showed disruptive behavior between 3 pm and 6 pm. Disruptive behavior at sunset is known as *sundowning* and is a recognized syndrome of dementia (Sharer 2008; Khachiyants et al 2011; Carson 2012). In Curran's study (n = 10), all patients who had been agitated before the lavender diffusion became calm after the lavender was diffused.

Another RJBA student (Trumbull 2003) used lavender *(Lavandula angustifolia)* applied to a ribbon. (This was before aromatherapy patches became available.) The ribbon was attached to the clothing of six residents in a long-term care facility in rural New Hampshire, United States, at 2 pm each day for 6 consecutive days. The outcomes were compared with the 6 previous days. Five of the six residents had reduced disruptive behavior. Denert (2005), another RJBA student, offered a 4 × 4 gauze swab with four drops of bergamot *(Citrus bergamia)* to disruptive patients during the 11 am to 7 pm nurses shift. This study is particularly interesting because one of the outcome measures was the number of pro re nata (prn, as required) medications used per patient. Of the 10 patients with disruptive or aggressive behavior (despite regular medication), none required prn medication after the bergamot intervention. This was a great improvement on the 12 prn medicines given in the baseline period.

Aromatherapy has also been found to be helpful for carers of patients with dementia (Atkins & Smith 2009). This British study explored the effect of a weekly aromatherapy massage on the stress and well-being of 12 carers of patients with

Alzheimer's disease over a period of 8 weeks. Outcome measures were taken at 1, 4, and 8 weeks. They included MYMOP2 (Measure Your Medical Outcome Profile), HADS (Hospital Anxiety and Depression Scale), and a VAS (visual analog scale). Results showed that aromatherapy reduced stress levels across all measures.

When a patient is unable to select an aroma, offer a choice of two different smells that are likely to be familiar. Suggestions for aromas to try are listed in Box 12-1 (listed in alphabetical order).

Preventing Falls in the Elderly

In many countries, fall prevention among older adults has become a major public health issue (Axer et al 2010; Quigley et al 2010; Chang et al 2013; Tchalla et al 2013). Odor is one of the strongest stimuli over a wide area of the cerebral cortex (Lopez & Blanke 2011), therefore it makes sense to offer an aroma and see if it reduces the number of falls. A Japanese study (Sakamoto et al 2012) found that inhaling lavender prevented falls in the elderly. In this RCT (n = 145), the experimental group wore a lavender patch attached to their clothes for continuous inhalation of lavender *(Lavandula angustifolia)*. There were fewer fallers in the lavender group (26) than in the placebo group (36). This is interesting because lavender is traditionally used to relax people. I have used peppermint on a gauze swab to help elderly people concentrate before they get up and it does seem to work. The only study I could find on aiding ambulation and peppermint was on mice (Umezu et al 2001). It would be interesting to do further studies in this area. Suggested essential oils would be rosemary, peppermint, rose, lemon, and of course lavender.

Skin Ulcers and Slow Healing Wounds

Aging slows down the body's ability to heal. Skin becomes thinner and more fragile, and the slightest knock can cause a deep bruise, especially if the person is taking

BOX 12-1 *Essential Oils for Dementia in Alphabetical Order*

Common Name	Botanical Name
Clary sage	*Slavia sclarea*
Eucalyptus	*Eucalyptus globulus*
Geranium	*Pelargonium graveolens*
Ginger	*Zingiber officinalis*
Lavender	*Lavandula angustifolia*
Mandarin	*Citrus reticulate*
Melissa	*Melissa officinalis*
Patchouli	*Pogostemon patchouli*
Peppermint	*Mentha piperita*
Rose	*Rosa damascena*
Rosemary	*Rosmarinus officinalis*
Sandalwood	*Santalum album*
Ylang ylang	*Cananga odorata* var. *genuine*

steroids. Very gentle massage with cold-pressed vegetable oils, such as oil of evening primrose, can aid the elasticity of aging skin, and certain essential oils can enhance the ability of aging skin to heal. Although most of the published research on essential oils in wound care is on animals (Orafidiya et al 2003; Suntar et al 2012; Tumen et al 2012), there are plenty of articles and case studies to show that aromatherapy is used in many counties for skin ulcers and slow healing wounds, for example, UK (Thorne 1996; Harris 2006; Clark 2011; Price 2012), United States (Ames 2006), Australia (Mercier & Knevitt 2005; Kerr 2006), South Africa (Nye 2005), and Canada (Tavares 2011).

Ames (2006) describes using essential oils on the chronic leg ulcer (Stage 2) of a 70-year-old diabetic woman. The ulcer measured 4 × 4 cm. Despite medical treatment, the ulcer had never resolved and she was referred to Ames (a nurse practitioner) for aromatherapy treatment. German chamomile 10% *(Matricaria recutita)* in grapeseed oil was applied twice a day and the wound completely healed in 13 days. Four years later, the wound remained healed.

Alan Barker, a clinical aromatherapist who was employed by the British National Health Service (NHS), used floral waters to irrigate wounds (Barker 1994). Floral waters are the byproduct of steam distillation and can be obtained from many essential oil suppliers. Slightly acidic, they are refreshing to use, smell lovely, and are excellent for skin care. (Floral waters are slightly acidic because they contain parts of the essential oil that are most soluble.) When using floral water, make sure the distributor can supply an analysis to prove the floral water is not contaminated with bacteria or fungi. Tellier (2005) explains how she used hydrosols to heal granulated scar tissue at a stoma site.

After irrigating the wound, a compress soaked in diluted (10% to 25%) essential oils can be applied to aid healing. The essential oils will reduce inflammation, encourage granulation, and reduce the chance of infection. Apply a fresh compress twice daily, or every 4 hours if the wound is infected. In another case study by Ames (2006), 10% tea tree *(Melaleuca alternifolia)* and frankincense *(Boswellia carterii)* in calendula-infused oil *(Calendula officinalis)* was applied directly to the wound cavity of a heel ulcer (3.5 × 5 × 2.2 cm in depth). It was then packed loosely with gauze soaked in the essential oil mixture, and a nonadhesive bandage was applied to hold it in place. This was a Stage 4 pressure ulcer so there was full thickness skin loss with extensive tissue destruction and necrosis. Multiple drug regimens and products had previously been used with no effect; in fact, the wound was increasing. However, the ulcer decreased to 0.8 cm in depth in only 14 days and went on to heal completely.

Kerr (2002, 2006), who has done much to introduce essential oils into wound care in Australia, writes about the use of essential oils to treat diabetic venous ulcers in a man aged 80 years. The wound started as a simple abrasion and slowly became worse. It ended up measuring 8 × 3 cm although mainly superficial. Conventional dressings, including compression bandages, plus antibiotics made no difference to the ulcer. Kerr used a 12% essential oil mixture: lavender *(Lavandula angustifolia)*, German chamomile *(Matricaria recutita)*, myrrh *(Commiphora molmol)*, and tea tree *(Melaleuca alternifolia)* mixed into fresh aloe vera gel. The pain subsided on the first application of the gel and the ulcer healed completely. A favorite mixture of mine for slow healing of wounds is lavender *(Lavandula angustifolia)*, helichrysum

TABLE 12-3 *Selection of Some Recent Published Studies on Aromatherapy of Arthritis*

Author	Year	Essential Oil	Method	Number of Participants
Kim et al	2005	Mixture*	Topical	40
Smith et al	2011	*Eucalyptus globulus*	Topical	43
Yip & Tam	2008	*Zingiber officinalis*	Topical	59

*Lavender, marjoram, eucalyptus, rosemary & peppermint

(*Helichrysum italicum*), tea tree (*Melaleuca alternifolia*), and frankincense (*Boswellia carterii*) in *Calophyllum inophyllum* (Tamanu).

Osteoarthritis and Hemorrhoids

No chapter on care of the elderly would be complete without a mention of osteo-arthritis and hemorrhoids. Although essential oils will not prevent osteoarthritis, topically applied essential oils such as ginger, black pepper, or peppermint can certainly help soothe the pain (Bliddel et al 2000; Cote 2002; Yip & Tam 2008). A small list of published research on arthritis can be found in Table 12-3. There is more information about essential oils for pain in the chapter on pain. In a different type of study, Joksimovic et al (2012) explored the effect of tea tree in an ointment (trade name Proctoial) on 36 patients with hemorrhoids in a double-blind RCT. Results showed that the tea tree ointment reduced all symptoms more than the placebo.

Finally, as I am now officially an elderly person myself, I would like to finish this chapter with the poem below.

The body it crumbles. Grace and vigor depart.
There is now a stone where I once had a heart.
But inside this old carcass, a young girl still dwells,
And now and again my battered heart swells.
I remember the pain, and I remember the joys,
And I'm living and loving all over again.
And I think of the years, all too few, gone too fast,
And accept the stark fact that nothing will last.
So open your eyes, nurse, open and see, not a crabbed old woman.
Look closer. See me.

Anonymous—found in a nursing home after the author's death. (cited in Montagu 1986)

REFERENCES

Alzheimers Society UK. 2012. http://www.alzheimers.org.uk. Accessed November 8, 2013.
Alzheimers Society USA. 2013. http://www.alz.org. Accessed November 8, 2013.
Ames D. 2006. Aromatic wound care in a health care system: a report from the USA. *Int J Clin Aromather.* 3(2):3–8.
Atkins R, Smith F. 2009. The use of aromatherapy massage with carers of dementia patient: a preliminary evaluation. *Int J Clin Aromather.* 6(2):9–14.

Axer H, Axer M, Sauer H, Witte O, Hagemann G. 2010. Falls and gait disorders in geriatric neurology. *Clin Neurol Neurosurg.* 112(4):265–74.

Ayers E, Verghese J. 2013. Locomotion, cognition and influences of nutrition in ageing. *Proc Nutr Soc.* 1:1–7.

Ballard C, O'Brien J, Reichelt K, Perry E. 2002. Aromatherapy as a safe and effective treatment for the management of agitation in severe dementia: the results of a double-blind, placebo-controlled trial with Melissa. *J Clin Psych.* 63(7):553–8.

Barat-Dupont J. 2008. Using essential oils in a French elderly care facility. *Int J Clin Aromather.* 5(1):26–28.

Barker A. 1994. Pressure sores. *Aromather Quarterly.* 41:5–7.

Berg A, Sadowski K, Beyrodt M, Hanns S, Zimmermann M et al. 2010. Snoezelen, structured reminiscence therapy and 10-minutes activation in long term care residents with dementia (WISDE): study protocol of a cluster randomized controlled trial. *BMC Geriatr.* 31;10:5. doi:10.1186/1471-2318-10-5. Accessed November 12, 2013.

Bliddel H, Rosetzsky A, Schlinchting P et al. 2000. A randomized placebo controlled cross-over study of ginger extracts and ibuprofen in osteoarthritis. *Osteoarthritis Cartilage.* 8(1):9–12.

Bowles E, Griffiths D, Quirk L, Brownrigg A, Croot K. 2002. Effects of essential oils and touch on resistance to nursing care procedures and other dementia-related behaviours in a residential care facility. *Int J Aromather.* 12(1):22–29.

Bowles E, Cheras P, Stevens J, Myers S. 2005. A survey of aromatherapy practices in aged care facilities in northern NSW, Australia. *Int J Aromather.* 15(1):42–50.

Bowles J. 2009. Investigating cognitive effects of aromatherapy on people with dementia living in residential care facilities. *Int J Clin Aromatherapy.* 6(1):26–36.

Brodaty H, Heffernan M, Kochan NA, Draper B, Trollor J et al. 2013. Mild cognitive impairment in a community sample: the Sydney Memory and Ageing Study. *Alz Dement.* 9(3):310–31.

Brook D. 2003. Frankincense for dementia. Unpublished dissertation for RJBA.

Brooker C. 2008. *Medical Dictionary.* Churchill Livingstone. London.

Burns A. 2000. Might olfactory dysfunction be a marker for early Alzheimer's disease? *Lancet.* 355(9198):84–85.

Burns A, Perry E, Holmes C, Francis P, Morris J et al. 2011. A double-blind placebo-controlled randomized trial of *Melissa officinalis* oil and donepezil for the treatment of agitation in Alzheimer's disease. *Dement Geriatr Cogn Disord.* 31(2):158–64.

Caley M, Sidhu K. 2011. Estimating the future healthcare costs of an aging population in the UK: expansion of morbidity and the need for preventative care. *J Public Health (Oxf).* 33(1):117–22.

Carson V. 2012. Sundowning in the Alzheimer's patient. *Caring.* 31(6):52–3.

Chang M, Lin C, Wu T, Chu M, Huang T, Chen H. 2013. Eight forms of moving meditation for preventing falls in community-dwelling middle-aged and older adults. *Forsch Komplementmed.* 20(5):345–52.

Chartsbin. 2011. http://chartsbin.com/view/1239. Accessed November 8, 2013.

Clark S. 2011. A holistic approach to wound healing. *In Essence.*10(1):18–21.

Cote S. 2002. The effects of essential oils of black pepper on arthritis. Unpublished RJBA dissertation.

Curran P. 2003. Effect of diffusing lavender at sunset on patient with dementia. Unpublished dissertation for RJBA.

Denert D. 2005. Inhaling bergamot for agitated patients with dementia. Unpublished dissertation for RJBA.

Eddes E. 2013. [Improving healthcare and its manageability]. *Ned Tijdschr Geneeskd.* 157(25):A6485.

Fu C, Moyle W, Cooke M. 2013. A randomised controlled trial of the use of aromatherapy and hand massage to reduce disruptive behaviour in people with dementia. *BMC Complement Altern Med.* 10;13:165. doi:10.1186/1472-6882-13-165.

Fujii M, Hatakeyama R, Fukuoka Y, Yamamoto T, Sasaki et al. 2008. Lavender aroma therapy for behavioral and psychological symptoms in dementia patients. *Geriatr Gerontol Int.* 8(2):136–8.

Fung J, Tsang H, Chung R. 2012. A systematic review of the use of aromatherapy in treatment of behavioral problems in dementia. *Geriatr Gerontol Int.* 12(3):372–82.

Green A, Cervantez M, Graves L, Morgan C, Murphy C. 2013. Age and apolipoprotein E ε4 effects on neural correlates of odor memory. *Behav Neurosci.* 127(3):339–49.

Grover A, Niecko-Najjum L. 2013. Building a health care workforce for the future: more physicians, professional reforms, and technological advances. *Health Aff (Millwood).* 32(11):1922–7.

Harris R. 2006. Aromatic approaches to wound care. *Int J Clin Aromather.* 3(2):9–18.

Ho C. 1996. Stirring memories through all the senses. *J Dementia Care.* 4(4):15.

Ikegama N, Anderson G. 2012. In Japan, all-payer rate setting under tight government control has proved to be an effective approach to containing costs. *Health Aff (Millwood)*. 31(5):1049–56.

Jimbo D, Kimura Y, Taniguchi M, Inoue M, Urakami K. 2009. Effect of aromatherapy on patients with Alzheimer's disease. *Psychogeriatrics*. 9:173–7.

Jimbo D, Inoue M, Taniguchi M, Urakami K. 2011. Specific feature of olfactory dysfunction with Alzheimer's disease inspected by the Odor Stick Identification Test. *Psychogeriatrics*. 11(4): 196–204.

Johannessen B. 2013. Nurses experience of aromatherapy use with dementia patients experiencing disturbed sleep patterns. An action research project. *Complement Ther Clin Pract*. 19(4):209–13.

Joksimovic N, Spasovski G, Joksimovic V, Andreevski V, Zuccari C, Omini C. 2012. Efficacy and tolerability of hyaluronic acid, teatree oil and methyl-sulfonyl-methane in a new gel medical device for treatment of haemorrhoids in a double-blind, placebo-controlled clinical trial. *Updates Surg*. 64(3):195–201.

Kerr J. 2002. The use of essential oils in healing wounds. *Int J Aromather*. 12(4):202–6.

Kerr J. 2006. Venous ulcer – healing with essential oils and aloe vera: a case-study. *Int J Clin Aromather*. 3(2):34–39.

Khachiyants N, Trinkle D, Son SJ, Kim KY. 2011. Sundown syndrome in persons with dementia: an update. *Psychiatry Investig*. 8(4):275–87.

Kim H, Moon M, Choi J, Park G, Kim A et al. 2013. Donepezil inhibits the amyloid-beta oligomer-induced microglial activation in vitro and in vivo. *Neurotoxicology*. doi:pii:S0161-813X(13)00159-9. Accessed November 8, 2013.

Kim M, Name E, Paik S. 2005. The effects of aromatherapy on pain, depression and life satisfaction of arthritis patients. *Taehan Kanho Hakhoe Chi*. 35(1):186–94.

Kimura T, Takamatsu J. 2013. Pilot study of pharmacological treatment for frontotemporal lobar degeneration: effect of lavender aroma therapy on behavioral and psychological symptoms. *Geriatr Gerontol Int*. 13(2):516–7.

Lin P, Chan W, Ng B, Lam L. 2007. Efficacy of aromatherapy *(Lavandula angustifolia)* as an intervention for agitated behaviours in Chinese older persons with dementia: a cross-over randomized trial. *Int J Geriatr Psychiatry*. 22(5):405–10.

Lofan M, Gold C. 2009. Meta-analysis of the effectiveness of individual intervention in the controlled multisensory environment (Snoezelen) for individuals with intellectual disability. *J Intellect Dev Disabil*. 34(3):207–15.

Lopez C, Blanke O. 2011. The thalamocortical vestibular system in animals and humans. *Brain Res Rev*. 67(1-2):119–46.

MacMohan S, Kermode S. 1998. A clinical trial of the effect of aromatherapy on motivational behavior in a dementia care setting using single subjects. *Austral J Holistic Nursing*. 5(2):47–9.

Mercier D, Knevitt A. 2005. Using topical aromatherapy for the management of fungating wounds in a palliative care unit. *J Wound Care*. 14(10):497-8, 500–1.

Mitka M. 2013. IOM report: aging US population, rising costs, and complexity of cases add up to crisis in cancer care. *JAMA*. 2013;310(15):1549–50.

Montagu A. 1986. *Touching: The Human Significance of Skin*. New York: Perennial.

Naudin M, Mondon K, Atanasova A. 2013. Alzheimer's disease and olfaction. *Geriatr Psychol Neuropsychiatr Vieil*. 11(3):287–93.

Nishimura M. 2004. Aromatherapy treatments in a hospital for the elderly – meeting many happy faces through aromatherapy. *Int J Clin Aromather*. 1(2):39–41.

Nye S. 2005. Aromatic intervention for decubitus ulcer: a case report from South Africa. *Int J Clin Aromather*. 3(2):25–28.

Omoumi A, Fok A, Greenwood T, Sadovnick A, Feldman H, Hsiung G. 2013. Evaluation of late-onset Alzheimer disease genetic susceptibility risks in a Canadian population. *Neurobiol Aging*. doi:pii:S0197-4580(13)00427-2. Accessed November 8, 2013.

Orafidiya L, Agbani E, Abereoje B, Awe T, Abudu A, Fakoya F. 2003. An investigation into the wound healing properties of essential oil of *Ocimum gratissimum* Linn. *J Wound Care*. 12(9):331–4.

Passant H. 1990. A holistic approach in the ward. *Nursing Times*. 86(4):26–8.

Powell 1973. Powell. A. 1973. Temporary Kings. William Heinemann Ltd. London.

Price P. 2012. Essential oils in wound care. *In Essence*. 11(2):20–3.

Quate D. 2002. Aromatherapy using the 'M' Technique on hands of dementia patients. Unpublished RJBA certification paper.

Quigley P, Bulat T, Kurtzman E, Olney R, Powell-Cope G, Rubenstein L. 2010. Fall prevention and injury protection for nursing home residents. *J Amer Dir Assoc*. 11(4):284–93.

Rho K-H, Han S-H, Kim K-S, Lee M. 2006. Effects of aromatherapy massage on anxiety and self-esteem in Korean elderly women: a pilot study. *Int J Neurosci*. 116(12):1447–55.

Sakamoto Y, Ebihara S, Ebihara T, Tomita N, Toba K et al. 2012. Fall prevention using olfactory stimulation with lavender odor in elderly nursing home residents: a randomized controlled trial. *J Am Geriatr Soc*. 60(6):1005–11.

Satou T, Chikama M, Chikama Y, Hachigo M, Urayama H et al. 2013. Effect of aromatherapy massage on elderly patients under long-term hospitalization in Japan. *J Altern Complement Med*. 19(3):235–7.

Sharer. 2008. Tackling sundowning in a patient with Alzheimer's disease. *Medsurg Nurs*. 17(1):27–9.

Smith. 1999. Aromatherapy for dementia. Unpublished dissertation for RJBA.

Smith D, Standing L, de Man A. 2002. Verbal memory elicited by ambient odor. *Percept Motor Skills* 74(2):339–43.

Smith D, Jacobson B. 2011. Effect of a blend of comfrey root extract (Symphytum officinale L.) and tannic acid creams in the treatment of osteoarthritis of the knee: randomized, placebo-controlled, double-blind, multiclinical trials. *J Chiropr Med*. 2011 Sep;10(3):147–56.

Snow L, Havanec L, Brandt J. 2004. A controlled trial of aromatherapy for agitation in nursing home patients with dementia. *J Altern Complement Med*. 10(3):431–7.

Staal J, Sacks A, Matheis R, Collier L, Calia T et al. 2007. The effects of Snoezelen (multi-sensory behavior therapy) and psychiatric care on agitation, apathy, and activities of daily living in dementia patients on a short term geriatric psychiatric inpatient unit. *Int J Psychiatry Med*. 37(4):357–70.

Suntar I, Tumen I, Ustun O, Keles H, Akkol E. 2012. Appraisal on the wound healing and anti-inflammatory activities of the essential oils obtained from the cones and needles of *Pinus* species by in vivo and in vitro experimental models. *J Ethnopharmacol*. 139(2):533–40.

Tavares M. 2011. Integrating clinical aromatherapy in specialist palliative care. Available from www.clinicalaromapac.ca.

Tellier E. 2005. Case-study. The use of hydrosols to heal granulated scar tissue at a stoma site. *Int J Clin Aromather*. 2(2):35–36.

Tchalla A, Lachal F, Cardinaud N, Saulnier I et al. 2013. Preventing and managing indoor falls with home-based technologies in mild and moderate Alzheimer's disease patients: pilot study in a community dwelling. *Dement Geriatr Cogn Disorder*. 36(3-4):251–61.

Thorne D. 1996. Healing ulcers using essential oils. *J Commun Nursing*. 10(9):14–16.

Trumbull A. 2003. Lavender and dementia patients of residential homes. Unpublished RJBA certification paper.

Tumen I, Süntar I, Keleş H, Küpeli Akkol E. 2012. Therapeutic approach for wound healing by using essential oils of *Cupressus* and *Juniperus* species growing in Turkey. *Evidence-Based Complement Altern Med*. 2012:728281. doi:10.1155/2012/728281. Accessed November 15, 2013.

Umezu T, Sakata A, Ito S. 2001. Ambulation-promoting effect of peppermint oil and identification of its active constituents. *Phamacol Biochem Behav*. 69(3-4):383–90.

Verboomen R. 2005. 5 essential oils and memories in the elderly. RJBA unpublished dissertation.

Webster J, Ma X. 2013. A balanced time perspective in adulthood: well-being and developmental effects. *Can J Aging*. 22:1–10.

Wijsman A, Westendorp G, Verhagen A, Catt M, Slagboom P et al. 2013. Effects of a web-based intervention on physical activity and metabolism in older adults: randomized controlled trial. *Med Internet Res*. 15(11):e233.

Yip Y, Tam A. 2008. An experimental study on the effectiveness of massage with aromatic ginger and orange essential oils for moderate-to-severe knee pain among the elderly in Hong Kong. *Comp Ther Med*. 16(3):131–8.

Chapter 13

Critical Care/ICU

"Feeling safe is an overall need for Critical Care/ICU patients, and safety is negatively affected by lack of control."

Brigid Lusk 2005

CHAPTER ASSETS

A search of the literature using the words ICU (intensive care unit) or critical care plus aromatherapy identified more articles on preventing and treating hospital acquired infection in the ICU than anything else, so this chapter will begin with specific infections in the ICU. General infection will be covered in the chapter on infection.

Despite the advances in critical care, the incidence of infection continues to rise (Kaye et al 2010). An international study of 1265 ICUs, found 60% of ICU patients were considered infected at the time of survey (Vincent et al 2009). Infection was a strong independent predictor for mortality (OR = 1.51, P < 0.001). Patients in critical care are more vulnerable to hospital-acquired infection (HAI) than any other hospital department (Mnatzaganian et al 2005), and this is a problem for many countries (Januel et al 2010; Kallel et al 2010; Kollef 2008; Honda et al 2010; Yamakawa et al 2011).

ICU-acquired infections account for significant morbidity, mortality, and expense. The most frequently identified infections are ventilator-associated pneumonia, bloodstream infections caused by use of a central venous catheter, and urinary tract infections (Rosenthal et al 2006; Starnes et al 2008; Vincent et al 2009; Yamakawa et al 2011). Many ICU pathogens are now drug resistant (Weinstein & Bonten 2005). These include methicillin-resistant *Staphylococcus aureus* (MRSA) and multidrug-resistant *Pseudomonas aeruginosa* (MDRPA). Gram-negative bacteria, such as *Pseudomonas*, are particularly difficult to treat (Neuhauser et al 2003) and *Clostridium difficile* has become more daunting during the last few years (Bobo et al 2011) (Table 13-1).

To exacerbate the situation, a new bacterial pathogen has appeared in the ICU: *Acinetobacter baumannii* (Acinetobacter B). Acinetobacter B is an aerobic gram-negative bacillus (similar in appearance to *Haemophilus influenzae* on Gram stain). This pathogen is appearing in more and more ICUs worldwide (Heo et al 2011) (Kong et al 2011). Very quickly it became drug resistant. Multidrug-resistant *Acinetobacter baumannii* (MDRAB) caused the closure of an ICU in France on four occasions during an epidemic (Landelle et al 2013). The cause of the outbreak was traced to the transfer of two patients from Tahiti. During the following 18 months, a further 84 ICU patients became infected. Cross-infection was thought to be from hands of health personnel, poor cleaning protocols, airborne spread, and contaminated water from sink traps.

TABLE 13-1 *Hospital-Acquired Infection in Critical Care*

Author	Year	N	Subject	Country
Januel et al	2010	3,450	Death from HAI	France
Luqman et al	2007	In vitro	Drug-resistant mutants of *Mycobacterium smegmatis*, *Escherichia coli* and *Candida albicans*	India
Kallel et al	2010	261	Site of infection Multidrug-resistant *P. aeruginosa*, Acinetobacter B	Tunisia
Erbay et al	2003	434	*Pseudomonas aeruginosa*, MRSA, Acinetobacter B	Turkey
Vincent et al	2009	13,796	Site of infection MRSA, Acinetobacter B *Pseudomonas*, and *Candida* spp.	75 countries
Honda et al	2010	5,161	MRSA precolonized patients	United States
Meric et al	2005	131	*Staphylococcus aureus*, Acinetobacter B	Turkey
Kaye et al	2010	470	Infected suction equipment in ICU	United States
Rosenthal et al	2006	21,069	Infected devices in ICU	United States
Trouillet et al	2002	135	*Pseudomonas pneumonia*	France
Yamakawa et al	2011	474	MRSA at admission	Japan
Heo et al	2011	30	MDR Acinetobacter B	Korea
Kollef	2013	15,314	*Clostridium difficile*	Canada

MDRAB and *Pseudomonas* A are very challenging to treat, and even the poly-myxin group of drugs (such as colistin), used as a last resort for treatment of gram-negative bacterial infections, are not always successful (Balaji et al 2011). The incidence of Acinetobacter B was reduced for a year following the structural reno-vation of an ICU in Japan. However, this appeared to be transient (Nah et al 2013). In Poland, MDRAB was brought under control by vaporizing hydrogen peroxide in two ICUs (Chmielarczyk et al 2012).

Some equipment used in critical care, such as suction regulators, can become compromised with bacteria (Kaye et al 2010). Rosenthal et al (2006) found that between 2002 and 2005, 21,069 patients who were hospitalized in ICUs in 55 separate intensive care units in eight developing countries acquired 3095 device-associated infections. Ventilator-associated pneumonia posed the greatest risk having caused 41% of all device-associated infections, followed by bloodstream infections associated with central vascular catheters (CVCs) (30%), and then fol-lowed by catheter-associated urinary tract infections (29%).

Boucher et al (2009) reports on the lack of new antibacterial drugs in the pipe-line against the most prevalent resistant bacteria: *Enterococcus faecium, Staphylococcus aureus, Klebsiella pneumoniae, Acinetobacter baumannii, Pseudomonas aeruginosa,* and *Enterobacter* species. However, for this chapter, emphasis will be on the drug-resistant pathogens in the ICU and a discussion of the best way forward. *Clostridium difficile (C. diff)*-associated diarrhea is increasing in ICUs (Kollef 2008). In a study by Dodek et al (2013), of 15,314 patients admitted to the ICUs during the study period, 236 developed *Clostridium difficile* infection (CDI) and this was associated with a longer stay in the ICU. Drug-resistant *C. diff* is also increasing and such is the severity that, in some instances, it is being treated with fecal transplantation (Nagy 2012).

AROMATHERAPY FOR DRUG-RESISTANT PATHOGENS IN CRITICAL CARE

Kon and Rai (2012) suggest that essential oils could be used as effective treatments against many bacterial pathogens, including methicillin-resistant *Staphylococcus aureus* (MRSA), vancomycin-resistant enterococci (VRE) plus resistant isolates of *Pseudomonas aeruginosa, Klebsiella pneumoniae* and others. They also suggest that certain essential oils may potentiate the effectiveness of antibiotics against MDR bac-teria. Fadli et al (2012) led a Moroccan study that explored the effect of combin-ing essential oils with conventional medicines against resistant bacteria involved in nosocomial infections. They explored the combined effects of two different species of thyme endemic to Morocco (*Thymus maroccanus* and *T. broussonetii*) plus con-ventional antibiotics such as ciprofloxacin, gentamicin, pristinamycin, and cefixime. Of the 80 combinations tested, 71% showed total synergism, 20% had partial synergy and 9% showed no effect. The combinations were more successful with gram-positive bacteria than gram-negative. Cavacrol, one of the main components in thyme, had an "interesting synergistic effect in combination with ciprofloxacin" (Fadli et al 2012). They concluded that their findings were "very promising" as this kind of combination treatment for nosocomial infections is likely to reduce the minimum effective dose needed of the antibiotic, thus minimizing any possible toxic side effects and reducing treatment cost. No mention is made of how the combination would be delivered.

Clearly some essential oils, such as horseradish, are not suitable for use with ICU patients (or probably anyone!) although they have been found to be effective against MRSA (Nedorostova et al 2011). However, as Table 13-2 shows, there are many other essential oils (such as *Eucalyptus globulus*) that are effective against resistant pathogens, and smell pleasant (Tohidpour et al 2010). Several other studies suggest combining essential oils with conventional antibiotics (Shin & Kim 2005; Rosato et al 2007; Saad et al 2010). Langeveld et al (2013) postulate on the synergistic ability of separate components within essential oils to potentiate conventional antibiotics. They suggest carvacrol, cinnamaldehyde, cinnamic acid, eugenol, and thymol could have a synergistic effect when used in combination with antibiotics.

TABLE 13-2 *Essential Oils for Resistant Infections*

Author	Year	Essential Oil	Pathogen	Method
Silva et al	2013	Thyme Oregano Pennyroyal	P. aeruginosa and E. faecalis	Agar diffusion
Duarte et al	2012	Coriandrum sativum	Acinetobacter baumannii	Improved effectiveness of ciprofloxacin, gentamicin, and tetracycline
Végh et al	2012	Lavandula vera L. intermedia L. pyrenaica L. stoechas	P. aeruginosa	Tube dilution containing 0.2% polysorbate 80
Hamoud et al	2012	Peppermint Olbas	MRSA VRE	Kill time assay
Lysakowska et al	2011	Thymus vulgaris	Acinetobacter baumannii	Agar diffusion
Tyagi et al	2010	Lemongrass Mentha arvensis Peppermint Eucalyptus globulus	P. aeruginosa	Vapour and liquid diffusion
Owlia	2009	Zataria multiflora Myrtle communis Eucalyptus camaldulensis	P. aeruginosa	Disk diffusion

Continued

TABLE 13-2 *Essential Oils for Resistant Infections—cont'd*

Author	Year	Essential Oil	Pathogen	Method
Roller et al	2009	*Lavandula angustifolia* L. latifolia L. stoechas L. luisieri	MRSA	Direct contact
Doran et al	2009	Lemongrass Geranium	MRSA VRE *A. baumannii C. difficile*	Diffused into air
Jazani et al	2009	Fennel: *Foeniculum vulgare*	*Acinetobacter baumannii*	48 isolates from humans. Disc diffusion
Hosseini et al	2008	Cumin	MDR *P. aeruginosa*	52 burn isolates from 2 hospitals
Chao et al	2008	Lemongrass Lemon myrtle Mountain savory, Cinnamon Melissa	MRSA	Disc diffusion
Dryden et al	2004	Tea tree	MRSA	Human study; 224 patients
Opalchenova	2003	Basil: *Ocimum basilicum*	MDR *P. aeruginosa* MRSA MDR *E. coli*	Kill time assay

In a separate paper, Saad et al (2010) found essential oils of two species of thyme potentiated the effect of amphotericin B and fluconazole B against *Candida*, a fungal infection now becoming more common in ICU. Rosato et al (2008) found several essential oils potentiated the effect of amphotericin B against Candida. And, in a later paper, Rosato et al (2009) found *Oreganum vulgar* (oregano) and *Pelargonium graveolens* (geranium) enhanced the effect of Per Google: Nystatin on *Candida*.

Chan et al (2010) suggest using polymeric nanoparticles (NPs) for drug delivery. The use of biodegradable microparticles for controlled drug delivery has shown great potential as they can target specific areas of the body and thus reduce toxicity. Ungaro et al (2012) explored the use of tiny dry particles containing antibiotics for the treatment of pulmonary infections. They concluded "aerosolized antibiotics offer an attractive way to deliver high drug concentrations directly to the site of infection, reducing the toxicity while improving the therapeutic potential of existing antimicrobial agents against resistant microorganisms." Ultrasonic diffusion will readily break up any essential oil into many tiny particles that can also be easily absorbed by the lung. This could be an area for exciting research.

Sometimes, the oldest medicines can still be effective. Olbas is an over-the-counter medicine that has been used for many years for respiratory infections. It contains a mixture of essential oils: peppermint, eucalyptus, cajuput oil plus small amounts of juniper berry oil and wintergreen oil. Hamoud et al (2012) evaluated the minimum inhibitory and minimum microbicidal concentrations of Olbas (and each of the single essential oils) on 17 species/strains of bacteria and fungi. Olbas displayed a high antimicrobial activity against all test strains used, including antibiotic-resistant MRSA (methicillin-resistant *Staphylococcus aureus*) and VRE (vancomycin-resistant *Enterococcus*). This study also compared the kill time of peppermint essential oil on its own and found it was comparable to that of the mixture.

An interest in the medical use of essential oils for infection has led to the application of several patents (Sienkiewicz et al 2012). However, not every essential oil will be effective against every resistant pathogen. A selection of some of the studies showing effective essential oils against specific resistant pathogens relevant to ICU can be found in Table 13-2.

Twelve years ago, Caelli et al (2000) found the effects of a 5% tea tree oil body wash combined with 4% tea tree oil nasal ointment was comparable to a standard triclosan body wash plus 2% mupirocin nasal ointment for the eradication of MRSA. As pathogens mutated to accommodate triclosan, hexachloraphine was introduced. Until about 3 years ago, patients in the ICU were sponge-bathed daily, initially with soap and water, which was superseded by a triclosan soap. Today, patients in many ICUs worldwide are wiped down every day with chlorhexidine instead of receiving a sponge bath. This is to reduce the acquisition of resistant pathogens (Climo et al 2009; Munoz-Price et al 2009; Borer et al 2007). In Climo's study, patients in six ICUs were wiped down daily with chlorhexidine for six months and the incidence of bloodstream infections with MRSA and VREC were monitored. MRSA decreased by 32% and VREC decreased by 50%. Munoz-Price (2009) found that daily 2% chlorhexidine "cleaning" reduced the incidence of CVC-associated bloodstream infections by 90%, but this did not reduce ventilator-associated pneumonia. Borer et al (2007) found 4% chlorhexidine wipes reduced the prevalence of Acinetobacter B bloodstream infections by 85%. In this study, all patients were screened for skin colonization with Acinetobacter B on admission to the medical ICU.

Although chlorhexidine is a common, topical antiseptic skin scrub in hospital and household settings in the United States, it does have some problems (Sivathasan & Vijayarajan 2010), (Sivathasan & Goodfellow 2011). In 2012, the Medicines and Healthcare Products Regulatory Agency (MHRA) UK issued a patient safety alert on the risk of anaphylactic reactions from medical devices and medicinal products containing chlorhexidine (MHRA 2012). A similar antiseptic action (with a much nicer smell and no sticky after feel) could be achieved by using a few drops of the relevant essential oil on a washcloth, and sponge-bathing the patient. This can also be achieved by using a soap/gel containing the relevant antibacterial essential oils.

If I was a patient in an ICU, I would prefer to have water on my skin instead of a chlorhexidine wipe with its sticky, unpleasant residue and horrible smell, especially if the essential oils gave me the same protection against resistant pathogens. There is more to giving a sponge bath to a patient in ICU than preventing infection; it is also about refreshing patients and helping them to feel as good as possible about their situation. If essential oils are as effective as chlorhexidine, why not use them? And if there is no research, why not do some?

Inoculation of the formerly sterile lower respiratory tract with pathogens typically arises from aspiration of secretions, colonization of the aerodigestive tract, or use of contaminated equipment or medications (Safdar et al 2005). It is possible that hospital-acquired respiratory tract infections could be reduced by a few simple ways with aromatherapy. Here are some ideas to reduce across-the-board infection in Critical Care/ICU:

1. Place a few drops of relevant essential oils on to a filter placed in the tubing that connects the ventilator to the patient. (Filters are common in the portable respirators.)
2. There is a one-way valve that connects the ventilator tubing from the heater to another piece of tubing that goes to the patient. (This is used to prevent patient's secretions from going into the heater.) Essential oil could be added to the side of the filter that faces the patient.
3. There is a filter that fits on a tracheostomy. This is used for patients who are only receiving oxygen through a tracheostomy. The filter is green and spongy. Essential oils could be added to the filter.
4. Suction is usually part of a closed system in the ICU and the canister that collects the secretions is changed every day. The canister could have a few drops of essential oil added to prevent any pathogen in the secretions from leaking into the air while it is changed.
5. A few drops of diluted essential oils could be applied around the central venous line insertion site twice a day.
6. A few drops of diluted essential oil could be added to the urinary drainage bag.
7. The air in an ICU could be tested for airborne infection on a weekly basis. This could be done simply with an empty glass jar and the identification of pathogens that developed within a 12-hour period. Once any airborne pathogens are identified, essential oils could be used in electric diffusers, or personal patches on the patient, to ensure the air immediately around the patient was kept pathogen-free.
8. A separate diffuser could be positioned near the nurses' station to reduce stress and/or encourage alertness, as well as preventing cross-infection.
9. ICU equipment could be wiped down twice daily with an essential oil mix. The mixtures should be changed weekly (either in percentage mix 2:3:1 to 3:1:2, or in combination of essential oils) to prevent pathogens becoming resistant.
10. The sink drains could be checked for infection weekly and treated with essential oils.

It is important to keep changing the mixture of essential oils. A study by McMahon et al (2007) found that, although tea tree was still effective against many pathogens, habitation to sub-lethal concentrations of tea tree caused the minimum inhibitory concentration (MIC) required to increase slightly. The implications of this are discussed in the infection chapter.

FEAR

Critical care and ICUs are places where sudden emergency situations can occur at any time. Patients often experience excessive noise, constant light, unpleasant odors, crisis situations, fear of infection, and fear of death. Patients in ICUs face more invasive and obnoxious procedures than in any other unit in a hospital. Invasive procedures are those such as the insertion of hemodynamic monitoring lines, thoracentesis, paracentesis, and chest-tube placement and removal. As well as the uncertainty and invasive procedures, patients experience many things that can make them fearful. They are surrounded by complicated (and often noisy) machinery and are unable to speak if they are ventilated. Their life depends on those who care for them, so replacing that fear with trust is hugely important. Some ICUs are dedicated to surgical or medical patients. Other ICUs have a mixture of patients: some with grave, long-term medical conditions with other patients who have had major surgery and may be discharged to another part of the hospital after a very short stay.

Two days after discharge from an ICU in England, 71 patients were asked to rank a list of stressful items (Cornock 1998). Top of the list was thirst, followed by tubes in the nose or mouth, inability to communicate and being unable to move. However, lack of control, not knowing the time, and fear of death were also listed. Fear should not be underestimated. It is a strong emotion that links most ICU patients and their relatives.

Over 20 years ago, in 1989, Ingham (an ICU nurse) suggested communication should be written in to a patient's care plan and Ashworth (1984), another ICU nurse, wrote of the importance in learning nonprocedural touch as a method of communicating and reassuring patients. This is still the case today, noting that many patients still suffer from anxiety and depression even after discharge from an ICU (Flaaten 2010). Touch is a communication skill that can enhance trust. Henricson et al (2009) wrote of the hope gained by ICU patients who had experienced gentle tactile touch from nurses. Almerud et al (2008) writes that "tools are useful, but technology can never replace the closeness and empathy of the human touch." Lusk (2005) wrote that ICU nurses should be physically present for their patients and when nurses were perceived as caring and competent, this reduced the patient's level of fear. Gentle touch is one of the simplest methods of reducing fear. O'Lynn and Krautscheid (2011) wrote "perhaps no aspect of care is as essential to nursing as touch. Nurses touch patients to perform clinical tasks, communicate caring and ensure comfort." How strange and sad that today not all nursing schools include any method of simple touch in their curriculum. The 'M' Technique® was created to fill such a vacuum and it is my deep hope that nurses will learn this gentle method of touch as a basic part of nursing education. Sometimes a nurse may overlook the stress of an ICU patient, because she/he is more concerned with maintaining the patient's hemodynamic stability. But I hope the day never comes when a nurse is too busy to touch a patient: it only takes a few minutes. Nursing schools that do include Watson's Theory of Transpersonal Caring are moving in this direction of holding a patient's hand, hand massage, and back rubs during evening care (Schmock et al 2009; Hills & Watson 2011).

Being a patient in an ICU can be a psychologically traumatic and socially isolating. An ICU nurse who experienced being intubated as a patient in an ICU described how "her worst nightmare came true." She felt "abandoned and longed for someone to reassure her." Following her experience she understood "why it was sometimes necessary to hold a patient's hand" (Urden 1997). It is greatly underestimated how important it is for ICU patients to feel trust and confidence in their caregivers. Nonprocedural touch and pleasant aromas can do much to relieve anxiety and give comfort in what is perceived by patients to be a "hostile environment" (Welsh 1997). Essential oils can be used in many ways in an ICU from aiding intravenous insertions (Kristiniak et al 2012) to alleviating bronchial spasm (Buckle 1998).

AROMATHERAPY IN ICU

Early studies of aromatherapy in the ICU (Woolfson & Hewitt 1992; Buckle 1993; Stevensen 1994; Dunn et al 1995) showed that massage using aromatherapy was an effective method of reducing patients' stress. The essential oil used was predominantly lavender, although Stevensen used neroli. The percentage used was low: 1% to 3%. Massage lasted between 15 and 30 minutes. Comments from patients were very encouraging: "Aromatherapy made me feel like a whole person." "I feel like you really cared about me." "I felt like I was important, not just a number, and that you really would take care of me." "Until you did that, I was really scared, but you made me feel it would be okay to relax." Nurses in the study said they felt empowered as aromatherapy helped their patients feel less afraid.

In my own study (Buckle 1993), one of my patients said to me "you were the first person who didn't hurt me." That really made me think; I hadn't gone into nursing to hurt people! But much of what happens in the ICU is painful or distressing. There is little pleasure. Waldman et al (1993) suggested the following essential oils were useful in ICU: lavender, clary sage, jasmine, peppermint, rose, rosemary, tea tree, and ylang ylang. The oils were used in a 2% massage or in electric burners. Other nurse/aromatherapists suggested neroli, Roman chamomile, sandalwood, lemon, lemongrass, and palma rosa. Mitchell (2002), a critical care nurse, chose frankincense, geranium, petitgrain, sweet marjoram, mandarin, juniper, and German chamomile. I would choose an aroma that was familiar to the patient. If it was impossible to know what that was because there were no relatives to ask, I would use a mixture of rose, frankincense, mandarin, and lavender.

Cho et al (2013) conducted a randomized, controlled study to measure the effects of aromatherapy on anxiety, vital signs and sleep on 55 patients receiving percutaneous coronary intervention (PCI). The essential oils used were lavender, Roman chamomile and neroli. Patients inhaled the mixture (using an aromastone that gently heated the essential oils and so made them vaporized) using 10 deep breaths both before and after PCI. Then the aromastone was placed under the patient's pillow until the following morning. Outcome measures were the Spielberger State-Trait Anxiety Inventory Form Korean YZ (STAI-KYZ) and the Korean translation form of the VSH Sleep Scale (Verran and Snyder-Halpern). The aromatherapy group showed significantly less anxiety ($P < 0.001$) and improved sleep quality ($P = 0.001$) than the group who received conventional nursing care. Interestingly, the blood pressure of the control group rose immediately before and during the intervention. This did not happen with the aromatherapy group.

Hsieh (2011) gave a presentation at the Sigma Theta Tau International Honor Society of Nursing 41st Biannual Conference in Grapevine, Texas. Her randomized, control study evaluated the effects of using aromatherapy on patients in a 50-bed ICU in Taiwan over a period of 1 week. The results indicated that aromatherapy improved physical and psychological problems, especially for leg edema ($P < 0.05$) and anxiety ($P < 0.05$). This study found an additional benefit: the patients' families could help with the aromatherapy, thus removing their own feelings of powerlessness and fear.

Moeini et al (2010) conducted a controlled study to assess the effect of lavender for insomnia on patients with ischemic heart disease in an ICU. Sixty-four patients took part in this Iranian study. Those in the aromatherapy group received 9 hours of lavender for 3 nights (two drops lavender oil on a piece of cotton placed within 20 cm of the patient's head). The control group received standard nursing care. There was a significant difference between the mean scores of sleep quality in the two groups ($P = 0.001$). Outcome measures also included a sleep quality questionnaire.

Each patient is someone's child, no matter how old he or she is. Most patients in ICUs are frightened, no matter how brave they try to appear. ICUs can be very frightening for relatives too. Mitchell (2002) writes that an ICU often stuns relatives, and how appreciative relatives are when their loved ones receive the loving care that aromatherapy provides.

I remember seeing my own father and brother-in-law in an ICU several years ago. I experienced the helplessness many relatives and visitors feel even though I had trained and worked in ICUs for many years. Often relatives feel there is nothing they can do except wait and pray. Aromatherapy presents a wonderful opportunity to give the family a simple way to contribute and provide comfort for their loved one.

The gentle, stroking movements of the 'M' Technique, which can be used with or without essential oils, are extremely simple to learn (Roberts & Campbell 2011; Rickerby & Cordell 2012; Buckle 2013). I showed the 'M' Technique to a 5-year-old granddaughter who spent almost an hour lovingly stroking her grandfather's hands. Her sad, cross little face softened as she sang gently under her breath, moving her hands in time to her lullaby. Her parents watched her as she worked, amazed at the transformation. This little girl knew she had been given an important task, one that not only empowered her, but was actually of therapeutic value.

Teaching relatives to touch in this way does not take very long, probably only 10 minutes. Everyone can find 10 minutes. Talking with relatives about aromas that their loved ones enjoyed before they came into the hospital allows dialogue on a safe subject. Choosing an aroma that relatives feel could help their loved ones gives them a way of becoming involved. It is best to offer just a few aromas known to have relaxing effects. The floral aromas are usually popular. The rose essential oil used on my brother-in-law in Papworth Hospital, Cambridge, England, produced a smile even though he was extremely ill and it was also appreciated by the staff who gravitated toward the lovely smell.

A study at Harris Methodist Medical Center, Texas, for RJBA certification by Pritchard (2012) evaluated the effect of aromatherapy on family members and friends of patients in the ICU following traumatic injury. This controlled study used bergamot in a hand 'M' Technique. Nurses took a few moments to teach the 'M' Technique to 30 relatives and friends. The relatives and friends then used their newly learned skill to administer to their loved one and afterward rated their own sense of anxiety and depression. The results showed a statistically significant reduction in anxiety and depression in the aromatherapy group (P = 0.0018). The study is being submitted for publication. Hopefully, other studies will follow, as this is a very simple, effective and inexpensive way to empower relatives and friends, soothe patients and help nursing staff.

ICU NURSES STRESS

Patients and relatives are not the only people to feel stress in an ICU—nurses do too.

Mealer et al (2012) conducted semi-structured interviews with 27 ICU nurses. Thirteen were "highly resilient" and 14 had posttraumatic stress disorder (PTSD). The differences were identified in four main areas: social network, worldview, cognitive flexibility and self-care. The resilient nurses used positive coping skills and psychological characteristics to help them cope. Yava et al (2010) explored the perceptions of stress of both nurses and patients in an ICU in Turkey and concluded that several factors could reduce the stressful perceptions. These included having familiar arrangements, a humane ICU environment and appropriate nursing interventions (Table 13-3).

Carayon and Gurses (2005) explored the relationship between workload and quality of life for ICU nurses for her PhD doctoral studies. Of the 300 nurses in 17 ICUs in seven hospitals, the results showed a clear correlation between workload and quality of life. Ulas (2012) investigated the effects of day and night shifts on the anxiety of 120 ICU nurses by measuring blood samples before and after shift for total antioxidant status. Interestingly there was no difference in day or night shifts. Her paper was published in 2005 (Carayon & Gurses).

Pemberton and Turpin (2008) carried out an innovative piece of research investigating the effects of aromatherapy on nurses in an ICU. This small pilot study was the first to evaluate the effect of a topical application of the essential oils *Lavandula angustifolia* and *Salvia sclaria* on the work-related stress of 14 nurses in an ICU

TABLE 13-3 *Published Studies on Nursing Stress in the ICU*

Author	Year	Number in Study	Outcome Measures	Country
Mealer et al	2012	27	Connor-Davidson Resilience Scale	USA
Yava et al	2011	152	ICU Environmental Stressor Scale	Turkey
Gurses	2005	300	Quality of Working Life	USA
Ulas et al	2012	120	Oxidative Stress and Anxiety Index	Turkey

setting. Results demonstrated decreased perception of stress level in the intervention group during their three 12-hour worked shifts. I am particularly proud of this study (and the one by Pritchard mentioned above) as they are published studies that were originally done for RJBA certification. Harris Methodist Medical Center, where Pemberton and Pritchard both work, has sponsored six RJBA practitioner courses (250 contact hours) during which more than 100 nurses and doctors have learned clinical aromatherapy. At the time of writing, 28 nurse aromatherapists are on staff. Other RJBA studies have looked at stress in nursing departments such as nurse management and night staff and will be covered in the stress chapter.

Clinical aromatherapy has much to offer ICU patients as it reveals the softer, more caring side of a hard, mechanistic world. In a place full of technical equipment, aromatherapy allows patients and nurses a chance to get in touch with their feelings, to trust, and to communicate. Human beings often forget how to "be" as they are programmed to "do." The transition from "*doing*" to "*being*" can be challenging because in ICU patients (and often relatives) are forced to *be*. Aromatherapy allows both patient and nurse to share in the healing process: it enables patients to feel better, as well as get better, and it allows nurses to do something pleasurable for their patients. That is the essence of holistic care. Anxiety, pain, insomnia, and stress are major areas where aromatherapy helps in a ICU. These have been covered in separate chapters, so please refer to the index for more information. The remaining part of this chapter will address other areas in ICU where aromatherapy can be helpful.

EXTUBATION

Extubation is an alarming procedure for a patient who needs to be awake enough to breathe without assistance, but sedated enough not to fight the endotracheal tube. Tremendous trust is needed. Aromatherapy using the 'M' Technique can help produce a deep level of trust in a very short period of time. Just because a patient is intubated does not mean aromatherapy will have no effect. Components within essential oils, such as linalyl acetate, can be absorbed through the skin much as drugs like fentanyl, scopolamine and clonidine. During extubation, fear of oversedation can be a common cause of inadequate pain and anxiety relief. Aromatherapy has no side effects and can actually facilitate extubation by promoting relaxation, decreasing anxiety, relieving pain, and promoting trust between patient and caregiver. After extubation, clearance of secretions can be greatly aided by the skilled use of mucolytic essential oils, such as *Eucalyptus globulus* or *Lavandula latifolia,* which can be inhaled by the patient. Mitchell, an ICU nurse (2002), found the use of the 'M' Technique and essential oils really helped the extubation process.

Mitchell, a nurse in critical care, found 2% *Lavandula angustifolia* given in a hand 'M' Technique calmed a patient before extubation. The patient appeared much calmer and less anxious than during previous attempts at extubation. Afterward the patient said she felt "able to trust" Mitchell and extubation was achieved. I remember doing the hand 'M' Technique with some rose essential oils in the ICU at Columbia Presbyterian Hospital, New York, and watching the O_2 saturations on the monitor go up as the patient relaxed.

Hedayat (2008) reports on an intubated and ventilated child who was restless despite sedation. The mother asked if she could give an aromatherapy massage to her 18-month-old daughter. A 7.5% mixture of Roman chamomile, sandalwood, and galbanum in jojoba oil was massaged on to the child's legs, arms and chest, every 8 hours by the mother. The child's vital signs went from 96 to 166 bpm (beats per minute) before the aromatherapy to 85 to 132 bpm after, and the Midazolam infusion was reduced by 50% within 2 hours.

Henneman et al (2002) suggest a collaborative weaning plan for patients requiring prolonged mechanical ventilation, which draws on a multidisciplinary team. Aromatherapy, using gentle touch, or just aroma, can be carried out by any member of the team.

Adding three or four drops of essential oils to a moistened face flannel can greatly improve the mood of patients (and nursing staff). Geranium, sweet orange, or mandarin are excellent choices as they can lift depression, reduce anxiety and can hide some of unpleasant odors that are found in the ICU. For an antiseptic sponge bath, use one of the essential oils in Table 13-2 and add geranium, lavender or mandarin to enhance the smell. Spritzing the room with a solution of *Eucalyptus citriadora, Ravansara aromatica* or *Citrus limon* will do much to improve the ambience as well as helping to cut down cross-infection and resistant organisms. Please see Table 13-2 for other essential oils to use. There is no reason why ICUs should not smell welcoming and pleasant, as well as being places where resistant pathogens are no longer welcome.

REFERENCES

Almerud S, Alapack RJ, Fridlund B, Ekebergh M. 2008. Beleaguered by technology: care in technologically intense environments. *Nurs Philos.* 9(1):55–61.

Ashworth P. 1984. Staff-patient communication in coronary care units. *J Adv Nurs.* 9(1) 35–42.

Balaji V, Jeremiah S, Baliga P. 2011. Polymyzins: antimicrobial susceptibility concerns and therapeutic options. *Indian J Med Microbiol.* 29(3):230–42.

Bobo J, Dubberke E, Kollef M. 2011. Clostridium difficile in the ICU: the struggle continues. *Chest.* 140(6):1643–53.

Borer A, Gilad J, Porat N, Megrelesvilli R, Saidel-Odes L et al. 2007. Impact of 4% chlorhexidine whole-body washing on multidrug-resistant Acinetobacter baumannii skin colonisation among patients in a medical intensive care unit. *J Hosp Infect.* 67(2):149–55.

Boucher H, Talbot G, Bradley J, Edwards J, Gilbert D. 2009. Bad bugs. No drugs. No ESKAPE. An update from the infectious Disease Society of America. *Clin Infect Dis.* 48(1):1–12.

Buckle J. 1993. Aromatherapy. *Nursing Times.* 89(20): 32–35.

Buckle J. 1998. Clinical aromatherapy and touch: complementary therapies for nursing practice. *Critical Care Nurse.* 18(5): 54–61.

Buckle J. 2013. Aromatherapy in *Holistic Nursing: A Handbook for Practice.* Ed Montgomery Dossey B and Keegan L. 6th edition. Pub Jones & Bartlett Burlington MA. 563–581.

Caelli M, Porteous J, Carson C, Heller R, Riley T. 2000. Teatree oil as an alternative topical decolonization agent or MRSA. *Journal of Hospital Infection.* 46(3): 236–237.

Carayon P, Gurses A. 2005. A human factors engineering conceptual framework of nursing workload and patient safety in intensive care units. *Intensive Crit Care Nurs.* 21(5):284–301.

Chan J, Valencia P, Zhang L, Langer R, Farokhzad O. 2010. Polymeric nanoparticles for drug delivery. *Methods Mol Biol.* 624:163–75.

Chao S, Young G, Oberg C, Nakaoka K. 2008. Inhibition of methicillin-resistant Staphylococcus aureus (MRSA) by essential oils. *Flavour and Fragrance Journal.* 23(6):444–449.

Chmielarczyk A, Higgins PG, Wojkowska-Mach J, Synowiec E, Zander E et al. 2012. Control of an outbreak of Acinetobacter baumannii infections using vaporized hydrogen peroxide. *J Hosp Infect.* 81(4):239–45.

Cho M-Y, Min E, Hur M-H. 2013. Effects of aromatherapy on the anxiety, vital signs and sleep quality of percutaneous coronary intervention patients in Intensive Care Units. *Evidence-Based Complementary and Alternative Medicine.* Article ID 381381, 6 pp http://dx.doi.org/10.1155/2013/381381. Accessed 18 March 2013.

Climo M, Sepkowitz K, Zuccotti G, Fraser V, Warren D et al. 2009. The effect of daily bathing with chlorhexidine on the acquisition of methicillin-resistant Staphylococcus aureus, vancomycin-resistant Enterococcus, and healthcare-associated bloodstream infections: results of a quasi-experimental multicenter trial. *Crit Care Med.* 37(6):1858.

Cornock M. 1998. Stress and the Intensive Care patient: perceptions of nurses and patients. *J Adv Nursing.* 27(3):518–27.

Dodek P, Norena M, Ayas N, Romney M, Wong H. 2013. Length of stay and mortality due to Clostridium difficile infection acquired in the intensive care unit. *J Crit Care.* Jan 18. doi:pii: S0883-9441(12)00475-3. 10.1016/j.jcrc.2012.11.008. [Epub ahead of print]

Doran A, Morden W, Dunn K, Edwards-Jones V. 2009. Vapour-phase activities of essential oils against antibiotic sensitive and resistant bacteria including MRSA. *Letters in Applied Microbiology.* 48(4): 387–392.

Duarte A, Ferreira S, Silva F, Domingues F. 2012. Synergistic activity of coriander oil and conventional antibiotics against Acinetobacter baumannii. *Phytomedicine.* 19(3-4): 236–8.

Dunn C, Sleep J, Collett D. 1995. Sensing an improvement: an experimental study to evaluate the use of aromatherapy, massage and periods of rest in an intensive care unit. *Journal of Advanced Nursing.* 21(1):34–40.

Dryden M, Dailly S, Crouch M. 2004. A randomised, controlled trial of tea tree topical preparations versus a standard topical regimen for the clearance of MRSA colonisation. *J Hospital Infection.* 56(4):283–286.

Erbay H, Yalcin A, Serin S, Turgut H, Tomatir E et al. 2003. Nosocomial infections in intensive care unit in a Turkish university hospital: a 2-year survey. *Intensive Care Med.* 29(9):1482–8.

Fadli M, Saad A, Savadi S, Chavakuer J, Mezrioui N, Pages J, Hassani L. 2012. Antibacterial activity of *Thymus maroccanus* and *Thymus broussonetii* essential oils against nosocomial infection - bacteria and their synergistic potential with antibiotics. *Phytomedicine.* 19(5):464–71.

Flaaten. 2010. Mental and physical disorders after ICU discharge. *Curr Opin Crit Care.* 16(5):510–5.

Hamoud R, Sporer F, Reichling J, Wink M. 2012. Antimicrobial activity of a traditionally used complex essential oil distillate (Olbas(®) Tropfen) in comparison to its individual essential oil ingredients. *Phytomedicine.*19(11):969–76.

Hedayat K. 2008. Essential oil diffusion for the treatment of persistent oxygen dependence in a three-year-old child with restrictive lung disease with respiratory syncytial virus pneumonia. *Explore (NY).* 4(4):264-6.

Henneman E, Dracup K, Ganz T et al. 2002. Using a collaborative weaning plan to decrease duration of mechanical ventilation and length of stay in the intensive care unit for patients receiving long-term ventilation. *American Journal of Critical Care.* 11(2):132–140.

Henricson M, Segesten K, Berglund AL, Määttä S. 2009. Enjoying tactile touch and gaining hope when being cared for in intensive care—a phenomenological hermeneutical study. *Intensive Crit Care Nurs.* 25(6):323–31.

Heo ST, Oh WS, Kim SJ, Bae IG, Ko KS, Lee JC. 2011. Clinical impacts of a single clone (sequence type 92) of multidrug-resistant Acinetobacter baumannii in intensive care units. *Microb Drug Resist.* 17(4):559–62.

Hills M, Watson J. 2011. *Creating a caring science curriculum: An Emancipatory pedagogy for nursing.* Springer Publishing: New York, USA.

Honda H, Krauss M, Coopersmith C, Kollef M, Richmond A et al. 2010. Staphyloccus aureus nasal colonization and subsequent infection in intensive care unit patients: does methicillin resistance matter? *Infect Control & Hosp Epidemiol.* 31(6):584–91.

Hosseini Jazani N, Zartoshti M, Shahabi S. 2008. Antibacterial effects of Iranian Cuminum cyminum essential oil on burn isolates of Pseudomonas aeruginosa. *International Journa of Pharmacology.* 4(2):157–159.

Hsieh M-H. 2011. The Impact of using aromatherapy for ICU Patients. Sigma Theta Tau International Honor Society of Nursing 41st Biennial Convention. Accessed. 18 March 2013. https://stti.confex.com/stti/bc41/webprogram/Paper48895.html.

Ingham A. 1989. A review of the literature relating to touch and its use in intensive care. *Intensive Care Nurse.* 5(2) 65–75.

Januel J, Harbarth S, Allard R, Voirin N, Lepape A et al. 2010. Estimating attributable mortality due to nosocomial infections acquired in intensive care units. *Inf Control & Hosp Edipemiology.* 31(4):388–94.

Jazani N, Zartoshti M, Babazadeh H, Ali-Daiee N. Zarrin S, Hosseini S. 2009. Antibacterial effects of Iranian fennel essential oil on isolates of Acinetobacter baumannii. *Pakistan Journal of Biological Sciences.* 12(9):738–741.

Kallel H, Dammak H, Bahloul M, Ksibi H, Chelly H et al. 2010. Risk factors and outcomes of intensive care unit-acquired infections in a Tunisian ICU. *Medical Science Monitor.* 16(8):PH69–75.

Kaye K, Marchaim D, Smialowicz C, Bentley L. 2010. Suction regulators: a potential vector for hospital-acquired pathogens. *Infect Control Hosp Epidemiol.* 31(7):772–4.

Kollef. 2008. SMART Approaches for reducing nosocomial infections in the ICU. *CHEST.* 134(2):447–456.

Kon K, Rai M. 2012. Plant essential oils and their constituents in coping with multidrug-resistant bacteria. *Expert Review of Anti-infective Therapy,* 10(7):775–790.

Kong B, Hanifah Y, Yusef M, Thong K. 2011. Antimicrobial susceptibility profiling and genomic diversity of multidrug-resistant Acinetobacter baumannii isolates from a teaching hospital in Malaysia. *Jpn J Infect Dis.* 64(4):337–40.

Kristiniak S, Harpel J, Breckenridge D, Buckle J. 2012. Black pepper essential oil to enhance intravenous catheter insertion in patients with poor vein visibility: a controlled study. *J Alt & Complemen Med.* 18(11):1003–7.

Landelle C, Legrand P, Lesprit P, Cizeau F, Ducellier D et al. 2013. Protracted outbreak of multidrug-resistant Acinetobacter baumannii after intercontinental transfer of colonized patients. *Inf Control Hosp Epidemiol.* 34(2):119–124.

Langeveld W, Veldhuizen E, Burt S. 2013. Synergy between essential oil components and antibiotics: a review. *Crit Rev Microbiol.* 2013 Feb 28. [Epub ahead of print] PMID: 23445470. Accessed 15 March 2013.

Luqman S, Dwivedi G, Daroker M, Kaira Khanuja S. 2007. Potential of rosemary oil to be used for drug-resistant infections. *Alt Ther Health & Med.* 13(5):54–9.

Lusk B. 2005. The Stress Response. Psychoneuroimmunology and stress among ICU patients. *Dimensions of Critical Care Nursing.* 24(1):25–31.

Lysakowska M, Denys A, Sienkiewicz M. 2011. The activity of thyme essential oil against Acinetobacter spp. *Central European Journal of Biology.* 6(3):405–413.

McMahon M, Blair I, Moore J, McDowell D. 2007. Habituation to sub-lethal concentrations of tea tree oil (*Melalueca alternifolia*) is associated with reduced susceptibility to antibiotics in human pathogens. *J Antimicrobial Chemotherapy.* 59(1): 125–127.

Mealer M, Jones J, Moss M. 2012. A qualitative study of resilience and post traumatic stress disorder in United States ICU nurses. *Intensive Care Medicine.* 38(9):1445–51.

Meric M, Wilke A, Caglavan C, Toker K. 2005. Intensive care unit-acquired infections: incidence, risk factors and associated mortality in a Turkish university hospital. *Jpn J Infect Dis.* 58(5):297–302.

Mitchell L. 2002. Personal communication.

Mnatzaganian G, Galai N, Sprung C, Zitser-Gurevich Y, Mandel M et al. 2005. Increased risk of bloodstream and urinary infections in intensive care unit patients compared with patients fitting ICU admission criteria treated in regular wards. *J Hosp Infect.* 59(4):331–342.

Moeini M, Khadibi M, Bekhradi R, Mahmoudian S, Nazari F. 2010. Effect of aromatherapy on the quality of sleep in ischemic heart disease patients hospitalized in intensive care units of heart hospitals of the Isfahan University of Medical Sciences. *Iran J Nurs Midwifery Res.* 15(4):234–239.

MHRA. 2012. Medical Device Alert: All medical devices and medicinal products containing chlorhexidine (MDA/2012/075). http://www.mhra.gov.uk/Publications/Safetywarnings/MedicalDeviceAlerts/CON197918. Accessed March 20, 2013.

Munoz-Price LS, Hota B, Stemer A, Weinstein RA. 2009. Prevention of bloodstream infections by use of daily chlorhexidine baths for patients at a long-term acute care hospital. *Infect Control Hosp Epidemiol.* 30(11):1031–5.

Nagy G, Várvölgyi C, Paragh G. 2012. Successful treatment of life-threatening, treatment resistant Clostridium difficile infection associated pseudomembranous colitis with faecal transplantation. *Orv Hetil.* 153(52):2077–83.

Nah SS, Park YH, Chung JW, Yoo S, Hong SB et al. 2013. Acinetobacter baumannii infection was decreased by the structural renovation of a medical intensive care unit. *J Crit Care.* 2013 Feb 18. doi:pii: S0883-9441(13)00005-1. 10.1016/j.jcrc.2012.12.013. [Epub ahead of print]. Accessed 15 March 2013.

Nedorostova L, Kloucek P, Urbanova K, Kokoska L, Smid J. 2011. Antibacterial effect of essential oil vapours against different strains of Staphylococcus aureus, including MRSA. *Flavour and Fragrance Journal.* 26(6):403–407.

Neuhauser M, Weinstein R, Rydman R, Danziger L, Karam G, Quinn J. 2003. Antibiotic resistance among gram-negative bacilli in US intensive care units: implications for fluoroquinolone use. *JAMA.* 289(7):885–8.

O'Lynn C, Krautscheid L. 2011. How Should I Touch You? A Qualitative Study of Attitudes on Intimate Touch in Nursing Care. *American J Nursing.* 11(3):24–31.

Opalchenova G, Obreshkova D. 2003. Comparative studies on the activity of basil—an essential oil from *Ocimum basilicum L.* – against multidrug resistant clinical isolates of the genera Staphylococcus, Enterococcus and Pseudomonas by using different test methods. *Journal of Microbiological Methods.* 54(1):105–110.

Owlia P, Saderi H, Rasooli I, Sefidkon F. 2009. Antimicrobial characteristics of some herbal oils on *Pseudomonas aeruginosa* with special reference to their chemical compositions. *Iranian Journal of Pharmaceutical Research.* 8(2):107–114.

Pemberton E, Turpin P. 2008. The effect of essential oils on work-related stress in intensive care unit nurses. *Holist Nurs Pract.* 22(2):97–102.

Pritchard C. 2012. Aromatherapy intervention to reduce the anxiety and depression levels of family members and friends of patients with traumatic injury in an ICU. RJBA unpublished dissertation.

Rickerby K, Cordell B. 2012. Application of the M Technique to 2 severely disabled children in Belarus. *Int J Palliative Nursing.* 18(7):355–359.

Roberts K, Campbell H. 2011. Using the M Technique as therapy for patients at the end of life: two case-studies. *Int J Palliative Nursing.* 17(3):114–118.

Roller S, Ernest N, Buckle J. 2009. The antimicrobial activity of high-necrodane and other lavender oils on methicillin-sensitive and -resistant Staphylococcus aureus (MSSA and MRSA). *Journal of Alternative and Complementary Medicine.* 15(3): 275–279.

Rosato A, Vitali C, De Laurentis N, Armenise A, Milillo M, 2007. Antibacterial effect of some essential oils administered alone or in combination with norfloxacin. *Phytomedicine.* 14, 727–732.

Rosato A. Vitali C, Gallo D, Balenrano L, Mallamaci R. 2008. The inhibition of Candida albicans by selected essential oils and their synergim with amphotericin B. *Phytomedicine.* 15, 635–638.

Rosato A, Vitali C, Piarulli M, Mazzotta M, Argentieri M, Mallamaci R. 2009. In vitro synergic efficacy of the combination of nystatin with the essential oils of *Origanum vulgare* and *Pelargonium graveolens* against some Candida species. *Phytomedicine.* 16, 972–975.

Rosenthal V, Maki D, Salomao R, Moreno C, Mehta Y et al. 2006. Device-associated nosocomial infections in 55 intensive care units of 8 developing countries. *Ann Intern Med.* 145(8):582–91.

Saad A, Fadli M, Bouaziz M, Benharref A, Mezrioui N, Hassani L. 2010. Anticandida activity of the essential oils of *Thymus maroccanus* and *Thymus broussonetii* and their synergism with amphtericin B and fluconazol. *Phytomedicine.* 17(13):1057–1060.

Safdar N, Crnich C, Maki D. 2005. The pathogenesis of ventilator-associated pneumonia: its relevance to developing effective strategies for prevention. *Respir Care.* 50:725-739; discussion 739–741.

Schmock B, Breckenridge D, Benedict K. 2009. Effect of sacred space environment on surgical patient outcomes: a pilot study. *Int J Human Caring.* 13(1):49–59.

Shin S, Kim J. 2005. In vitro inhibitory activities of essential oils from two Korean Thymus species against antibiotic-resistant pathogens. *Arch Pharmacol Res.* 28:897–901.

Sienkiewicz M, Kowalczyk E, Wasiela M. 2012. Recent patents regarding essential oils and the significance of their constituents in human health and treatment. *Recent Pat Antiinfect Drug Discov.* 7(2):133–40.

Silva N, Alves S, Gonçalves A, Amaral J, Poeta P. 2013. Antimicrobial activity of essential oils from mediterranean aromatic plants against several foodborne and spoilage bacteria. *Food Sci Technol Int.* 2013 Feb 26. [Epub ahead of print]. Accessed 15 March 2013.

Sivathasan N, Vijayarajan L. 2010. Chlorhexidine's complications. *Journal of perioperative practice.* 20(8):300–1.

Sivathasan N, Goodfellow P. 2011. Skin Cleansers: The Risks of Chlorhexidine. *The Journal of Clinical Pharmacology.* 51(5):785–6.

Starnes M, Brown C, Morales I, Hadjizacharia P, Salim A. 2008. Evolving pathogens in the surgical intensive care unit: A 6-year experience. *Journal of Critical Care.* 23(4):507–512.

Stevensen C. 1994. The psychophysical effects of aromatherapy massage following cardiac surgery. *Complementary Therapies in Medicine.* 2(1):27–35.

Tohidpour A, Sattari M, Omidbaigi R, Yadegar A, Nazemi J. 2010. Antibacterial effect of essential oils from two medicinal plants against Methicillin-resistant Staphylococcus aureus (MRSA). *Phytomedicine.* 17(2):142–145.

Trouillet J, Vuagnat A, Combes A, Kassis N, Chastre J, Gilbert C. 2002. Pseudomonas aeruginosa ventilator-assisted pneumonia: comparison of episodes due to piperacillin-resistnat versus piperacillin-susceptible organisms. *Clin Infect Dis.* 34(8):1047–54.

Tyagi A, Malik A. 2010. Antimicrobial action of essential oil vapours and negative air ions against Pseudomonas fluorescens. *International Journal of Food Microbiology.* 143(3):205–210.

Ungaro F, d'Angelo I, Coletta C, d'Emmanuele di Villa Bianca R, Sorrentino R et al. 2012. Dry powders based on PLGA nanoparticles for pulmonary delivery of antibiotics: Modulation of encapsulation efficiency, release rate and lung deposition pattern by hydrophyilic polymers. *Journal of Controlled Release,* 157(1):149–159.

Urden L. 1997. From the patient's eyes. *Critical Care Nurse.* 17(1):104–105.

Ulas T, Buyukhatipoglu H, Kirhan I, Dal M, Eren M et al. 2012. The effect of day and night shifts on oxidative stress and anxiety of nurses. *Eur Rev Med Pharmacol Sci.*16(5):594–9.

Végh A, Bencsik T, Molnár P, Böszörményi A, Lemberkovics E et al. 1012. Composition and antip-seudomonal effect of essential oils isolated from different lavender species. *Nat Prod Commun.* 7(10):1393–6.

Vincent J, Rello J, Marshall J, Silva E, Anzueto A et al. 2009. International study of the prevalence and outcomes of infection in intensive care units. *JAMA.* 302(21):2323–9.

Waldman C, Tseng P, Meulman P, et al. 1993. Aromatherapy in the intensive care unit. *Care of the Critically Ill.* 9(4):170–174.

Weinstein R, Bonten M. 2005. Controlling antibiotic-resistant bacteria: what's an intensivist to do? *Crit Care Med.* 33(10):2446–2447.

Welsh C. 1997. Tissue viability. Touch with oils: a pertinent part of holistic hospice care. *American Journal of Hospital Palliative Care.* 14(1):42–44.

Woolfson A, Hewitt D. 1992. Intensive aromacare. International Journal of Aromatherapy. 4(2):12–13.

Yamakawa K, Tasaki O, Fukuyama M, Kitayama J, Matsuda H. 2011. Assessment of risk factors related to healthcare-associated methicillin-resistant Staphylococcus aureus infection at patient admission to an intensive care unit in Japan. *BMC Infect Dis.* Nov 1;11:303. doi: 10.1186/1471-2334-11-303. Accessed 16 March 2013.

Yava A, Tosun N, Ünver V, Çiçek H. 2010. Patient and nurse perceptions of stressors in the intensive care unit. *Stress and Health.* 27:e36–e47.

Chapter 14

Dermatology

In the castle of my skin.

George Lamming, 1942

CHAPTER ASSETS

Increasingly, transdermal therapeutic systems (TTS) are used as an alternative to oral and parenteral pharmaceuticals. The skin, and therefore the care of skin (dermatology), has become an important part of new drug delivery (Aggarwal & Aggarwal 2010). Some essential oils and the isolated components from essential oils (such as nerolidol, limonene, cineole, pinene, and carvone) are used to enhance drug delivery (Krishnaiah et al 2006; Krishnaiah et al 2008; Ahad et al 2011; Buckle 2010; Valgimigli et al 2012; Shen et al 2013). Essential oil components appear to enhance drug absorption by interacting with the polar domain of the skin lipids (Chen et al 2013). Some components, like carvone, can also reverse the permeation enhancement effect, so that vital skin barrier function is restored and not permanently changed after the application of dermal enhancers (Kang et al 2007; Aggarwal et al 2012). Some components enhance the permeation of other components: limonene enhances absorption of citronellol and eugenol (Schmitt et al 2009).

The skin is the largest organ of the body. It is also a stress barometer that provides the outside world with an indication of the serenity or confusion within. Much of dermatology is concerned with putting topical drugs onto the skin. However, skin problems may be linked to stress and diet (Chida et al 2007; Ro et al 2002). Possibly three of the most common skin conditions suitable for aromatherapy are acne, herpes, and onychomycosis. With the increased drive for perpetual youth, wrinkles seem a relevant issue to touch on in this chapter.

ACNE

Acne vulgaris is a common dermatologic disorder that affects adolescents (more boys than girls), but can occur at any age. Female acne is becoming more and more common between the ages of 40 and 50 (Preneau & Dreno 2012). Approximately 45 million people in the United States have acne (Decker & Graber 2012). However, acne is common in many countries such as China (Shen 2012), Africa (Yahya 2009), India (Nikaliji et al 2012), and the United Kingdom (Ozolins et al 2005).

According to the medical dictionary (Brooker 2008 p 4), the "pilosebaceous units are overstimulated by circulating androgens and the excessive sebum is trapped by a plug of keratin. Acne is one of the top three reasons why people seek a dermatologist (Decker & Graber 2012). Current conventional treatments include systemic antibiotics, creams containing antibiotics such as clindamycin phosphate and benzoyl peroxide, or laser to destroy the bacteria. In a study of 649 people aged 12 to 39, topical antimicrobial therapies performed at least as well as oral antibiotics in terms of clinical efficacy. Benzoyl peroxide was the most cost-effective and minocycline the least cost-effective therapy for facial acne (Ozolins et al 2005). A 2012 Cochrane systemic review decided that minocycline **was** an effective treatment for moderate severely acne vulgaris, but concluded there was no evidence it was better than any other commonly used acne treatments (Garner et al 2012).

Due to convenience, lower cost, and difficulty getting an appointment with a dermatologist, the use of over-the-counter (OTC) acne treatments is increasing (Decker & Graber 2012) and many people use both prescriptive and OTC medicines. There are five different kinds of OTC acne therapies: 1) cleansers, 2) leave-on products, 3) mechanical treatments, 4) essential oils and 5) vitamins (this includes retinol obtained from vitamin A) (Kligman & Gans 2000).

Acne is graded into four levels of severity: mild, moderate, severe and very severe (Katsambas et al 2004). Mild acne usually includes comedones with a few mild pustules. Moderate acne includes many comedones and pustules with a few small nodules but no scarring. In severe acne there are many pustules and nodules with marked inflammation and scarring. In very severe acne there are also sinus tracts with many deeply located nodules. *Propionibacterium acnes* is the main bacterium cited in acne vulgaris and many in vitro studies look at kill times against this bacteria (Viyoch et al 2006, Fu et al 2007, Lerysatitthanakorn et al 2010). Some studies such as Gavini et al (2005) have investigated how to encapsulate an essential oil (in this case juniper) inside a solid lipid microparticle (SLM) for longevity. However, propionbacterium is a commensal that lives happily just below the surface of the skin and keeps it healthy. It is only when the sebaceous glands become overactive that the pores can become blocked and cause propionbacterium to multiply. Therefore, for essential oils to be effective against acne, they need to have antiseptic,

TABLE 14-1 *Published Research on Essential Oils and Acne*

Author	Year	Number	Essential Oil	Condition
Gavini et al	2005	In vitro	Juniper	Acne
Lertsatitthanakorn	2006	In vitro	Lemongrass	Acne
Viyoch et al	2006	In vitro	Basil	Acne
Fu et al	2007	In vitro	Rosemary	Acne
Kim et al	2008	In vitro	Geumgamja Cheonyahagyul	Acne
Oh et al	2009	In vitro	*Thymus quinquecostatus*	Acne
Wylde	2009	Review	Grapefruit	Acne
Lertsatithanakorn et al	2010	In vitro	Citronella	Acne
Matiz et al	2012	28	Sweet orange Sweet basil	Acne
Azimi et al	2012	Review	Several	Acne
da Silva et al	2012	10	Copaiba	Acne

antibacterial, antiinflammatory, citratrisant, keratolytic, and antiscarring properties. (Keratolytic agents help remove the hardened comedone.)

Many of the 11 studies listed in Table 14-1 are in vitro studies. Although an in vitro study is a good starting point, it does not mean the essential oil (or component) will be effective (or that someone will want to use it) in a human study. What is encouraging is the range of essential oils that have been tested. Of the human studies, Matiz et al (2012) is worth mentioning. This was a controlled study on 28 volunteers with acne. Treatment was applied daily for 8 weeks. The essential oils used were sweet orange *(Citrus sinensis)* and sweet basil *(Ocimum basilicum)*. There was a 43% to 75% in reduction of lesions. This was thought to be a result of their joint antiseptic and keratolytic activity. Side effects (burning and redness) disappeared within a few minutes of applying the essential oils.

In another placebo-controlled study, a lesser-known essential oil (copaiba) from Brazil was applied twice a day for 21 days in 1% gel to 10 volunteers with acne (da Silva et al 2012). The placebo gel was applied similarly to other areas with acne, so each volunteer acted as his or her own control. There was a significant reduction in acne ($P = 0.0001$) where copaiba was applied. Copaiba is a resin from the diesel tree *(Copaifera langsdorffii)*. It is high in sesquiterpenes such as B caryophyllene and bisabolene, and in diterpenes. Sesquiterpenes are traditionally thought to be antiinflammatory. The gels were weighed before and after the study to ensure compliance.

Minaglou (2006) gives an extremely helpful and informative overview of his experience of treating acne with essential oils. This scholarly article is interesting reading for anyone interested in this condition. The principles of Minaglou's treatment are:

1) Use of keratolytic agents to help remove comedone plug
2) Antibacterial essential oils

3) Reduction and control of excessive sebum
4) Antiinflammatory essential oils
5) Tissue support for regeneration (antioxidant essential oils)

ATHLETE'S FOOT AND ONYCHOMYCOSIS

Athlete's foot *(tinea pedis)* is the most common form of superficial dermatophyte infection in the developed world and infects approximately 70% of adults (Pau et al 2010, Peréz-González 2009, Watanabe 2010). It is more common in adults aged 15 to 40 years and in men rather than women (Skerlev & Miklic 2010). Onychomycosis (sometimes called *tinea unguium*) is a fungal infection that destroys the entire nail unit. It is a cousin of *tinea pedis*, which causes athlete's foot (fungal infection between the toes). Onychomycosis is less contagious than athlete's foot, but when contracted, it is extremely difficult to remove completely (Walling et al 2009). Symptoms are a thickened nail that becomes discolored, brittle, or chalky and ultimately disintegrates. Medical treatment is topical or systemic antifungals (Table 14-2).

Tinea pedis can be treated with topical or systemic prescription drugs such as griseofulvin, itraconazole, ketoconazole and terbinafine, however, these carry the possibility of adverse reactions such as diarrhea. There are many OTC treatments available in creams, powders, and gels. Unfortunately, many toenail infections and athlete's foot infections recur. It is worth trying antifungal essential oils. The added bonus is that are most are safe to use topically on children under 12 years, unlike some OTC products.

Buck et al (1994) carried out one of the earliest multicentered, double-blind, randomized and controlled studies on onychomycosis that compared *Melaleuca alternifolia* (tea tree) to clotrimazole. One-hundred seventeen patients with onychomycosis under the toenail (proven by culture) took part in the study. Patients received either twice-daily applications of clotrimazole solution or 100% tea tree. Debridement took place at 0, 1, 3, and 6 months. Topical use of tea tree produced a similar result to oral doses of clotrimazole, with 55% of the clotrimazole group and 56% of the tea tree group reporting improvement or resolution after 3 months. The number of adverse reactions was similar: three out of 53 for the clotrimazole group and five out of 64 in the tea tree group.

Four years later, Syed et al (1999) carried out a randomized, double-blind, placebo-controlled study to examine the clinical efficacy and tolerability of 5% *Melaleuca alternifolia* with 2% butenafine hydrochloride incorporated in a cream. Sixty patients took part in the study. There were 39 men and 21 women, and the average age was 29 years. Each participant had a history of onychomycosis for 6 to 36 months. After using the cream for 16 weeks, 80% of the participants in the experimental group were cured. No participant was cured in the placebo group. Four participants in the experimental group experienced mild inflammation but did not discontinue treatment. During follow-up, no relapse occurred in the cured patients, and no improvement was seen in the medication-resistant and placebo participants.

TABLE 14-2 *Published Studies on Athlete's Foot/Toenail Fungus*

Author	Year	Number	Essential Oil	Condition
Buck et al	1994	117	Tea tree	Onychomycosis
Syed et al	1999	60	Tea tree	Onychomycosis
Gayoso et al	2005	In vitro	*Eugenia cariophyllata* 1%, 4%	Onychomycosis
Satchell et al	2002	158	Tea tree 25%, 50%	Tinea pedis
Inouye et al	2001	In vitro vapor	Cinnamon Citron Lemongrass Thyme Perilla Lavender Tea tree	*Trichophyton mentagrophytes*
Inouye et al	2006	In vitro vapor	Oregano Perilla Tea tree Lavender Clove Geranium	*Trichophyton mentagrophytes*
Inouye et al	2007	In vitro using salt bath	Oregano Thyme Cinnamon Lemongrass Clove Palma rosa Peppermint Lavender Geranium Tea tree	*Trichophyton mentagrophytes*

Satchell et al (2002) conducted a randomized, placebo-controlled study on 158 patients with interdigital athlete's foot *(tinea pedis)* using 25% and 50% tea tree essential oil. Patients applied tea tree twice a day to the affected areas for 4 weeks and were reviewed after 2 and 4 weeks of treatment. There was a marked clinical response seen in 68% of the 50% tea tree oil group and 72% of the 25% tea tree oil group, compared to 39% in the placebo group. Interestingly, the lower percentage appeared to be more successful. However, the mycological cure rate was 64% in the 50% tea tree oil group, compared to 31% in the placebo group.

An RJBA student, Elsethager (2000), investigated the combined effect of two essential oils (lemongrass and tea tree) on 12 study participants who had onychomycosis for a minimum duration of 1 year. One participant had it for more than 10 years. Participants rubbed a mixture of 2% tea tree and 3% lemongrass in grapeseed

oil into the affected nail bed twice a day for 2 months. Only four people continued treatment for the whole 2 months. All participants said their nails were less
discolored and cracked. Two of the four had previously used OTC medications
(Tinactin and Dr. Scholl's) with no success. One of the four participants had been
offered an oral course of griseofulvin, which she had declined because she was concerned about the side effects. Garg and Dengre (1988) found *Cymbopogon citratus*
(West Indian lemongrass) effective against *Trichophyton mentagrophytes*. The most
active component of lemongrass was citral (70% to 80%), which is thought to be
responsible for the antifungal activity of this plant. *Lippia alba,* which grows widely
in Central and South America, also has strong antifungal activity against *Trichophyton mentagrophyes* var. *interdigitale.* Several chemotypes of the plant exist, and
the essential oil from the plant grown in Aruba is thought to be most suitable as it
contains 64% citral (Fun & Svendsen 1990).

Even at the low concentrations, several essential oils can show very significant
antimycotic activity against *Trichophyton mentagrophytes* (Rai & Mares 2003). Sahi
et al (1999) compared *Eucalyptus citriadora* with commercial antifungal drugs and
found minimal concentration of the oil completely inhibited all the tested pathogens
(*Microsporum nanum, Trichophyton mentagrophytes,* and *Trichophyton rubrum*).
Eucalyptus citriadora contains up to 80% citronellal—an aldehyde. Romagna et al
(1994) reported the antifungal effects of alpha-terthienyl from *Tagetes patula* on
five dermatophytes. Rai and Acharya (1999) found *Tagetes erecta, T. patula,* and
Eupatorium triplinerve to be an effective topical antimycotic.

A Japanese research team led by Professor Inouye conducted several studies.
The 2001 study explored the effects of essential oil vapor in a closed airtight box
and found that citron oil *(Citron medica)* showed the greatest Minimum Inhibitory Dose (MID) and interestingly it was 320 times greater than cinnamon bark
essential oil. The citron fruit is different to the lemon and comprises mainly a very
thick, white rind. Lemongrass, thyme, and perilla essential oils killed the fungus and
prevented germination at lower concentrations in the air than lavender. Thyme and
perilla essential oil vapors were also effective in vivo (in guinea pigs infected with
T. mentagrophytes).

Five years later Inouye et al (2006) published a study using other essential oils—
again in a closed airtight box. This time oregano, perilla, tea tree, clove, lavender, and
geranium were tested against *Trichophyton mentagrophytes*. The results were interesting as tea tree was the least effective of the essential oils. Although the vapor of the
essential oils had a marked effect on the fungus after 3 hours, it needed 15 hours of
exposure before irreversible damage was done. A year later, Inouye et al (2007) published their work on 11 essential oils in a heated footbath (with or without added
salt). This was also an in vitro study. Agar blocks implanted with *T. mentagrophytes*
were immersed in 0.1% aqueous agar that contained essential oils at various temperatures for 10 and 20 minutes. The results showed the fungicidal activity of the
11 essential oils in order of effectiveness was oregano, thyme CT thymol, cinnamon
bark, lemongrass, clove, palmarose, peppermint, lavender, geranium, tea tree, and
thyme CT geraniol. Again, tea tree is near the bottom for effectiveness.

Moericke (2005), an RJBA student, conducted a study on 10 participants with toenail fungal infection. She used undiluted tea tree applied to the nail bed and under the nail twice a day for 6 months and found it either removed or very substantially reduced toenail fungal infection. Outcome measures were photographs. Some participants had had toenail fungal infections for 20 years. During this study, participants were asked to fumigate their shoes with tea tree inserted into the shoes (while the shoes were in double plastic bags) overnight to remove spores. Clearly more studies are needed, perhaps using a combination of essential oils and a generous percentage and not forgetting to fumigate the shoes of participants so the spores do not reinfect their feet.

HERPES

Cases of herpes simplex Type 1 (HSV-1) and Type 2 (HSV-2) reached epidemic proportions in the 1980s. Initially, HSV-1 was thought to only affect the mouth (cold sores) and that HSV-2 caused genital herpes. However, now it is recognized that HSV-1 can also cause genital herpes (Wald et al 2006, Garceau et al 2012). Herpes is prevalent worldwide (Leroux-Roels 2013). HSV-2 is one of the most common sexually transmitted infections in the world and the primary cause of genital and neonatal herpes and genital ulcer disease (Center for Disease Control USA 2010). The World Health Organization found that globally 314 million women and 220 million men had HSV-2 (Looker et al 2008). It is possible to have herpes and be asymptomatic, but this does not stop transmission of the virus to another person (Tronstein et al 2011). HSV-2 antibody tests are now commercially available. Attempts to create a vaccine have not yet been successful (Coleman & Shukler 2013).

HSV-1 and HSV-2 infect and replicate in cells at the site of entry. The painful blister(s) reappear, usually in the same area, with agonizing regularity and the patient is infected for life (Schnitzler et al 2008). Outbreaks can be triggered by sexual activity, stress, heat, hormonal changes (so attacks are often linked to the menstrual cycle), diet, and low immunity. The blisters can occur in the genital area (either internally or externally) and may also be found on the thighs and buttocks. Extremely contagious at the blister stage, herpes can remain dormant for months or years in the spinal cord, ready to migrate down the sensory nerves to the skin.

Orthodox treatment for herpes is with nucleoside analogues, such as acyclovir (ACV) and penciclovir (PCV) with their respective prodrugs valaciclovir and famciclovir that introduce intracellular impediment to viral replication (Vadlapudi et al 2013). These medications are taken orally (although they can be given intravenously or topically) and often leave a metal-like after taste. Some HSV drugs are associated with toxicities that limit their use. Though effective, long-term use has led to drug-resistant viral isolates (Andrei et al 2013).

Essential oils found effective against herpes in research are shown in Table 14-3. Fifteen published studies used essential oils on HSV-1 and seven on HSV-2. They were all in vitro. Some of the studies looked at both HSV-1 and HSV-2. Fourteen

TABLE 14-3 *Published Studies on Essential Oils/Components and Herpes*

Author	Year	Number	Essential Oil	Herpes Type
Zolfaghari et al	1997	80	Myrtle 10%	HSV-1
Armaka et al	1999	In vitro	Isoborneol	HSV-1
Benencia & Courreges	2000	In vitro	Eugenol	HSV-1
Schnitzler et al	2001	In vitro	Tea tree Eucalyptus	HSV-1, HSV-2
Minami et al	2003	In vitro	Lemongrass Ravansara	HSV-1
Sinico et al	2005	In vitro	Wormwood: *Artemesia arborenscens*	HSV-1
Tragoolpua & Jatisatienr	2007	In vitro	Clove: *Eugenia caryophyllus*	HSV-1, HSV-2
Saddi et al	2007	In vitro	Tree wormwood: *Artemesia arborescens*	HSV-1, HSV-2
Schnitzler et al	2007	In vitro	Ginger Thyme Hyssop Sandalwood	Acyclovir-resistant HSV-1
Loizzo et al	2008	In vitro	*Cedrus libani*	HSV-1
Koch et al	2008	In vitro	Anise Thyme Hyssop Ginger Chamomile Sandalwood Dwarf pine	HSV-2
Schnitzler et al	2008	In vitro	*Melissa officinalis*	HSV-1, HSV-2
Garozzo et al	2009	In vitro	Tea tree	Not effective HSV-1 or HSV-2
Astani et al	2010	In vitro	Tea tree Eucalyptus Thyme	HSV-1, HSV-2
Astani et al	2011	In vitro	Star anise	HSV-1
Lai et al	2012	In vitro	Thymol Cavacrol	HSV-1
Astani et al	2012	In vitro	*Melissa officinalis*	HSV-1
Orhan et al	2012	In vitro	Peppermint Spearmint Lavender Basil Oregano Marjoram Rosemary Sage	HSV-1, HSV-2

studies found certain essential oils were very successful against HSV-1. Interestingly, Garozzo et al (2009) found the major components in tea tree were not effective when used on their own, and the whole essential oil was only slightly effective (0.125%v/v). However, a German study (Astani et al 2010) found the major components of tea tree (and the whole essential oil) reduced viral infectivity of HSV-1 by >80% and >96% respectively. This agrees with a previous German study (Schnitzler et al 2001). Astani found essential oils of eucalyptus, tea tree and thyme (as well as their major monoterpene compounds: alpha-terpinene, gamma-terpinene, alpha-pinene, p-cymene, terpinen-4-ol, alpha-terpineol, thymol, citral and 1,8-cineole) were able to reduce viral infectivity. Aastani also states that mixtures of different components present in natural tea tree showed a 10 times higher selectivity index and lower toxicity than isolated components. Clearly, synergy plays a key role in aromatherapy and will be discussed more in the chapter on evolutionary pharmacology.

20 years ago, Wolbling and Leonhardt (1994) conducted a randomized, controlled, multicentered study on 115 patients and found the aqueous extract of *Melissa* was effective in treating herpes. On the final day (fifth day) of treatment, 24 patients in the *Melissa* group were symptom free versus 15 symptom-free patients in the placebo control group. Scabbing and swelling were more reduced in the *Melissa* group, indicating reduced cell damage and accelerated healing. The method of treatment was a proprietary-brand cream (Lomaherpan) that contains 1% *Melissa* extract. The control was an identical cream base without *Melissa*. The site of the herpes treated was the lips in 34 in the *Melissa* group and 33 in the control group and on the genitals in four in the *Melissa* group and six in the control group. A subgroup of 67 patients tested positive for herpes labialis (Type 2, on the lips). The decline of the lesions remained statistically faster in the *Melissa* group than the placebo group.

Five years later, a second study also found 1% *Melissa* aqueous extract effective at treating recurring herpes labialis (Koytchev et al 1999). This was a double-blind, placebo-controlled, randomized trial on 66 patients who had a history of four episodes of herpes labialis per year. The *Melissa* cream was applied four times a day. There was significant reduction in size of affected area and blisters at day two in the *Melissa* group and a rapid ameliorating effect on typical symptoms, reduction in healing time, and prolonged periods between occurrences.

Both these studies used an aqueous extract. This is not the same as an essential oil. I have found essential oil of *Melissa* effective both against HSV-1 and HSV-2. However, because *Melissa* is so expensive (and frequently adulterated with synthetics, lemongrass, or citronella that may have a worsening effect on abraded lesions) it was pertinent to try other essential oils.

It is surprising there is little in the literature on ravansara or ravintsara. I have found both these essential oils have excellent results on HSV-1 and HSV-2. There has been much confusion between the taxonomy of these two essential oils over the last 10 years (Behra 2001, Juliani et al 2005, Juliani et al 2006, Andrianoelisoa et al 2008). However, despite the difference in chemistry, both are excellent for HSV-1 and HSV-2. *Ravansara aromatica* is sometimes confused with *Ravansara anisata*

TABLE 14-4 *Protocol for Using Essential Oils in Treating Herpes*

Symptom	Topical Application	Frequency
Tingling	Undiluted essential oil	Every hour
Redness and swelling	Undiluted essential oil	Every 2 hours
Pustule formation	Undiluted essential oil	Every 2 hours
Broken pustule, raw skin	25% diluted essential oil*	Every 4 hours
Raw skin	5% diluted essential oil	Every 4 hours

*Dilute in a cold-pressed vegetable oil, like sweet almond or olive oil, or in aloe vera gel.

or *Cinnamomum camphora,* ct *cineole* (commonly known as ravintsara). *Ravansara aromatica* and *Ravansara anisata* are essential oils from the same tree: the leaf produces *Ravansara aromatica* and the bark produces *Ravansara anisata.* The only way to be absolutely sure of what you have is to check the smell and the chemistry. *Ravansara aromatica*: leaves contains up to 6% 1,8 cineole and it smells similar to rosemary or eucalyptus, but softer and sweeter. If the essential oil smells like licorice you have *Ravansara anisata*: This contains two phenolic ethers, methyl chavicol (estragole) and anethole that give the licorice smell (Theron et al 1994). Essential oil of ravintsara is obtained from the leaves of *Cinnamomum camphora* and was introduced to Madagascar from Taiwan as an ornamental tree. Ravintsara (*Cinnamomum camphora*) has often been misreported and traded as *Ravansara aromatica* (Juliani et al 2005). It has a strong eucalyptus smell and identification is possible through spectroscopy (Juliani et al 2006) and contains up to 60% cineole.

Twenty years of clinical experience has confirmed that ravansara or ravintsara applied to the area when the tingling begins can actually prevent herpes blisters from forming. And, when the essential oil is applied directly to the blisters, the pain and itching are greatly relieved. Severity, duration, and frequency of herpes outbreaks have decreased substantially with their use. For instance, monthly breakouts have been reduced to once a year. Outbreaks that lasted 10 days have been reduced to 3 days. Severity has gone from an 8 (0 to 10 scale) to a 4. A suggested protocol for application is shown in Table 14-4.

Each person will have his or her own individual response to a particular essential oil, or mix of oils. The reason the essential oils work is because they are lipophyllic and appear to dissolve the lipid capsule (or capsid) of the virus. There are also some excellent aromatherapy products available for herpes that contain a mixture of essential oils such as Oil of Mercy available from http://www.oilofmercy.com.

WRINKLES

In a world obsessed with staying young, the removal or reduction of wrinkles has become part of dermatology. Some RJBA student studies attempted to measure the effects of diluted essential oils on the skin (Tables 14-5 and 14-6). Several used one half of the face as a control. Kunz (2000) used 4% frankincense in evening

TABLE 14-5 *Published Studies on Wrinkles and Essential Oils*

Author	Year	Number	Essential Oil	Condition
Tsukahara et al	2006	Rat/mouse skin	*Zingiber officinalis* (extract)	Wrinkles
Calabrese et al	2000	In vitro	Rosemary	Antiaging
Jung et al	2007	30	*Camellia japonica*	Antiaging
Almada	2004	Patent application	*Commiphora wightii*	Wrinkles
Pedretti et al	2009	15	*Boswellia serrata*	Antiaging

TABLE 14-6 *R.J. Buckle Student Dermatology Studies*

Name	Year	State	Symptom	Number	Essential Oil
May	2000	MA	Acne	6	Helichrysum/angelica
Baker	2001	MN	Acne	10	Tea tree
Alexander	2001	IN	Acne	5	Tea tree
Drach	2005	WI	Acne	8	Sandalwood/tea tree/lavender
Scott	2010	WI	Acne	10	Tea tree
Elsethager	2001	WA	Toenail fungus	4	Lemongrass/tea tree
Moericke	2005	WI	Toenail fungus	10	Tea tree
Kunz	2003	MN	Wrinkles	12	Frankincense
Andreski	2003	MN	Wrinkles	10	Frankincense
Schoenengerger	2005	WI	Wrinkles	20	Lavender/frankincense and geranium/myrrh
Corcoran	2005	VA	Wrinkles	11	Frankincense
Bochte	2007	WI	Wrinkles	10	Frankincense or lavender
Kinkela	2008	TX	Psoriasis	10	German chamomile
Tomaszewski	2005	WI	Spider veins	10	Lavender
Reams	2008	PA	Spider veins	10	Helichrysum, geranium, cypress, sandalwood and ylang ylang
Rollo	2001	NY	Varicose veins	6	Cypress, patchouli
Garbin	2002	PA	Varicose veins	8	Geranium

primrose carrier oil on one side of the face of 12 women every evening for 30 consecutive nights. The side to which the frankincense was applied appeared to have fewer wrinkles. Andreski (2003) diluted her 4% frankincense in aloe vera on 10 women but found there was little difference (this was thought to be the effect of aloe). Schoenengerger (2005) used a 5% mixture of essential oils that contained frankincense, geranium, myrrh and lavender in jojoba oil every evening and morning for 30 consecutive days. This study (n = 20) had a separate control group. All 10 of the aromatherapy group felt their wrinkles were improved. Only three of the control group (jojoba only) thought their wrinkles were improved. Corcoran (2005) used 4% frankincense in evening primrose on the left eye wrinkles only. Outcome measures were photographs that were scrutinized by a former Estee Lauder skin specialist who was blinded to who had a greater reduction than the wrinkles treated with evening primrose only. It was good to have an expert opinion, as photographs can be hard to judge without specialized cameras and lighting.

Finally, here are two articles that might be of interest. Christian Dior registered a patent (U.S. patent number: 6630177) in 2003 for the use of novel constituents discovered in *Commiphora* (Myrrh species) particularly *Commiphora wightii* (Almada 2004). An Italian randomized split-face controlled study by Perdretti et al (2009) explored the effects of *Boswellia seratta*. In the study, 15 women with sun damaged skin used a cream containing a 0.5% Indian frankincense gum resin extract from *Boswellia serrata* once a day for 30 days. They had reduced wrinkles compared to baseline.

REFERENCES

Aggarwal S, Aggarwal A. 2010. Randomized, cross-over, comparative bioavailability trial of matrix type transdermal delivery system (TDS) of carvedilol and hydrochlorothiozide in healthy, human volunteers: a pilot study. *Contem Clin Trials*. 34(4):272-8.

Aggarwal G, Dhawan S, HariKumar S. 2012. Natural oils as skin permeation enhancers for transdermal delivery of olanzipine: in vitro and in vivo evaluation. *Curr Drug Deliv*. 9(2):172-81.

Ahad A, Aqil M, Kohli K, Sultana Y, Mujeeb M, Ali A. 2011. Interactions between novel terpenes and main components of rat and human skin: mechanistic view for transdermal delivery of propranolol hydrochloride. *Curr Drug Deliv*. 8(2):213-24.

Alexander L. 2001. Teatree for various skin conditions. Unpublished dissertation for RJ Buckle Associates.

Almada A. 2004. Gum guggul extract as an anti-wrinkle agent. *HerbalGram*: 61;36.

Andrei G, Georgala A, Topalis D, Fiton P, Aoun N et al. 2013. Heterogeneity and Evolution of Thymidine Kinase and DNA Polymerase Mutants of Herpes Simplex Virus Type 1: Implications for Antiviral Therapy. *J Infect Dis*. Feb 1. [Epub ahead of print]. Accessed 7/3/2013.

Andrianoelisoa H, Menut C, de Chatelperron P, Saracco et al. 2008. Intraspecific chemical variability and highlighting of chemotypes of leaf essential oils from Ravansara aromatica Sonnerat, a tree endemic to Madagascar. *Flav Frag Journal*. 21(5):833-838.

Armaka M, Papanikolaou E, Sivropoulou A et al. 1999. Antiviral properties of isoborneol, a potent inhibitor of herpes simples virus type 1. *Antiviral Research*. 43(2):79-92.

Astani A, Reichling J, Schnitzler P. 2010. Comparative study on the antiviral activity of selected monoterpenes derived from essential oils. *Phytotherapy Res*. 24(5):673-9.

Astani A, Reichling J, Schnitzler P. 2011. Screening for antiviral activities of isolated compounds from essential oils. *Evid Based Complement Alternat*. 2011, 2011:253643. Accessed 7/2/2013.

Astani A, Reichling J, Schnitzler P. 2012. Melissa officinalis extract inhibits attachment of herpes simplex virus in vitro. *Chemotherapy*. 58(1):70-7.

Azimi H, Fallah-Tafti M, Khakshur A, Abdollahi M. 2012. A review of phytotherapy of acne vulgaris: Perspective of new pharmacological treatments. *Fitoterapia*. 83(8):1306-17.

Baker L. 2001. Teatree for teenage acne. Unpublished dissertation for RJ Buckle Associates.

Behra O. 2001. Ravintsara v Ravansara: a Taxonomic Clarification. *Int J Arom*. 11(1):5-7.

Benencia F, Courreges M. 2000. In vitro and in vivo activity of eugenol on human herpes virus. *Phytotherapy Res.* 14:495-500.

Brooker C. 2008. *The Medical Dictionary*, 16th edition. Churchill Livingstone.

Bochte S. 2007. Frankincense versus lavender for wrinkles. Unpublished dissertation for RJ Buckle Associates.

Buck D, Nidorf D, Addino J. 1994. Comparison of two topical preparations for the treatment of onychomycosis: *Melaleuca alternifolia* (tea tree) oil and clotrimazole. *J Fam Prac.* 38(6):601-605.

Buckle J. 2010. Aromatherapy: is there a role for essential oils in current and future healthcare? *Bulletin Technique Foundation Gattefosse*, France. 95-101.

Calabrese V, Scapagnini G, Catalano C, Dinotta F, Geraci D, Morganti P. 2000. Biochemical studies of a natural antioxidant isolated from rosemary and its application in cosmetic dermatology. *Int J Tissue React.* 22(1):5-13.

Centers for Disease Control and Prevention (CDC). 2010. Seroprevalence of herpes simplex virus type 2 among persons aged 14-49 years—United States, 2005-2008. *MMWR Morb Mortal Wkly Rep.* 59(15):456-459.

Chen Y, Wang J, Cun D, Wang M, Jiang J et al. 2013. Effect of unsaturated menthol analogues on the in vitro penetration of 5-fluorouracil through rat skin. *Int J Pharm.* A 16;443(1-2).

Chida Y, Steptoe A, Hirakawa N, Sudo N, Kubo C. 2007. The effects of psychological intervention on atopic dermatitis. A systematic review and meta-analysis. *Int Arch Allergy Immunol.* 144(1):1-9.

Coleman J, Shukler D. 2013. Recent advances in vaccine development for herpes simplex virus types I and II. *Hum Vaccin Immunother.* 26;9(4). Accessed ahead of print. 7/3/2013.

Corcoran W. 2005. Frankincense for wrinkles. Unpublished RJBA Dissertation.

da Silva A, Puziol P de F, Leitao R, Gomes T, Scherer R, et al. 2012. Application of the essential oil from copaiba (Copaifera langsdori) for acne vulgaris: a double-blind, placebo controlled clinical trial. *Altern Med Rev.* 17(1):69-75.

Decker A, Graber EM. 2012. Over-the-counter Acne Treatments: A Review. *J Clin Aesthet Dermatol.* 5(5): 32-40.

Drach W. 2005. Sandalwood, teatree and lavender for acne. Unpublished dissertation for RJ Buckle Associates.

Elsethager T. 2001. The use of lemongrass and tea tree for fungal infections of feet and nails. Unpublished RJBA dissertation.

Fu Y, Zu Y, Chen L, Efferth T, Liang H et al. 2007. Investigation of antibacterial activity of rosemary essential oil against propionibacterium acnes with atomic force microscopy. *Planta Medica.* 73(12):1275-80.

Fun C, Svendsen A. 1990. The essential oils of *Lippia alba. J Ess Oil Res.* 2(5) 265-267.

Garbin C. 2002. Geranium for varicose veins. Unpublished dissertation for RJ Buckle Associates.

Garceau R, Leblanc D, Thibault L, Girouard G, Mallet M. 2012. Herpes simplex virus type 1 is the leading cause of genital herpes in New Brunswick. *Can J Infect Dis Med Microbiol.* 23(1):15-8.

Garg S, Dengre S. 1988. Antifungal activity of some essential oils. *Pharmacie.* 43(2) 141-142.

Garner S, Eady A, Bennett C, Newton J, Thomas K, Popescu C. 2012. Minocycline for acne vulgaris: efficacy and safety. *Cochrane Database Syst Rev.*15; 8:CD002086.

Garozzo A, Timpanaro R, Bisignano B, Furneri P, Bisignano G, Castro A. 2009. In vitro antiviral activity of Melaleuca alternifolia essential oil. *Lett App Microbiol.* 49(6):806-808.

Gavini E, Sanna V, Sharma R, Juliano C, Usai M et al. 2005. Solid lipid microparticles (SLM) containing juniper oil as anti-acne topical carriers: preliminary studies. *Pharm Dev Technol.* 10(4):479-87.

Gayoso C, Lima E, Oliviera V, Pereira F, Souza E et al. 2005. Sensitivity of fungi isolated from onychomycosis to Eugenia cariophyllata essential oil and eugenol. *Fitoterapia.* 76(2):247-9.

Inouye S, Uchida K, Yamaguchi H. 2001. In-vitro and in-vivo anti-Trichophyton activity of essential oils by vapour contact. *Mycoses.* 44(3-4):99-107.

Inouye S, Nishiyama Y, Uchida K, Hasumi Y, Yamaguchi H, Abe S. 2006. The vapor activity of oregano, perilla, tea tree, lavender, clove, and geranium oils against a Trichophyton mentagrophytes in a closed box. *J Infect Chemother.* 12(6):349-54.

Inouye S, Uchida K, Nishiyama Y, Hasumi Y, Yamaguchi H, Abe S. 2007. Combined effect of heat, essential oils and salt on fungicidal activity against Tricophyton mentagrophytes in a foot bath. *Nihon Ishinkin Gakkai Zasshi.* 48(1):27-36.

Juliani H, Behra O, Moharram H, Ranarivelo L, Ralijerson B, Andriantsiferana M et al. 2005. Searching for the real ravansara (*Ravansara aromatica* Sonn.) essential oil: a case study for *Natiora*: the Malagasy natural product label. *Perf Flavor* 30, 60-65.

Juliani H, Kapteyn J, Jones D, Koroch A, Wang M, Carles D, Simon J. 2006. Application of near-infrared spectroscopy in quality control and determination of adulteration of African essential oils. *Pytochem Anal.* 17:121-128.

Jung E, Kim S, Hur S, Park D, Koh J et al. 2007. Effect of Camillia japonica on human type 1 procollagen production and skin barrier function. *J Ethnopharm.* 112(1):127-131.

Kang L, Poh A, Fan S, Ho P, Chan Y, Chan S. 2007. Reversible effects of permeation enhancers on human skin. *Eur J Pharm Biopharm.* 67(1):149-55.

Katsambas A, Stefanaki C, Cunliffe W. 2004. Guidelines for treating acne. *Clin Dermatol.* 22(5):439-44.

Kinkela J. 2008. German chamomile for psoriasis. Unpublished dissertation for RJ Buckle Associates.

Kim S, Baik J, Oh T, Yoon W, Lee N, Hyun C. 2008. Biological activities of Korean Citrus obovoides and Citrus natsudaidai essential oils against acne-inducing bacteria. *Biosci, Biotech Biochem.* 72(10):2507-13.

Kligman L, Gans E. 2000. Re-emergence of topical retinol in dermatology. *J Dermatol Treat.* 11:47-52.

Koch C, Reichling J, Kehm R, Sharaf M, Zentgraf H, Schneele J, Schnitzler P. 2008a. Efficacy of anise oil, dwarf-pine oil and chamomile oil against thymidine-kinase-positive and thymidine-kinase-negative herpes viruses. *J Pharm Pharmacol.* 60(11):1545-50.

Koch C, Reichling J, Schneele J, Schnitzler P. 2008b. Inhibitory effect of essential oils against herpes simplex virus type 2. *Phytomedicine.* 15(1-2):71-8.

Koytchev R, Alken R, Dundarov S. 1999. Balm mint extract (Lo-701) for topical treatment for recurring herpes labialis. *Phytomedicine.* 6(4):225–230.

Krishnaiah Y, Al-Saidan S, Jayaram B. 2006. Effect of nerodilol, carvone and anethole on the in vitro transdermal delivery of selegiline hydrochloride. *Pharmazie.* 61(1):46-53.

Krishnaiah Y, Raju V, Shiva Kumar M, Rama B, Raghumurthy V, Ramana Murthy K. 2008. Studies on optimizing in vitro transdermal permeation of ondansetron hydrochloride using nerodiol, carvone and limonene as penetration enhances. *Pharm Dev Technol.* 13(3):177-85.

Kunz J. 2003. Frankincense for wrinkles. Unpubellished RJBA dissertation.

Lai W, Chuang H, Lee M, Wei C, Lin C, Tsai Y. 2012. Inhibition of herpes simplex virus type 1 by thymol-related monoterpenoids. *Planta Medica.* 78(15):1636-8.

Leroux-Roels G, Clement F, Vandepapeliere P, Fourneau M, Heineman T, Dubin G. 2013. Immunogenicity and safety of different formulations of an adjuvanted glycoprotein D genital herpes vaccine in healthy adults: A double-blind randomized trial. *Human Vaccin Immunother* 22(9):6. Accessed 4/3/2013. http://www.ncbi.nlm.nih.gov/pubmed/23434737.

Lertsatitthanakorn P, Aromdee C, Khunkitti W, Taweechaisupapong S, Arunyanart C. 2010. Effect of Citronella Oil on Time Kill Profile, Leakage and Morphological Changes of Propionibacterium acne. *J Ess Oil Res.* 22(3):270-274.

Lertsatitthanakorn S, Taweechaisupapong S, Aromdee C, Khunkitti W. 2006. In vitro bioactivities of essential oils used for acne control. *Int J Aromatherapy.* 16(1):43-49.

Loizzo M, Saab A, Tundis R, Statti G, Lampronti I et al. 2008. Phytochemical analysis and in vitro evaluation of the biological activity against herpes simplex virus type 1 (HSV-1) of Cedrus libani. *Phytomedicine.* 15(1-2):79-83.

Looker K, Garnett G, Schmid G. 2008. An estimate of the global prevalence of herpes simplex virus type 2 infection. *Bull World Health Org.* 86(10):805-812.

Matiz G, Osorio M, Camacho F, Atencia M, Herazo J. 2012. Effectiveness of antimicrobial formulations for acne based on orange (Citrus sinensis) and sweet basil (Ocimum basilicum L) essential oils. *Biomédica: Revista Del Instituto Nacional De Salud.* 32(1): 125-33.

May C. 2000. Helichrysum and angelica topically applied for adolescent acne. Unpublished dissertation for RJ Buckle Associates.

Minaglou F. 2006. The use of phyto-aromatherapy in the treatment of non-severe acne vulgaris. *Int J Clin Aroma.* 3(1):3-8.

Minami M, Kita M, Nakaya T, Yamamoto T, Kuriyama H, Imanishi J. 2003. The inhibitory effect of essential oils on herpes simplex virus type-1 replication in vitro. *Microbiol Immunol.* 47(9):681-4.

Moericke B. 2005. Unpublished RJBA Dissertation. Tea tree for toenail fungal infection.

Nikalji N, Godse K, Sakhiya J, Patil S, Nadkarni N. 2012 Complications of medium depth and deep chemical peels. *J Cutan Aesthet Surg.* 5(4):254-60.

Oh T, Kim S, Yoon W, Kim J, Yang E, Lee N, Hyun C. 2009. Chemical composition and biological activities of Jeju Thymus quinquecostatus essential oils against Propionibacterium species inducing acne. *J Gen Appl Microbiol.* 55(1):63-8.

Orhan İ, Erdoğan Ö, Berrin K, Murat K. 2012. Antimicrobial and antiviral effects of essential oils from selected Umbelliferae and Labiatae plants and individual essential oil components. *Turkish J Biol.* 36(3):39-246.

Ozolins M, Eady E, Avery A, Cunliffe W, O'Neill C et al. 2005. Randomised controlled multiple treatment comparison to provide a cost-effectiveness rationale for the selection of antimicrobial therapy in acne. *Health Technol Assess.* 9(1):iii-212.

Pau M, Atzori L, Aste N, et al. 2010. Epidemiology of tinea pedis in Cagliari, Italy. *G Ital Dermatol Venereol.* 145:1-5.

Pedretti A, Capezzera R, Zane C, Facchinetti E, Calzavara-Pinton P. 2009. Effects of topical boswellic acid on photo and age-damaged skin: clinical, biophysical, and echographic evaluations in a double-blind, randomized, split-face study. *Planta Med.* 76(6):555-60.

Peréz-Gonsáles M, Torres-Rodriguez J, Martines-Roig A, Segura S, Griera G. 2009. Prevalence of tinea pedis, tinea unguium of toenails and tinea capitis in school children from Barcelona. *Rev Iberoam Micol.* 26(4): 228-32.

Preneau S, Dreno B. 2012. Female acne - a different subtype of teenager acne? *J Eur Acad Dermatol Venereol.* 26(3):277-82.

Rai M, Acharya D, 1999. Screening of some Asteraceae plants for antimycotic activity. Compositae Newletter. 34:37-43.

Rai M, Mares M (Eds.) 2003. *Plant Derived Antimycotics.* Binghamton, NY: Haworth.

Ream J. 2008. Helichrysum, geranium, cypress, sandalwood and ylang ylang for spider veins. Unpublished dissertation for RJ Buckle Associates.

Ro Y, Ha H, Kim C, Yeom H. 2002. The effects of aromatherapy on pruritus in patients undergoing hemodialysis. *DermatolNurs.* 14(4): 231-4, 237-9, 256.

Rollo P. 2001. Cypress and patchouli for varicose veins. Unpublished dissertation for RJ Buckle Associates.

Romagna C, Mares D, Fasulo M et al. 1994. Antifungal effects of alpha-terthienyl from *Tagetes patula* on five dermatophytes. *Phyto Res.* 8(6):332-336.

Saddi M, Sanna A, Cottiglia F, Chisu L, Casu L et al. 2007. Antiherpevirus activity of Artemisia arborescens essential oil and inhibition of lateral diffusion in Vero cells. *Ann Clin Microbiol Antimicrob.* 26(6):10.

Sahi S, Shukla A, Bajaj A et al. 1999. Broad spectrum antimycotic drug for the control of fungal infections in human beings. *Curr Sci.* 76(6):836-939.

Satchell A, Sauragen A, Bell C, Barnetson R. 2002. Treatment of interdigital tinea pedis with 25% and 50% tea tree oil solution: a randomized, placebo-controlled, blinded study. *Australas J Dermatol.* 43(3):175-8.

Schmitt S, Schaefer U, Doebler L, Reichling J. 2009. Cooperative interaction of monoterpenes and phenylpropanoids on the in vitro human skin permeation of complex composed essential oils. *Planta Med.* 75(13):1381-5.

Schnitzler P, Schön K, Reichling J. 2001. Antiviral activity of Australian tea tree oil and eucalyptus oil against herpes simplex virus in cell culture. *Die Pharmazie [Pharmazie].* 56(4):343-7.

Schnitzler P, Koch C, Reichling J. 2007. Susceptibility of drug-resistant clinical herpes simplex virus type 1 strains to essential oils of ginger, thyme, hyssop, and sandalwood. *Antimicrob Agents Chemother.* 51(5):1859-62.

Schnitzler P, Schuhmacher A, Astani A, Reichling J. 2008. Melissa officinalis oil affects infectivity of enveloped herpesviruses. *Phytomed.* 15(9):734-40.

Schoenengerger R. 2005. RJBA Dissertation. Essential oil mix for wrinkles.

Scott K. 2010. Teatree for acne. Unpublished dissertation for RJ Buckle Associates.

Shen Y, Wang T, Zhou C, Wang X, Ding X et al. 2012. Prevalence of acne vulgaris in Chinese adolescents and adults: a community-based study of 17,345 subjects in six cities. *Acta Derm Venereol.* 92(1):40-4.

Shen T, Zu H, Went W, Zhang J. 2013. Development of a reservoir-type transdermal delivery system containing eucalyptus oil for tetramethylpyrazine. *Drug Del.* 20(1):19-24.

Sinico C, De Logu A, Lai F, Valenti D, Manconi M. 2005. Liposomal incorporation of Artemisia arborescens L. essential oil and in vitro antiviral activity. *Eur J Pharm Biopharm.* 59(1): 161-8.

Skerlev M, Miklic P. 2010. The changing face of *Microsporum* spp infections. *Clin Dermatol.* 28:146-150.

Syed T, Qureshi Z, Ali S et al. 1999. Treatment of toenail onychomycosis with 2% butenafine and 5% *Melaleuca alternifolia* (tea tree in cream). *Trop Med and Int Health.* 4(4):284-287.

Theron E, Holeman M, Potin Gautier M, Pinel R. 1994. Authentication of Ravansara aromatica and Ravansara anisata. *Planta Med.* 60(5):489-491.

Tomaszewski E. 2005. Lavender for spider veins. Unpublished dissertation for RJ Buckle Associates.

Tragoolpua Y, Jatisatienr A. 2007. Anti-herpes simplex virus activities of Eugenia caryophyllus (Spreng.) Bullock & S. G. Harrison and essential oil, eugenol. *Phytother Res.* 21(12):1153-8.

Tronstein E, Johnston C, Huang M, Selke S, Magaret A et al. 2011. Genital Shedding of Herpes Simplex Virus Among Symptomatic and Asymptomatic Persons With HSV-2 Infection. *JAMA.* 305(14): 1441-1449.

Tsukahara K, Nakagawa H, Moriwaki S, Takema Y, Fujimura T, Imokawa G. 2006. Inhibition of ultraviolet-B-induced wrinkle formation by an elastase-inhibiting herbal extract: implication for the mechanism underlying elastase-associated wrinkles. *In J Dermatol.* 45(4):460-8.

Vadlapudi A, Vadlapatia R, Mitra A. 2013. Update On Emerging Antivirals For The Management Of Herpes Simplex Virus Infections: A Patenting Perspective. *Recent Pat Anitinfect Drug Discov.* Jan 15. [Epub ahead of print]. Accessed 7/3/2013.

Valgimigli L, Gabbanini S, Berlini E, Lucchi E, Beltramini C, Bertarelli Y. 2012. Lemon (Citrus limon, Burm.f.) essential oil enhances the trans-epidermal release of lipid-(A, E) and water-(B6, C) soluble vitamins from topical emulsions in reconstructed human epidermis. *Int J Cosmet Sci.* 34(4):347-56.

Viyoch J, Pisutthanan N, Faikreua A, Nupangta K, Wangtorpol K, Ngokkuen J. 2006. Evaluation of in vitro antimicrobial activity of Thai basil oils and their micro-emulsion formulas against Propionibacterium acne. *Internat J Cos Sci.* 28(2):125-33.

Wald A. 2006. Genital HSV-1 Infections. *Sex Transm Infect.* 82(3):189-90.

Walling H. 2009. Subclinical onychomycosis is associated with tinea pedis. *Br J Dermatol.* 161:746-749.

Watanabe S, Harada T, Hiruma M, et al. 2010. Epidemiological survey of foot diseases in Japan: results of 30,000 foot checks by dermatologists. *J Dermatol.* 37:397-406.

Wolbling R, Leonhardt K. 1994. Local therapy of herpes simplex with dried extract from *Melissa officinalis. Phytomed.* 1:24-31.

Wylde B. 2009. Grapefruit's bittersweet reality. *Alive: Canada's Natural Health and Wellness Magazine.* 325:107-107.

Yahya H. 2009. Acne vulgaris in Nigerian adolescents – prevalence, severity, beliefs, perceptions, and practices. *Int J Dermatol.* 48(5):498-505.

Zolfaghari M, Salamian P, Riazi A, Khaksa G. 1997. Clinical Efficacy of myrtle oil in Herpes simplex. *Iranian J Med Sci.* 22(3-4):134-137.

Chapter 15

Mental Health

"The mind is ever a tourist, wanting to touch and buy new things then toss them into an already filled closet."

Hafiz, The Gift, p 132

CHAPTER ASSETS

There is no suggestion that anyone on medication for a mental illness should stop taking *them* and replace *them* with aromatherapy. However, smell does impact the brain and aromatherapy could play a role in ameliorating mental symptoms. Pickover (1998) quotes Hippocrates, who wrote, "Men ought to know that from nothing else but the brain come joys, delights, laughter, sorrows, griefs, despondency and lamentations."

SCHIZOPHRENIA

Over 40 years ago, Wiener (1966) of the New York Medical College suggested our bodies had an internal and external communicating system that used our nervous system without alerting us to its existence. Such a system, he suggested, was made up of chemicals that interacted with the other systems in the body **by means of**

odor. Subsequent to his theory was the discovery that people with schizophrenia gave out a persistent aroma discernible to dogs and rats. This aroma became more pronounced when they were in crisis (Smith & Sines 1960).

In 2001, a report in the *Journal of the American Medical Association* suggested a study of smell could shed light on some of the symptoms of schizophrenia (O'Neil 2001). Dr. Daniel O'Leary from the University of Iowa Hospitals and Clinics exposed 18 people with schizophrenia and 15 healthy volunteers to a pleasant smell (vanilla) and an unpleasant smell. An imaging device was used to track blood flow to different areas of the brain, and subjects were asked to rate each smell. The mental imaging showed big differences between the two groups in the mental processing of the unpleasant smell. The limbic system appeared to be highly active in healthy subjects but largely unused with people with schizophrenia. The latter depended more on frontal cortical areas usually reserved for functions such as decision making. This misuse of brain circuits could play a role in paranoia.

A recent systematic review by Schecklmann et al (2013) found there were specific changes in olfactory function in people with mental illness. Olfactory function was a biomarker in adult neuropsychiatric disorders. This was particularly so in children/adolescents with disorders that involved dopamine transmission (e.g., attention-deficit hyperactivity disorder, autism, schizophrenia, 22q11 deletion syndrome).

Humans have approximately 1000 different olfactory receptor types, each tuned to a particular kind of odor, that together contribute to our perception of smell (Yeshurun & Sobel 2010). When humans lose their sense of smell (anosmia), there is a risk of depression (Douek 1988, Smeets et al 2009, Irani et al 2010). Aristotle noted that just the thought of smell could affect us (Caston 1998). Smell is the most potent trigger for flashbacks suffered in posttraumatic stress (PTSD) (McCormick 2013, Abramovitz & Lichtenberg 2009). Smell affects what we crave, what we become addicted to, what we find pleasure in, and even the will to live (Shepherd 2011). A familiar smell that has good memories allows us to feel safe.

The use of psychoactive products evolved along two related paths: for religious or recreational pursuits, and to modify normal behavior (Alexander 2001). The effects of aromas on the brain were first tested in 1966 (Moncrieff 1966). He used an electroencephalograph (EEG) to monitor changes in brainwave patterns. Moncrieff later found that basil, black pepper, cardamom, and rosemary induced mainly beta patterns. Jasmine, neroli, and rose induced mainly delta patterns (Moncrieff 1977). Beta brain patterns (13 to 40 cycles per second) are concerned with attention and alertness. Delta brain patterns (0 to 4 cycles per second) are concerned with euphoria and calmness (Thorsten et al 2001). Dodd and Van Toller (1983) compared the action of chemical components found in essential oils to the action of psychotropic drugs such as antidepressants. Torii et al (1988) reported on the electrical changes of the brain and the similarities between emotion and the sense of smell. King (1988) explored the relationship between odor and anxiety. Hirata et al (2002) showed that cerebral blood flow to the prefrontal cortex increased when fragrance was inhaled. Since then, considerable research on the effects of aroma (and some

TABLE 15-1 *Selection of Published Articles on Animals*

Author	Year	Animal	Neurochemical or Addictive Chemical	Essential oil/ Component	
Zhao et al	2005	Rats	Nicotine	*Angelica gigas*	+ve
Norte et al	2005	Rats	Depression	Methyl eugenol	+ve
Komiya et al	2006	Mice	5-HT & DA	Lemon	+ve
Ito et al	2007	Mice	Depression	l-Perillaldehyde (PAH)	+ve
Karimzadeh et al	2012	Rats	Inhibition of synaptic plasticity in epilepsy	*Pimpenella anisum*	+ve
Costa et al	2011	Mice	GABA(A) receptor-benzodiazepine complex	Lemongrass *Cymbopogon citratus*	+ve
Fukada et al	2012	Rats	HPA axis	Rose	+ve

of their components) on brain function and brain disorders has been published. A selection is listed in Table 15-1.

During intense stress, bereavement, or when the dark dog of despair descends, links with reality can become blurred. Familiar smells that are reminders of a safe world and reassuring touch may operate like beacons in the fog, illuminating the way back to reality. Patients with mental health problems can be a reminder of just how fragile sanity is.

AROMATHERAPY AND MENTAL ILLNESS

Essential oils affect how we feel (Burnett et al 2004). This means that components within essential oils have the capacity to alter brain chemistry. As long ago as 1992, Sugano suggested that natural fragrances could provide a cost-effective and efficient alternative to some stimulants and sedatives. Tisserand (1988) suggested that olfactory "ecstasy" was discovered by man at a very early age. Buchbauer and Jirovetz (1994) wrote that essential oils could be viewed as medicines.

Most synthetic psychotropic medications have limited efficacy and significant side effects. Preliminary findings suggest several treatments based on natural substances are as effective and safe as the synthetic pharmaceuticals in current use (Lake 2000, Uehleke et al 2012).

Obviously, strong sedatives and antipsychotic medicines can become essential when the condition of a patient is unmanageable. However, it could be argued that there are some patients who have poor coping mechanisms. This could be due to genetics, environmental issues, or just one of those unexplainable things. There is a large group of people in mental healthcare programs for whom aromatherapy could be beneficial. It could also be useful in psychiatric centers, when a patient becomes agitated and needs to calm down.

Fowler (2004), an R.J. Buckle student, carried out such a study in a step-down residential center for adolescents with DSM-1 (Diagnostic and Statistical Manual of Mental Disorders). Patients were offered a "calming blend" (3% ylang ylang, sweet marjoram, and bergamot in jojoba oil) instead of medication when necessary (prn) for agitation. The calming blend was given in a 5-minute hand 'M' Technique. All nurses were on the unit were taught the hand 'M' Technique. Parents signed consent forms and patients gave informed consent. The number of prn interventions (oral, IM or restraint) for the 3 months before the aromatherapy study began was compared with the duration of the 3-month study. There were significant reductions in the number of prn interventions for agitation during the aromatherapy study. The number of injections decreased from 43 to 31 and oral medications decreased from 631 to 397. Additionally, the number of seclusion and restraint interventions decreased from 29 to 20. This could be from the essential oils, the 'M' Technique or the novelty of something new. But this kind of drug (and nurse time) saving is worth investigating further. Fowler published her findings in 2006 (Fowler 2006). Butje et al (2008) discuss the low cost and low side effect appeal of aromatherapy for mental health in their article.

ADDICTION

"Addiction is a condition that results in significant harm to the individual and to society more generally" (Capps et al 2012). Society "judges" addiction, feeling it to be a bad *choice* that an individual makes. However, recent brain research challenges that there is a choice, with the suggestion that addiction could be a brain disease (Rahman 2011): a brain disease that could be treatable. It is known that an individual's inherited genetic makeup can influence his or her addiction risk. A growing body of preclinical and clinical data appears to suggest that nicotinic acetylcholine receptors (nAChRs) in the human brain play a pivotal role in drug addiction, including nicotine and alcohol dependence (Rahman 2011).

Today's society is an addictive one, and it often rewards socially acceptable addictions like workaholism, accepts shopaholics and nicotine addiction, condones alcohol addiction, and prosecutes drug addiction. Yet the ethos behind addiction—instant gratification—is at the very core of today's society. People want things instantly. Texting and emails have replaced letters, faxes and, to an extent, phone calls. In addition to this, we live in a world where people who are unable to cope with the pace of life are often isolated, ridiculed, or forgotten. It is hardly surprising that addiction is on the increase.

Results of the 2010 National Survey on Drug Use and Health (NSDUH) showed an estimated 22.6 million Americans (8.9%) aged 12 or older were current or past month illicit drug users (Manchikanti 2012). There is a huge increase in adolescents (13 to 18 years) developing Substance Use Disorder (SUD) (Merikangas & McClair 2012). This increase in substance abuse is a global phenomenon and covers alcohol, nicotine, cannabis, and cocaine (Degenhardt 2008). This statement is supported by studies from Korea (Kim et al 2012), Taiwan (Wang et al 2012), Brazil (Madruga et al 2012), and France (Mura et al 2012), as well as many other countries.

In 2008, the number of deaths by poisoning exceeded the number of those dying in a car accident. Poisoning was the leading cause of "injury death" in the United States (Warner et al 2011). A total of 90% of deaths by poisoning were from drug overdose, with the vast majority being unintentional (Shah et al 2008). In addition, many illicit drugs, e.g., amphetamines, cocaine, ecstasy, heroin, lysergic acid diethylamide, marijuana and phencyclidine, have been linked to major cardiovascular events such as strokes (Esse et al 2011).

While there are many detox programs available in the United States (Polsky et al 2010) and in other countries such as Canada (Li et al 2008) and Australia (McAvoy 2008), much depends on the person being able to withstand the cravings during, and after, withdrawal.

There are three stages to drug detox (Praveen et al 2011)—primary stage is stabilization, second stage is withdrawal, and third stage is preventing relapse by improving well-being. Ernst (2012) debunks the idea of any alternative detox. However, it may be that some complementary therapies, such as aromatherapy, may help in the process. According to studies carried out by R.J. Buckle students, aromatherapy appears to reduce cravings (Table 15-2). Aromatherapy alleviated the withdrawal process during the second stage. Aromatherapy can also improve hard hyph well-being (third stage). However, there is no suggestion aromatherapy should **replace** conventional drug detox treatment. However, for those wanting to cut down on cigarettes, inhaling essential oils (through a personal inhaler) might help reduce craving. For those wanting to cut down gradually on sleeping tablets or antidepressants, a protocol (that has been used successfully for the last 15 years) can be found in Table 15-3 and Box 15-1. More recently, a similar protocol has been used by Komori et al (2006). The mixture of essential oils (sandalwood [35%], juniper berry [12%], rose [8%], and orris [6%]) was first tested on rats and then on 42 outpatients with low-dose dependence on hypnotic benzodiazepines. Sedation was reduced 25% each week while the participant inhaled the essential oil mixture at bedtime: 26 participants reduced the dosage and 12 subjects were weaned off completely.

Nicotine Addiction

The idea that an olfactory stimulus might reduce craving for nicotine was explored by Seyette and Parrott (1999). They found that both negative and positive aromas decreased cravings against a nonodoriferous control in nicotine addiction. The sense of smell is lessened in a heavy smoker nevertheless, aromatherapy has achieved some modest success. R.J. Buckle students have conducted several studies as listed in Table 15-2. DaCosta (1999) was one of the first R.J. Buckle students to explore the effect of inhaled essential oils as a means to reduce the craving of nicotine withdrawal. The three essential oils DaCosta used were lavender (*Lavandula angustifolia*), *Helichrysum italicum*, and *Angelica archangelica*. Four male subjects who smoked at least 10 cigarettes a day and had tried unsuccessfully to stop smoking in the past were recruited. The period immediately after breakfast, lunch and supper were chosen as those were the hardest times to abstain from smoking.

TABLE 15-2 *RJ Buckle Student Studies on Addiction*

Name	Year	State	Number	Method	Addiction	Essential Oil
DaCosta	2000	MA	4	Inhaled	Nicotine	Three different oils*
Caldwell	2001	MN	5	Inhaled	Substance	Ylang ylang
Newsham	2001	NY	170	Inhaled	Nicotine	Lavender plus acupuncture
Barrett	2002	WA	16	Topical	Alcohol	Lavender/Roman chamomile
Carino[†]	2003	NY	16	Inhaled	Alcohol	Bergamot
McMahon	2003	NY	7	Inhaled	Nicotine	Angelica/Black pepper
West	2003	MN	15	Inhaled	Nicotine	Three different oils[‡]
Cordell[§]	2004	TX	20	Inhaled	Nicotine	Angelica/black pepper
Hood	2005	WI	30	Inhaled	Food	Mandarin/lavender
Chalifour[†]	2005	MA	8	Inhaled	Opiates	Peppermint
Gryniewski	2005	MN	10	Inhaled	Nicotine	Angelica
Romero	2006	MN	4	Inhaled	Nicotine	Angelica
Herring	2006	AZ	21	Topical	Food	Fennel
Drumm[†]	2006	NJ	10	Inhaled	Nicotine	Angelica/ *Helichrysum*
Walker	2007	IN	20	Inhaled	Nicotine	Angelica
Paine	2008	NJ	10	Inhaled	Nicotine	Black pepper
Logue	2010	NJ	20	Inhaled	Nicotine	Black pepper/ *E. globulus*
Sirignano	2011	MA	11	Inhaled	Nicotine	*Helichrysum*/black pepper
Katseres	2011	MA	5	Inhaled	Nicotine	Black pepper/ lavender
Biesecker	2011	MA	12	Inhaled	Nicotine	Black pepper

*Three different oils: angelica, *Helichrysum*, and lavender.
[†]Carino, Chalifour and Drumm carried out studies on in-patients in hospitals.
[‡]Dr. Cordell's research was carried out on a college campus, and later published (2012).
[§]A mixture of three different oils: angelica, *Helichrysum*, and German chamomile.

The normal period the test subjects could wait before smoking (baseline) was minimal, less than 2 minutes. Each essential oil was then tested separately for 5 consecutive days, divided by a dry-out period of 2 days, and the subjects timed how long they could last without a cigarette. Angelica root appeared to be the most helpful, with subjects able to wait an average of 53 minutes before having a cigarette. This was a considerable improvement on 2 minutes, although inhaling angelica did not prevent them from smoking after 53 minutes.

TABLE 15-3 *RJ Buckle Student Studies on* DEPRESSION

Name	Year	State	Number	Method	Type	Essential Oil
Charleton	1999	WA	14	Topical	Postnatal	Roman chamomile
Templeton	2002	WA	10	Bath	General	Bergamot
Martine	2002	WA	12	Inhaled	SAD	Bergamot
Kane	2004	AZ	18	Inhaled	Cardiac rehab	Petitgrain
Krieger	2010	NY	12	Diffused	Pediatric	Mandarin

BOX 15-1 *Protocol for Coming off Benzodiazepine or Night Sedation with Aromatherapy*

Week 1	Choose aroma(s) from a selection of six.
	Choose touch or nontouch application. Apply oil in office.
	Give written instructions on when and how to use aromatherapy.
Week 2	Reduce medication by 25%.
Week 3	Reduce medication by further 25%.
Week 4	Remain on 50% medication.
Week 5	Reduce medication to 25%.
Week 6	Remain on 25% medication.
Week 7	25% medication alternate days.
Week 8	Remain on 25% medication alternate days.
Week 9	25% medication twice a week.
Week 10	25% medication once a week.

Since then, there have been 13 further pilot studies conducted by R.J. Buckle students. Most of them used inhaled essential oils. Many of them chose black pepper because of the study by Rose and Behm (1994). Rose and Behm hypothesized that clients needed to experience the respiratory-tract sensations that accompany cigarette smoking in order to quit successfully. They believed black pepper essential oil could simulate those sensations. When they tested their theory, the found "the vapor of black pepper essential oil, when inhaled, partially reproduces the respiratory tract sensations experienced when smoking, thereby reducing the craving for cigarettes."

In the RJBA studies, angelica appeared to make the craving more bearable and therefore the person could wait longer before smoking, or smoke fewer cigarettes. This essential oil is from the root of *Angelica archangelica*. I have found it extremely useful to empower people in difficult situations where they need to stay in control—for example, at a funeral of a loved one. I am not sure how to describe that intrinsic property—but it does appear to work in addiction withdrawal.

Cordell explored the effect of inhaled aromas on a university campus. This study compared the effect of inhaling black pepper to angelica. What is interesting about this study is that while the subjects were all trying to quit tobacco, their use of tobacco ranged from smoking cigarettes to chewing tobacco or using snuff. Black pepper appeared to reduce craving across the board, but angelica allowed a longer period of time before using the tobacco product.

Finally, aromatherapy appeared to enhance motivation during conventional nicotine dependence treatment (Koszwoski et al 2005). This would occur even if black pepper or angelica or any other essential oil did not reduce the actual craving itself.

Substance Addiction

Caldwell (2001) explored the effects of ylang ylang *(Cananga odorata)* in a small, controlled study of 10 women suffering from cravings following withdrawal of substance abuse. All women were taking orthodox medication. The participants were randomly split into two groups: an experimental group and a control group. The experimental group was given essential oil of ylang ylang to inhale and the control group received plain almond oil. Both groups were told that they were using something. The participants were self-selecting and limited to women dealing with chemical addiction. All 10 participants had either stopped using and were still experiencing cravings, or were trying to stop using and were experiencing cravings.

Each participant put two drops of the oil on a cotton square and put the square in her pillowcase every night for 7 nights. The participants were also asked to put two to three drops of oil on a cotton hanky, carry the hanky with them for 7 days, and smell it if they experienced a craving. The participants were asked to record the number of cravings, their intensity, and any other comments.

The results showed the number of cravings for the essential oil group went down more than for the control group. However, ylang did not prevent cravings completely. Four out of five women in the experimental group believed "smelling the oil relieved the stress and anxiety of that moment." None of the participants using the almond oil expressed this feeling. Caldwell (2001) notes that ylang ylang's positive effect might be enhanced by using a diffuser at night.

Chalifour (2005) looked at reducing the nausea experienced in patients withdrawing from opiate and crack at the Cooley Dickenson Hospital, Northampton, Massachusetts. Eight patients were given peppermint to inhale for nausea. Subjects rated their nausea using a CIWA form (Clinical Institute Withdrawal Assessment). This scale was used before meals (breakfast and lunch). Peppermint was given 30 minutes before meals. There appeared to be a 100% reduction in nausea.

Alcohol Addiction

Olfactory loss is common in alcoholics (Shear et al 1992) as well as cocaine users (Schwartz et al 1998), and heroin addicts (Perl et al 1997). Loss of smell is not thought to affect the transfer of the volatile molecules unless there is damage to the olfactory nerve. Loss of smell in addicts is thought to be due to damage to the cortical and subcortical brain regions (Shear et al 1992), but it is possible there is nerve damage due to snorting or sniffing cocaine, heroin, and glue.

A search of the literature only produced one piece of research on alcohol addiction and aromatherapy (Kunz et al 2007). This randomized, controlled study compared aromatherapy to auricular acupuncture in alcohol addiction for 5 days. There were 99 participants: 54 randomized to the aromatherapy group and 55 to the acupuncture group. The main rating scale was assessment of alcohol withdrawal syndrome (AWS scale). There was a fairly high dropout factor. Only 36 patients completed acupuncture and 38 patients completed aromatherapy. Both groups appeared to have the same reduction in the craving and withdrawal symptoms. Thus aromatherapy was as successful as acupuncture in this instance.

Barrett (2002) explored the effects of aromatherapy on alcohol addiction withdrawal at Highline Community Medical Center for her RJBA certification. This facility offers hospital-based treatment for chemical dependency at its Tukwila, Washington, location and had been treating addiction for 40 years. HRS Highline operates 12 beds for medical detoxification and 18 beds for brief inpatient stabilization. In addition, approximately 100 patients are treated concurrently on an outpatient basis. Barrett created both protocol and policy and then introduced an aromatherapy program to support the detox process.

Participants rated their symptoms on a scale of 0 to 4 (0 = no symptoms, 4 = extreme symptoms). A medicine cup containing 5 mL diluted essential oils was given to the participant by a nurse at bedtime. The essential oils were 5% Roman chamomile, lavender and ylang ylang in sunflower oil. The patient rubbed the mixture into their throat and chest area and the nurse documented the use of aromatherapy in the progress notes. The following morning, participants ranked their symptoms again while the nurse took their vital signs (respiration, blood pressure). The nurse also noted any difference in mood the patient reported. The study was carried out over a 3-week period in 2002.

The scent of the mixture appealed to more women than men and there was less compliance in the male sector. However, there appeared to be a positive change of more than 50% in terms of feeling less restless. It also reduced their anxiety and increased their ability to go to sleep. Barrett's most recent thoughts are that inhaled aromas might be an easier method, especially now there are personal inhalers, packets and pouches available (personal communication, January 2013).

Food Addiction

Obesity and its undisputed links to hypertension, diabetes and many other health conditions is increasing rapidly. Currently, approximately 70% of adult Americans are overweight or obese. This figure is replicated throughout much of the Western world. More UK, South Asian, black African-Caribbean and white European children are becoming obese (Nightingale et al 2011). Fast food has been named the culprit. As early as 2007, there was growing concern about corn syrup, with one study even suggesting the intense sweetness of corn syrup was as addictive as cocaine (Lenoir et al 2007). Three years later, some researchers still felt there was no evidence that any food or food ingredient (including sucrose) was addictive (Benton 2010). Current research says that bingeing on food that is crammed with sugar/sweeteners (as fast food is) increases extracellular dopamine in the striatum, and this is what gives it an addictive potential (Fortuna 2012).

Dopamine plays an important role in addiction as it produces both feel good and reward sensations (Saddoris et al 2013). When blood glucose levels rise, they increase absorption of tryptophan (through the large neutral amino acid [LNAA] complex). Trytophan is then converted into serotonin, a mood elevator (Fortuna 2012). Today, the medical system worldwide is having to deal with epidemic of those wanting to "overcome food addiction and reverse proinflammatory states of illhealth" (Shriner 2012).

Interestingly, the olfactory cortex has been shown to be the site in the brain that monitors the consumption of essential amino acids in the diet (Shepherd 2010). If there are insufficient essential amino acids in the food presented to a rat, it will stop eating it (Gietzen & Rogers 2006). There is some evidence the same mechanism may act in humans (Neville & Haberly 2004, Wilson & Linster 2008).

In today's society, large portions of food are expected, even if they cannot be eaten. Everything must be big. It is as though people feel too small in a world that undervalues them. It may be that people feel they have a "hole in their wholeness" and are hungry for anything that will stop that feeling of emptiness. There have been various attempts to help people eat smaller portions of food. These have ranged from sprinkling food with crystals to make the food taste more filling, to a "smart" fork that vibrates when you eat too fast. These inventions may not be a bad idea, but if some food is addictive, there will be withdrawal symptoms. Inhaling an essential oil may help those withdrawal symptoms. The best method would be to use an individual inhaler, packet or patch.

RJBA students carried out two studies on reducing food intake, Table 15-2. Hood (2005) randomly allocated her 30 volunteers into three groups. Each volunteer was at least 10 pounds overweight and had been unable to lose weight. There were two experimental groups (mandarin or lavender) and one control group (grapeseed oil). The participants were asked to smell the oil (a) before meals and (b) when food cravings came. Participants were asked not to alter their normal eating habits and not to try to diet. The study lasted 6 weeks. The mandarin group had average weight loss of 2.4 pounds. The lavender group had average weight loss of 5.3 pounds. The control group had average weight loss of 1.2 pounds.

Herring (2006) chose fennel *(Foeniculum vulgare)* for her study. Her 21 volunteers were people who had been trying unsuccessfully to reduce their carbohydrate intake and thus lower their weight. Volunteers were randomly allocated to the experimental or control group. The experimental group applied diluted 3% fennel to their wrists three times a day. (In addition, they could also apply it prn.) The study lasted 2 weeks. Participants recorded the number of times they applied the fennel mixture and rated their cravings on a 0 to 10 scale. Weight was recorded at the beginning and end of the study. It appeared that as applications of the fennel increased so craving decreased. There was no correlation between the control group application and craving. The average weight loss was 3.51 pounds in the fennel group and 2.81 pounds in the control group.

Sleeping Pill and Benzodiazepine Addiction

According to the British Freedom of Information Act, in 2011 approximately 15.3 million sleeping pill prescriptions were handed out by the NHS at a cost to the UK government of nearly £50 million. The most popular sleeping pill was zopiclone. It was prescribed to more than 5.2 million patients nationally, making it the most popular sleeping tablet. In the United States, 1 in 10 Americans take sleeping pills. Insomnia has a chapter dedicated to it in this book, so suffice to go straight to the protocol to enable patients to get off sleeping pills (Box 15-1).

Benzodiazepine addiction has the same protocol. There is a nice Japanese piece of research in the literature (Komori et al 2006) that used a very similar protocol. Forty-two outpatients from Department of Psychiatry, Mie University Graduate School of Medicine took part in the study. Initially, participants were asked to try and reduce their benzodiazepine dose by 25% per week, without any essential oils: 29 subjects failed. These patients were then invited to retry, using essential oils. Participants inhaled a mixture of sandalwood (35%), juniper berry (12%), rose (8%) and orris (6%). Twenty-six out of 29 reduced their dose and 12 managed to come off the drug completely.

DEPRESSION

The number of people taking antidepressant drugs in the Western world has increased exponentially. According to the Center for Disease Control and Prevention (CDC), the increase is 400% since 1998. However, some people may confuse being depressed with what is really an inability to cope, or loneliness. In the words of Patch Adams, a medical doctor who is also a famous clown (1997), "Prozac has replaced a hug." It is in this shadowy area of mild depression where aromatherapy may help. Although all the hi-tech advances in the world cannot rewire the brain, something as simple as an essential oil may enable the brain to reregulate itself (Alexander 2001).

There are been several published studies on aromatherapy and depression in humans: Table 15-4. Most of these studies have involved massage. Most of them have looked at depression as a symptom of a specific illness such as cancer or in hospice patients. There is a lack of evidence for using inhaled essential oils in depression in a clinical way. This is surprising as it has been shown that inhaled aroma has a rapid effect on mood and this effect is measurable by EEG (Diego et al 1998). Itai et al's study (2000) concluded that inhaled aroma was an effective, noninvasive way of treating depression. Perry and Perry (2006) wrote in their review of aromatherapy in mental health that there were some promising results and suggested concentrating on inhaled aromas studies for depression. Van der Watt also asks for more inhalation studies to support the use of aromatherapy in mental healthcare (2008). Dobetsberger and Buchbauer (2010), several years later, state that research proves that essential oils can influence the central nervous system, but again calls for more research.

TABLE 15-4 *Published Articles on Depression in Humans*

Author	Year	Number	Depression	Essential Oil	Method	Result
Kite et al	1998	58	Oncology	Various	T	+ve
Louise & Kowalski	2002	17	Hospice	Lavender	I	+ve
Graham et al	2003	313	Radiotherapy	Lavender, bergamot, cedarwood	I	-ve
Soden et al	2004	42	Hospice	Lavender	T	+ve
Kim et al	2005	40	Arthritis	Mixture*	T	+ve
Lee & Lee	2006	42	College students	Lavender	T	+ve
Wilkinson et al	2007	288	Oncology	Various	T	+ve[†]
De Watt et al	2008	Review	Various	Various	I	+ve
Yim et al	2009	Review	Various	Various	T	+ve

+ve, positive; -ve, negative.
*A mixture of lavender, marjoram, eucalyptus, rosemary and peppermint in the ratio 2:1:2:1:1.
[†]Positive at 6 weeks but not at 10 weeks.

Clearly, inhaled essential oils for depression would be an exciting area of study. It would also be interesting to explore how an inhaled essential oil might impact a conventional antidepressant drug. It would be possible to add ambient aroma to psychotherapy counseling and give the patient the same aroma to inhale on a regular basis to measure if this enhanced the therapy session. Another idea would be to use the individual aroma pouches that are now available or to explore the impact of using a diffuser at night on prn medication.

Essential oils applied topically (but without massage) have also been shown to affect mood. Hongratanaworakit and Buchbauer (2006) found that ylang ylang applied to the skin had a relaxing effect. Two years earlier, these two scientists had evaluated the effect of ylang ylang when inhaled (Hongratanaworakit & Buchbauer 2004).

Depression has been linked to the inability to give up smoking in a Korean study (Kim et al 2013), so inhaling a mixture of specific essential oils could be an excellent way to reduce both depression and smoking.

Okomoto et al (2005) explored the effect of aromatherapy massage on mild depression. Five patients (aged 31 to 59) who had a diagnosis of depression took part in the study. No patient was taking antidepressants or receiving psychotherapy. Each patient was given a 30-minute aromatherapy massage with a mixture of essential oils (geranium, basil and sweet orange) twice a week for 4 weeks (eight massages in total). Outcome measures were Hamilton Depression Rating (HDR) scale and Profile of Mood (POM) scale. The measures were taken before the first session and after the eighth session. Data was examined using Wilcoxin matched pairs test. Ham score and the confusion-bewilderment (C-B) score that are part of POMs were significantly improved (P = 0.039 and 0.043, respectively). This suggests that there was both subjective and objective improvement.

Bipolar Disorder

"Bipolar disorder is responsible for the loss of more disability-adjusted life years (DALYs) than all forms of cancer, or than major neurologic conditions such as epilepsy and Alzheimer's disease" (Merinkangas et al 2011). The incidence of bipolar disorder appears to be increasing. This could be because there is more, or because it is recognized and diagnosed more often. There are different intensities of bipolar. The NIMH (National Institute of Mental Health) defines these as:

Bipolar 2 Disorder: pattern of depressive episodes shifting back and forth with hypomanic episodes, but no full-blown manic or mixed episodes.

Bipolar 1 Disorder: mainly defined by manic or mixed episodes that last at least 7 days, or by severe manic symptoms that require immediate hospital care.

Approximately 2.5 million Americans are diagnosed with bipolar disorder. The United States has the highest lifetime and 12-month prevalence of bipolar (bipolar 1 = 4.4%, bipolar 2 = 2.8%) while India has the lowest (0.1%,) for both categories (Merinkangas et al 2011). Bipolar disorder can cause serious problems with work, social life, and relationships unless the person is stabilized with drugs and psychotherapy (Maiera 2012).

There is a distinct lack of information about the use of aromatherapy in bipolar disorder (Andreescu et al 2008) and there is no suggestion that anyone with bipolar disorder should come off their stabilizing drugs. However, aromas may prove useful as an adjunctive therapy. Hardy et al (2012) found the sense of smell was heightened during the depressive stage of bipolar disorder, and reduced during the manic stage (P = 0.024). They tested 64 people (20 with bipolar disorder and 44 controls).

Originally named manic-depression, bipolar disorder was discovered by German psychiatrist Emil Kraepelin after carefully observing many patients in the nineteenth century (Zivanovic & Nedic 2012). Kraepelin found patients had spontaneous remission of symptoms that could last for months or years before relapsing. The patients who had suffered episodic periods of illness in their 20s were more likely to have them in their 40s. Bipolar disorder is a relapsing illness that may recur more frequently as the patient ages. Bipolar disorder is thought to run in families, and chromosome 18 is thought to be the gene responsible (Stine et al 1995, Mulle et al 2007, Howrigan et al 2011).

Conventional drug treatment is with lithium and divalproex (Depakote). However, they both have significant side effects. The National Institutes of Mental Health states that people with bipolar disorder often have thyroid gland problems but lithium treatment may also cause low thyroid levels. It also states that divalproex (sometimes called valproic acid) can increase levels of testosterone in teenage girls and lead to polycystic ovaries if medication commences before age 20.

BOX 15-2 *Commonly Used Medications for Bipolar Disorder: Benefits and Common Side Effects*

Lithium	Pure mania, history of depression, family history of bipolar disorder, previous favorable response to lithium, few previous episodes, full relief between symptoms	May correct chemical imbalance in brains' transmission of nerve impulses that influence mood and behavior	Weight gain, dry mouth, confusion, poor concentration, shakiness, tremor, increased urination
Depakote	Mixed mania, nonfavorable response to lithium, mood swings, adverse effects less severe, attention deficit hyperactivity disorder, substance abuse	Increases gamma aminobutyric acid, which inhibits nerve transmission to parts of the brain	Loss of appetite, nausea, diarrhea, tremor, unusual weight gain (or loss), menstrual changes
Carbamazepine	No family history of bipolar disorder, bipolar disorder is a secondary condition, lack of response to other medication	Analgesic, anticonvulsant	Dizziness, blurred vision, headaches, back-and-forth eye movement (nystogmus)

The anticonvulsant lamotrigine (Lamictal) has recently been approved for bipolar disease (Box 15-2).

Many neurologic problems are a function of altered brain pattern and a change in neurochemicals. The human body is controlled by extremely delicate mechanisms that rely on hormonal and chemical communication. Each person has a slightly different body chemistry that requires different things to achieve homeostasis. Like herbs, essential oils are therapeutically multifaceted. Therefore, the components within an essential oil may produce a different reaction in one person than in another, depending on the availability of receptor sites (Mills 1991). For example, an essential oil may work to reduce blood pressure (acting as a hypotensor) if that is what is required for homeostasis, or it may not if the blood pressure is normal for that person. When a plant has the ability to change function it is called adaptogenic. Many essential oils also have a balancing effect on the emotions.

Various antipsychotic agents have antagonistic interactions toward a whole selection of receptor sites including serotoninic, adrenergic, and histaminic. Therefore their ongoing effects on the autonomic nervous system are complex and unpredictable (Alexander 2001). This is the case with each of the hundreds of components in essential oils that interact with many receptor sites. While antidepressants work by making the neurotransmitter serotonin linger in the gaps between brain cells, essential oils are thought to work as serotonin agonists, which can push the serotonin system into overdrive. This makes the brain more sensitive, rather like turning up the volume on a radio so very weak stations can be heard.

BOX 15-3 *Essential Oils That May Be Useful in Bipolar Disorder*

Common Name	Botanical Name
Geranium	*Pelargonium graveolens*
Lavender	*Lavandula angustifolia*
Sandalwood	*Santalum album*
Angelica root	*Angelica archangelica*
Rose	*Rosa damascena*
Patchouli	*Pogostemon cablin*
Ylang ylang	*Cananga odorata* var. *genuina*
Valerian	*Valeriana fauriei*
Vetiver	*Vetiveria zizanoides*
Spikenard	*Nardostachys jatamansi*
Melissa	*Melissa officinalis*
Bergamot	*Citrus bergamia*
Clary sage	*Salvia sclarea*

BOX 15-4 *Essential Oils to Avoid in Bipolar Disorder*

Essential Oil	Suspect Component	Amount (approximate)
White camphor	Camphor	30%-50%
Hyssop	Pinocamphone	70%
Nutmeg	Myristicin	3%-14%
	Elemicin	0.1%-4.6%
Pennyroyal	Pulegone	55%-95%
Tansy	Thujone	66%-81%

I want to emphasize that there is no suggestion that patients with bipolar disorder should give up medication in favor of aromatherapy.

There is little if anything published on bipolar disorder and aromatherapy. However, essential oils may enhance orthodox medication so dosages may be kept sufficiently low and thus reduce side effects. However, a few psychiatric nurses (who were my students) have had some success with stabilizing patients using aromatherapy. As these were case studies it is difficult to say whether the patients' stability would have happened anyway. Other case studies by psychiatric nurses have indicated aromatherapy may help reduce the level of orthodox medication and still retain stability. Box 15-3 lists recommended essential oils and Box 15-4 details essential oils to avoid.

Stress exacerbates the number of relapses with bipolar disorder (type 2). Psychotherapy has been shown to reduce the number of relapses and improve the quality of life of these patients (Maiera 2012). A psychotherapy session may be a safe situation where a set aromatherapy ritual or protocol could be worked out with the patient. The aromas would be experienced for the first time in a stable, calm, balanced situation, with supervision. The protocol would include what essential oil(s) to use, when, where, and how, and this could form part of the therapy. When this pattern is well established, the essential oils could be experienced in the patient's own setting. This is akin to preparing a "psychological comfort blanket." This setting of a psychological trigger is similar to Bett's research (1994) with epilepsy. He found massage with ylang ylang set a precedent so strong, that ultimately, patients had only to think about the aroma of ylang ylang to prevent a seizure occurring. Perhaps psychotherapy for bipolar patients could be underpinned by scent (in the form of essential oils) in a similar way?

REFERENCES

Abramovitz E, Lichtenberg P. 2009. Hypnotherapeutic olfactory conditioning (HOC): case-studies of needle phobia, pain disorder and combat-induced PTSD. *Int J Clinical Experimental Hypnosis.* 57(2):184–187.

Alexander M. 2001. *How Aromatherapy Works.* Odessa, FL: Whole Spectrum Books.

Andreescu C, Mulsant B, Emanuel J. 2008. Complementary and alternative medicine in the treatment of bipolar disorder—a review of the evidence. *J Affect Disord.* 110(1-2):16–26.

Barrett D. 2002. Aromatherapy to alleviate addiction withdrawal in hospitalised patients. RJBA unpublished dissertation.

Benton 2010. The plausibility of sugar addiction and its role in obesity and eating disorders *Clin Nutrition.* 29(3):288–303.

Biesecker B. 2011. Black pepper for nicotine withdrawal. Unpublished dissertation for RJ Buckle Associates.

Buchbauer G, Jirovetz L 1994. Aromatherapy—use of fragrances and essential oils as medicants, *Flav Frag J.* 9:217–222.

Burnett K, Solterbeck L, Strapp C. 2004. Scent and mood state following an anxiety-provoking task. *Psychol Rep.* 95(2):707–722.

Butje A, Repede E, Shattell M. 2008. Healing scents: An overview of clinical aromatherapy for emotional distress. *Journal of Psychosocial Nursing.* 46(10):46–52.

Caldwell N. 2001. Effects of ylang ylang on cravings of women with substance abuse: RJBA unpublished dissertation.

Capps B, Hall W, Carter A. 2012. *Encyclopedia of Applied Ethics (Second Edition), Pages 21.*

Carino E. 2003. Bergamot for alcohol withdrawal. Unpublished dissertation for RJ Buckle Associates.

Caston V. 1998. Aristotle and the problem of intentionality. *Philosophy and Phenomenological Research.* 58(2):249–298.

Chalifour M. Peppermint in opiate-withdrawal in a locked hospital unit. Unpublished dissertation for RJ Buckle Associates.

Charleton C. 1999. Roman chamomile for post-natal depression. Unpublished dissertation for RJ Buckle Associates.

Cordell B. 2004. Effects of aromatherapy on nicotine withdrawal. RJBA Unpublished dissertation.

Cordell B, Buckle J. 2012. The effects of aromatherapy on nicotine craving on a US campus: a small comparison study. *J Alt Comp Med.* 19(8):709–713.

Costa CA, Kohn DO, de Lima VM, Gargano AC, Flório JC, Costa M. 2011. The GABAergic system contributes to the anxiolytic-like effect of essential oil from Cymbopogon citratus (lemongrass). *J Ethnopharmacol.* 137(1):828–36

DaCosta R. 2000. Angelica, helicrysum and lavender for nicotine withdrawal. Unpublished dissertation for RJ Buckle Associates.

Degenhardt L, Chiu W, Sampson N, Kessler R, Anthony J. 2008. Towards a global view of alcohol, tobacco, cannabis and cocaine use: findings from WHO World Mental Surveys. *PLoS Med.* 5(7):e141.

De Watt G, Janca A. 2008. Aromatherapy in nursing and mental health care. *J Austr Prof.* 30(1): 69–75.

Diego M, Jones N, Field T, Hernandez-Reif M, Schanberg S et al. 1998. Aromatherapy positively affects mood, EEG patterns of alertness and math computations. *Int J Neurosci*. 96(3-4):217–224.

Dobetsberger C. Buchbauer G. 2010. Actions of essential oils on the central nervous system: an undated review. *Flav Frag J*. 26:300–316.

Dodd G, Van Toller S. 1983. The biology and psychology of perfumery. *Perfumer & Flavorist*. 8:1–14.

Douek E. 1988. Abnormalities of smell. In Van Toller S, Dodd G (eds.), *Perfumery: The Psychology and Biology of Fragrance*. London: Chapman and Hall, xvii-3.

Drumm 2006. Angelica and helicrysum for nicotine withdrawal in a Mental Health hospital. Bergamot for alcohol withdrawal. Unpublished dissertation for RJ Buckle Associates.

Ernst E. 2012. Alternative Detox. *Br Med Bull*.101:33–8.

Esse K, Fossati-Bellani M, Traylor A, Martin-Schild S. 2011. Epidemic of illicit drug use, mechanisms of action/addiction and stroke as a health hazard. *Brain Behav*. 1(1):44–54.

Fortuna J. 2012. The obesity epidemic and food addiction: clinical similarities to drug dependence. *J Psychoactive Drugs*. 44(1):56–63.

Fowler N. 2004. Aromatherapy for Crisis Management in hospitalized adolescents. RJBA Unpublished dissertation.

Fowler N. 2006. Aromatherapy, used as an integrative tool for crisis management by adolescents in a residential treatment center. *J Child Adoles Psych Nursing*, 19:69–76.

Fukada M, Kano E, Miyoshi M, Komaki R, Watanabe T. 2011. Effect of rose essential oil inhalation on stress-induced skin-barrier disruption in rats and humans. *Chem Senses*. 37(4):347–56.

Gietzen D, Rogers Q. 2006. Nutritional homeostasis and indispensable amino acid sensing: A new solution to an old puzzle. *Trends Neurosci*. 29(2):91–99.

Graham P, Browne L, Cox H, Graham J. 2003. Inhalation aromatherapy during radiotherapy, results of a placebo-controlled double-blind randomized trial. *J Clin Oncol*. 21(12):2372–6.

Gryniewski 2005. Angelica in nicotine withdrawal. Bergamot for alcohol withdrawal. Unpublished dissertation for RJ Buckle Associates.

Hardy C, Rosedale M, Messinger J, Kleinhaus K, Aujero N et al. 2012. Olfactory acuity is associated with mood and function in a pilot study of stable bipolar disorder patients. *Bipolar Disord*. 14(1):109–17.

Herring. 2006. RJBA. Aromatherapy to reduce food craving. RJBA Unpublished dissertation.

Hirata K, Tanaka H, Arai M et al. 2002. The cerebral blood flow change by fragrance: an evaluation using near-infrared spectroscopic topography. *Japan J Pharmaco-EEG*. 4:43–47.

Hongratanaworakit T, Buchbauer G. 2004. Evaluation of the harmonizing effect of ylang ylang oil on humans after inhalation. *Plant Med 2004*. 70(7):632–6.

Hongratanaworakit T, Buchbauer G. 2006. Relaxing effect of ylang ylang oil on humans after transdermal absorption. *Phytother Res*. 20(9):758–63.

Hood. 2005. RJBA Aromatherapy to reduce food craving. Unpublished dissertation.

Howrigan D, Laird N, Smoller J, Devlin B, McQueen M. 2011. Using linkage information to weight a genome-wide association of bipolar disorder. *Am J Med Genet B Neuropsychiatr Genet*. 156B(4):462–71.

Irani S, Thomasius M, Schmid-Mahler C, Holzmann D, Goetzmann L et al. 2010. Olfactory performance before and after lung transplantation: quantitative assessment and impact on quality of life. *J Heart Lung Transplant*. 29(3):265–72.

Itai T, Amayasu H, Kuribayashi M, Kawamura N, Okada M et al. 2000. Psychological effects of aromatherapy on chronic hemodialysis patients. *Psychiatry Clin Neuroscience*. 54(4):393–7

Ito N, Nagai T, Oikawa T, Yamada H, Hanawa T. 2007. Antidepressant-like effect of l-perillaldehyde in stress-induced depression-like model mice through regulation of the olfactory nervous system. *Evidence-Based Complementary and Alternative Medicine*. 2011;2011:512697.

Kane 2004. Petitgrain for depression in cardiac rehabilitation. Unpublished dissertation for RJ Buckle Associates.

Karimzadeh F, Hosseini M, Mangeng D, Alavi H, Hassanzadeh G et al. 2012. Anticonvulsant and neuroprotective effects of Pimpinella anisum in rat brain. *BMC Complement Altern Med*. 18;12:76.

Katseres J. 2011. Black pepper and lavender for nicotine withdrawal. Unpublished dissertation for RJ Buckle Associates.

Kim M, Nam E, Paik S. 2005. The effects of aromatherapy on pain, depression and life satisfaction of arthritis patients. *Daehan Ganho Hagheji.* 35(1):186–94

Kim J, In S, Choi H, Lee S. 2012. Illegal use of benzodiazepines and/or zolpidem proved by hair analysis. *J Forensic Sci.* 27. doi:10.1111/1556-4029.12034. Accessed 4/1/2013.

Kim S, Park J, Lee J, Lee S, Kim T et al. 2013. Smoking in elderly Koreans: prevalence and factors associated with smoking cessation. *Arch Gerontol Geriatr.*56(1):214–9.

King J. 1988. Anxiety reduction using fragrances. In Van Toller S, Dodd G (eds.), Perfumery: The Psychology and Biology of Fragrance. London: Chapman and Hall, 147–167.

Kite S, Maher E, Anderson K, Young T, Young J et al. 1998. Development of an aromatherapy service at a cancer centre. *Palliative Medicine.* 12(3):171–180.

Komiya M, Takeuchi T, Hareda E. 2006. Lemon oil vapor causes an anti-stress effect via modulating the 5-HT and DA activities in mice. *Behav Brain Res.* 25;172(2):240–9.

Komori T, Matsumoto T, Yamamoto M, Motomura E, Shiroyama T, Okazaki Y. 2006. Application of fragrance in discontinuing the long-term use of hypnotic benzodiazepines. *Int J Aromatherapy.* 16(1):3–7.

Koszwoski B, Goniewicz M, Cgogala J. 2005. Alternative methods of nicotine dependence treatment. *Przegl Lek.* 62(10):1176–9.

Krieger S. 2010. Mandarin for depression in children. Unpublished dissertation for RJ Buckle Associates.

Kunz S, Schultz M, Lewitzky M, Driessen M, Rau H. 2007. Ear acupuncture for alcohol withdrawal in comparison with aromatherapy: a randomized, controlled trial. *Alcoholism: Clin Exp Res.* 31(3): 436–42.

Lake J. 2000. Psychotropic medications from natural products: a review of promising research and recommendations. *Alt Therap Health Med.* 6(3):36–60.

Lee I, Lee G. 2006. Effects of lavender on insomnia and depression in women college students. *Daehan Ganho Hagheji.* 36(1): 136–143.

Lenoir M, Serre F, Cantin L, Ahmed S. 2007. Intense sweetness surpasses cocaine reward. *PLoS One.* 1;2(8):e698. Accessed 14/1/2013.

Li X, Sun H, Marsh D, Anis A. 2008. Factors associated with seeking readmission among clients admitted to medical withdrawal management. *Subst Abus.* 29(4):65–72.

Louise M, Kolowski S. 2002. Use of aromatherapy with hospice patients to decrease pain, anxiety and depression and to promote an increased sense of wellbeing. *Am J Hospice Palliative Medicine.* 19(6):381–6.

MacMahon E. 2003. Angelica and black pepper for nicotine withdrawal. Unpublished dissertation for RJ Buckle Associates.

Madruga C, Laranjeira R, Caetano R, Pinksy I, Zaleski M, Ferri C. 2012. Use of licit and illicit substances among adolescents in Brazil—a national survey. *Addict Behav.* 37(10):1171–5.

Maiera E. 2012. Psychopharmacological treatment and psychoeducational management in bipolar disease. *Psychiatr Danube.* 24 Suppl 1:S56–8.

Manchikanti L, Helm S 2nd, Fellows B, Janata J, Pampati V et al. 2012. Opioid epidemic in the United States. *Pain Physician.* 15(3 Suppl):ES9–38.

Martine J. 2002. Bergamot for Seasonal Affective Disorder. Unpublished dissertation for RJ Buckle Associates.

McAvoy B. 2008. Addiction and addiction medicine: exploring opportunities for the general practitioner. *Med J Aust.* 21;189(2):115–7.

McCormick E. 2013. Personal communication.

Merikangas K, McClair V. 2012. Epidemiology of substance use disorders. *Hum Genet.* 131(6):779–89.

Merinkangas K, Jin R, Jian-Ping H, Kessler R, Sing L. 2011. Prevalence and Correlates of Bipolar Spectrum Disorder in the World Mental Health Survey Initiative. *Arch Gen Psychiatry.* 68(3):241–251.

Mills S. 1991. *Out of the Earth.* London: Viking Arkana.

Moncrieff R. 1966. *Odor Preferences.* New York: Wiley.

Moncrieff R. 1977. Emotional response to odors. *Soap, Perfumery and Cosmetics.* 50:24–25.

Mulle J, Fallin M, Lasseter V, McGrath J, Wolyniec P. 2007. Dense SNP association study for bipolar I disorder on chromosome 18p11 suggests two loci with excess paternal transmission. *Mol Psychiatry.* 12(4):367–75

Mura P, Saussereau E, Brunet B, Goullé J. 2012. Workplace testing of drugs of abuse and psychotropic drugs. *Ann Farm Fr.* 70(3):120–32.

Neville K, Haberly L. 2004. Olfactory cortex. In: Shepherd G.M., editor. *In The Synaptic Organization of the Brain.* New York: Oxford University Press; pp. 415–54

Newsham G. 2001. Lavender plus acupuncture for nicotine withdrawal. Unpublished dissertation for RJ Buckle Associates.

Nightingale C, Rudnicka A, Owen C, Cook D, Whincup P. 2011. Patterns of body size and adiposity among UK children of South Asian, black African-Caribbean and white European origin: Child Heart and Health Study in England (CHASE Study). *Int J Epidemiol.* 40(1):33–44.

Norte M, Cosentino R, Lazarini C. 2005. Effects of methyl-eugenol administration on behavioral models related to depression and anxiety, in rats. *Phytomedicine.* 12(4):294–8.

Okamoto A, Kuriyama H, Watanabe S, Aihara Y, Tadai T, Imanishi J, Fukui J. 2005. The effect of aromatherapy massage on mild depression: a pilot study. *Psych Clin Neurosci.* 59: 363.

O'Neil J. Jan. 2001. Smells used to explore schizophrenia. www.schizophrenia.com.

Paine S. 2008. Black pepper for nicotine withdrawal. Unpublished dissertation for RJ Buckle Associates.

Perl E, Shufman E, Vas A et al. 1997. Taste and odor reactivity in heroin addicts. *Israel J Psych Related Sci.* 34(4) 290–299.

Perry N and Perry E. 2006. Aromatherapy in the management of psychiatric disorders: clinical and neuropharmacological perspectives. *CNS Drugs* 20(4):257–280.

Pickover C. 1998. *Strange Brains and Genius.* New York: Plenum.

Polsky D, Glick H, Yang J, Subramaniam G, Poole S, Woody G. 2010. Cost-effectiveness of extended buprenorphine-naloxone treatment for opioid-dependent youth: data from a randomized trial. *Addiction.* 105(9):1616–24.

Praveen KT, Law F, O'Shea J, Melichar J. 2011. Opioid Dependence. *Clin Evid (Online).* Sep 20;2011. doi:pii:1015. PMID: 21929827. Accessed Jan 4, 2013.

Rahman S. 2011. Brain Nicotinic Receptors as Emerging Targets for Drug Addiction: Neurobiology to Translational Research. *Prog Molec Biol Transl Sci,* 98:349–365.

Romero M. 2006. Angelica for nicotine withdrawal.

Rose J, Behm F. 1994. Inhalation of vapor from black pepper extract reduces smoking withdrawal symptoms. *Drug and Alcohol Dependence.* 34(3) 225–229.

Saddoris M, Sugam J, Cacciapaglia F, Carelli R. 2013. Rapid dopamine dynamics in the accumbens core and shell: Learning and action. *Front Biosci (Elite Ed).*1(5):273–88.

Schecklmann M, Schwenck C, Taurines R, Freitag C, Warnke A. 2013. A systematic review on olfaction in child and adolescent psychiatric disorders. *J Neural Transm.* 120(1):121–30.

Schwartz R, Estroff T, Fairbanks D et al. 1998. Nasal symptoms associated with cocaine abuse during adolescence. *Archives of Otolaryngology-Head & Neck Surgery.* 115(1) 63–64.

Seyette M, Parrott D. 1999. Effects of olfactory stimuli on urge reduction in smokers. *Experimental and Clinical Psychopharmacology.* 7(2) 151–159.

Shah N, Lathrop S, Reichard R, Landen M. 2008 Unintentional drug overdose death trends in New Mexico, USA, 1990-2005: combinations of heroin, cocaine, prescription opioids and alcohol. *Addiction* 103(1):126–136.

Shear P, Butters N, Jernigan T et al. 1992. Olfactory loss in alcoholics: correlations with cortical and subcortical MRI indices. *Alcohol.* 9(3) 247–255.

Shepherd G. 2010. New Perspectives on Olfactory Processing and Human Smell in *The Neurobiology of Olfaction.* Menini A. (Ed). Boca Raton: CRC Press.

Shepherd G. 2011. *Neurogastronomy: How the Brain Creates Flavor and Why It Matters.* New York: Columbia University Press..

Shriner R. 2012. Food addiction: Detox and abstinence reinterpreted? *Exp Gerantol.* pii: S0531–5565(12)00318-X. doi:10.1016/j.exger.2012.12.005. Accessed 14/1/203.

Sirignano L. 2011. Helicrysum and black pepper for nicotine withdrawal. Unpublished dissertation for RJ Buckle Associates.

Smeets M, Veldhuizen M, Galle S, Gouweloos J, de Haan A et al. 2009. Sense of smell disorder and health-related quality of life. *Rehab Psychol.* 54(4):404–12.

Smith K, Sines J. 1960. Demonstration of a peculiar odor in the sweat of schizophrenic patients. *Archives of General Psychiatry.* 2:184.

Soden K, Vincent K, Craske S, Lucas C, Ashley S. 2004. A randomized controlled trial of aromatherapy massage in a hospice setting. *Palliative Medicine.* 18(2):87–92.

Stine O, Xu J, Koskela R, et al. 1995. Evidence for linkage of bipolar disorder to chromosome 18 with a parent-or-origin effect. *Am J Human Genetics.* 57(6) 1384–1394.

Sugano H. 1992. Psychophysical studies of fragrances. In Dodd G, Van Toller S (eds.), *Fragrance: The Psychology and Biology of Perfume.* London: Elsevier Science, 227.

Templeton J. 2002. Bergamot for depression of no specific aetiology. Unpublished dissertation for RJ Buckle Associates.

Thorsten F, Kissler J, Moratti S, Vienbruch C, Rochstroh B. 2001. Source distribution of neuromagnetic slow waves and MEG-delta activity in schizophrenic patients. Biological Psychiatry. 50(2):108–116.

Tisserand R. 1988. Essential oils as psychotherapeutic agents. In Van Toller S, Dodd G (eds.), *Perfumery: The Psychology and Biology of Fragrance.* London: Chapman and Hall, 167–180.

Torii S, Fukada H, Kanemoto H et al. 1988. Contingent negative variation (CNV) and the psychological effects of odor. In Van Toller S, Dodd G (eds.), *Perfumery: The Psychology and Biology of Fragrance.* London: Chapman and Hall, 107–118.

Uehleke B, Schaper S, Dienel A, Schlaefke S, Stange R. 2012. Phase II trial on the effects of Silexan in patients with neurasthenia, post-traumatic stress disorder or somatization disorder. *Phytomedicine.*19(8–9):665-71.

Van der Watt G, Janca A. 2008. Aromatherapy in nursing and mental health care. *Contemporary Nurse.* 30(1):69–71.

Walker A. 2007. Angelica for nicotine withdrawal. Unpublished dissertation for RJ Buckle Associates.

Wang K, Cheng M, Hsieh C, Hsu J, Wu J, Lee C. 2012. Determination of nimetazepam and 7-aminonimetazepam in human urine by using liquid chromatography-tandem mass spectrometry. *Forensic Sci Int.* Dec 11. doi:pii:S0379-0738(12)00516-6.10.1016/j.forsciint.2012.11.001. Accessed 4/1/2013.

Warner M, Chen L, Makuc D, Anderson R, Miniño A. 2011. Drug poisoning deaths in the United States, 1980-2008. *NCHS Data Brief.* 81):1–8.

West L. 2003. Angelica, helicrysum and German chamomile for nicotine withdrawal. Unpublished dissertation for RJ Buckle Associates.

Wiener H. 1966. External chemical messengers I. *New York State Journal of Medicine.* 66:3153.

Wilson D, Linster C. 2008. Neurobiology of a simple memory. *J Neurophysiol.* 100(1):2–7.

Wilkinson S, Love S, Westcombe A, Gambles M Burgess C et al. 2007. Effectiveness of aromatherapy massage in the management of anxiety and depression in patients with cancer: a multicenter, randomized, controlled trial. *J Clinical Oncology.* 25(5): 532–539.

Yeshurun Y, Sobel N. 2010. An odor is not worth a thousand words: from multidimensional odors to unidimensional odor objects. *Annu Rev Psychol.* 61:219–41.

Yim V, Ng A, Tsan H, Leung A. 2009. A review of the effects of aromatherapy for patients with depressive symptoms. *J Alternative Complementary Med.* 15(2):187–95.

Zhao R, Koo B, Kim G, Jang E, Lee J et al. 2005. The essential oil from Angelica gigas NAKAI suppresses nicotine sensitization. *Biol Pharm Bull.* 28(12):2323–6.

Zivanovic O, Nedic A. 2012. Kraepelin's concept of manic-depressive insanity: one hundred years later. *J Affect Disord.* 137(1-3):15–24

Chapter **16**

Oncology

Better to light one small candle than to curse the darkness.

Buddha

An estimate of the prevalence of cancer worldwide (measured over a 5-year period) was 28.8 million in 2008 (Bray et al 2013). Almost half of those with cancer lived in highly developed areas. Breast cancer was the most common overall. Prostate cancer was most prevalent in the United States and Europe. Stomach cancer was most prevalent in Asia, notably in China. Cervical cancer was most prevalent in Africa and parts of Asia. The incidence of oral cancer was highest in India. More than 3.5 million nonmelanoma skin cancers were treated in 2006 (Fleming et al 2013). The incidence of human papillomavirus (HPV) is increasing and has been identified as a precursor to cancer (Forman et al 2012). However, more people die from lung cancer in the United States than any other type of cancer (CDC 2013). In the United States in 2009, 205,974 people were diagnosed with lung cancer, and 158,081 people died from it (USCS—United States Cancer Statistics 2013). In the UK in 2010, there were 157,275 deaths from cancer overall (Cancer Research UK 2013). The predicted number of deaths from cancer within the European Union in 2013 is 1,314,296 (737,747 men and 576,489 women) (Malvezzi et al 2013).

The cost of treatment for cancer varies according to the site of the cancer, but in fee-paying countries the patient is often faced with worryingly large bills. For example, the cost of treating pancreatic cancer was estimated as $65,500 per person (O'Neill et al 2012) and an estimate of the cost of breast cancer treatment (over a lifetime) ranged from $US20,000 to $US100,000 (Campbell & Ramsey 2009). Prevention can be as expensive as treatment. Goulart et al (2012) state that the cost of screening to avoid one lung cancer death is $240,000.

The possible causes of cancer are many and range from electromagnetic (Hardell & Sage 2008) or chemical pollution (Poirier 2012) to genetic predisposition (Fleming et al 2013) and severe psychological stress (Cabaniols et al 2011). Many cancer patients suffer symptoms such as pain, nausea, and emotional distress that conventional medicine is unable to treat satisfactorily. Recently, it was found that some cancer cells have become drug resistant (He et al 2013). Cancer has been around for a million years; traces of it were found in mummies from the Great Pyramid at Giza (Lewis & Elvin-Lewis 1977). Humans do not have a monopoly on the disease, as higher-order animals also suffer from cancer.

The three main orthodox treatments for cancer are surgery, radiation, and chemotherapy. These treatments save lives but can be hard to endure—some patients saying the treatment is worse than the cancer it is supposed to treat. Cancer-drug research has had its share of bad publicity. In 2008, four Italian academics analyzed all the randomized clinical trials on cancer treatments that had been published during the previous 11 years and that were stopped early (Goldacre 2012). Eighty-six percent of the trials that were stopped early were to bring a new cancer drug on to the market. A review published in the *Journal of the American Medical Association* (*JAMA*) found that 100 clinical trials had been stopped early to show the test drug in the most positive light and that the effects of the drug were consequently overstated (Bassler et al 2010).

AROMATHERAPY AND CANCER TREATMENT

Plant materials have been used to treat malignant diseases for centuries. It is fascinating how the same plants are cited all over the world for the treatment of cancer. For example, Dr. Fell completed a study of 25 cases of breast cancer using the herb bloodwort at the Middlesex Hospital in London in 1857. He chose bloodwort (*Sanguinaria canadensis*) because it had been used by American Indians. Fell found that all his cases went into remission (Fell 1857). It is difficult to establish whether this really happened, although *Sanguinaria* also has a long history of use in Russia for the treatment of cancer (Lewis & Elvin-Lewis 1977).

Madagascan periwinkle *(Catharanthus roseus)* contains the alkaloids vinblastine and vincristine that have been useful in treating cancer (Dewick 1989). However, recently some renal carcinoma cells have become vinblastine resistant (Long et al 2013) and some laryngeal cancers are now vincristine resistant (Yin et al 2013). Interestingly, some plants can enhance the effect of conventional anticancer drugs on resistant cancer cells. For example, curcumin reverses the multidrug resistance of human colon cancer cells in vitro and in vivo (Lu et al 2013).

Ironically, the uses of plants and plant extracts are now called "novel approaches" (Park et al 2012). Indeed, a search on PubMed using the words *antitumor drug* and *herb* produced 203 hits. These include honokiol from magnolia (Zheng et al 2013), corilagin from *Phyllanthus niruri* (Jia et al 2013) and fenugreek (Al-Daghri et al 2012).

Some essential oils, or components found within essential oils, have been found to have antitumoral activity. An in vitro cytotoxicity assay (using MTT— microtube-targeting) indicated that the essential oil of *Melissa officinalis* was very effective against a series of human cancer cell lines (A549, MCF-7, Caco-2, HL-60, K562) (de Sousa et al 2004). Sclareol, a diterpenol in *Salvia sclarea* (clary sage), was found to kill cell lines of human leukemia and had an inhibitory concentration of lower than 20 µg/mL (Dimas et al 1999). Recent research found sclareol reduced tumor size and enhanced the effect of cancer therapy (Noori et al 2013). Delora et al (1994) found myrrh had an anticarcinogenic effect on tumors induced in mice. Recent Chinese research found that sesquiterpenoids from myrrh inhibited human prostate cancer cells and suggested they could be developed as novel therapeutic agents for treating prostate cancer (Wang et al 2011). Bergamottin, a furanocoumarin found in bergamot (5%) and lemon (0.2%), was one of several coumarins found to inhibit in vitro tumor promoters (Miyake et al 1999). Recent Korean research has confirmed the antitumoral properties of bergamottin (Hwang et al 2010), and bergamot essential oil was found to induce multiple death pathways in cancer cells in an Italian study by Russo et al (2013). What is interesting about the Italian study is that the individual chemical constituents (linalyl acetate, limonene, linalool, and bergapten) did not produce cancer cell death—only when they were combined together as they would be in the whole essential oil (Table 16-1).

CANCER AND CONVENTIONAL SIDE EFFECTS

The side effects of some conventional treatments for cancer can be very hard to endure. A few of my close friends have died from cancer recently and I have other friends and relatives who are cancer survivors. In the 1980s, I had a small aromatherapy private practice in England. My patients came by doctor's referral or word of mouth. Almost half of them had cancer, and the role of aromatherapy in their treatment was one of support. The cancer patients were mainly undergoing chemotherapy and radiation therapy following surgery and, without exception, they found the going very tough. Many expressed their despair that conventional medicine did not adequately address the unpleasant side effects of the cancer treatment. Twenty years later, aromatherapy has become the main complementary therapy used in the UK to support oncology patients (Harris 2012).

Clinical aromatherapy is now frequently used as a supportive complementary therapy in several large cancer hospitals in the UK, such as The Royal Marsden in London, The Christie in Manchester and The Clatterbridge Cancer Center in Wirral and Liverpool. In the United States, several centers use clinical aromatherapy, such as the Penny George Institute for Health & Healing (PGIHH), America's largest hospital-based integrative care program (Kinney 2012), and the Columbia University

TABLE 16-1 *Published Studies on Essential Oils with Antitumoral Properties*

Author	Year	Essential Oil	Common Name	Target
Al Kalaldeh et al	2010	*Origanum vulgare* *Origanum syriacum* *Salvia triloba*	Origanum Lebanese oregano Greek sage	Apoptosis of breast adenocarcinoma cells
Loizo et al	2010	*Salvia leriifolia* *Salvia acetabulosa*	No known common name No known common name	Apoptosis of cancer cells
Greay et al	2010	*Melaleuca alternifolia*	Tea tree	Subcutaneous murine cancer cells
Di Sotto et al	2011	*Lavandula angustifolia*	Lavender	Lymphocytes
Ngo et al	2011	*Rosmarinus officinalis*	Rosemary	Suppression of cancer cells
Soeur et al	2011	*Aniba rosaeodora*	Brazilian rosewood	Epidermoid cancer cells
Sertel et al	2011	*Thymus vulgaris*	Thyme	Human oral cavity squamous cell carcinoma
Bostancioglu et al	2012	*Origanum onites*	Turkish oregano	Apoptosis of 5RP7 cells
Kathirvel et al	2012	*Ocimum basilicum*	Basil	HeLa and HEp-2 cancer cells
Ao & Shiodo	2012	*Cupressus sempervirens* *Thujopsis dolabrata*	Cypress Hiba	Apoptosis of SBC-3, A549, MEWO, and G-361 human cancer cell lines

Medical Center, New York (Kelly 2012). Several large U.S. hospitals such as the Texas Health Harris Methodist Hospital, Fort Worth, Texas; the Aurora Medical System, Wisconsin; and the Cooley-Dickinsen, Massachusetts also have robust and expanding clinical aromatherapy programs for patients—please see the list in the resource section.

In Canada and Australia, aromatherapy is frequently offered to patients in oncology departments. Other countries such as Japan, Korea, China, and India are rapidly catching up and there is tremendous interest in how aromatherapy can be used clinically to alleviate some of the distressing symptoms caused by conventional medicine (Koyama 2012, Hongkeun 2012, Shioda 2012, Imanishi 2012). As one patient said to me, "Conventional medicine saved my life, but clinical aromatherapy saved my sanity and made the process much more bearable."

TABLE 16-2 *Essential Oils and Spritzers for Radiation Burns*

Common Name	Botanical Name
Blue chamomile	*Matricaria recutita*
Everlasting	*Helichrysum italicum*
Lavender	*Lavandula angustifolia*
Niaouli	*Melaleuca viridiflora*
Rose	*Rosa damascena*
Blue tansy	*Tanacetum annuum*
Yarrow	*Achillea millefolium*

Postradiation Burns

Most radiologists request nothing to be put on the skin during radiation. This is to ensure the marks for radiation will not be removed as it is extremely important that radiotherapy is accurate. Some patients choose to have tiny tattoos that mark the radiation site. Many radiologists now understand that preparing the skin before radiotherapy reduces the severity of burns and skin irritation. In the weeks before radiation begins, the skin can be prepared with undiluted niaouli *(Melaleuca viridiflora)*. This seems to toughen the skin and results in fewer and less severe burns. Apply niaouli to the area three times a day for a week. Roulier (1990) and Franchomme and Penoel (1990) both suggest using 50% niaouli immediately before each radiation session and 50% niaouli in a St. John's wort-infused oil, or rosehip carrier oil, after each session. Sheppard-Hanger (2000) also used spritzers of everlasting *(Helichrysum italicum)* and blue tansy *(Tanacetum annuum)* immediately following each radiation treatment. Blue tansy is dark blue in color and high in chamazulene, hence it is an excellent antiinflammatory essential oil. Do not mistakenly use *Tanacetum vulgare,* another species of *Tanacetum. Tanacetum vulgare* is yellow to pale blue in color and contains 60% thujone, a ketone, which is not recommended for use in oncology or aromatherapy in general. Waghmare (2013) suggests that aloe vera is effective as a mild steroidal cream and has no side effects. Aloe vera squeezed straight from the living plant can be very useful either on its own, or with essential oils added to it, immediately after each radiotherapy session. A good present to anyone about to undergo radiotherapy would be a nice healthy *Aloe* plant.

My patients have used tansy *(Tanacetum annuum)* and everlasting *(Helichrysum italicum)* in spritzers and also spritzers of lavender *(Lavandula angustifolia)* plus rose *(Rosa damascena)* with good results. Yarrow *(Achillea millefolium)* and blue chamomile *(Matricaria recutita)* are also good choices. Table 16-2 lists suggested essential oils that can be used in postradiation spritzers. To make a spritzer, add 4 mL of essential oils to 4 oz of water and put in a spray bottle. Shake well before using. Take care not to use anything on the skin that has been stored in an aluminum container (such as antiperspirants) or that contains aluminum because aluminum can interfere with radiation treatment.

When radiation therapy is finished, apply a compress. Mix antiinflammatory essential oils like German chamomile, frankincense, or rose into a base of either aloe vera gel or tamanu *(Calophyllum inophyllum)*. An infused oil of gotu kola *(Centella asiatica)* or comfrey *(Symphytum officinale)* can also bring rapid relief and help promote healing.

Maiche et al (1990) carried out a controlled, single-blind study on 50 women aged from 30 to 79, who had been operated on for breast cancer and who had received radiation therapy. Kamillosan ointment, a proprietary cream that contains chamomile, is widely available in Europe. It was applied 30 minutes before radiation and just before bed. Measurements were made by an oncologist using a four-point scale (no change–moist desquamation). A comparison between the control group and the Kamillosan group showed no statistical significant changes overall, but skin deterioration appeared to happen later in the Kamillosan group, and there were fewer patients who presented with Grade 2 (dark erythema) reactions. In a further controlled study on leg ulcers, Kamillosan appeared to enhance the standard treatment of corticosteroids and antihistamines (Nasemann 1975). Kamillosan can also be helpful with the canker sores that appear during radiation.

A small, controlled, pilot study carried out at the Texas Health Harris Methodist Hospital found dilute essential oils topically applied had comparable effects to triaminolone cream (Shields 2004). Fourteen patients comprised the convenience sample. They were patch tested. Then 5% lavender *(Lavandula angustifolia)* and German chamomile *(Matricaria recutita)* in 20% tamanu plus 80% sweet almond oil was applied twice a day to the right side of the irradiated breast. Triamcinolone cream was applied to the left side of the breast. A RTOG acute skin toxicity grading tool was used. Five patients withdrew from the study because they disliked the smell. One withdrew after a rash appeared. Eight patients completed the study. Of these, five patients had comparable results to triamcinolone and the essential oil mixture seemed to delay the onset of skin radiation damage in the other three patients. These modest results are encouraging. Better compliance (and therefore better results) might occur by replacing blue chamomile *(Matricaria recutita)* with blue tansy *(Tanacetum annuum)*, Helichrysum *(Helichrysum italicum)*, and frankincense *(Boswellia carteri)* because the mixture would smell better. The added antiinflammatory effect of the additional essential oils would probably enhance the results.

Chemo-Induced Nausea

Chemo-induced nausea is covered in Chapter 9: Nausea and Vomiting. However, I have included a small table of published studies on chemo-induced nausea in this chapter for quick review. Please see Table 16-3. The best methods of application for chemo-induced nausea are individual aromasticks or aromapackets. Please see Chapter 2: How Essential Oils Work. Drinking ginger tea may also help, as may slowly chewing oranges.

TABLE 16-3 *Published Studies on Essential Oils for Chemo-Induced Nausea*

Author	Year	Number	Essential Oil	Method
Stringer & Donald	2011	123	Peppermint/lemon	Inhaled
Tayarani-Najaran et al	2013	200	Peppermint, spearmint	Essential oils taken orally in capsules
Haniadka et al	2012	Review	Ginger	Various

BOX 16-1 *The Oral Mucositis Assessment Scale (OMAS)*

Ulceration in Oral Cavity		Erythema in Oral Cavity	
Grade 0	No lesion	Grade 0	None
Grade 1	Lesion < 1 cm^2	Grade 1	Not severe
Grade 2	Lesion 1-3 cm^2	Grade 2	Severe
Grade 3	Lesion > 3 cm^2		

Radiation-Induced Mucositis

Almost 75% of cancer patients receive radiation (Radvansky et al 2013), and xerostomia (dry mouth) and mucositis are common adverse effects of radiation to the neck and head (Scarpace et al 2009). Xerostomia and mucositis, as well as being uncomfortable, also expose the mouth and throat to infection. Canker sores can occur. Topical application of lavender *(Lavandula angustifolia)* can be helpful in these instances (Baccaglini 2013). There are several scales used to measure oral mucositis:

1) World Health Organization (WHO) Handbook for reporting results of cancer treatment (1979)
2) National Cancer Institute—Common Terminology Criteria for Adverse Events (CTCAE)
3) Radiation Therapy Oncology Group (RTOG) Criteria
4) The Oral Mucositis Assessment Scale (OMAS) (Box 16-1)

Daily chlorhexidine mouthwash is often recommended for preventing chemotherapy-induced or radiotherapy-induced oral mucositis (Potting et al 2006). In a meta-analysis of three randomized controlled trials, patients complained about the negative side effects of chlorhexidine. These included teeth discoloration and alteration of taste in two of the five studies. Much worse, however, was that the results of the meta-analysis did not support the use of chlorhexidine mouthwash to prevent oral mucositis (Potting et al 2006).

Mouthwashes containing essential oils can help reduce the pain of mucositis, improve oral hygiene, promote salivation, prevent further mucosal breakdown, and prevent (or treat) oral infections (Harris 2012). For mouth care to be effective, it is important for the mouthwash containing the essential oils to be kept in the mouth

TABLE 16-4 *Essential Oils for Mucositis*

Peppermint	*Mentha × piperita*
Spearmint	*Mentha × spicata*
Myrrh	*Commiphora molmol*
Lemon	*Citrus limon*
Thyme	*Thymus vulgaris* CT thymol

for as long as possible before spitting it out (some essential oil mouthwashes can be swallowed). Encourage the patient not to eat, drink, or clean their teeth for at least 30 minutes after using the essential oil mouthwash. Dover Hospital, NJ, uses mouthwashes containing *Cymbopogon martinii* (palma rosa). An added advantage of using palma rosa is it reduces mouth odor and helps the mouth smell nice, as well as addressing the pain of mucositis, and treating and/or reducing oral infections. Buckingham (2010) reports on a mixture used by a UK hospital that contains myrrh *(Commiphora molmol)*, spearmint *(Mentha spicata)*, and sweet orange *(Citrus sinensis)* in a hydrolat (floral water) of lavender and chamomile. Maddocks-Jennings et al (2009) used manuka *(Leptospermum scoparium)* and kunuka *(Kunzea ericoides)*—both essential oils from New Zealand—in their randomized, controlled feasibility study. Nineteen adult patients took part in the study. The aromatherapy group used a gargle containing two drops of a 1:1 mix of the essential oils of manuka *(Leptospermum scoparium)* and kanuka *(Kunzea ericoides)* in water. The control group gargled with plain water. Both groups received conventional nursing care. Participants in the essential oil gargle group had a delayed onset of mucositis and their pain and oral symptoms were less than participants in the placebo (gargling with water) or the control ("usual care") groups.

Suggested essential oils for mouthwashes can be found in Table 16-4.

Chemo-Induced Peripheral Neuropathy

Peripheral neuropathies induced by chemotherapy (CIPN) are an increasingly frequent problem (Grisold et al 2012, Mir et al 2012), and one of the main reasons why patients stop treatment early. It is not absolutely clear what the cancer drugs actually do to cause CIPN, but it is thought the cytotoxic drugs increase oxidative stress and this activates the ion channel TRPA1 expressed by nociceptors (Trevisan et al 2013). This means nerves can become sensitized because the concentration of salts in the fluid surrounding them changes, or because the channels that use these salts to trigger nerve impulses become dysfunctional and this causes the patient to feel more pain (NCI 2010). Symptoms vary from an increased sensation to heat, cold, and pressure to stabbing pains and difficulty with balance (Harris 2012).

Some CIPNs are partially reversible during posttreatment nerve recovery (Englander 2013). Amifostine and antidepressants are often prescribed in an attempt to improve the quality of life, but these have limited efficacy and can produce other side effects. A review of 24 studies by Schloss et al (2013) concludes that currently no supplement such as vitamin B6, vitamin E, or others, showed solid beneficial evidence for the treatment of CIPN. It is certainly worth trying topically applied peppermint *(Mentha x piperta)* and cornmint *(Mentha arvensis)* in a gel—using a low percentage of 1 to 5%. Colvin et al (2008) and Storey et al (2010) found menthol (the main component in these two mints) effective in reversing bortezo-mib-induced neuropathic pain. Harris (2012) suggests applying dilute essential oils to the sacral area for lower limbs and the cervical area for upper limbs—as well as applying it to the limbs themselves. Her suggestions for a 5% mixture can be found in Table 16-5.

Lymphedema

Lymphedema occurs frequently following mastectomy but is also fairly common following lumpectomy if there has been removal of lymph glands. The risk of arm edema increases when axillary dissection and axillary radiation therapy are used. The incidence of arm lymphedema following breast surgery is 8% to 30% (Card et al 2012) and appears to increase up to 2 years after diagnosis or surgery of breast cancer (DiSipio et al 2013). Lymphatic cording, sometimes called axillary web syn-drome (AWS), can also be a problem. Lymphatic cording means a rope-like struc-ture that develops in the axilla area and can extend to the elbow (Tilley et al 2009).

When lymph pathways are reduced, either due to surgery or due to trauma, it is more difficult to return excess interstitial fluid to the blood. Lymph accumu-lates in the subcutaneous tissue causing the affected limb to become swollen and tender. Lymph contains large protein molecules, and buildup of protein in the tis-sue leads to chronic inflammation and, over a period of time, thickened leathery looking skin. After the initial phase of soft skin and pitting, chronic lymphedema is characteristically nonpitting. Because of chronic inflammation, local immunity is compromised, with subsequent bouts of cellulitis and poor resistance to insect bites or minor cuts.

The large lymphatic vessel walls are contractile (so progress is in one direction only). This is why the Vodder method of manual lymphatic drainage (MLD) can be so beneficial. The pressure of MLD is light and always in the direction of the lymph. Although not trained in the method, I have had success using "tramlines"—one of the MLD strokes—running my fingers gently, slowly, and repeatedly in the direc-tion of the lymph. With a bit of practice it was possible to feel the lymph move. It

TABLE 16-5 *Essential Oils for Chemo-Induced Peripheral Neuropathy*

Common Name	Botanical Name
Peppermint	*Mentha piperita*
Sweet marjoram	*Origanum majorana*
Spike lavender	*Lavandula latifolia*
Thai ginger	*Zingiber cassumunar*
Indian wintergreen	*Gaultheria fragrantissima*

helped that the very light pressure is similar to the pressure used in my own 'M' Technique.

Essential oils can be added to MLD and aromatherapy can play an important role when the skin loses its elasticity and infections become more frequent. Choose a nice-smelling mixture of essential oils and avoid those with an astringent action like *Cupressus sempervirens* (cypress) or those high in phenols that may be too agressive. I was unable to find any published studies on lymphedema and aromatherapy, which is surprising and an area definitely worth exploring. An R.J. Buckle student, Judy Ryan (2007), conducted a small case series using essential oils on three patients receiving MLD. Outcome measures were infrared temperature, limb measurement, muscle testing, and pain VAS (0 to 10). The study lasted 12 weeks. During the first 2 weeks baseline was established. The following 9 weeks comprised the aromatherapy intervention and the last week was the control/washout. During weeks 3 and 4, antiinflammatory essential oils were used. A different selection of essential oils was chosen for each patient depending on his or her requirements. The antiinflammatory essential oils were the most effective and appeared to reduce tissue congestion. This small case series helped set a new standard of care within the clinic where Ryan works in the United States.

AROMATHERAPY AS A GENERAL SUPPORTIVE ROLE

Aromatherapy is one of the most popular complementary therapies offered to cancer patients in the UK. An NHS survey of 142 CAM cancer units in the UK found counseling was the most widely provided (82%) with aromatherapy coming second, and was provided 59% of the time (Agan et al 2012). Velindre is one of the 10 largest regional clinical oncology units in the UK and the largest in Wales. The center deals with 5000 new referrals a year and 50,000 new outpatient appointments (Green 2012). Aromatherapy is offered as a complementary therapy and the service is audited using the MYCAW (Measure Yourself Concerns and Wellbeing) tool. Inhaled essential oils, using diffusers or aromasticks, are popular as well as aromatherapy massage. The center offers both inpatient and outpatient care.

The Christie HNS Foundation Trust in Manchester is the largest acute cancer center in the UK. At this hospital, clinical aromatherapy is used to support the side effects of treatment, but also to calm and support the patients. The hospital has raised the profile of aromasticks by instigating their use in 2006, and since then, by auditing and publishing several articles about their use (Stringer & Donald 2011, Carter et al 2011). In this hospital, aromasticks are used for (in order of importance): anxiety, nausea, sleep disturbance, a distressing procedure, smoking cessation, low mood, pain, and odor issues. The Royal Marsden Hospital, London, also offers aromatherapy to its cancer patients (Dyer et al 2008) through aromasticks and through aromatherapy massage.

In other parts of the world, aromatherapy is beginning to become integrated into cancer care for survivors, as well as in palliative or hospice support for cancer patients. In 2010, the first funded complementary therapy program in Canada was instigated at Mackenzie Richmond Hill Hospital in the Greater Toronto area

(Tavares 2012). This was no small feat, as Canada has a widely accepted fragrance-free culture and aromatherapy is less known about than in the UK, United States, or Australia. Aromatherapy in Canada is predominantly massage based. In the United States, aromatherapy is an integral part of patient care at the Penny George Institue for Health and Healing (PGIHH) and this includes an aromatherapy department (Kinney 2013). Aromatherapy is given through massage and by inhalation.

Globally, most studies of aromatherapy in oncology have involved massage (Wilkinson et al 2008). Some examples are: in the UK (Wilkinson et al 2007), Korea (Chang 2008), United States (Myers et al 2008, Russell et al 2008), and Japan (Kohara et al 2004, Imanishi et al 2009). In Japan, a survey of 300 patients with cancer found 44% were using complementary therapies and this included aroma-therapy (Koyama 2012) (Table 16-6).

Most studies appear to target palliative, hospice, or end of life cancer care (Nakano et al 2012). Few studies have used inhalation or spritzers but there are some. For example, Graham et al (2003) explored the use of inhaled essential oils of lavender, bergamot, and cedarwood during radiotherapy and Dyer et al (2008a) explored the effect of neroli and peppermint hydrolat on hot flushes in breast cancer patients.

Perhaps because many countries are fee paying, there is little information in the literature about the supportive role of aromatherapy in cancer care outside the UK. However, aromatherapy is part of a package of complementary therapies that have significantly reduced the use (and therefore the cost) of antiemetic, anxiolytic, and

TABLE 16-6 *Sample of Published Aromatherapy Studies in Cancer Patients*

Author	Year	N	Symptom	Essential Oil	Method
Chang	2008	28	Pain, anxiety, depression	Bergamot, lavender, and frankincense	Hand massage
Imanishi et al	2007	12	Anxiety	Lavender, sweet orange, and sandalwood	Hand massage
Dyer et al	2008	44	Hot flushes in breast cancer	Neroli, peppermint	Spritzer
Graham et al	2003	313	Anxiety during radiation	Lavender, bergamot, and cedarwood	Inhalation
Ndao et al	2012	37	Nausea – stem cell infusion	Bergamot	Inhalation
Stringer & Donald	2011	123	Nausea, sleep disturbance, low mood, anxiety	Peppermint, lemon	Aromasticks
Hackman et al	2012	75	Relaxation, coping	Several blends – not specified	Aromasticks

hypnotic medication at the oncology inpatient department of Beth Israel Medical Center, New York (Kligler et al 2011).

Oncology patients prefer a very light touch. Thus the 'M' Technique can be really valuable, because it is so quick to learn (and to do) and can be shown to family, friends, and volunteers. The 'M' Technique is used by many nurses in the United States as part of holistic nursing care. There follows a case study from Valley Hospital, Ridgewood, NJ, where nurses use clinical aromatherapy and the 'M' Technique in the oncology unit, as well as in many other areas of the hospital.

Alice (not her real name) is a 17-year-old female, diagnosed with a metastatic yolk sac tumor. Following aggressive surgical debulking and S/P chemotherapy, she became severely anemic/neutropenic and her platelet count plummeted to 5 (normal is 150 to 400). She was admitted to the ICU with pleural effusion where chest tubes were inserted. She was intubated and a nasogastric tube was passed for nutritional maintenance. Alice's kidney and liver function was affected and she presented with fungicemia. Consultation with the holistic nursing service was a request for comfort. The 'M' Technique was provided to the patient's hands using a dilute lavender cream mix. She was also given aromasticks (inhalers) for relaxation (lavender/mandarin combo), nausea control (ginger/lavender/peppermint/spearmint combo), and to support her emotions and digestion (lemon). At the time of writing, Alice was doing well enough to be discharged to a rehabilitation facility for strengthening before she could be considered for another round of chemotherapy. Alice personally requested fresh inhalers before discharge and uses them on a continuous basis. They give her a sense of well-being and control in a situation that has been life threatening, and will be challenging for the foreseeable future (Mazzer 2013).

An R.J. Buckle student, Judith Dibartolo (2011), carried out a small study on 10 patients in New York, using a case-study format. Patients were given an aromastick containing ylang ylang. The aromastick was held in front of the patient's nose, not inserted into the nostrils. Three interviews were conducted with the participants—before, during, and after the study. The first interview was face to face, the second and third were by phone. Eighty-six percent of patients reported less anxiety after using the inhaler compared to week 1, but this feeling dissipated during the next 2 weeks (Table 16-7).

ESSENTIAL OILS TO AVOID IN ONCOLOGY

A recent study found that plant-based phytoestrogens have both estrogenic and antiestrogenic properties that may be important in breast carcinogenesis (Xie et al 2013). This study involved lignans. While essential oils do not contain lignans, it might be prudent to avoid essential oils that are thought to have estrogen-like properties in tumors that are estrogen dependent. Estrogen-dependent cancers are breast, uterine, and ovarian cancer. Essential oils thought to have an estrogen-like effect include fennel and aniseed as they contain anethole (Albert-Pulco 1980). Anethole is a phenol methyl ether. Sclareol (found in clary sage) and viridifloral (found in niaouli) are other components of essential oils

TABLE 16-7 *R.J. Buckle Student Studies on Cancer Patients*

Name	Year	State	Number	Condition	Essential Oil
Ogden	2002	MI	1	Thyroid cancer	Peppermint, frank-incense, rose
Figuenick	1999	MA	9	Chemo nausea	Peppermint
Conrad	2000	AZ	12	Anxiety	Lavender, frankincense, mandarin
Willee	2003	MN	8	Anxiety before breast biopsy	Lavender
Shields	2004	TX	14	Radiation burns	German chamomile, lavender
Irby	2006	MN	8	Chemo nausea	Peppermint
Lowdermilk	2007	WI	10	Chemo nausea	Peppermint, ginger
Ryan	2007	PA	3	Lymphedema	Several mixtures
Dibartolo	2011	NY	7	Anxiety	Ylang ylang

that have structures similar to estrogen (Franchomme & Penoel 1990). The link to geranium and rose is really too tenuous, and both essential oils should be fine to use in estrogen-dependent tumors. Two Chinese studies (Wang et al 2009, Huang 2011) measured the levels of seven sex hormones in essential oils. Wang measured estradiol-17β, estriol, estrone, testosterone, methyl-testosterone, progesterone, and diethylstilbestrol and Huang measured estriol, estradiol, estrone, ethinyloestradiol, dienestrol, hexestrol, and diethylstilbestrol. Unfortunately, because both papers are in Chinese, it is impossible to discover what essential oils contained what sex hormone and in what quantities. Hopefully, these two papers will be translated soon! For more research, please see Tisserand's latest book on Essential Oils Safety.

In vitro studies on rat skin indicated that some essential oils enhance the penetration of 5-fluorouracil (5FU) (Abdullah et al 1996). Peppermint increased penetration by 46 times, and *Eucalyptus globulus* increased penetration by 60 times. Therefore, peppermint and eucalyptus should not be used topically near an intravenous catheter site if the chemotherapy agent used is 5FU.

REFERENCES

Abdullah D, Ping Q, Liu G. 1996. Enhancing the effect of essential oils on the penetration of 5-fluorouracil through rat skin. *Yao Xue Xue Bao*. 31(3):214–221.

Agan B, Gage H, Hood J, Poole K, McDowell C et al. 2012. Availability of complementary and alternative medicine for people with cancer in the British National Health Service: results of a national survey. *Complement Ther Clin Practice*. 18(2):75–80.

Albert-Puleo M. 1980. Fennel and anise as estrogenic agents. *Journal of Ethnopharmacology*. 2(4): 337–344.

Al-Daghri N, Alokail M, Alkharfy K, Mohammed A, Abd-Alrahman S et al 2012. Fenugreek extract as an inducer of cellular death via autophagy in human T lymphoma Jurkat cells. *BMC Complement Altern Med.* Oct 30; 12:202.

Al Kalaldeh J, Abu Dahab R, Afifi F. 2010. Volatile oil composition and antiproliferative activity of *Laurus nobilis, Origanum syriacum, Origanum vulgare,* and *Salvia triloba* against human breast adenocarcinoma cells. *Nutrition Research,* 30(4):271–278.

Ao Y, Shioda S. 2012. Cytotoxic effect of some essential oils on Human Cancer Cells. *Conference Proceedings. 1st International Congress of Aromatherapy. J Japanese Soc Aromatherapy.* 11. Suppl: 32–37.

Baccaglini L. 2013. There is limited evidence that topical lavender oil is effective for palliative treatment of recurrent aphthous stomatitis. *J Evid Based Dent Pract.* 13(2):47–9.

Bassler D, Briel M, Montori V, Glaziou P, Zhou Q et al. 2010. Stopping randomized trials early for benefit and estimation of treatment effects: systematic review and meta-regression analysis. JAMA. 303(12):1180–7.

Bostancioglu R, Kurkcuoglu M, Baser K, Koparal A. 2012. Assessment of anti-angiogenic and anti-tumoral potentials of *Origanum onites* L. essential oil. *Food and Chemical Toxicology,* 50(6):2002–2008.

Bray F, Ren J, Masuyer E, Ferlay J. 2013. Global estimates of cancer prevalence in 27 sites in the adult population in 2008. *Int J Cancer.* 132(5):1133–45.

Buckingham L. 2010. Managing mucositis: a case-study. *Intern J Clinical Aromatherapy.* 7(2):31–33.

Cabaniols C, Giorgi R, Chinot O, Ferahta N, Spinelli V et al. 2011. Links between private habits, psychological stress and brain cancer: a case-control pilot study in France. *J Neurooncol.* 103(2):307–16.

Campbell J, Ramsey S. 2009. The costs of treating breast cancer in the US: a synthesis of published evidence. *Pharmacoeconomics.* 27(3):199–209.

Card A, Crosby M, Liu J, Lindstrom W, Lucci A, Chang D. 2012. Reduced incidence of breast cancer-related lymphedema following mastectomy and breast reconstruction versus mastectomy alone. *Plast Reconstr Surg.* 130(6):1169–78.

Carter A, Maycock P, Mackereth P. 2011. Aromasticks in clinical practice. *In Essence.* 10(2):16–19.

Cancer Research UK. 2013. http://www.cancerresearchuk.org/cancer-info/cancerstats/mortality/uk-cancer-mortality-statistics. Accessed June 24, 2013.

CDC. 2013. Centers for Disease Control. USA. http://apps.nccd.cdc.gov/uscs/. Accessed 24 June 2013.

Chang S. 2008. Effects of aroma hand massage on pain, state anxiety and depression in hospice patients with terminal cancer. *Taehan Kanho Hakhoe Chi.* 38(4):493–502.

Colvin L, Johnson P, Mitchell R, Fleetwood-Walker S, Fallon M. 2008. From bench to bedside: a case of rapid reversal of bortezomib-induced neuropathic pain by the TRPM8 activator, menthol. *J Clin Oncology.* 20;26(27):4519–20.

Conrad P. Aromatherapy for cancer support – anxiety and patient satisfaction. Unpublished dissertation for RJ Buckle Associates.

Delora P, Luceri C, Gherlandini C et al. 1994. Anticarcinogenic effect of *Commiphora molmol* on solid tumors induced by Ehrlich carcinoma cells in mice. *Chemotherapy.* 40:337–347.

De Sousa AC, Alviano DS, Blank AF, Alves PB, Alviano C et al. 2004. *Melissa officinalis* L. essential oil: antitumoral and antioxidant activities. *Pharm Pharmacol.* 56(5):677–81.

Dewick P. 1989. Tumour inhibitors from plants. In Evans W (ed.), *Trease and Evan's Pharmacognosy,* 13th ed. London: Bailliere Tindall, 634–656.

Dibartolo J. 2011. Dissertation for RJ Buckle Associates LLC.

Dimas K, Kokkinopoulos D, Demetzos C et al. 1999. The effect of sclareol on growth and cell cycle progression of human leukemic cell lines. *Leukemia Research.* 23(3):217–234.

DiSipio T, Rye S, Newman B, Hayes S. 2013. Incidence of unilateral arm lymphoedema after breast cancer: a systematic review and meta-analysis. *Lancet Oncol.* 14(6):500–15.

Di Sotto A, Mazzanti G, Carbone F, Hrelia P, Maffei F. 2011. Genotoxicity of lavender oil, linalyl acetate, and linalool on human lymphocytes in vitro. *Environmental and Molecular Mutagenesis,* 52(1):69–71.

Dyer J, Ashley S, Shaw C. 2008a. A study to look at the effects of a hydrolat spray on hot flushes in women being treated for breast cancer. *Complementary Therapies in Clinical Practice,* 14(4):273–279.

Dyer J, McNeill S, Ragsdale Low M, Tratt L. 2008. A snap-shot survey of current practice: the use of aromasticks for symptom management. *Int J Clin Aroma.* 5(2):17–21.

Englander. 2013. DNA damage response in peripheral nervous system: coping with cancer therapy-induced DNA lesions. DNA Repair (Amst). 16. doi:pii: S1568–7864(13)00101-8. 10.1016/j.dnarep.2013.04.020. [Epub ahead of print]

Fell J. 1857. *A Treatise on Cancer and Its Treatment.* London: J & A Churchill.

Figuenick R. 1990. Peppermint for chemo-induced nausea. Unpublished dissertation for RJ Buckle Associates.

Fleming J, Dworkin A, Allain D, Fernandez S, Wei L et al. 2013. Allele-specific imbalance mapping identifies HDAC9 as a candidate gene for cutaneous squamous cell carcinoma. *Int J Cancer.* 2013 Jun 20. doi: 10.1002/ijc.28339. [Epub ahead of print]

Forman D, de Martel C, Lacey CJ, Soerjomataram I, Lortet-Tieulent J et al. 2012. Global burden of human papillomavirus and related diseases. *Vaccine.* 20(30): Suppl 5:F12–23.

Franchomme P, Penoel D. 1990. *Aromatherapie Exactement.* Limoges, France: Jollois.

Goldacre B. 2012. Bad Pharma. Fourth Estate London.

Goulart B, Bensink M, Mummy D, Ramsey S. 2012. Lung cancer screening with low-dose computed tomography: costs, national expenditures, and cost-effectiveness. *J Natl Compr Canc Netw.* 118(20):5132–9.

Graham P, Browne L, Cox H, Graham J. 2003. Inhalation aromatherapy during radiotherapy: results of a placebo-controlled double-blind randomized trial. *Journal of Clinical Oncology.* 21(12): 2372–2376.

Greay S, Ireland D, Kissick H, Heenam P, Carson C et al. 2010. Inhibition of established subcutaneous murine tumour growth with topical *Melaleuca alternifolia* (tea tree) oil. *Cancer Chemotherapy and Pharmacology,* 66(6):1095–1102.

Green A. 2012. Complementary cancer care in south east Wales: an interview with Angela Green. *Int J Clinical Aromatherapy.* 8(1):27–29.

Grisold W, Cavaletti G, Windebank A. 2012. Peripheral neuropathies from chemotherapeutics and targeted agents: diagnosis, treatment, and prevention. *Neuro Oncol.* 14 Suppl 4:iv45–54.

Hackman E, Mackereth P, Maycock P, Orrett L, Stringer J. 2012. Expanding the use of aromasticks for surgical and day care patients. *Int J Clinical Aromatherapy.* 8(1):10–15.

Haniadka R, Rajeev A, Palatty P, Arora R, Baliga M. 2012. *Zingiber officinale* (ginger) as an anti-emetic in cancer chemotherapy: a review. *J Altern Complement Med.* 18(5):440–4.

Hardell L, Sage C. 2008. Biological effects from electromagnetic field exposure and public exposure standards. *Biomed Pharmacother.* 62(2):104–9.

Harris R. 2012. Making a difference in cancer and palliative care: a spotlight on key interventions and essential oils in cancer and palliative care settings. *Journal of Japanese Society of Aromatherapy.* 11 Suppl. S2–1. Page 82. Available: www.aroma-jsa.jp.

He K, Xu T, Xu Y, Ring A, Kahn M, Goldkorn A. 2013. Cancer cells acquire a drug resistant, highly tumorigenic, cancer stem-like phenotype through modulation of the PI3K/Akt/β-catenin/CBP pathway. *Int J Cancer.* 2013 Jun 20. doi: 10.1002/ijc.28341. [Epub ahead of print]

Hongkeun O. 2012. Aromatherapy in Korea. *Journal of Japanese Society of Aromatherapy.* 11 Suppl. S1–5. Page 81. Available: www.aroma-jsa.jp.

Huang B, Han Z, Xu X, Cai Z, Jiang W et al. 2011. Simultaneous determination of 7 female sex hormones in essential oil by high performance liquid chromatography–tandem mass spectrometry with isotope dilution. *Se Pu.* 29(1):20–5.

Hwang Y, Yun H, Choi J, Kang K, Jeong H. 2010. Suppression of phorbol-12-myristate-13-acetate-induced tumor cell invasion by bergamottin via the inhibition of protein kinase Cdelta/p38 mitogen-activated protein kinase and JNK/nuclear factor-kappaB-dependent matrix metalloproteinase-9 expression. *Mol Nutr Food Res.* 54(7):977–90.

Imanishi J, Kuriyama H, Shigemori I, Watanabe S, Aihara Y et al. 2009. Anxiolytic effect of aromatherapy massage in patients with breast cancer. *Evid Based Complement Alternat Med.* 6(1):123–8.

Imanishi 2012. Usefulness of integrative medicine including aromatherapy in cancer care. *Conference Proceedings from the 1st International Conference of Aromatherapy.* Kyoto, Japan. Page 12. Available: www.aroma-jsa.jp.

Irby S. 2006. Peppermint for chemo-induced nausea. Unpublished dissertation for RJ Buckle Associates.

Jia L, Jin H, Zhou J, Chen L, Lu Y et al. 2013. A potential anti-tumor herbal medicine, corilagin, inhibits ovarian cancer cell growth through blocking the TGF-β signaling pathways. *BMC Complement Altern Med.* 15;13:33.

Kathirvel P, Ravi S. 2012. Chemical composition of the essential oil from basil (*Ocimum basilicum* Linn.) and it's in vitro cytotoxicity against HeLa and HEp-2 human cancer cell lines and NIH 3T3 mouse embryonic fibroblasts. *Natural Product Research*, 26(12):1112–1118.

Kelly K. 2012. Conducting research on aromatherapy for management of cancer-related symptoms: focus on research challenges, successes and resources in clinical research. *Journal of Japanese Society of Aromatherapy.* 11 Suppl. S2–5. Page 86. Available: www.aroma-jsa.jp.

Kinney M. 2012. Clinical Aromatherapy and Inpatient Oncology – Insights on Integrative Health a Large United States Health Care System. Conference proceedings. *Journal of Japanese Society of Aromatherapy.* 11 Suppl. S2–3. Page 84. Available: www.aroma-jsa.jp.

Kligler B, Homel P, Harrison L, Levenson H, Kenney J, Merrell W. 2011. Cost-savings in inpatient oncology through an integrative medicine approach. *Am J Manag Care.* 17(12):779–84.

Kohara M, Miyauchi T, Suehiro Y, Ueoka H, Takeyama H, Morita T. 2004. Combined modality treatment of aromatherapy, foot soak, and reflexology relieves fatigue in patients with cancer. *J Palliative Med.* 7(6):791–6.

Koyama M. 2012. Cancer and aromatherapy – for their development into clinical practice. *Journal of Japanese Society of Aromatherapy.* 11 Suppl. S2–2. page 83. Available: www.aroma-jsa.jp.

Lewis W, Elvin-Lewis M. 1977. *Medical Botany.* New York: Wiley Interscience.

Loizo M, Menichini F, Tundis R, Bonesi M, Nadjafi F, Saab A, Menichini F. 2010. Comparative chemical composition and antiproliferative activity of aerial parts of *Salvia leriifolia* Benth. and *Salvia acetabulosa* L essential oils against human tumor cell in vitro models. *Journal of Medicinal Food.* 13(1):62–29.

Long Q, Zhou M, Liu X, Du Y, Fan J et al. 2013. Interaction of CCN1 with αvβ3 integrin induces P-glycoprotein and confers vinblastine resistance in renal cell carcinoma cells. *Anticancer Drugs.* Jun 5. [Epub ahead of print]

Lowdermilk G. 2007. Peppermint and ginger to reduce chemo-nausea. Unpublished dissertation for RJ Buckle Associates.

Lu W, Qin Y, Yang C, Li L. 2013. Effect of curcumin on human colon cancer multidrug resistance in vitro and in vivo. *Clinics (Sao Paulo).* May;68(5). doi:pii: S1807–59322013000500694.

Maddocks-Jennings W, Wilkinson J, Cavanagh M, Shillington D. 2009. Evaluation the effects of the essential oils of *Leptospermum scoparium* (manuka) and *Kunzea ericoides* (kanuka) on radiotherapy-induced mucositis: a randomized, placebo-controlled feasibility study. *European Journal of Oncology Nursing.* 13(2):87–93.

Maiche A, Grohn P, Maki-Hokkonen H. 1990. Effect of chamomile cream and almond ointment on acute radiation skin reaction. Acta Oncologica. 30(3):395–396.

Malvezzi M, Bertuccio P, Levi F, La Vecchia C, Negri E. 2013. European Cancer Mortality Predictions for 2013. *Annals of Oncology.* doi: 10.1093/annonc/mdt010. Accessed. June 24, 2013.

Mazzer M. 2013. Personal communication.

Mir O, Boudou-Rouquette P, Giroux J, Chapron J, Alexandre J et al. 2012. Pemetrexed, oxaliplatin and bevacizumab as first-line treatment in patients with stage IV non-small cell lung cancer. *Lung Cancer.* 77(1):104–9.

Miyake Y, Murakami A, Sugiyama Y et al. 1999. Identification of coumarins from lemon fruit (*Citrus limon*) as inhibitors of in vitro tumor promotion and superoxide and nitric oxide generation. *Journal of Agricultural and Food Chemistry.* 47(8):3151–3157.

Myers C, Walton D, Bratsman L, Wilson J, Small B. 2008. Massage modalities and symptoms reported by cancer patients: narrative review. *J Soc Integr Oncology.* 6(1):19–28.

Nakano K, Sato K, Katayma H, Miyashita M. 2012. Living with pleasure in daily life at the end of life: recommended care strategy for cancer patients from the perspective of physicians and nurses. *Palliat Support Care.* Jul 6:1–9. [Epub ahead of print]. Accessed July 11, 2013.

Nasemann T. 1975. Kamillosan therapy in dermatology. *Z Allgemeinmed.* 25:1105–1106.

NCI. National Cancer Institute USA. 2010. 7(4): http://www.cancer.gov/aboutnci/ncicancerbulletin/archive/2010/022310/page6. Accessed June 27, 2013.

Ndao D, Ladas E, Cheng B, Sands S, Snyder K et al 2012. Inhalation aromatherapy in children and adolescents undergoing stem cell infusion: results of a placebo-controlled double-blind trial. *Psychooncology.* 21(3):247–54.

Ngo S, Williams D, Head R. 2011. Rosemary and cancer prevention: preclinical perspectives. *Critical Reviews in Food Science and Nutrition.* 51(10):946–954.

Noori S, Hassan ZM, Salehian O. 2013. Sclareol reduces CD4+ CD25+ FoxP3+ Treg cells in a breast cancer model in vivo. *Iran J Immunol.* 10(1):10–21.

Ogden C. Peppermint, frankincense and rose for cancer support – a survivor's case-story. Unpublished dissertation for RJ Buckle Associates.

O'Neill C, Atoria C, O'Reilly E, LaFemina J, Henman M et al 2012. Costs and trends in pancreatic cancer treatment. *Cancer.* 118(20):5132–9.

Park B, Jung K, Son M, Seo J, Lee H et al. 2012. Antitumor activity of *Pulsatilla koreana* extract in anaplastic thyroid cancer via apoptosis and anti-angiogenesis. *Mol Med Rep.* Nov 5. doi: 10.3892/mmr.2012.1166.

Poirier M. 2012. Chemical-induced DNA damage and human cancer risk. *Disc Med.* 14(77):283–8.

Potting CM, Uitterhoeve R, Op Reimer WS, Van Achterberg T. 2006. The effectiveness of commonly used mouthwashes for the prevention of chemotherapy-induced oral mucositis – a systematic review. *Eur J Cancer Care (Engl).* 15(5):431–9.

Radvansky L, Pace M, Siddiqui A. 2013. Prevention and management of radiation-induced dermatitis, mucositis, and xerostomia. *Am J Health Syst Pharm.* 15;70(12):1025–1032.

Roulier G. 1990. *Les Huiles Essentielles Pour Votre Sante.* St. Jean-de-Braye, France: Dangles.

Russell N, Sumler S, Beinhorn C, Frenkel M. 2008. Role of massage therapy in cancer care. *J Altern Complement Med.* 14(2):209–14.

Russo R, Ciociaro A, Berliocchi L, Cassiano M, Rombolà L et al. 2013. Implication of limonene and linalyl acetate in cytotoxicity induced by bergamot essential oil in human neuroblastoma cells. *Fitoterapia.* 23 (89C):48–57.

Ryan J. 2007. Dissertation for RJ Buckle Associates.

Scarpace S, Brodzik F, Mehdi S, Belgam R. 2009. Treatment of head and neck cancers: issues for clinical pharmacists. *Pharmacotherapy.* 29(5):578–92.

Schloss J, Colosimo M, Airey C, Masci P, Linnane AW, Vitetta L. 2013. Nutraceuticals and chemotherapy induced peripheral neuropathy (CIPN): a systematic review. *Clin Nutr.* 13. doi:pii: S0261–5614 (13)00107-6. Accessed 26 June 2013.

Sertel S, Eichhorn T, Plinkert P, Efferth T. 2011. Cytotoxicity of *Thymus vulgaris* essential oil towards human oral cavity squamous cell carcinoma. *Anticancer Research.* 31(1):81–87.

Sheppard-Hanger S. 2000. Use of essential oils and natural extracts to help counter side effects of radiation during cancer treatment. Proceedings of the 3rd Scientific Wholistic Aromatherapy Conference. San Francisco. Nov 10-12, 174–191.

Shields S. 2004. Comparison study of triamcinolone and essential oils to prevent post radiation burns. RJ Buckle Associates certification study.

Shioda S. 2012. Past, present and future outlook for aromatherapy in Japan. *Journal of Japanese Society of Aromatherapy.* 11 Suppl. S1–1. Page 77. Available: www.aroma-jsa.jp.

Soeur J, Marrot L, Perez P, Iraqui I, Kienda G et al. 2011. Selective cytotoxicity of *Aniba rosaeodora* essential oil towards epidermoid cancer cells through induction of apoptosis. *Mutation Research.* 718(1-2):24–32.

Storey D, Colvin L, MacKean M, Mitchell R, Fleetwood-Walker S, Fallon M. 2010. Reversal of dose-limiting carboplatin-induced peripheral neuropathy with TRPM8 activator, menthol, enables further effective chemotherapy delivery. *J Pain Symptom Management.* 39(6):e2–4.

Stringer J, Donald G. 2011. Aromasticks in cancer care: an innovation not to be sniffed at. *Complementary Therapies in Clinical Practice.* 17(2):116–121.

Tavares M. 2012. Aromatherapy makes its mark in Canadian palliative care. *Int J Clin Aroma.* 9(1):30–37.

Tayarani-Najaran Z, Talasaz-Firoozi E, Nasiri R, Jalali N, Hassanzadeh M. 2013. Antiemetic activity of volatile oil from *Mentha spicata* and *Mentha × piperita* in chemotherapy-induced nausea and vomiting. *Ecancermedicalscience*. 7:290. [Epub 2013 Jan 31]. Accessed July 15, 2013.

Tilley A, Thomas-MacLean R, Kwan W. 2009. Lymphatic cording or axillary web syndrome after breast cancer surgery. *Can J Surg*. 52(4): E105–E106.

Trevisan G, Materazzi S, Fusi C, Altomare A, Aldini G et al. 2013. Novel therapeutic strategy to prevent chemotherapy-induced persistent sensory neuropathy by TRPA1 blockade. *Cancer Res*. 73(10): 3120–3131.

USCS. 2013. United States Cancer Statistics. http://www.cdc.gov/cancer/npcr/uscs/qa.htm. Accessed July 16, 2013.

Waghmare CM. 2013. Radiation burns: from mechanism to management. *Burns*. 39(2):212–219.

Wang X, Kong F, Shen T, Young C, Lou H et al. 2011. Sesquiterpenoids from myrrh inhibit androgen receptor expression and function in human prostate cancer cells. *Acta Pharmacol Sin*. 32(3):338–44.

Wang X, Zeng W, Wang J, Ren R. 2009. Simultaneous determination of seven sexual hormones in essential oil by high performance liquid chromatography with diode array and fluorescence detectors. *Se Pu*. 27(3):328–32.

Wilkinson S, Barnes K, Storey L. 2008. Massage for symptom relief in patients with cancer: systematic review. *J Adv Nurs*. 63(5):430–9.

Wilkinson S, Love S, Westcombe A, Gambles M, Burgess C et al. 2007. Effectiveness of aromatherapy massage in the management of anxiety and depression in patients with cancer: a multicenter randomized controlled trial. *J Clin Oncol*. 25(5):532–9.

Willee C. Lavender to reduce anxiety prior to breast biopsy for cancer. Unpublished dissertation for RJ Buckle Associates.

Xie J, Tworoger S, Franke A, Terry K, Rice M et al. 2013. Plasma enterolactone and breast cancer risk in the Nurses' Health Study II. *Breast Cancer Res Treat*. 139(3):801–9.

Yin W, Wang P, Wang X, Song W, Cui X et al. 2013. Identification of microRNAs and mRNAs associated with multidrug resistance of human laryngeal cancer Hep-2 cells. *Braz J Med Biol Res*. 2013 June. [Epub ahead of print]

Zheng J, Tang Y, Sun M, Zhao Y, Li Q, Zhou J, Wang Y. 2013. Characterization, pharmacokinetics, tissue distribution and antitumor activity of honokiol submicron lipid emulsions in tumor-burdened mice. *Pharmazie*. 68(1):41–6.

Chapter 17

Palliative, Hospice, and End-of-Life Care

"Death is not the worst evil, but rather when we wish to die and cannot."

Sophocles (496–406 BC)

CHAPTER ASSETS

Although palliative care may ultimately lead to hospice care and hospice care may lead to care of the dying, they can be viewed as separate specialties and are defined differently in the Medical Dictionary (Brooker 2008). Palliative care is defined as the "multidisciplinary specialty of symptom relief with the care and support of the patient, family and friends" (Brooker 2008, p 352). Patients in palliative care may have several years to live. Hospice care is defined as "care for those with chronic or terminal illness and their family—at home, in a day unit or hospice" (Brooker 2008, p 226). Hospice care is centered around individualized symptom relief—particularly pain, usually in the last 6 months of life. Patients in a hospice may be receiving respite care as well as end-of-life care. End-of-life care is defined as the "care given at the very end of life, during the last week, days, or hours" (Brooker 2008, p 158). End-of-life patients may or may not have received palliative care and may or may not be in a hospice.

The terms 'palliative', 'hospice', and 'end-of-life' care are often used as if they are synonyms. However, a search on the database PubMed in August, 2013 produced different results, depending on which word was used. Palliative care plus aromatherapy produced 45 hits, hospice care plus aromatherapy produced 17 hits, and end-of-life care plus aromatherapy produced 7 hits. The Help the Hospices UK website gives different definitions for hospice and palliative care (www.helpthehospices.org.uk). Palliative care in the UK is provided by the National Health Service (NHS) with referrals for admission to a hospice via a doctor. Hospice care in the UK is funded by charitable organizations; hospices receive small financial support from the NHS.

PALLIATIVE CARE

Palliative care is the active, total care of the patient whose disease is not responsive to curative treatment (Radbruch & Payne 2009). There have been several attempts to measure palliative care globally (Clark & Centeno 2006, Martin-Marino et al 2008, Wright et al 2008). In 2011, 136 out of the world's 234 countries (58%) had at least one palliative care service—an increase of 21 countries (up by 9%) from 2006, with the largest increase in Africa (Lynch et al 2013). Advanced integration of palliative care has only been achieved in 20 countries (Lynch et al 2013), namely Australia, Austria, Belgium, Canada, France, Germany, Hong Kong, Iceland, Ireland, Italy, Japan, Norway, Poland, Romania, Singapore, Sweden, Switzerland, Uganda, UK, and the United States.

One of the greatest emotional shocks a person can receive is the knowledge that he or she has a terminal illness. This sets off an internal process of mourning, with the associated feelings of denial/numbness, anger, bargaining, depression, and finally acceptance (Axelrod 2006). Many patients remain stuck in the anger stage with the question "why me?" or they displace their anger and sense of unfairness onto others and make their lives miserable (Kubler-Ross 1978). Perhaps the answer to this dilemma could be found in the following quotation:

The Pathless Path

There is no answer.

There never has been an answer.

There never will be an answer.

That's the answer. (Gertrude Stein 1925)

Western society does little to honor the process of mourning for anything other than death. There is no rite of passage for divorce, failure, or a terminal prognosis. However, patients in palliative care are mourning the death of their future. They know there will be no happy ending. The sudden knowledge of the close proximity of death comes as a bitter blow to many patients. There is no way of knowing (outside a hospital) if someone has a limited time to live. They don't wear an armband to state it. So, unless he or she chooses to share this knowledge, we don't know. Many don't share the information because they don't want pity or forced joviality. This can keep patients locked in a world of their own, unwilling to communicate at a time when communication is important and time is limited.

Gentle touch and beautiful smells can cross these barriers. Touch communicates a sense of acceptance to such patients, many of whom may have feelings of self-disapproval (Pratt & Mason 1981, Olson & Keegan 2013). Touch and smell often penetrate the despondency of a patient who is struggling to accept that life is no longer going to be as he or she had hoped. Touch is an important commodity during palliative care because patients can often feel more "skin hunger" (Simon 1976, Jackson & Latini 2013). Touch opens up dialogue, while smells nudge memories.

Together they can help patients who may struggle with feelings of anger, denial, guilt, and frustration by allowing them to verbalize those feelings and communicate at a deeper level.

Palliative care should embrace the whole family, who may be trying to "remain brave." Smells are not easily hidden, and beautiful smells are an easy way to begin dialogue with family members. It is not unusual for aromatherapy to act as the catalyst, allowing patients and their relatives to begin talking to one another at a useful level. This period before a patient enters the terminal stage is important for a peaceful death. It is a time to clear old scores and resolve past disagreements. It is a time of completion, so the process of dying, when it finally occurs, can be as serene and dignified as possible.

AROMATHERAPY IN PALLIATIVE CARE

Many countries use aromatherapy in palliative care, for example, Italy (Latina et al 2012), Germany (Warnke et al 2004), the United States (Kozak et al 2008, Schwan & Ash 2004), UK (Horrigan 2004, Kyle 2006; Harris 2013), Australia (Knevitt 2004), Japan (Kawamura et al 2013), and Korea (Chang 2008). Most of the studies on aromatherapy in palliative care are centered on cancer care. There is a dearth of studies on other chronic diseases in palliative care such as multiple sclerosis (MS), ischemic heart disease, stroke, and so on. However, aromatherapy has ameliorated symptoms of MS (Esmonde & Long 2008), ischemic heart disease (Moeini et al 2010), and stroke (Shin & Lee 2007). Definitive research on the use of aromatherapy for these conditions in palliative care could prove interesting. Most of the current published studies in palliative care focus on depression or anxiety. A list of some of the published studies can be found in Table 17-1.

TABLE 17-1 *Published Articles on Aromatherapy in Palliative Care*

Author	Year	Essential Oil	Common Name	Number of Participants	Method
Louis & Kowalski	2002	*Lavandula angustifolia*	Lavender	17	Diffused
Wilcock et al	2004	*Lavandula angustfolia Chamaemelum nobile*	Lavender Roman chamomile	46	Massage
Kyle	2006	*Santalum album*	Sandalwood 1%	34	Massage
Soden et al	2004	*Lavandula angustifolia*	Lavender	42	Massage
Wilkinson et al	2007	20 essential oils (not listed)		288	Massage
Serfaty et al	2012	20 essential oils (not listed)		39	Massage

Fungating Wounds

Malignant fungating wounds (MFW) are the result of cutaneous infiltration by cancerous cells (da Costa Santos et al 2010) and present a multidimensional challenge in palliative care (Merz et al 2011). MFW are complex wounds that become malodorous as a result of infection (Lo et al 2012). They may also bleed, are often painful, and cause physical and psychological distress because the smell of a fungating wound is usually offensive (Fleck 2006, Gibson & Green 2013). Conventional treatment is with a metronidazole and Mesalt® dressing (da Costa Santos et al 2010) or 6% miltefosine solution (Adderley & Smith 2007). Foam dressings that include silver (Kalemikerakis et al 2012) or activated carbon dressing with curcumin ointment (da Costa Santos et al 2010) are also used. Some success has been found using ghee and honey (Udwadia 2011). The most expensive treatment is metronidazole cream (Mercier & Knevitt 2005).

An Australian team, Mercier and Knevitt (2005), found that essential oils used in creams ameliorated the bad smell of the fungating wound and also helped the wound. Between 2003 and 2005, they used aromatherapy successfully in 13 patients with fungating wounds. This work resulted in a nursing protocol for using essential oils in fungating wound care in the state of New South Wales, Australia. The article presents three detailed case studies with some helpful hints. They suggest that if odor is only present during dressing changes, then essential oils need just be diffused during the procedure. If the odor of the wound is detectable (but not too offensive apart from dressing change), a few drops of the chosen oils can be applied to the outside of the dressing. Only if the odor becomes too distressing are essential oils applied directly to the fungating wound. When this does happen, the patient's choice of essential oil can be mixed with an equal amount of tea tree oil *(Melaleuca alternifolia)* in a water-based cream at 2.5% to 5% dilution and applied directly to the wound. Slight stinging may occur initially. Enough cream is applied to prevent the dressing from sticking to the wound, to avoid inadvertent disturbance in dressing changes.

Tavares (2011), a UK-trained nurse, outlines another protocol for using essential oils for fungating malodorous wounds in her self-published booklet "Integrating Clinical Aromatherapy into Specialist Palliative Care." Her booklet is based on 9 years' experience working in palliative care in the UK before she moved to Canada. Tavares recommends using tea tree and lavender combined in equal proportions in either aloe vera gel or infused *Calendula officinalis*.

In another Australian study, Warnke et al (2006) conducted a case series ($n = 30$) using an essential oil mix on the fungating wounds of patients with inoperable squamous cell carcinomas (head and neck). The same essential oil mixture was used for each person. The mix contained (per g) 70 mg eucalyptus, 50 mg tea tree, 45 mg lemongrass, 45 mg lemon, 7 mg clove leaf, and 3 mg thyme essential oils in a 40% ethanol base. The ulcers were rinsed with 5 mL of the mixture twice a day. All patients experienced complete removal of the malodor by the fourth day. Some patients also had wound healing and a few achieved complete reepithelialization. This report includes three detailed case studies with clear photographic evidence of wound improvement.

TABLE 17-2 *Published Studies on Fungating Wounds*

Author	Year	Essential Oil	Common Name	Number of Participants
Warnke et al	2004	*Melaleuca alternifolia,* Citrus paradisi Eucalyptus globulus	Tea tree Grapefruit Eucalyptus	25
Ames	2006	*Thymus vulgaris* CT linalool *Boswellia carterii*	Thyme Frankincense	Case studies
Mercier & Knevitt	2005	*Melaleuca alternifolia* + patient's chosen essential oil	Tea tree	Case studies

My own choice of essential oils for fungating wounds would be tea tree, eucalyptus, geranium, and frankincense in aloe vera. A small selection of pertinent, published fungating wound studies can be found in Table 17-2.

Giving Comfort During Palliative Care

Aromatherapy can aid the management of symptom control, but perhaps aromatherapy's greatest strength in palliative care lies in its ability to facilitate communication at an emotional and spiritual level, as well as giving feelings of comfort and relaxation. For this reason, the choice of essential oils should rest with the patient. Concentrate on offering the patient a selection that could be relaxing or relevant to how they are feeling. If he or she is particularly withdrawn or depressed, an uplifting essential oil known for its gentle antidepressant properties, such as bergamot *(Citrus bergamia)* or frankincense *(Boswellia carterii)*, would be appropriate. Familiar aromas that give pleasure can relax a patient sufficiently to allow him or her to open up. Aromatherapy in combination with the 'M' Technique allows a patient to experience pleasure, relaxation, and acceptance simultaneously. The 'M' Technique is a simple method of gentle, structured stroking. For more information, please see the relevant chapter. Trust can occur at a deep level between caregiver and patient with the use of aromatherapy. This level of intimacy allows caregivers to show their profound love of humanity in a deeply moving way and provide real "comfort care" to their patients (Kolcaba 1995). A growing number of healthcare professionals desire to give this level of care (Montgomery 1996).

HOSPICE CARE

Hospice care is intended for the whole person, aiming to meet all needs—physical, emotional, social, and spiritual—at home, in day care, and in the hospice itself (Radbruch & Payne 2009). The hospice movement was founded in the UK by Dame Cecily Saunders in 1967 with the opening of the first hospice, St. Christopher's, in south London. The hospice movement in the UK has since then expanded rapidly; today, there are over 100 hospices (NHS UK 2013). Two teams of specialist nurses—the Macmillan nurses and the Marie Curie nurses—support the work of the hospice movement. Macmillan nurses are trained in palliative care and pain management in oncology (Leadbeater 2013) and mainly give advice and support. Marie Curie nurses are trained in cancer care (particularly end-of-life care) and can give hands-on help at home for people at the end stages of life. They will stay overnight if needed to give the family a break (www.mariecurie.org.uk/).

In Germany, the hospice movement had a rocky start after a documentary about St. Christopher's hospice in London was shown on television, sparking a heated debate about assisted suicide versus palliative care and if the two could coexist (Muller-Busch 2009). However, the debate has not deterred excellent palliative care. Today, end-of-life care in Germany is managed mainly by doctors in general practice with help from specialists in palliative care with the result that over one third of patients in palliative care die in hospices (Heese et al 2013). There are hospices in many other European countries such as Italy (Partinico et al 2013), Austria, and Poland (Centeno et al 2007). In Belgium, Luxembourg, and The Netherlands (where euthanasia and physician-assisted suicide [PAS] are accepted) there are robust hospice movements (Thulesius et al 2013). In France, the hospice model is slightly different with mobile teams supporting the terminally ill at home (Centeno et al 2007).

In the United States, there are more than 4700 hospice programs. In 2007, these hospice programs cared for nearly 1.4 million people (Hospice Foundation of America 2013). Care is provided through Medicare and other health insurance providers and 80% of hospice care is provided in the patient's home or in a nursing home. The United States allows PAS in three States (Oregon, Montana, and Washington). However, this has not impacted the level or acceptance of hospice care (Thulesius et al 2013).

In countries such as Japan, Korea, and Taiwan, the hospice movement is only just emerging (Glass et al 2011, Kao et al 2013). In Africa, there is a need to develop both palliative and hospice care (Onyeka et al 2013). In Australia, there is a growing hospice movement (Yoong et al 2013).

AROMATHERAPY IN HOSPICE CARE

Dame Cicely Sounders, the founder of the hospice movement wrote, "we do not have to cure to heal." In using aromatherapy in hospice care, there is no attempt to cure, but there is a great attempt to ameliorate symptoms, provide support, and enable the patient to have the best quality of life for the time they have left. Many countries use aromatherapy in hospice care, however, an Italian study found that only five hospices offered aromatherapy and this could be attributed to lack of training, knowledge, and funding (Latina et al 2012). In the United States, 86% of Washington State hospices offered aromatherapy (Kozak et al 2008). Most U.S. hospices allow aromatherapy and some have their own aromatherapy programs. The San Diego Hospice even has its own hospice blends—these include a mix for comfort (lavender, rose, Roman chamomile), serenity (sandalwood, rose, bergamot), and grief (rose, frankincense, cypress, helichrysum) (Schwan & Ash 2004). Almost every UK hospice uses aromatherapy.

Mouth Care

Mouth problems such as dry mouth, cracked lips, painful mouth, ulcers, and swallowing difficulties are common in all three areas—palliative, hospice, and end-of-life care. However, dry mouth is particularly relevant in end-of-life care and can result from many causes such as mouth breathing, the use of drugs such as opiates and sedatives, oxygen therapy, radiotherapy, chemotherapy, and dehydration (Tavares 2011). An Australian study demonstrated that dry mouth and mouth ulcers significantly impacted the physical, social, and psychological well-being of terminally ill patients (Rohr et al 2010). Dry mouth was one of the eight most distressing symptoms in a Taiwanese study of palliative care (Tsai et al 2007).

A study to explore the use of essential oils to improve oral health in hospice patients was carried out by Kang et al (2010). In this Korean study, 43 patients with terminal cancer were randomly allocated to the aromatherapy group ($n = 22$) or the control group ($n = 21$). The essential oil mixture included geranium, lavender, peppermint, and tea tree. The control group received 0.9% saline. Mouth care was given twice a day for 1 week to both groups. The outcome measures were: (a) reduction in discomfort; (b) improvement in the state of the mouth; and (c) reduction of any presence of *Candida albicans*. The results demonstrated that the presence of *Candida albicans* was significantly decreased, discomfort was reduced, and the state of the patient's mouth was improved in the aromatherapy group compared to the control group. The reduction in *Candida albicans* is important because this fungal infection is very common in advanced cancer, and although Bagg et al (2006) found that tea tree was effective to reduce the infection, the addition of lavender, peppermint, and geranium would make the taste and smell more acceptable.

Palma rosa *(Cymbopogon martinii)* can also be very useful in mouth care: it is high in alcohols but safe to use orally; the taste is acceptable, therefore compliance among patients is high; it is easy to administer so compliance by nurses is high; it is inexpensive and therefore attractive for hospital use; and, it makes the patient's breath smell pleasant. It is also antifungal, antibacterial, and antiviral so it can clear up any nasty infections. Palma rosa mouth care is used with acceptance and great success in the palliative care departments of some hospitals in the United States (Surrette 2006).

END-OF-LIFE CARE

The physical process of dying is recognizable (Keegan & Drick 2011). Bodily functions cease, and the peripheral temperature drops as circulation fails. This means the hands/arms and feet/legs become cold and the skin begins to look mottled and discolored. Thirst is often the last craving, with food refused. Many dying patients breathe through their mouths, which become dry and cracked. Often their eyes remain open, even though the patient may be asleep or unconscious. However, most patients can hear right up until the moment of death. This was the case with a dear friend of mine who died recently at a famous London hospital. The consultant said "the most important thing about end of life care is pain management." He was speaking in a loud voice, right across my dying friend, to her husband who was sitting on the opposite side of the bed (actually doing the hand M Technique). "She can hear you!" the husband said. And my friend, eyes half closed and glazed over, mouth open, nodded twice. She died less than 4 hours later.

PEACE AND SERENITY AT THE END OF LIFE

One of the most important goals of end-of-life care is achieving a good death (Hirai et al 2006). To many doctors, this means adequate pain management. However, there is much more to a good death than lack of pain (Buckley 2008; Knapp-Hayes 2014). The challenge is to minimize end-of-life symptoms while improving the quality during the final hours of life. Aromatherapy can be helpful in both reducing symptoms, such as terminal agitation and fear, and improving the quality of life with beautiful smells and gentle touch. Each person deserves the dignity to die surrounded by family or, if there are no relatives and friends, to die surrounded by caring people (Keegan & Drick 2011).

This brings us to think of the word "care" and what it really means, as well as if healthcare actually includes care. Perhaps, a better term to describe healthcare might be disease management! End-of-life care is sympathetic and is hard to teach to another person because caring involves feelings. A person feels sympathy or they don't. I think the majority of those working in palliative, hospice, and end-of-life care do genuinely care. Hopefully, governments will learn the importance of quality of care at the end of life and allow healthcare professionals the time, resources, and support to be able to give that care. A feature in the *Royal College of Nursing Bulletin* about nursing in Wales was entitled "Time to Care" (RCN 2013, p 11). In the UK, the cuts to the NHS have resulted in there not being enough nurses or physicians in many hospitals. Caring takes time and it is hard to quantify for budgets yet it is quantifiable in family satisfaction and in cherishing the honor and care given at the end of life. The idea of a Golden Room (Keegan & Drick 2011), where someone can choose to go and experience the best death he or she can achieve, is a great concept and worthy of integrating into healthcare systems globally. (I really hope this will be available when my time comes.) If this were not possible, then following some of the suggestions in *Gentle Dying* (Warner 2008) would help improve the quality of death.

Most of us would like to die at home, or at least, in the place of our choice. However, for many people, this may not be possible and the alternatives can be frightening. A comparison study of England, Canada, Germany, and the United States found that many patients did not die in their preferred location (Klinger et al 2013). In Canada more than 50% of end-of-life patients were being treated "aggressively" rather than palliatively (Hu et al 2013), and although most Canadian people wanted to die at home, few were actually allowed to do so (Topf et al 2013). Aromatherapy, using familiar smells and a gentle touch like the 'M' Technique, can help with fear and anxiety in the last few days/hours of life.

END-OF-LIFE CARE WITH THE 'M' TECHNIQUE AND AROMATHERAPY

Many people have a fear of dying alone. When patients are at the point of death, they may have been unconscious for some time, but it is still important to be really "present" for them. They will probably still be able to hear you, so talk gently to them or play their favorite music. Tell them you are there for them, but give them permission to go. Touch using the 'M' Technique is a wonderful way to say goodbye and to soothe the dying person.

The 'M' Technique has been used successfully on both pain and agitation at the end of life on two patients at St. Richard's Hospice in Worcester, UK (Roberts & Campbell 2011). The first patient had MS and the second patient had cerebral palsy (CP). The MS patient scored her pain as 10 on the 0-10 pain scale despite having patient-controlled analgesia and recent, additional, subcutaneous morphine. The 'M' Technique appeared to have a very rapid relaxation effect and the patient died peacefully within 24 hours. The second patient was extremely agitated—kicking, very restless, and not sleeping for days. After 10 minutes of the 'M' Technique, the patient appeared relaxed and the jerking movements stopped. When the 'M' Technique was completed on both his hands and feet, the patient fell asleep and slept for 3 hours. It only takes a few moments to show the hand 'M' Technique to a relative. This can empower the relative and soothe their loved one.

R.J. Buckle students have completed studies using the 'M' Technique plus essential oils on end-of-life patients (Table 17-3). The most frequently used essential oil was frankincense, followed by lavender. However, the one essential oil I always take with me when I visit terminally ill patients is rose. The aroma is instantly recognized, accepted, and universally liked. Rose has a deep calming effect that is readily apparent in the change in breathing and body relaxation. Neroli hydrolat is also effective when sprayed on pillows and sheets. These, plus the hand 'M' Technique can soothe and calm at the end of life.

One of the first R.J. Buckle student studies was carried out by Katz (1999). This was a study of 20 patients in the active dying process, who were showing terminal agitation, at her hospice in Pennsylvania. Katz applied 1% *Lavandula angustifolia* with the 'M' Technique to hands and feet. All the patients had reduction in pulse

TABLE 17-3 *R.J. Buckle Student Studies on Hospice and End-of-Life Care*

Name	Year	State	Number of Participants	Essential Oil	Method
Katz	1999	PA	15	Lavender	'M' Technique
O'Keefe	2000	AZ	10	Frankincense/lavender	'M' Technique
Ocampo	2000	NY	6	Frankincense	'M' Technique
Anderson	2004	AZ	13	Mixture*	'M' Technique
Eaton	2008	MI	9	Frankincense	'M' Technique
Donadson-Steverson	2007	TX	30	Frankincense/clary sage	'M' Technique
Sullivan	2008	TX	4	Frankincense/lavender	'M' Technique

*Lavender, frankincense, and sandalwood 1%.

and respiration, and all demonstrated reduction of agitation by unclenching their hands. In 75% of cases, family members verbalized that they had observed a decrease in agitation. Two comments from her study are haunting: from a patient—"There is a sense of peace I haven't felt since the diagnosis was made"; from a 5-year-old— "My granny feels better, and I helped" (she had been shown how to do the hand 'M' Technique).

O'Keefe (2000) carried out a study on 10 patients using frankincense in a foot and leg 'M' Technique and a drop of lavender on a pillow at her hospice in Arizona. All patients were in the active stage of dying, and some of them died within hours. After treatment, the restlessness of nine of the patients decreased. For most, their respiration slowed and became deeper as they became quieter. Most of them slept peacefully following the treatment. The response of the patients' relatives was one of deep appreciation for this level of caring.

Ocampo (2000) carried out a controlled study on six terminally ill patients experiencing moderate to severe pain at her hospice in New York. Eight volunteers were trained in the 'M' Technique and performed it on patients' hands. All patients receiving the 'M' Technique experienced considerable reduction in their pain perception, according to a visual analog. The treatment group slept for longer periods than the control group.

Eaton (2008) conducted a small, controlled, pilot study in a hospice in Wisconsin ($n = 9$). Patients were given the 'M' Technique with frankincense or with plain grapeseed oil. Outcome measurements were respiration, blood pressure (BP), and psychological changes. Decreases in BP occurred in both groups. All patients said they felt calmer. The control group did not have changes in respiration. The aroma group appeared to have a greater psychological effect. The entire frankincense group had a positive response whereas 50% of the control group had a positive effect.

Donadson-Steverson (2008) conducted a pilot study ($n = 30$) in Addison, Texas, on the effects of 5% frankincense *(Boswellia carteri)* and clary sage *(Salvia sclarea)* while using the hand 'M' Technique during the dying process. The 'M' Technique was completed every 2 to 4 hours by a family member who had been previously shown the 'M' Technique by a nurse. Each time the technique and essential oil mixture were applied, the family member would write down the date, time, symptoms, and responses to the therapy. Outcome measurements were changes in comfort levels as shown by changes in facial grimacing, grunting, and restlessness. Twenty-seven of the 30 (90%) patients had some symptom relief. The other three patients died before the 'M' Technique could be given. Sullivan (2008) conducted a separate study (also in Texas) on the effects of 5% lavender *(Lavandula angustifolia)* and frankincense *(Boswellia carteri)* given in a hand and foot 'M' Technique for end-of-life agitation. Again, positive effects on the agitation of dying were observed.

I feel that the soul does not die but moves on, and just as a newborn child is helped into this world, so should a soul be helped in its transition out of this world. Whatever the healthcare provider believes, by caring for a dying patient in this way, the transition from life to death is supported in the most holistic way possible.

Using familiar smells and gentle touch are two of the tools we can use. When I have used the 'M' Technique and essential oils on a dying patient, as I did very recently, I have felt an enormous sense of gratitude to be able to do something that gives peace and comfort to the patient, the relatives, and to myself. This sense of gratitude is expressed in the following poem.

Thank you, my friend
For sharing your dying.
I can be with you
To catch a glimpse of the life you are leaving
And the life to which you return.
In the process, I can accompany your tumult,
Your fear, resistance,
And hope.
Thank you my friend
For sharing your soul. (Dorothea Hover-Kramer, 1993; reproduced with the kind permission of the author)

REFERENCES

Adderley U, Smith R. 2007. Topical agents and dressings for fungating wounds. *Cochrane Database Syst Rev.* (2):CD003948.

Ames D. 2006. Aromatic wound care in a healthcare system: a report from USA. *Int J Clin Aromather.* 3(2):3-18.

Anderson C 2004. Lavender, sandalwood and frankincense in the M Technique to reduce restlessness in hospice patients. Unpublished dissertation for RJ Buckle Associates.

Axelrod J. 2006. The 5 stages of loss and grief. *Psych Central.* http://psychcentral.com/lib/the-5-stages-of-loss-and-grief/000617. Accessed August 8, 2013.

Bagg J, Jackson M, Petrina Sweeney M, Ramage G, Davies A. 2006. Susceptibility to *Melaleuca alternifolia* (tea tree) oil of yeasts isolated from the mouths of patients with advanced cancer. *Oral Oncol.* 42(5):487-492.

Brooker C. 2008. *Churchill Livingstone's Medical Dictionary.* Churchill Livingstone, Elsevier. London.

Buckley J. 2008. *Palliative Care: An Integrated Approach.* Wiley-Blackwell. London.

Centeno C, Clark D, Lynch T, Rocafort J, Prall D et al. 2007. Facts and indicators on palliative care development in 52 countries of the WHO European region: results of an EAPC Task Force. *Palliat Med.* 21(6):463-71.

Chang S. 2008. Effect of aroma hand massage on pain, state, anxiety and depression in hospice patients with terminal cancer. *Taehan Kanho Hakhoe Chi.* 38(4):493-502.

Clark D, Centeno C. 2006. Palliative care in Europe: an emerging approach to comparative analysis. *Clin Med.* 6(2):197-201.

da Costa Santos C, de Mattos Pimenta C, Nobre M. 2010. A systematic review of topical treatments to control the odor of malignant fungating wounds. *J Pain Symptom Manage.* 39(6):1065-76.

Donadson-Steverson A. 2008. Does aromatherapy plus the 'M' technique enhance the dying process? Unpublished dissertation. RJ Buckle Associates.

Eaton K. 2008. Does frankincense and the 'M' Technique enhance the dying process? Unpublished dissertation. RJ Buckle Associates.

Esmonde L, Long A. 2008. Complementary therapy use by persons with multiple sclerosis: benefits and research priorities. *Complement Ther Clin Pract.* 14(3):176-84.

Fleck C. 2006. Palliative dilemmas: wound odour. *Wound Care Canada.* 4(3):10-14.

Gibson S, Green J. 2013. Review of patients' experiences with fungating wounds and associated quality of life. *J Wound Care.* 22(5):265-6.

Glass A, Chen L, Hwang E, Ono Y, Nahapetyan L et al. 2011. A cross-cultural comparison of hospice development in Japan, South Korea, and Taiwan. *J Cross Cult Gerontol.* 25(1):1-19.

Harris R. 2013. Making a difference in cancer and palliative care: a spotlight on key interventions and essential oils in cancer and palliative care settings. 2012 Conference Proceedings. *J Japan Soc Aromather.* 11(Suppl):48-54.

Heese O, Vogeler E, Martens T, Schnell O, Tonn J et al. 2013. End-of-life caregivers' perception of medical and psychological support during the final weeks of glioma patients: a questionnaire-based survey. *Neuro Oncol.* Jun 28. [Epub ahead of print]. PMID:23814266. Accessed August 5, 2013.

Hirai K, Miyahita M, Morita T, Sanjo M, Uchitomi Y. 2006. Good death in Japanese cancer care: a qualitative study. *J Pain Symptom Manage.* 31(2):140-7.

Horrigan C. 2004. The benefits and possibilities for the use of aromatherapy in palliative care. *Int J Clin Aromather.* 1(2):23-7.

Hospice Foundation of America. 2013. http://www.hospicefoundation.org/whatishospice. Accessed August 5, 2013.

Hover-Kramer D. 1993. Thank you my friend. *J Holistic Nursing.* 11(1):115-6.

Hu W, Yasui Y, White J, Winget M. 2013. Aggressiveness of end-of-life care for patients with colorectal cancer in Alberta, Canada: 2006-2009. *J Pain Symptom Manage.* Jul 16. doi: pii: S0885-3924(13)00312-6. Accessed August 5, 2013.

Jackson C, Latini C. 2013. Touch and hand-mediated therapies. In *Holistic Nursing: A Handbook for Practice.* Ed Montgomery-Dossey B, Keegan L. Jones & Bartlett, Boston, USA pp 417-37.

Kang H, Na S, Kim Y. 2010. Effects of oral care with essential oil on improvement in oral health status of hospice patients. *J Korean Acad Nurs.* 40(4):473-81.

Kao C, Cheng S, Chiu T, Chen C, Hu W. 2013. Does the awareness of terminal illness influence cancer patients' psycho-spiritual state, and their DNR signing: a survey in Taiwan. *Jpn J Clin Oncol.* 2013 Jul 25. [Epub ahead of print]. Accessed August 5, 2013.

Katz J. 1999. Does aromatherapy enhance the dying process? Unpublished dissertation. RJ Buckle Associates.

Kawamura K, Maeda R, Yoshimatu K, Ishida N, Yamada K, Ikeuchi M. 2013. Stress abatement effect of aromatherapy treatment for terminally ill cancer patients. 2012 Conference Proceedings. *J Japan Soc Aromather.* 11(Suppl):106.

Kalemikerakis J, Vardaki Z, Fouka G, Vlachou E, Gkovina U et al. 2012. Comparison of foam dressings with silver versus foam dressings without silver in the care of malodorous malignant fungating wounds. *J BUON.* 17(3):560-4.

Keegan L, Drick C-A. 2011. *End of Life: Nursing Solutions for Death with Dignity.* Singer. New York.

Klinger C, Howell D, Zakus D, Deber R. 2013. Barriers and facilitators to care for the terminally ill: a cross-country case comparison study of Canada, England, Germany, and the United States. *Palliat Med.* 28(2):111-20.

Knevitt A. 2004. Therapeutic aromatherapy in a palliative setting. *Int J Clin Aromather.* 1(2):46-50.

Knapp-Hayes M. 2014. Complementary Nursing in End of Life Care. Kicozo-Knowledge Insitute for Complementary Care. http://www.kicoxo.nl.

Kolcaba K. 1995. Comfort as process and product, merged in holistic nursing art. *Journal of Holistic Nursing.* 11(1):115-116.

Kozak L, Kayes L, McCarty R, Walkinshaw C, Congdon S et al. 2008. Use of complementary and alternative medicine (CAM) by Washington State hospices. *Am J Hosp Palliat Care.* 25(6):463-8.

Kubler-Ross E. 1978. *To Live Until We Say Good-Bye.* London: Prentice Hall.

Kyle G. 2006. Evaluating the effectiveness of aromatherapy in reducing levels of anxiety in palliative care patients: results of a pilot study. *Complement Ther Clin Pract.* 12(2):148-55.

Latina R, Mastroianni C, Sansoni J, Piredda M, Casale G. 2012. The use of complementary therapies for chronic pain in Italian hospices. *Prof Inferm.* 65(4):244-50.

Leadbeater M. 2013. The role of a community palliative care specialist nurse team in caring for people with metastatic breast cancer. *Int J Palliat Nurs.* 19(2):93-7.

Lo S, Hayter M, Hu W, Tai C, Hsu M, Li Y. 2012. Symptom burden and quality of life in patients with malignant fungating wounds *J Adv Nurs.* 68(6):1312-21.

Louis M, Kowalski S. 2002. Use of aromatherapy with hospice patients to decrease pain, anxiety and depression and to promote an increased sense of well-being. *Am J Hospice & Palliative Care.* 19(6):381-6.

Lynch T, Connor S, Clark D. 2013. Mapping levels of palliative care development: a global update. *J Pain Symptom Manage.* 45(6):1094-106.

Martin-Moreno J, Harris M, Gorgojo L et al. 2008. *Palliative Care in the European Union.* European Parliament Economic and Scientific Policy Department. *www.lse.ac.uk/LSEHealthAndSocialCare*

Mercier D, Knevitt A. 2005. Using topical aromatherapy for the management of fungating wounds in a palliative care unit. *J Wound Care.* 14(10):497-8.

Merz T, Klein C, Uebach B, Kern M, Ostgathe C, Bükki J. 2011. Fungating wounds – multidimensional challenge in palliative care. *Breast Care (Basel).* 6(1):21-4.

Moeini M, Khadibi M, Bekhradi R, Mahmoudian S, Nazari F. 2010. Effect of aromatherapy on the quality of sleep in ischemic heart disease patients hospitalized in intensive care units of heart hospitals of the Isfahan University of Medical Sciences. *Iran J Nurs Midwifery Res.* 15(4):234-9.

Montgomery C. 1996. The care-giving relationship: paradoxical and transcendent aspects. *Alternative Therapies.* 2(2):52-57.

Muller-Busch C. 2009. DGP: Germany aims to offer specialist palliative care to all who need it. *Eur J Palliative Care.* 16(6):308-310.

NHS UK. 2013. http://www.nhs.uk/CarersDirect/guide/bereavement/Pages/finding-a-hospice.aspx. Accessed Aug 7, 2014.

O'Keefe M. 2000. The effects of *Boswellia carteri* and *Lavandula angustifolia* on the dying process. Unpublished dissertation for RJ Buckle Associates.

Ocampo A. 2000. The effect of frankincense of alternation of pain perception in hospice patients. Unpublished dissertation. Unpublished dissertation for RJ Buckle Associates.

Olson M, Keegan L. 2013. Dying in peace. In *Holistic Nursing: A Handbook for Practice.* Ed Montgomery-Dossey & Keegan. Jones & Bartlett. Boston, USA. pp 463-84.

Onyeka T, Velijanashvili M, Abdissa S, Manase F, Kordzaia D. 2013. Twenty-first century palliative care: a tale of four nations. *Eur J Cancer Care (Engl).* 2013 May 6. PMID: 23647421. Accessed August 5, 2013.

Partinico M, Corà A, Ghisi M, Ouimet AJ, Visentin M. 2013. A new Italian questionnaire to assess caregivers of cancer patients' satisfaction with palliative care: multicenter validation of the Post Mortem Questionnaire-Short Form. *J Pain Symptom Manage.* S0885-3924(13) 00307-2.

Pratt J, Mason A. 1981. *The Caring Touch.* Heyden, London.

Radbruch L, Payne S. 2009. White paper on standards and norms for hospice and palliative care in Europe: Part 1. *Eur J Palliative Care.* 16(6):278-89.

RCN 2013. Time to care. http://www.rcn.org.uk/aboutus/wales/time_to_care. Accessed December 14, 2013.

Roberts K, Campbell H. 2011. Using the M technique as therapy for patients at the end of life: two case studies. *Int J Palliat Nurs.* 17(3):114-8.

Rohr Y, Adams J, Young L. 2010. Oral discomfort in palliative care: results of an exploratory study of the experiences of terminally ill patients. *Int J Palliat Nurs.* 16(9):439-44.

Schwan R, Ash P. 2004. Integrative palliative aromatherapy care program at San Diego Hospice and Palliative Care. *Int J Clin Aromather.* 1(2):5-9.

Serfaty M, Wilkinson S, Freeman C, Mannix K, King M. 2012. The ToT Study: helping with Touch or Talk (ToT): a pilot randomised controlled trial to examine the clinical effectiveness of aromatherapy massage versus cognitive behaviour therapy for emotional distress in patients in cancer/palliative care. *Psychooncology.* 21(5):563-9.

Shin B, Lee M. 2007. Effects of aromatherapy acupressure on hemiplegic shoulder pain and motor power in stroke patients: a pilot study. *J Altern Complement Med.* 13(2):247-51.

Simon S. 1976. *Caring, Feeling, Touching.* Argus Communication. London

Soden K, Vincent K, Craske S, Lucas C, Ashley S. 2004. A randomized controlled trial of aromatherapy massage in a hospice setting. *Palliative Medicine.* 18(2):87-92.

Stein G. 1925. The pathless path. In Dossey L. (ed.). 1995. *Healing Words.* San Francisco: Harper San Francisco.

Sullivan V. 2008. Lavender and frankincense in the M Technique to reduce agitation at the end of life. Unpublished dissertation for RJ Buckle Associates.

Surrette B. 2006. Personal communication and testimonial. www.rjbuckle.com.

Tavares M. 2011. Integrating clinical aromatherapy into specialist palliative care. Available from http://www.naha.org/bookstore/integrating-clinical-aromatherapy-in-specialist-palliative-care/. Accessed. August 7, 2014.

Thulesius H, Scott H, Helgesson G, Lynöe N. 2013. De-tabooing dying control – a grounded theory study. *BMC Palliat Care.* 12:13. doi: 10.1186/1472-684X-12-13. Accessed August 5, 2013.

Topf L, Robinson C, Bottorff J. 2013. When a desired home death does not occur: the consequences of broken promises. *J Palliat Med.* 16(8):875-80.

Tsai L, Li I, Lai Y, Liu C, Chang T, Tu C. 2007. Fatigue and its associated factors in hospice cancer patients in Taiwan. *Cancer Nurs.* 30(1):24-30.

Udwadia T. 2011. Ghee and honey dressing for infected wounds. *Indian J Surg.* 73(4):278-83.

Warnke P, Sherry E, Russo P, Aeil Y et al. 2006. Antibacterial essential oils in malodorous cancer patients: clinical observations in 30 patients. *Phytomedicine.* 13:463-7.

Warnke P, Terheyden H, Ac Y, Springer I, Sherry E, Reynolds M et al. 2004. Tumor smell reduction with antibacterial essential oils. *Int J Clin Aromather.* 1(2):21-22.

Warner F. 2008. *Gentle Dying. The Simple Guide to Achieving a Peaceful Death.* Hay House, London.

Wilcock A, Manderson C, Weller R, Walker G, Carr D et al. 2004. Does aromatherapy massage benefit patients with cancer attending a specialist palliative care day centre? *Palliat Med.* 18(4):287-90.

Wilkinson S, Love S, Westcombe A, Gables M, Burgess C et al. 2007. Effectiveness of aromatherapy massage in the management of anxiety and depression in patients with cancer: a multicenter, randomized, controlled trial. *J Clin Oncol.* 25(5):532-9.

Wright M, Wood J, Lynch T, Clark D. 2008. Mapping levels of palliative care development: a global view. *J Pain Symptom Manage.* 35(5):469-85.

Yoong J, Boughey M, Leung S. 2013. Investigating trends in discharge destinations and impact on allied health service utilization in an Australian hospice. *Am J Hosp Palliat Care.* 2013 Jul 8. Accessed August 5, 2013.

Chapter 18

Pediatrics

"Childhood is measured out by sounds and smells and sights, before the dark hour of reason grows."

John Betjeman

CHAPTER ASSETS

There is a Chinese saying that "children get sick easily, and sickness can quickly become serious," and another says "children easily ill, easily cured." There is no doubt that children in the hospital are very vulnerable. They deteriorate or improve rapidly and they need a tremendous amount of love and support, particularly if their families cannot visit. Although children are more adaptable than adults and often face intimidating procedures with interest and no apparent fear, some may display behavioral problems when they become institutionalized.

Some of the most distressing aspects of hospitalization are invasive medical procedures, such as venipuncture and the placing of nasogastric tubes. Aromatherapy can help soothe the child before these interventions. A few moments of hand or foot 'M' Technique can help relax a child while you explain what is going to happen, how long it will last, and how it will help him/her. Anxiety about being hurt, or having lasting pain, has been identified as one of a child's greatest fears (Foster & Park 2012, Logan et al 2012). A systematic review did not find that conventional preoperative analgesia was useful in children (Ashley et al 2012). Although these findings were about dental surgery, they could be extrapolated to cover other kinds of operations. Therefore, it is pertinent to explore if aromatherapy could help reduce pediatric pain. van Dijk (2001) discusses the problems of pain assessment in neonates and infants in her excellent PhD thesis *Pain Unheard?* She has generously allowed this to be available to everyone and it can be

Alleviating pediatric pain has been central to Dr. van Dijk's ongoing research at both the Red Cross War Memorial Children's Hospital in Cape Town, South Africa, and Erasmus Medical Centre-Sophia Children's Hospital, Rotterdam, The Netherlands. To this end, her team uses topical application of essential oils and the 'M' Technique with good results (O'Flaherty et al 2012).

Sweet orange oil was found to be helpful in the induction of 120 unpremedicated children aged 5 to 14 years in a study by Mehta et al (1998). Children in the essential oil group were significantly more likely to say they would be willing to have a similar anesthetic technique again in the future ($P < 0.05$). A South African discussion article by Daniels and O'Flaherty (2010) reported on the positive combination of aromatherapy and the 'M' Technique on reducing anxiety in the burns unit of the Red Cross Memorial Children's Hospital in Cape Town. The aromatherapy oils used were a 1% mixture of lavender, German chamomile, and neroli. A second paper expanded on this observational pilot study (O'Flaherty et al 2012) and covers 126 massage sessions on 71 burns patients between January and October 2009. Although this was not a randomized controlled study, statistical evidence of improvement was achieved, such that a major randomized controlled trial (RCT) in that setting started in April 2013.

Disappointingly, in an RCT published by De Jong et al (2012) and carried out at the Erasmus Medical Centre, mandarin did not appear to reduce infants' distress when used after major craniofacial surgery. Sixty children aged 3 to 36 months were randomly allocated to one of three groups: (1) 'M' Technique with plain carrier oil; (2) 'M' Technique with mandarin; or (3) standard postoperative care. Primary outcome measures were changes in COMFORT behavior scores and Numeric Rating Scale pain and Numeric Rating Scale distress scores assessed on videotape by an observer blinded for the condition. Several reasons were given for the lack of success. However, the hospital continues to use both the 'M' Technique and aromatherapy in many wards because they have both been found to soothe and calm the children. The primary reason for the lack of success was that the intervention was given too soon after surgery when the anesthetic had not yet worn off. Secondly, the patient group was toddlers who were potentially fearful of strangers; also, as a result of swollen eyes following surgery, they were even more scared of unfamiliar noises, voices, and smells.

Aromatherapy is a natural thing to a child, whose early life revolves around smell and touch. Babies identify their mothers through the mother's smell (Russell 1976) because a baby is born with a structurally mature olfactory system (Humphrey 1940). Schaal et al (2000) demonstrated that the human fetus can detect and record aromatic information gleaned from maternal intake, before birth. Twenty-four pregnant women were randomly allocated to one of two groups. Babies born to mothers who had consumed anise-flavored products during the last 2 weeks of pregnancy displayed positive oro-facial responses (at just 8 hours and 4 days after birth) when offered anise-flavored aroma. Babies born to mothers in the control group, whose mothers had not ingested anise-flavored products, displayed aversive or neutral oro-facial responses. A later study by

Sevelinges et al (2009) found that odorization of a mother's nipples with banana or almond solution from birth to weaning resulted in impairment at adulthood of conditioned odor aversion (COA).

Young children up to the age of 5 years are not repelled by smells that most adults dislike, such as feces. However, by the age of 7 years, many children are beginning to establish similar "tastes" in smells to adults (Engen 1974). Children also display the facility of "learned memory" early on, gravitating toward the smell of a perfume worn by their mother, rather than another unknown perfume (Schleidt & Genzel 1990). Therefore, familiar smells are more acceptable to children in a hospital environment. Children from other cultures may respond (and prefer) different aromas than a Western child (Fitzgerald et al 2010). Children can be extremely sensitive to smell and it is possible to test odor identification using a "smell wheel" (Cameron & Doty 2012). A familiar scent can be a useful way of calming a child and is an extension to the "favorite blanket" that many young children carry around as security. However, babies and children are exposed to more and more scented products such as baby perfumes, scented nappies, and fragranced toys (Harris 2005). These aromas are usually synthetic and are linked to the increasing number of allergies in children (Mazuck et al 2011).

Most of us find it an instinctive action to cuddle and stroke a child. Aromatherapy takes that instinct a little further and adds some extra therapeutic value. Parents and relatives can be taught very easily how to use the 'M' Technique on a sick child, and they relish the feeling of being empowered to do something in a situation most parents fear. This experience of empowerment can be made more potent by the addition of an aroma that both mother or father and child are familiar with and like. Gentle aromas can soothe a child, but the emphasis is on gentleness. It is necessary to use only half the normal number of drops of an essential oil required for an adult. Please see Table 18-1 for dosage recommendations for children.

When children may have been subjected to previous abuse and will not be receptive to touch, using a soothing aroma can still be beneficial. Children like to be involved in choosing an aroma, especially if the choice is small. More than four essential oils will demand too much effort from a sick child. Sometimes a choice of just two will make aromatherapy acceptable, whereas if only one smell is offered it

TABLE 18-1 *Doses for Children and Babies**

Preemies	Floral waters only	N/A
Newborn to 6 months	1 drop in 20 mL	0.25%
6 months to 2 years	1 drop in 10 mL	0.5%
2 to 5 years	1 drop in 5 mL	1%
5 to 10 years	1 to 2 drops in 5 mL	1% to 2%
More than 10 years	1 to 5 drops in 5 mL	1% to 5%

*Unless treating specific infections, for example, onychomycosis (toenail fungus) or hair lice.
N/A = nonapplicable.

might be refused. However, it is important never to insist; children are patients with patient rights, no matter how old they are.

So, it is easy to see that aromatherapy could have an important supportive role in pediatrics. Aromatherapy can bring comfort to both child and parent and give a sense of empowerment to staff. Caring for sick children is an emotionally draining experience, and caring for a dying child is one of the most challenging tasks faced by any health professional (Hodson 1995, Youngblut & Brooten 2012).

HYPERACTIVITY

Every child will have a unique response to being hospitalized. Some children become withdrawn, some become placatory, and others become hyperactive. It is the hyperactive children who can become a source of irritation to staff and other children. Aromatherapy can often help calm children down (O'Flaherty et al 2012). The cause underlying the behavior may be the strange environment (and smells) that make the child feel threatened. Hyperactivity may be a means of asking for more attention or a means of communicating a child's sense of ill ease. The 'M' Technique on its own, or with a familiar smell, can soothe a child and reduce his/her hyperactivity (Daniels & O'Flaherty 2010). Sometimes mixing aromas to produce a new but faintly familiar aroma can also be beneficial (Worwood 2000) (Table 18-2).

A foot or hand 'M' Technique is usually acceptable to a sick child. Teaching parents to help their sick children is one of the most rewarding things I have ever done. A mother's touch, no matter how unfamiliar she is with any technique or stroke, is what a child will usually recognize and respond to. However, parents do experience a great deal of stress and anxiety when their child is admitted to a pediatric intensive care unit and some parents may be too tense to practice the 'M' Technique. In those cases, the nurse can temporarily perform the 'M' Technique until the parents feel ready to do it. Gentleness and slow strokes are what matters. The slowness can be quite challenging to a stressed parent. Both gentleness and slow speed are particularly important to remember if the child is unconscious. If the mother wears a lot of bracelets, do not ask her to remove them, as her child will remember how they sounded and how they felt.

TABLE 18-2 *Essential Oils to Relax a Hyperactive Child in Hospital*

Common Name	Botanical Name
Roman chamomile	*Chamaemelum nobile*
Mandarin	*Citrus reticulata*
Lavender	*Lavandula angustifolia*
Neroli	*Citrus aurantium* var amara (flos)
Rose	*Rosa damascena*
Geranium	*Pelargonium graveolens*
Sweet marjoram	*Origanum majorana*

ATTENTION DEFICIT/HYPERACTIVITY DISORDER

Attention deficit/hyperactivity disorder (ADHD) is a combination of inattention, hyperactivity, and impulsive behavior that is classified as a disorder when these behaviors are severe. ADHD is thought to be a developmental failure in the brain circuitry that underlies inhibition and self-control (Tucker 1999). More recent work has linked ADHD to poor neuronal activity within the basal ganglia and cerebellar loops within the prefrontal cortex (Leisman & Melillo 2012).

Children with ADHD have poor social skills, yet mechanisms for this remain unclear (van Eck et al 2012). During the last 20 years, an increasing number of children have been diagnosed with attention deficit disorder (ADD) or ADHD. It is the most commonly diagnosed behavioral disorder in children and the fastest growing disorder in adults. Since 1990, the number of children in the United States diagnosed with ADHD has increased from 900,000 to more than 5.5 million ADD/ADHD Research and ADD/ADHD Online Support Group. 2014. ADHD is thought to affect 5% to 10% of all school-aged children. One and a half million adults also have been diagnosed with ADHD. Similar patterns have emerged in Germany (Garbe et al 2012), Italy (Ruggiero et al 2012), Canada (Patten et al 2012), and Australia (Johnstone et al 2012). A systematic review of worldwide prevalence found that geography did not play a significant part in the prevalence of ADHD (Polanczyk et al 2009).

Charles Bradley first noticed that amphetamine (Benzedrine) calmed hyperactive children in 1937 (Gainetdinov & Caron 2001). Numerous studies have shown that stimulants such as amphetamines interact with plasma membrane monoamine transporters (dopamine, serotonin, and norepinephrine transporters) (Gainetdinov et al 1999). Stimulants are believed to work by increasing dopamine levels in the brain. Dopamine is a neurotransmitter associated with motivation, pleasure, and attention. The stimulants used to treat ADHD are Ritalin, Adderall, and Dexidrine. Ritalin is thought to work by altering levels of dopamine. However, studies with rats found that Ritalin boosted serotonin levels in the brain, not dopamine. The researchers concluded that ADHD may occur when the chemical balance between dopamine and serotonin is thrown off (Caron 1999). Sales of Ritalin have increased 700% since 1990 (Haislip 2002). Little is known about the long-term effect of stimulants on brain chemistry, and there is concern about the long-term use of Ritalin (Breggin 1998). Another drug called Strattera (atomoxetine) is a nonstimulant medication for ADD/ADH. Strattera boosts the levels of norepinephrine (not dopamine).

There is no single medical, physical, or other test for diagnosing ADD/ADHD. There have been various hypotheses on the cause of ADHD with suggestions that many different contributing factors are involved, including sensitivity to the yellow dye tartrazine. Tartrazine is derived from coal tar and often marketed as FD&C yellow 5, E102, or C.I. 19140. It is used in many products targeting children.

However, no definite cause for the disorder has been found although research at Harvard and Massachusetts General Hospital found that adults with longstanding ADHD had an abnormal elevation in dopamine.

About 15 years ago, I found that children with ADHD became more stimulated with sedative essential oils such as Roman chamomile and lavender. So, I tried essential oils with stimulant properties and found they had a relaxing effect. Following this, two of my students carried out two separate studies on ADHD using two different essential oils (Table 18-3). The first study, by Sorenson (1999), was very simple and involved observing four children with ADHD who were attending piano lessons. When lavender *(Lavandula angustifolia)* was diffused into the air, all four children became more inattentive and restless. When rosemary *(Rosmarinus officinalis)* was diffused into the air, three of the four children became more attentive and less restless.

Spitzer (2000) carried out a study on 10 children (aged 7 to 9 years) attending a school for children with special needs. Children who were prone to seizures were excluded from the study. Two occupational therapists conducted the experiment at the school and used a Likert scale for analysis. Baseline data were recorded for four separate visits. This included the number of times the children (a) got out of their chairs, (b) needed directions repeated, (c) engaged in self stimulation (rocking), and (d) the number of minutes the children sustained attention to a particular task. During the experimental stage, two drops of *Rosmarinus officinalis* were placed on an aromastone before each of the four occupational therapy sessions. (An aromastone is a ceramic stone that uses electricity to gently heat a few drops of essential oil placed on the stone.)

TABLE 18-3 *Pediatric Studies Carried out by RJ Buckle Students*

Name	Year	State	Number of Participants	Symptom	Essential Oil
Sorenson	1999	NM	10	ADHD	Rosemary
Barger	1998	TX	2	Hyperactivity	Mandarin
Knuteson	2000	IN	8	Insomnia	Mandarin
Spitzer	2000	NY	10	ADHD	Rosemary
Romano	2003	MA	5	Concentration for homework	Lavender
Schauer	2006	MN	10	Infant sleep	Lavender
Fandrich	2007	WI	9	Insomnia	Mandarin
Hosler	2007	OH	12	Gender preference of aromas	Selection*
Hynson and Gilbert	2009	TX	32	ADHD	Lavender
Trox	2009	TX	22	School cross-infection	Eucalyptus
Krieger	2010	NY	12	Depression	Mandarin
Blyth	2011	WI	10	Autism	Lavender

*Selection = mandarin, frankincense, geranium.
ADHD = attention deficit/hyperactivity disorder.

Because each child was so different, the data were examined individually. In the best-case scenario, Child 6 managed to focus with rosemary and sustained attention for up to 23 minutes, instead of 18 minutes without the oil. Child 1 sustained focused attention for 9 minutes instead of 3 minutes. Child 3 was able to remain seated the longest. Child 4, who was prone to tantrums, did not have any tantrums during the aromatherapy sessions. Child 5 did not have any self-regulating problems, and therefore there was no room for improvement. Three other children had slight improvements overall, two children had no difference, and one child performed worse. Although this study is inconclusive, both occupational therapists felt the findings warranted further study.

Pitman (2000) invited a group of 11 children with ADHD to choose three essential oils from a selection of 15 oils that included stimulant and sedative essential oils. The three were then mixed together, diluted in vegetable oil, and applied to the children's wrists. The same mixture was sometimes used at home in a bath or diffused into the air. The oils appeared to relax the children, increase their concentration in class, and decrease disruptions, and the children all appeared calmer. The parents said the essential oil mixtures had helped their children calm down, although one parent said their child became hyperactive when a citrus aroma was vaporized for too long.

However, in another study a calming essential oil was beneficial for ADHD. Hynson and Gilbert (2009) conducted an interesting 6-week study on 23 children diagnosed with moderate to severe ADHD who were enrolled in special horse-riding classes for ADHD children. Ages ranged from 7 to 13 years, with 17 female and 15 male children. Aromatherapy was introduced during the regular 5-minute period where horse and rider became accustomed to each other at the start of the lesson. Each child inhaled three drops of *Lavandula angustifolia* (on a cotton ball) for 5 minutes. The cotton ball was renewed each week. The ability to focus on the riding lesson was measured using a 0-10 scale. The children rated themselves, and they were also rated by their parents and by their teacher. The results suggested that lavender calmed the children and, in so doing, improved their focus.

PEDICULOSIS (HEAD LICE)

Head lice have become endemic worldwide (Canyon & Speare 2007, Doulgeraki & Valari 2011, AlBashtawy & Hasna 2012, Gutiérrez et al 2012, Smith & Goldman 2012). Over the last 10 years, the head louse *Pediculus humanus capitis* has become resistant to pyrethrins or pyrethroids (Toloza et al 2010). Despite this, most people with pediculosis will still be treated with neurotoxic pediculicides containing pyrethrins or pyrethroids (Marcoux et al 2010). Resistance to permethrin, malathion, and N,N-diethyl-3-methylbenzamide (DEET), and doubts about the safety of these pesticides, have encouraged other methods of control. Early attempts at "home remedies" using mayonnaise and olive oil failed (Takano-Lee et al 2004). Wet-combing and dry-on suffocation, while awkward and time-consuming, yielded better success (Izri et al 2010). Essential oils are an attractive alternative and, over the last 10 years, many essential oils and their components have been tested against head lice and found to be effective. A sample of them can be found in Table 18-4.

Many pediculicides are only partially ovicidal, resulting in another batch of new lice after 10 days. It is important that a special lice comb is used and all the eggs are removed after treatment, because some nits can remain glued onto the hair for several months, even if they are dead.

The fight against hair lice infestation begins with creating a product that repels the hair louse. If the product fails and infestation occurs, treatment needs to be effective against (1) the crawling stage (lousicidal efficacy) and (2) the eggs (ovicidal efficacy). However, lousicidal and ovicidal efficacy are often combined in clinical trials, and it can be difficult to extrapolate the different information (Barker & Altman 2011).

A study to test the repellant activity of essential oils was conducted by Canyon & Speare (2007). In this study, tea tree proved more effective at repelling head lice than peppermint or lavender essential oil. All three essential oils were more effective than DEET. Citronella was found to be an effective repellent during a 4-month randomized, placebo-controlled, double-blind clinical study conducted on 198 children in four elementary schools in Israel (Mumcuoglu et al 2004).

TABLE 18-4 *Published Research on Essential Oils and Head Lice*

Essential Oil	Year	Author	Number of Participants	Result
Cintronella	2004	Mumcuoglu et al	198	+ve
(+)-Terpinen-4-ol, nerolidol	2006	Priestley et al	In vitro	+ve
Cinnamomum zeylanicum bark	2005	Yang et al	In vitro	+ve
Tea tree, peppermint, lavender	2007	Canyon & Speare	In vitro	+ve
Peppermint, lavender, *Eucalyptus globulus*	2007	Gonzales et al	In vitro	+ve
Tea tree, lavender	2010	Barker & Altman	123	+ve
Clove, *Eucalyptus globulus*	2010	Choi et al	In vitro	+ve
Eucalyptus sideroxylon, Eucalyptus globulus	2010	Toloza et al	In vitro	+ve
1,8-Cineole	2010	Toloza et al	In vitro	+ve
Tea tree, lavender, eucalyptus, lemon tea tree	2011	Barker & Altman	92	+ve

+ve, positive result; −ve, negative result.

Barker and Altman (2011) conducted a trial that was specially designed to rank the clinical effectiveness of two different combinations of essential oils against eggs. Eggs were collected (pretreatment and posttreatment) from the hair of participants. The researchers selected participants with different types of hair, different colored hair, and hair of different lengths. Ninety-two participants with hair lice were randomly assigned to one of three groups: (a) the control group, who received a conventional "suffocation" agent; (b) the tea tree plus lavender group; and (c) the eucalyptus and lemon tea tree oil group. One hair was taken from the participant before the intervention and the eggs incubated for 14 days. The participant then received the intervention (control or one of the two essential oil combinations). Following this, the hair was examined again and another strand of hair with attached eggs was taken. Those eggs were incubated for a further 14 days. The results showed that "suffocation" pediculicide had 68.3% efficacy against the eggs. Tea tree plus lavender oil was 44.4% effective but the eucalyptus plus lemon tea tree oil (Leptospermum petersonii) only had 3.3% effectiveness. In this case, the essential oils were not as effective as the sufficant; however, the study drew attention to the number of different tea tree and eucalyptus essential oils available.

In Australia, a randomized, assessor-blind, parallel-group comparative-efficacy trial found that essential oils were an effective treatment (Barker and Altman 2010). In this study, 41/42 (97.6%) of the children were louse-free following treatment with a product containing tea tree and lavender essential oils. The control group (who received treatment with a proprietary suffocation product) had exactly the same outcome. However, only 10/40 (25.0%) of the group treated with pyrethrins and piperonyl butoxide were louse free.

Five different species of eucalyptus were tested against hair lice in a study by Toloza et al (2010). The most effective species were Eucalyptus sideroxylon, Eucalyptus globulus ssp. globulus, and Eucalyptus globulus ssp. maidenii, with knockdown time 50% [KT(50)] values of 24.75, 27.73, and 31.39 minutes. A linear regression analysis between percentage of 1,8-cineole and KT(50) values of the essential oils showed significant correlation at $P < 0.01$. This suggests that other essential oils high in 1,8-cineole may also be effective pediculicides.

Several pharmaceutical companies have shown interest in the active pediculicidal components within essential oils. For example, GlaxoSmithKline conducted a study in 2006 and found that (+)-terpinen-4-ol was the most effective compound against adult lice, whereas nerolidol was particularly lethal to eggs, but ineffective against adult lice (Priestley et al 2006). Another study by Gonzalez-Audino et al (2011) found that citronellol and geraniol had the highest knockdown and mortality effect (>60%) on nits. Pulegone, linalool, and citral showed knockdown percentages between 42% and 55% and mortality percentages between 47% and 53%.

An Argentinian study showed the effectiveness of lavender, peppermint, and eucalyptus (Gonzalez et al 2007) against permethrin-resistant Pediculus humanus capitis. In this study, two experimental lotions were studied. The first one contained lavender, peppermint, and eucalyptus oils in a 5% dilution. The second one contained eucalyptus and peppermint in a 10% dilution. Both mixtures were diluted in a 50% ethanol/isopropanol mix (1:1) in water. The lotion containing peppermint and eucalyptus oil at 10% dilution was as effective as the commercial lotion.

Some essential oils may be effective against hair lice but inappropriate to use with children. For example, Lahlou et al (2000) investigated the effectiveness of 24 essential oils and 15 of their isolated compounds against human head lice in vitro using microatmosphere and direct application. *Mentha pulegium* (pennyroyal), *Thymus broussonetti*, *Chenopodium ambrosioides* (American wormseed), and *Ruta chalepensis* were found to be the most effective. The lice died within 15 minutes of direct application of the essential oils. The nits were a little more difficult. At a 1:4 dilution of *Thymus broussonetti* applied directly, 20% of the nits hatched. None of these essential oils are suitable for children. However, of the isolated components, phenols, phenolic ethers, ketones, and 1,8-cineole were the most effective. These components can be found in many safe essential oils.

A word of caution: Waldman (2011) reports on a seizure caused by dermal application of over-the-counter eucalyptus oil head lice preparation. Initial symptoms were vomiting, lethargy, and ataxia followed by a grand mal seizure. Recovery occurred rapidly after the skin was washed. There was no indication the child had been patch tested. If this had been done, perhaps this allergic reaction may have been averted.

INFANTILE COLIC

Infantile colic is a common condition that can affect up to 28% of infants in the first few months of life. In a Brazilian study, 30 babies aged between 15 and 60 days old were randomly allocated to receive either peppermint oil or simethicone (Alves et al 2012). Simethicone is a mixture of polydimethylsiloxanes that reduce the surface tension of air bubbles; it is widely used for infant colic in many countries (Hall et al 2012). Simethicone is thought to be relatively safe because it is not absorbed into the bloodstream. In this crossover double-blind study, each baby received one drop of *Mentha piperita* per kilogram body weight for 7 days and 2.5 mg simethicone per kilogram body weight for 7 days. The two 7-day stages of the study were separated by a 3-day interval. All mothers reported a decrease in the frequency and length of infantile colic and there were no differences between responses to *Mentha piperita* and simethicone.

Fennel seed oil was found to be effective in reducing infant colic (Alexandrovish et al 2004). One hundred and twenty-five infants were enrolled in the study and randomly allocated to the treatment group (fennel seed oil) or placebo. Fennel emulsion or placebo was given up to four times a day before meals with consumption limited to 12 mg/kg/day. (This dose was chosen because it was well below the toxic level for animals.) Fennel seed oil eliminated colic in 65% of children in the treatment group but only 24% in the control group. The fennel seed oil emulsion was supplied by Lev Laboratories (Glencoe, IL, USA).

Savino et al (2005) explored the effect of a mixture of *Matricariae recutita*, *Foeniculum vulgare*, and *Melissa officinalis* (ColiMil) in the treatment of 90 breastfed colicky infants. However, in this study, herbal extracts were used, not essential oils.

BABY BATHS WITH LAVENDER

Lavender essential oil in a bath was found to have a soothing influence on babies (Field et al 2008). In this study, mothers and babies were randomly allocated to receive a bath with lavender or a bath without lavender. The results were videotaped, and in addition, saliva cortisol levels were measured. Mothers in the lavender bath oil group were more relaxed and touched their infants more during bath time than the control group. Their infants cried less and slept better. The cortisol levels of mothers and infants in the lavender group decreased significantly.

BABY APNEA, PEDIATRIC VIRAL PNEUMONIA, AND REDUCTION OF SEDATION DURING MECHANICAL VENTILATION OF A YOUNG CHILD

Vanilla aroma appeared to reduce apnea in premature infants (Marlier et al 2005). In this study, vanilla aroma was diffused inside the incubators of 14 preterm newborns (24 to 28 gestational weeks). These babies had recurrent apnea despite caffeine and doxapram therapy. (Vanilla was chosen because there had been previous research on vanilla with babies, but it should be possible to replicate this study using lavender.) Apnea was reduced by more than a third in 12 out of the 14 babies. The idea that essential oils might help a baby, or child, breathe more easily was the basis for a case study by Hedayat (2008a). This involved a 3-year-old girl with central core disorder who had an 18-day history of requiring high-flow oxygen for a persistent left upper lobe atelectasis caused by a viral infection. Hedayat, her physician, who had trained in clinical aromatherapy, diffused a mixture of four essential oils in her room (Spike lavender, peppermint, Spanish marjoram, and Fir Balsam). The mixture was renewed every 6 hours. Within 12 hours, her oxygen requirement was reduced by 50%, falling to 0.25 liters per minute (LPM) on the second day the essential oil mixture was used.

Hedayat (2008b) published another interesting case study—this time involving a critically ill 18-month-old girl with respiratory distress secondary to adenovirus pneumonia. The child required a tracheostomy and had been ventilated for 8 days. Extubation was proving difficult. A bispectral index (BIS) monitor was placed to measure her level of sedation (this is standard procedure because she was receiving drugs that paralyzed her so that she would not fight the use of the ventilator). Despite high doses of midazolam and morphine, her BIS score remained too high.

Her mother then used a 7.5% mixture of Roman chamomile, sandalwood, and galbanum in jojoba and massaged her daughter's arms, legs, and chest; 2.5 mL were applied every 6 to 8 hours. This appeared to soothe her daughter because her BIS declined, her sedation was reduced, and she was able to be successfully extubated.

This result could have been attributed purely to the massage. However, essential oils are absorbed through the skin and, in my experience, massage with essential oils (especially in children) does have more beneficial effects.

Orange essential oil helped induction of anesthesia in children (Mehta et al 1998). In another study, diffusion of essential oils of lavender and lemon helped reduce the perception of pain when dressings were changed (Kane et al 2004). For further reading, the *International Journal of Clinical Aromatherapy* 2005, Volume 2, Issue 2 is dedicated to pediatrics and contains some excellent material, including a very useful article by the editor, Rhiannon Lewis. Plese see www.ijca.net.

Finally, children may find the small bottles that contain essential oils appealing and want to play with them. This is not a good idea. Essential oils are very concentrated. Peppermint oil is not the same thing as gripe water. While aromatherapy is more common now and, hopefully, understanding is increasing, there have been several published articles about children who have poisoned themselves with essential oils (Davis & Livingstone 1986, Hartnoll et al 1993, Webb & Pitt 1993, Beccara 1995, Darben et al 1998). Anyone using essential oils needs to store them well away from little fingers. When clinical aromatherapy is used correctly, there is very little danger of side effects or of poisoning.

REFERENCES

ADD/ADHD Research and ADD/ADHD Online Support Group. www.adders.org. Accessed August 7, 2014.

Alexandrovish I, Rakovitskaya O, Kolmo E, Sidorova T, Shushunov S. 2004. The effect of fennel *(Foeniculum vulgare)* seed oil emulsion in infantile colic: a randomized placebo controlled study. *Int J Clin Aromather.* 1(1):42-6.

AlBashtawy M, Hasna F. 2012. Pediculosis capitis among primary-school children in Mafraq Governorate, Jordan. *East Med. Health J.* 18(1):43-8.

Alves J, de Brito R, Calcarth T. 2012. Effectiveness of *Mentha piperita* in the treatment of infantile colic: a crossover study. *Evid Based Complement Altern Med.* 21981352. Accessed December 23, 2012.

Ashley P, Parekh S, Moles D, Anand P, Behbehani A. 2012. Preoperative analgesics for additional pain relief in children and adolescents having dental treatment. *Cochrane Database Syst Rev.* http://www.ncbi.nlm.nih.gov/pubmed/22972120. Accessed December 11, 2012.

Barker SC, Altman PM. 2010. A randomised, assessor blind, parallel group comparative efficacy trial of three products for the treatment of head lice in children—melaleuca oil and lavender oil, pyrethrins and piperonyl butoxide, and a "suffocation" product. *BMC Dermatol.* 10:6. http://www.ncbi.nlm.nih.gov/pmc/articles/PMC2933647/. Accessed December 2012.

Barker SC, Altman PM. 2011. An ex vivo, assessor blind, randomised, parallel group, comparative efficacy trial of the ovicidal activity of three pediculicides after a single application—melaleuca oil and lavender oil, eucalyptus oil and lemon tea tree oil, and a "suffocation" pediculicide. *BMC Dermatol.* 11:14. http://www.ncbi.nlm.nih.gov/pmc/articles/PMC3182970/. Accessed December 2012.

Beccara M. 1995. Melaleuca poisoning in a 17 month old. *Vet Human Toxicol (Manhattan).* 37(6):557-8.

Blyth G. 2011. Lavender for children with autism. Unpublished dissertation for RJ Buckle Associates.

Breggin P. 1998. Report to the plenary session of the NIH consensus conference on ADHD and its treatment. www.breggin.com.

Cameron E, Doty R. 2012. Odor identification testing in children and young adults using the smell wheel. *Int J Pediatr Otorhinolaryngol.* pii: S0165-5876(12)00648-9. doi: 10.1016/j.ijporl.2012.11.022. [Epub ahead of print]. Accessed December 23, 2012.

Canyon DV, Speare R. 2007. A comparison of botanical and synthetic substances commonly used to prevent head lice *(Pediculus humanus* var. *capitis)* infestation. *Int J Dermatol.* 46(4):422-6.

Caron M. 1999. Role of serotonin in the paradoxical calming effect of psychostimulants on hyperactivity. *Science.* 283:397-401.

Choi H, Yang Y, Lee S, Clark J, Ahn J. 2010. Efficacy of spray formulations containing binary mixtures of clove and eucalyptus oils against susceptible and pyrethroid/malathion-resistant head lice (Anoplura: Pediculidae). *J Med Entomol.* 47(3):387-91.

Daniels R, O'Flaherty L. 2010. Aromatherapy at the Red Cross War Memorial Children's Hospital. *Int J Clin Aromather.* 7(2):1-4.

Darben T, Cominos B, Lee C. 1998. Topical eucalyptus oil poisoning. *Austral J Dermatol.* 39:265-7.

Davis S, Livingstone A. 1986. Respiratory collapse and karvol capsules. *Austral J Hosp Pharm.* 16(4):273-4.

De Jong M, Lucas C, Bredero B, van Adrichem L, Tibboel D, van Dick M. 2012. Does post operative 'M' technique massage with or without mandarin oil reduce infant's distress after major craniofacial surgery? *J Adv Nurs.* 68(8):1748-57.

Doulgeraki A, Valari M. 2011. Parental attitudes towards head lice infestation in Greece. *Int J Dermatol.* 50(6):689-92.

Engen T. 1974. Method and theory in the study of odor preferences. In Johnston J (ed.), *Human Response to Environmental Odors.* New York: Academic Press, pp 121-141.

Fandrich M. 2007. Mandarin for children with insomnia. Unpublished dissertation for RJ Buckle Associates.

Field T, Cullen C, Largie S, Diego M, Schanberg S, Kuch C. 2008. Lavender bath oil reduces stress and crying and enhances sleep in very young infants. *Early Hum Dev.* 84(6):399-401.

Fitzgerald M, Culbert T, Finkelstein M, Green M, Liu M. 2010. The effect of gender and ethnicity on children's attitudes and preferences for essential oils: a follow up study. *Explore.* 6(3):172.

Foster R, Park J. 2012. An integrative review of literature examining psychometric properties of instruments measuring anxiety or fear in hospitalized children. *Pain Manag Nurs.* 13(2):94-106.

Gainetdinov R, Wetzel W, Jones S et al. 1999. Role of serotonin in the paradoxical calming effect of psychostimulants on hyperactivity. *Science.* 283(5400):397-401.

Gainetdinov R, Caron M. 2001. Genetics of childhood disorders: XXIV, Part 8: Hyperdopaminergic mice as an animal model of ADHD. *J Am Acad Child Psych.* 40(3):380-2.

Garbe E, Mikolajczyk RT, Banaschewski T, Petermann U, Petermann F et al. 2012. Drug treatment patterns of attention-deficit/hyperactivity disorder in children and adolescents in Germany: results from a large population-based cohort study. *J Child Adolesc Psychopharmacol.* 22(6):452-8.

Gonzalez Audino P, Vassena C, Zerba E, Picollo M. 2007. Effectiveness of lotions based on essential oils from aromatic plants against permethrin resistant *Pediculus humanus* capitis. *Arch Dematol Res.* 299(8):389-92.

Gonzalez-Audino P, Picollo M, Gallardo A, Toloza A, Vassena C, Mougabure-Cueto G. 2011. Comparative toxicity of oxygenated monoterpenoids in experimental hydroalcoholic lotions to permethrin-resistant adult head lice. *Arch Dermatol Res.* 303(5):361-6.

Gutiérrez M, González J, Stefanazzi N, Serralunga G, Yañez L, Ferrero A. 2012. Prevalence of *Pediculus humanus capitis* infestation among kindergarten children in Bahía Blanca city, Argentina. *Parasitol Res.* 111(3):1309-13. doi: 10.1007/s00436-012-2966-y. Accessed December 11, 2012.

Hall B, Chesters J, Robinson A. 2012. Infantile colic: a systematic review of medical and conventional therapies. *J Paed Child Health.* 48:128-37.

Hartnoll G, Moore D, Douck D. 1993. Near fatal ingestion of oil of cloves. *Arch Dis Childhood (London).* 69:392-3.

Haislip G. 2002. Ritalin: the smart drug? www.vanderbilt.edu/AnS/psychology. Accessed September 2002.

Harris. R. 2005. The use of essential oils in child care. *Int J Clin Aromather.* 2(2):26-34.

Hedayat K. 2008a. Essential oil diffusion for the treatment of persistent oxygen dependence in a three-year-old child with restrictive lung disease and respiratory syncytial virus pneumonia. *EXPLORE.* 4(4):264-6.

Hedayat K. 2008b. Reduction of benzodiazepine requirements during mechanical ventilation in a child by topical application of essential oils. *EXPLORE.* 4(2):136-8.

Hodson D. 1995. The special needs of children and adolescents. In Penson J, Fisher R (eds.), *Palliative Care for People with Cancer,* 2nd ed. London: Edward Arnold, pp 198-229.

Hosler R. 2007. Boy and girl preferences for aromas. Unpublished dissertation for RJ Buckle Associates.

Humphrey T. 1940. The development of the olfactory and the accessory olfactory formations in human embryos and fetuses. *J Comp Neurol.* 73:431-68.

Hynson B, Gilbert J. 2009. Unpublished dissertation. RJ Buckle Associates.

Izri A, Uzzan B, Maigret M, Gordon M, Bouges-Michel C. 2010. Clinical efficacy and safety in head lice infection by *Pediculus humanis capitis* De Geer (Anoplura: Pediculidae) of a capillary spray containing a siucon-oil complex. *Parasite.* 17(4):329-35.

Johnstone S, Barry R, Clarke A. 2012. Ten years on: a follow-up review of ERP research in attention-deficit/hyperactivity disorder. *Clin Neurophysiol.* doi:pii: S1388-2457(12)00628-1. 10.1016/j.clinph. 2012.09.006. Accessed December 23, 2012.

Kane F, Brodie E, Coull A, Coyne L, Howd A et al. 2004. The analgesic effect of odour and music upon dressing change. *Br J Nursing.* 10;13(19):S4-12.

Knuteson R. 2000. Mandarin for children with insomnia. Unpublished dissertation for RJ Buckle Associates.

Kreiger K. 2010. Mandarin for children with depression. Unpublished dissertation for RJ Buckle Associates.

Lahlou M, Berrada R, Agoumi A et al. 2000. The potential effectiveness of essential oils in the control of human head lice in Morocco. *Int J Aromather.* 10(3/4):108-23.

Leisman G, Melillo G. 2012. The basal ganglia: motor and cognitive relationships in a clinical neurobe-havioral context. *Rev Neurosci.* 14:1-17. doi: 10.1515/revneuro-2012-0067. [Epub ahead of print]. Accessed December 23, 2012.

Logan D, Conroy C, Sieberg C, Simons L. 2012. Changes in willingness to self-manage pain among children and adolescents and their parents enrolled in an intensive interdisciplinary pediatric pain treatment program. *Pain.* 153(9):1863-70.

Marcoux D, Palma K, Kaul N, Hodgdon H, Van Geest A et al. 2010. Pyrethroid pediculicide resistance of head lice in Canada evaluated by serial invasive signal amplification reaction. *J Cutan Med Surg.* 14(3):115-8.

Marlier L, Gaugler C, Messer J. 2005. Olfactory stimulation prevents apnea in premature newborns. *Pediatrics.* 115(1):83-8.

Mazuck I, Hutzler C, Luch A. 2011. Estimation of dermal and oral exposure of children to scented toys: analysis of the migration of fragrance allergens by dynamic headspace GC-MS. *J Sep Sci.* 34(19):2686-96.

Mehta S, Stone D, Whitehead H. 1998. Use of essential oil to promote induction of anesthesia in children. *Anaesthesia.* 53(7):720-1.

Mumcuoglu K, Magdassi S, Miller J, Ben-Ishai F, Zentner G, et al. 2004. Repellency of citronella for head lice: double-blind randomized trial of efficacy and safety. *Israel Med Assoc J.* 6(12):756-9.

O'Flaherty LA, van Dijk M, Albetyn R, Miller A, Rode H. 2012. Aromatherapy massage seems to enhance relaxation in children with burns: an observational pilot study. *Burns.* 38(6):840-5.

Patten SB, Waheed W, Bresee L. 2012. A review of pharmacoepidemiologic studies of antipsychotic use in children and adolescents. *Can J Psychiatry.* 57(12):717-21.

Pitman V. 2000. Aromatherapy and children with learning difficulties. *Aromather Today.* 15:20-3.

Polanczyk G, de Lima M, Horta B, Biederman J, Rohde L. 2009. The worldwide prevalence of ADHD: a systematic review and metaregression analysis. *Am J Psychiatry.* 164(6):942-8.

Priestley CM, Burgess IF, Williamson EM. 2006. Lethality of essential oil constituents towards the human louse, *Pediculus humanus*, and its eggs. *Fitoterapia.* 77(4):303-9.

Romano 2003. Lavender to help concentration of children with their homework. Unpublished dissertation for RJ Buckle Associates.

Ruggiero S, Rafaniello C, Bravaccio C, Grimaldi G, Granato R et al. 2012. Safety of attention-deficit/hyperactivity disorder medications in children: an intensive pharmacosurveillance monitoring study. *J Child Adolesc Psychopharmacol.* 22(6):415-22.

Russell M. 1976. Human olfactory communication. *Nature.* 260:520-2.

Savino F, Cresi F, Castagno E, Silvestro L, Oggero R. 2005. A randomized double-blind placebo-controlled trial of a standardized extract of *Matricariae recutita, Foeniculum vulgare* and *Melissa officinalis* (ColiMil) in the treatment of breastfed colicky infants. *Phytother Res.* 19(4):335-40.

Schaal B, Marlier L, Soussignan R. 2000. Human foetuses learn odours from their pregnant mother's diet. *Chemical Senses.* 13:729-37.

Schleidt M, Genzel C. 1990. The significance of mother's perfume for infants in the first weeks of their life. *Ethol Sociobiol.* 11(1):145-50.

Sevelinges Y, Lévy F, Mouly A, Ferreira G. 2009. Rearing with artificially scented mothers attenuates conditioned odor aversion in adulthood but not its amygdala dependency. *Behav Brain Res.* 198(2):313-20.

Smith C, Goldman R. 2012. An incurable itch: head lice. *Can Fam Physician.* 58(8):839-41.

Sorenson K. 1999. Effects of aroma with poor attention span in music lessons. Unpublished dissertation. RJ Buckle Associates.

Spitzer H. 2000. Special needs children and aromatherapy: rosemary oil. Unpublished dissertation. RJ Buckle Associates.

Takano-Lee M, Edman J, Mullens B, Clark J. 2004. Home remedies to control head lice: assessment of home remedies to control the human head louse, *Pediculus humanus capitis* (Anoplura: Pediculidae). *J Pediat Nurs.* 19(6):393-8.

Toloza AC, Lucia A, Zerba E, Masuh H, Picollo MI. 2010. Eucalyptus essential oil toxicity against permethrin-resistant *Pediculus humanus capitis* (Phthiraptera: Pediculidae). *Parasitol Res.* 106(2): 409-14.

Trox M. 2009. Eucalyptus to prevent school cross infection. Unpublished dissertation for RJ Buckle Associates.

Tucker S. 1999. Attention deficit hyperactivity disorder. *J Royal Soc Med.* 92(5):217-9.

van Dijk M. 2001. *Pain Unheard: Postoperative Pain Assessment in Neonates and Infants.* ISBN 90-73235-41-3. Erasmus University, Rotterdam.

van Eck K, Flory K, Malone P. 2012. A longitudinal assessment of the associations among response access, attention problems, and aggression during childhood. *J Abnorm Child Psychol.* [Epub ahead of print]. PMID:23179290. Accessed December 23, 2012.

Waldman N. 2011. Seizure caused by dermal application of over-the-counter eucalyptus oil head lice preparation. *Clin Toxicol.* 49(8):750-1.

Webb N, Pitt W. 1993. Eucalyptus oil poisoning in childhood: 41 cases in south east Queensland. *J Pediat Child Health.* 29:368-71.

Worwood V. 2000. *Aromatherapy for the Healthy Child.* Navato, CA: New World Library.

Yang Y, Lee H, Lee S, Clark J, Ahn Y. 2005. Ovicidal and adulticidal activities of *Cinnamomum zeylanicum* bark essential oil compounds and related compounds against *Pediculus humanus capitis* (Anoplura: Pediculicidae). *Int J Parasitol.* 35(14):1595-600.

Youngblut J, Brooten D. 2012. Perinatal and pediatric issues in palliative and end-of-life care from the 2011 Summit on the Science of Compassion. *Nurs Outlook.* 60(6):343-50.

Chapter 19

Respiratory Care

"Every breath we take, every step we make, can be filled with peace, joy and serenity."
Thich Nhat Hanh

CHAPTER ASSETS

RESPIRATORY DISEASE

Chronic bronchitis, asthma, emphysema, and chronic obstructive pulmonary disease (COPD) are a group of inflammatory lung diseases where airway resistance is increased and airflow impaired (Brooker 2008). However, these are different diseases (Forey et al 2011) and may be distinct disorders (Allen-Ramey et al 2012). In a survey of 75,000 people in the United States, data obtained from the 2010 U.S. National Health and Wellness Survey (NHWS), respondents categorized themselves with COPD ($N = 970$), emphysema ($N = 399$), or chronic bronchitis ($N = 2071$). The study found that patients with chronic bronchitis were younger than patients with emphysema, more likely to be employed, and most were female. They were also less likely to be a current or former smoker. Different respiratory complaints are sometimes recognized as separate diseases therefore I have divided this chapter in a similar way, although parts of each section may overlap.

According to a comprehensive study by The European Respiratory Society (ERS) of mortality rates in 28 European Union (EU) countries, lung disease kills 1 in 10 Europeans (Lancet Respiratory Medicine 2013). The causes of death were listed as COPD, lung cancer, tuberculosis, and pneumonia. This means one million people in Europe die from lung disease annually and yearly loss of 10 million

DALYs (disability-adjusted life-years) because of chronic lung disease. The ERS suggests the percentage rate will rise to one in every five deaths by 2030. Currently, approximately 5% of deaths in EU countries are attributed to respiratory disease: 5.8% to lung cancer, 3.5% to pneumonia, and 3.4% to COPD. The highest mortality rate for lung conditions was in Belgium and Denmark (117 deaths per 100,000) and the highest rate from respiratory diseases was found in UK.

In the United States, a 2011 study (Behavioral Risk Factor Surveillance System [BRFSS] survey) found that approximately 20.5 million (8.8%) adults and 8.6% children had asthma and, of those, about 14.7 million adults (6.4 %) had been diagnosed with COPD (Centers for Disease Control & Prevention 2013). The World Health Organization (WHO) stated that in 2007, 300 million people had asthma, 210 million had COPD, and millions of others had sinusitis or other undiagnosed chronic respiratory diseases (CRDs), including tuberculosis (TB). The prevalence of CRDs is increasing globally and more than 50% of those with CRDs live in low and middle-income countries where the cost of medicines is high (WHO 2007). The economic and social impact of CRDs is huge.

Aromatherapy for General Respiratory Care

Respiratory care is one of the most obvious targets of clinical aromatherapy; when you inhale to breathe, you invariably smell as well. Why bother with the potentially hazardous oral intake of essential oils and "first pass" (metabolizing them via the liver) when inhaled oils will get straight to the site of the presumed problem? The most obvious method for using essential oils for respiratory complaints is inhalation, using one of the many different inhalation methods described in the Applications chapter. Bardeau (1976) used essential oils to "purify" the air nearly 40 years ago. Recently, pharmaceutical researchers have begun targeting the lungs as a portal for drug delivery in TB and other chronic respiratory complaints (Misra et al 2011). By delivering a drug directly to the lungs, researchers feel they can target alveolar macrophages that harbor bacilli, as well as keep a high concentration of drug in the lung tissue.

Vicks VapoRub is a strong childhood memory for me. When I had a cough, cold, or chest infection, my parents would rub Vicks onto my chest and back. They would also smear it on my bedclothes. It was comforting and warming; it relieved a stuffy nose and reduced my bouts of coughing. Research has shown that Vicks really did reduce these symptoms (Berger et al 1978) and Lunsford Richardson (1854–1919), the founder of Vicks, would be delighted that Vicks is still a household remedy so many years later. Vicks worked because it contains certain aromatic compounds: eucalyptol, camphor, and menthol. Eucalyptol is another name for 1,8-cineole, however, eucalyptol does sound like it comes from eucalyptus, which has a long history of use in folk medicine for respiratory complaints. Components of eucalyptus, such as 1,8-cineole, are contained in several proprietary medicines used for respiratory complaints (Sadlon et al 2010, Hamoud 2012, Hasani 2003).

A list of essential oils for respiratory infections is given in Table 19-1. Many of those listed contain large amounts of 1,8-cineole: an oxide with antitussive, mucolytic (reduces respiratory secretions) and bronchodilatory properties (Harris 2007).

TABLE 19-1 *Essential Oils for General Respiratory Tract Infections*

Common Name	Botanical Name
Eucalyptus, Blue gum	*Eucalyptus globulus*
Eucalyptus, Narrow Leaved	*Eucalyptus radiata*
Eucalyptus, Gully gum	*Eucalyptus smithi*
Lavender spike	*Lavandula latifolia*
Myrtle	*Myrtus communis*
Niaouli	*Melaleuca viridiflora*
Peppermint	*Mentha piperita*
Ravansara	*Ravansara aromatica*
Ravintsara	*Cinnamomomu camphora* CT cineole
Rosemary	*Rosmarinus officinalis* CT cineole
Thyme, Spanish	*Thymus mastachina*
Scots pine	*Pinus sylvestris*
Tea tree	*Melaleuca alternifolia*

The antitussive (cough suppressant) property of *Eucalyptus globulus* was explored by Packman and London in 1980 (European Medicines Agency 2013). They induced a cough in healthy participants and then evaluated the antitussive effect of eucalyptus. However, the reason why eucalyptus has cough-suppressant activity was not discovered until several years later. Takaishi et al (2012) found that 1,8-cineole was a TRPM8 agonist as well as being a "rare natural antagonist" of human TRPA1. This made it an ideal effective analgesic as well as an effective antitussive. As the largest single component in *Eucalyptus globulus*, approximately 34% to 65% (Kumar et al 2012, Stewart 2005), 1,8-cineole is also an effective expectorant (Begrow 2012). In Germany 1,8-cineole (in enteric-coated tablets) is available as a licensed medicine (Soledum) for oral use for chest complaints (Harris 2007). Camporese et al (2013) discuss the use of inhaled *Eucalyptus smithii* and juniper *(Juniperus communis)* in chronic recurrent respiratory tract infections.

A randomized double-blind, placebo-controlled trial of a spray containing five essential oils (*Eucalyptus citriodora, Eucalyptus globulus, Mentha piperita, Origanum syriacum,* and *Rosmarinus officinalis*) was conducted on patients with upper respiratory tract infection at six primary care clinics in Israel (Ben-Ayre et al 2011). The aromatic, or placebo, spray was used five times a day for 3 days in a dosage of four sprayings each time, directed at the back of the throat. Patients assessed their own worst symptom. The spray was much more effective than the placebo, but the soothing effect only lasted 20 minutes. It would be interesting to repeat this study with a personal inhaler to get the essential oil mix deeper into the respiratory tract. A German multicentered study by Kamin and Kieser (2007) measured the tolerability of Pinimenthol ointment and found the treatment effect was judged to be "good" by 88.3% of patients (*N* = 3060). Pinimenthol ointment contains eucalyptus and pine essential oil. I have personally found Pinimenthol pastilles to be very effective against troubling tickle coughs. One of the added bonuses of using essential oils for respiratory complaints is that many essential oils can actually prevent viral, fungal, or bacterial infections (Kilina & Kolesnikova 2011, Khan et al 2011) as well as treat them (Hamoud et al 2012, Sadlon & Lamson 2010).

Alpha pinene is one of the components found in myrtol standardized (Gelomyrtol forte), a German proprietary medicine made from essential oils for acute bronchitis (Gillissen et al 2013). Falk et al (1990) found 60% of α-pinene was absorbed through inhalation, but only 8% was exhaled. The rest was excreted in the urine. Some essential oils taken by mouth are exhaled. Some essential oils given rectally are excreted through respiration. Pulmonary excretion of 1,8-cineole, menthol, and thymol was demonstrated following rectal application in rats, although the percentage exhaled was extremely small (Grisk & Fischer 1969). Rectal suppositories are a common form of treating respiratory problems in France: one rectal formula for acute bronchitis contains myrtol (*Myrtus communis* CE cineole), tea tree *(Melaleuca alternifolia)*, thyme *(Thymus vulgaris)*, Roman chamomile *(Chamaemelum nobile)*, and inula *(Inula graveolens)* (Baudoux 2007).

Air pollution has become more prevalent, especially in cities during the summer months. The World Health Organization has linked air pollution to lung cancer and chronic respiratory diseases (Straif et al 2013). Essential oils are not able to reduce air pollution, but they can alleviate the symptoms of chronic respiratory disease.

CHRONIC BRONCHITIS

Chronic bronchitis is defined as a "cough that produces sputum for at least 3 consecutive months in 2 consecutive years" (Holm et al 2012). There is an increase of goblet cells that secrete mucus and a loss of ciliated cells that prevent mucus accumulation. Chronic bronchitis (CB) can lead to COPD or pulmonary emphysema. In the latter, there is a reduction of the number of alveoli and therefore reduced gas exchange in the lungs (Brooker 2008). A Swedish study (Holm et al 2012) found smoking and occupational exposure to welding fumes were both associated with an increased risk of CB. However, there are other causes such a postnasal drip, gastroesophageal reflux disease (GERD), chronic infection (viral or bacterial), or chronic allergic inflammation.

Aromatherapy for Chronic Bronchitis

Essential oils have been used in cough medicines for treatment of bronchitis for many years (Boyd 1954). Clearly, the actions needed are expectorant: to cough up the mucus; mucolytic: to dissolve the mucus and make it easier to cough up; and antiinflammatory: to soothe the inflamed mucus membrane from all the coughing. Therefore, a mixture of essential oils with these properties is best. The most direct way of applying them is through inhalation. Steam inhalation can be very effective and may also produce vigorous coughing. Rectal suppositories also can work well (Bardoux 2007). A gentler method would be to use a personal inhaler, patch, or packet. Sucking a lozenge containing essential oil components such as a pinelyptus pastille can be very soothing.

Eucalyptus globulus, spike lavender *(Lavandula latifolia), Ravensara aromatica,* and Scots pine *(Pinus sylvestris)* are essential oils that can work well to combat the infection and the symptoms of the infection. *Eucalyptus radiata* and *Styrax benzoin* (benzoin) have been used by health professionals to treat respiratory infections for many years (Stevenson 1995). As mentioned earlier, essential oils that are high in 1,8-cineole really come into their element for chronic bronchitis, summarized well in Harris (2007). That entire issue of that journal is dedicated to respiratory issues and makes excellent reading.

An R.J. Buckle student, Charron (1997), carried out an exploratory study on 40 patients with chronic bronchitis. Patients inhaled two drops of spike lavender floating in a bowl of hot water. All patients cleared their mucus immediately with results lasting from 20 minutes to 2 hours. Some patients who had been taking yearly repeat antibiotics no longer needed them (Table 19-2).

TABLE 19-2 *RJ Buckle Student Studies on Respiratory Conditions*

Name	Year	State	Number	Condition	Essential Oil
Charron	1997	WA	28	Chronic bronchitis	Spike lavender
Spear	1999	AK	8	Asthma	Spike lavender, frankincense
Rudansky	2000	NY	1	Cystic fibrosis	*Eucalyptus globulus*
Lockhard	2000	AZ	8	Asthma	Frankincense
Pitcher	2000	NY	20	Sinusitis	Peppermint
Machon	2000	NY	8	Sinusitis	*Eucalyptus globulus Ravansara aromatica Pinus sylvestris*
Elshoff	2001	IN	10	Sinusitis	Spike lavender, Roman chamomile
Ballenger	2002	WA	8	Chest infection	*Ravansara aromatica*
May	2003	NY	10	Sinusitis	Peppermint
Crawford	2003	MN	12	Sinusitis	*Eucalyptus globulus*
Dunster	2007	CT	19	Rhinitis	Tea tree, eucalyptus, *Ravansara aromatica*
Coon	2007	CT	20	FVLC*	Peppermint
Lawrence	2012	MN	10	Respiratory congestion	*Melaleuca alternifolia Eucalyptus citriadora*
Latimer	2012	IN	15	Seasonal rhinitis	Frankincense, peppermint, *Eucalyptus globulus,* Spike lavender

ASTHMA

Asthma causes characteristic paroxysmal wheezing and difficulty in breathing out (Booker 2008). This difficulty is caused by the bronchial tubes going into spasm. Asthma is thought to be an immune response. It leads to hyperactivity of the bronchial wall and narrowing of the bronchioles, leading to more difficulty in breathing. According to WHO, 235 million people were diagnosed with asthma in 2011 (WHO 2011).

Aromatherapy and Asthma

Very occasionally, asthma can be exacerbated by components within essential oils that the person has become allergic to. Guarneri et al (2008) reports on a male 40-year-old citrus fruit picker who became allergic to D-limonene and citronellol (as shown with Hayes test) and manifested asthma. However, generally, clinical aromatherapy can help asthma. Essential oils to avoid in asthma are those high in α-pinene, as this essential oil component was found to cause airway and breathing discomfort during a study by Filipsson (1996). Rohr et al (2002) found α-pinene and D-limonene limited upper airway flow in mice. Wolkoff (2008) also found that D-limonene reduced upper airway flow. Scots pine *(Pinus sylvestris)*, often thought to be a useful essential oil for many respiratory complaints, is high in α-pinene (42%) and therefore may need to be avoided in asthma.

Twenty years ago, Singh and Agrawal (1991) found holy basil *(Ocimum sanctus)* had antiasthma properties. A few years later, Tamaoki et al (1995) published results of their 4-week study on menthol, a component of peppermint. They found menthol was effective in calming asthma symptoms. *Eucalyptus globulus* is a popular choice for people with asthma because it has mucolytic, bronchodilating, and antiinflammatory effects. One of the main constituents of eucalyptus is 1,8-cineole. Juergens et al (1998 and 2003) found 1,8-cineole could be useful in asthma. Worth and Dethlefsen (2012) conducted a double-blind, placebo-controlled study to explore the effects of 1,8-cineole (given orally) to 247 patients with confirmed asthma. Patients in this multicentered study were randomly allocated groups that received either 200 mg of 1,8-cineole or a placebo, three times per day for 6 months. Outcome measures included measuring lung function, asthma symptoms and quality of life. Results showed patients who received the 1,8-cineole had significantly more improvements than patients in the placebo group (P = 0.0027).

Gilani et al (2009) found essential oil of *Nepeta cataria* (catnip) had antiasthmatic properties. El Gazzar et al (2006) found thymoquinone, one of the main components of *Nigella sativa* (black cumin), had antiasthmatic properties. The essential oil of *Artemisia maritime* (sea wormwood) was found to have antispasmodic and bronchodilator activities by Shah et al (2011). Finally, a Korean study (Lee et al 2010) found frankincense *(Boswellia carteri)* reduced allergic asthma in mice and a study by Podlogar et al (2012) found components within ginger essential oil reduced proinflammatory chemokine interleukin-8 (IL-8) secretion in human bronchial epithelial cells. Therefore, it is worth trying ginger and frankincense (Table 19-3).

TABLE 19-3 *Recent Published Studies on Essential Oils/Components and Asthma*

Author	Year	Common Name	Essential Oil	Method	Target
Juergens et al	2003	1,8-Cineole	1,8-cineole	Human oral	$N = 32$
Görnemann et al	2008	Aztec sweet herb	*Lippia dulcis*	In vitro	Pig bronchial assay
Fenu et al	2008	Myrtle	*Myrtus communis*	In vitro	Human nasal mucosa
Gilani et al	2009	Catnip	*Nepata cataria*	In vitro	Guinea pig
Ogunlesi et al	2009	Asthma plant	*Euphorbia hirta*	Review	
Lee et al	2010	Frankincense	*Boswellia carteri*	Nebulized	Mouse model
Shah et al	2011	Sea worm-wood	*Artemisia maritima*	In vitro	Isolated tracheal strips
Worth & Dethlefsen	2012	1,8-Cineole	*Eucalyptus globulus*	Human oral	$N = 247$
Fathy Balaha et al	2012		*Nigella sativa*	Oral	Mice
Boskabady & Khatami	2003	Fennel	*Foeniculus vulgare*	In vitro	Guinea pig

An R.J. Buckle student, Spear (1999) used a 3% solution of frankincense *(Boswellia carteri)*, spike lavender *(Lavandula latifolia)*, and lavender *(Lavandula angustifolia)* in an exploratory study of eight patients with asthma in Alaska. Twice daily topical application was self-applied to the chest, neck, and back. The age of patients ranged from 14 to 70 years. Outcome measurement was by questionnaire using the scale: no change, slight improvement, moderate improvement, noticeable improvement. Three patients said their symptoms were noticeably improved and four patients registered a moderate improvement. No patient became worse, but one patient noticed no improvement.

Another R.J. Buckle student, Lockhard (2000) used inhaled essential oil of frankincense on eight subjects aged 20 to 52 years of age (five females and three males), for 6 weeks. Following patch testing and assessment for allergies, the subjects were given a bottle of undiluted essential oil to inhale for 2 to 5 minutes when they felt an asthma attack coming. A Likert scale (strongly agree, agree, neither agree nor disagree, disagree, strongly disagree) was used at the end of 6 weeks. All subjects strongly agreed that their anxiety levels decreased when they inhaled frankincense.

All subjects verbally stated they were able to reduce the use of their normal steroid inhalers.

Fedeles and Butje (2007) give a detailed account of a 53-year-old male with exercise and allergy-induced asthma (oak tree pollen, mold, and dust). The patient also responded badly to changes in the weather and had been on medication since 1986. His prescription included prednisone, Astelin (for sinus decongestion), Advair inhaler (two puffs a day twice a day) plus a Maxair inhaler for emergencies. Two essential oil mixtures were to be used concurrently. One mixture was to be applied topically. This included frankincense, laurel leaf, opoponax, ravintsara, and German chamomile. The second mixture was to be inhaled. This mixture included all of the above plus helichrysum and vetiver. The lotion was applied morning and night. The inhaler was used every 4 to 6 hours. Six months later the patient (who was a pharmacist) was off all prescribed medications. The withdrawal had been cautious, slow, and steady, although he said he had experienced a "profound relief from the essential oils almost immediately." Subsequent computerized breathing test and air flow meter conducted by his pulmonologist were "the best scores he had ever achieved."

CHRONIC OBSTRUCTIVE PULMONARY DISEASE

COPD is also called chronic airflow limitation or chronic obstructive airways disease and is a group of diseases that includes emphysema, chronic bronchitis, and occasionally asthma (Brooker 2008). Diagnosis is based on forced expiry volume (<80% in 1 second) and forced vital capacity (<70%). COPD has been linked to smoking but is also linked to genetic predisposition. Up to 20% of the population in the United States has clinical criteria for COPD (Tilert et al 2013). Particular symptoms are difficulty in breathing in the morning with a very productive cough (Roche et al 2013). Increased mucus secretion often appears as the first symptom (Harris 2007). Patients with COPD often find it hard to keep to medication schedules (Bryant et al 2013). However, studies show that many patients are comfortable using complementary medicine (CAM) for COPD. The country with the highest population using CAM for COPD was Turkey where over 70% of such COPD patients used it. The most common CAM chosen was deep inhalation with aromatic herbs (Akinci et al 2011). A British study (Hasani et al 2003) explored the effect of aromatics (Vicks VapoRub) on 11 patients with chronic airway obstruction. This single-blind, placebo-controlled study found Vicks enhanced lung mucus clearance (measured by a standard radioaerosol technique) at two time points: 30 ($P < 0.05$) and 60 ($P < 0.02$) minutes postradioaerosol inhalation.

Mattys et al (2000) carried out a randomized, double-blind study to explore the effects of Myrtol. Myrtol is a standardized distillate marketed under the brand name Gelomyrtol and contains α-pinene, 1,8-cineole, and D-limonene. Patients, 676 in total, were allocated to four groups. The experimental group received myrtol orally (4 × 300 mg daily) for 2 weeks. The two control groups received either cefuroxine (2 × 250 mg daily) or ambroxol (a mucolytic agent), and the fourth group received placebo capsules (four daily) for 14 days. Patients receiving myrtol experienced a similar reduction in coughing to those receiving cefuroxine or ambroxol. Lung auscultation improved similarly.

A German study (Rantzsch 2009) found myrtol, eucalyptus, and orange essential oil reduced cytokine release and reactive oxygen species (ROS) production of alveolar macrophages obtained from patients with COPD. This indicates these essential oils had an antiinflammatory action in lung alveolar.

SINUSITIS

Sinusitis is inflammation of the paranasal sinuses (Brooker 2008). What happens is at least 30% of ciliated cells convert to mucus-secreting cells and the ciliated beat frequency is reduced (Harris 2007). This reduces mucociliary movement, increases mucus secretion and blocks drainage, producing the characteristic pressure and pain. Acute sinusitis lasts less than 4 weeks. Chronic sinusitis lasts longer than 8 weeks. Although some forms of chronic sinusitis are not caused by infection, many are. Viral upper respiratory tract infections frequently precede bacterial invasion of the sinuses. These can be caused by *Streptococcus pneumoniae, Haemophilus influenzae,* or *Moraxella catarrhalis* (Slavin et al 2005). Sinusitis is one of the most common medical conditions. Approximately 10% to 25% of people in Western societies have sinusitis, affecting 31 million patients annually in the United States (Dykewicz & Hamilos 2010). The combined cost of treating acute and chronic sinusitis in the United States is estimated at $7.3 billion per annum (Rosenfeld et al 2007).

Treatment includes antibiotics, steroids, and sometimes surgery. Although chronic sinusitis is not life threatening, it typically causes misery and reduces quality of life. Cigarette smoking, either active or passive, increases the risk of chronic sinusitis (Reh et al 2012).

Aromatherapy and Sinusitis

Peppermint *(Mentha piperita)* is the first essential oil that comes to mind for sinusitis. It is the essential oil the U.S. Navy used to test gas masks and if anything can penetrate a mucus-blocked sinus, peppermint will! There are several studies on menthol (one of the main active components in peppermint) and "upper airway congestion" (Pereira et al 2013, Millqvist et al 2013; Smith & Boden 2012). Scots pine *(Pinus sylvestris)* and rosemary *(Rosmarinus officinalis)* increased secretory response in the airways of rats (Nicolato et al 2009), suggesting these may not be useful in sinusitis. Scots pine essential oil inhalation significantly increased the surface fluid in the middle portion of the trachea and the increase was visible at both 5 and 10 minutes. A lesser secretory response was detected after rosemary essential oil inhalation. This response was significant at 10 minutes. This study used MRI (magnetic resonance imaging) as the measurement tool. However, peppermint *(Mentha piperita)* produced no secretory response at 5 and 10 minutes. This study was partly funded by the Italian Cystic Fibrosis Research Foundation.

Many over-the-counter products for sinusitis contain menthol and it is recognized as suitable for this purpose (Scholar 2007). Menthol is often combined with benzoin or eucalyptus oil for sinusitis. If we translate this information into using whole essential oils for clinical aromatherapy, it suggests using peppermint *(Mentha piperita),* benzoin *(Styrax benzoin)* and eucalyptus *(Eucalyptus globulus)*. This combination can be used via inhalation or applied topically in a lotion to the chest. Use extreme caution when using peppermint or eucalyptus essential oils near the nostrils of infants or young children, as these have caused a few instances of respiratory distress (Melis et al 1989, Tisserand 2013).

Any essential oil containing large amounts of 1,8-cineole might be useful in sinusitis. Kehrl et al (2004) conducted a double-blind, randomized, placebo-controlled study on the effects of 1,8-cineole on 152 patients with sinusitis. Participants in the experimental group took gelatin, enteric-coated capsules containing 100 mg of 1,8-cineole three times a day for 7 days. Participants in the control group took placebo capsules. At the beginning, the mean symptoms-sum-score was 15.6 in both treatment groups. After 4 days, the mean values for the symptoms-sum-scores were 6.9 ± 2.9 for the cineole group and 12.2 ± 2.5 for the placebo group. After 7 days, the symptom-sum-scores in the cineole group were 3.0 ± 2.8 and for the placebo group 9.2 ± 3.0.

In another study, manuka *(Leptospermum scoparium)*, tea tree *(Melaleuca alternifolia)* and niaouli *(Melaleuca quinquenervia)* were more effective in vitro against *Moraxella catarrhalis* than myrtol (Christoph et al 2001). Myrtol is accepted as an effective treatment for sinusitis (Rantzsch et al 2009).

An R.J. Buckle student, Machon (2001), conducted a controlled study to evaluate the effects of a mixture of *Eucalyptus globulus, Ravansara aromatica, Pinus sylvestris,* and *Mentha piperita* essential oils on sinus infections. Eight subjects (five females and three males) used three drops of the mixture via steam inhalation for 10 minutes, three times a day for 5 days. Three subjects (one male and two females) acted as controls and received only steam inhalation. Baseline measurements of pain, sense of wellness, color of mucus, and amount of mucus were recorded using a 0 to 10 visual analog scale. The essential oil group was consistently more improved with three of the five members completely clear of congestion and two nearly free. By the fifth day, their mucus was clear. In the control group, the congestion remained the same, and the mucus remained green. (Peppermint has antibacterial and antiviral properties and so may help combat any underlying sinus infection.)

Another R.J. Buckle student, Pitcher (2001), studied the effects of inhaled *Mentha piperita* on 20 adult patients (age range 18 to 90) with chronic sinusitis. Five of the 20 patients had a history of medically diagnosed asthma. Four patients used inhalers daily. No patients were using prescription decongestants daily, although 12 patients used over-the-counter decongestants as necessary. Smokers were excluded from the study. Undiluted peppermint was inhaled for 10 minutes at a time. A small cushion with two drops of peppermint was kept close to the bedside to assist with night breathing. Measurements of nasal congestion, sense of smell, headache, and postnasal drip were taken (scale 0 to 5). There was a noticeable improvement in all symptoms, particularly nasal congestion (average before treatment 3.2; average after treatment 1.35) and cough (average before treatment 3.0, average after treatment 1.4). Those who used an inhaler said they reduced the number of times they used their inhaler. No side effects were reported.

CYSTIC FIBROSIS

Cystic fibrosis (CF) is a generic, autosomal recessive disorder that affects the exocrine glands (Brooker 2008). This condition coats the lungs and the digestive system with sticky mucus leading to a persistent cough, recurrent lung infections, and poor weight gain because of food malabsorption. Current treatment includes intensive physiotherapy and long-term antibiotics. The United States CF Foundation recently proposed the term CF transmembrane conductance regulator-related metabolic syndrome (CRMS) to describe infants with elevated immunoreactive trypsinogen (IRT) who do not meet diagnostic criteria for CF (Ren et al 2011). A cross-sectional database analysis of European and non-European countries found a lower proportion of patients with CF in non-EU countries than in EU countries (McCormick et al 2010). The authors suggest this difference could be because of underdiagnosis and premature childhood mortality. The number of patients with CF in the United States has been increasing (Razvi et al 2009); however, the availability of genetic counseling and prenatal testing to parents who already have a child with CF may be starting to cause the prevalence of CF to begin to decline (Massie et al 2010). Patients with CF are very prone to lung infections with *Pseudomonas aeruginosa*.

AROMATHERAPY AND CYSTIC FIBROSIS

Bergamot *(Citrus bergamia)* and its component, bergapten, reduce some of the cytokines and chemokines that cause the inflammatory response in CF (Borgatti et al 2011). The results showed that bergapten had an inhibitory effect on IL-8 (IL-8 mRNA levels in TNF-α treated IB3-1 cells at IC_{50} concentration). IL-8 is a chemokine and its production is classically elevated in patients with CF (Vij et al 2008). Morise et al (2010) found that menthol, derived from peppermint *(Mentha piperita)*, activated the CF transmembrane conductance regulator (CFTR) and suggests that the unique effects of menthol may have the potential to ameliorate several lung conditions, including CF. Therefore, peppermint and bergamot might be useful essential oils to try.

An RJBA student, who was also a licensed massage therapist, used *Eucalyptus globulus* to good effect to aid expectoration in a patient with CF (Rudansky 2000). The patient, a 36-year-old woman with CF, had pneumonia, plural edema, was being treated with intravenous antibiotics (6 weeks on and 3 weeks off), and was dependent on an oxygen-concentrator machine. Her mucus was thick, dense, and flecked with blood. Following consultation with the woman's physician, regular inhalations of *Eucalyptus globulus* and massage with eucalyptus were given to help the patient relax, breathe, and expectorate. This appeared to increase her lung elasticity and reduce her oxygen demand. Her usual intravenous antibiotics were reduced, and she was able to go without them for several months at a time. The heaviness in her lungs decreased substantially, and she began sleeping better.

Baudoux (2007) suggests inhaling essential oils through ultrasonic nebulision as a way to ease breathing and reduce the risk of infection in patients with CF. However, he does caution that this should only be attempted in a hospital environment with medical supervision.

TUBERCULOSIS

Tuberculosis (TB) is the most ancient epidemic disease in the world and a serious opportunistic disease in HIV/AIDS patients (Bueno et al 2011). It is a chronic granulomatous infection caused by *Mycobacterium tuberculosis* (Brooker 2008). In humans, there are three types of TB (Dye 2007).
1) Pulmonary: spread by droplet infection.
2) Disseminated or Miliary: spread through the bloodstream and common in HIV-positive patients.
3) Meningitis.
Bovine tuberculosis is endemic in cattle and may be transmitted to humans through the consumption of infected milk (Brooker 2008). Bone, brain, liver, lung, spleen, and the genitourinary tract can become infected with TB (Brooker 2008).

TB was relatively well-controlled in the Western world by the BCG vaccine (Bacille Calmette-Guerin) and infection numbers fell to 10 in 100,000 people by the end of the 1980s (MacSween & Whaley 1992). However, this has changed dramatically and today about two billion people are thought to have latent TB: approximately one in three people (Buhner 2012, Kerr 2013). According to the World Health Organization (2013), an estimated 8.8 million people fell ill with TB in 2010, including 1.1 million cases among people with HIV. There are three million deaths annually (Siddiqui et al 2012) and of these 95% are in developing countries (NIAID 2013). The incidence of multidrug resistant TB (MDRTB) is rising in Asia, Africa, and Eastern Europe (Brooker 2008) and 2% of the world's population (approximately 40 million people) currently has untreatable MDRTB (Harrod Buhner 2012).

Before the arrival of antibiotics, patients with TB were sent to sanatoriums, often located high in the mountains and frequently close to Scots pine forests, because it was thought that breathing mountain air laced with pine "essence" would aid recuperation. Sanatorium windows contained no glass so sunlight (UV radiation kills TB bacteria) and air could flow freely through the facility. Scots pine contains over 50% α-pinene and over 20% β-pinene: two terpenes thought to have beneficial effects on the lungs (Lima et al 2010).

AROMATHERAPY AND TB

Several essential oils have been shown to have antimycobacterial activity in vitro, and some increase the antimycobacterial activity of orthodox medicines. Valnet (1990) was one of the first physicians to document the use of aromatherapy in the treatment of TB. He found essential oil of hyssop stopped TB bacillus multiplying at a concentration of 0.2 parts per 1000 (Valnet 1993). Hyssop is eliminated through the lungs. The high percentage of the ketones iso-pinocamphone and pinocamphone (70%) means that this essential oil requires caution and many feel it is contraindicated in patients with epilepsy.

Lawal et al (2012) explored the effect of two species of Eucalyptus (*camaldulensis* and *torelliana*) on TB using the microplate alamar blue assay (MABA) method and concludes, "the anti-TB activities of these plants on *M. tuberculosis* H37Rv support their use in traditional medicine for the treatment of coughs associated with TB."

A Russian paper reported the results of a 2-month study on the effects of inhaled essential oils on humans. The symptoms of 81.8% to 95.6% patients disappeared and their body masses increased (Petrosian et al 1999). Petrosian has published more recent articles on TB (in Russian) but none using essential oils. Lall and Meyer (1999) found 14 out of 20 South African plant extracts (extracted with acetone or water) showed inhibitory activity at a concentration of 0.5 mg/mL against isoniazid- and rifampin-resistant strains of TB, using the agar-plate method. Eight of the plants showed activity against the resistant strain at 1.0 mg/mL. One of the plants belonged to the *Helichrysum* genus (spp. *melanacme*), although the other plants were unfamiliar. A rapid radiometric method confirmed the inhibitory activity. Masoko and Nxumalo (2013) validated this study using microdilution assay and bioautography and ρ-iodonitrotetrazolium violet (INT) as indicator. The range of MIC (0.14 to 0.47) indicated that several South African aromatic plants had anti-TB activity (Table 19-4).

Nye, a nurse-trained naturopathic doctor, writes a very informative article on how aromatherapy is used in the TB ward of a South African Community Outreach program (2007). The standard mixture of essential oils used at Brooklyn Chest hospital in South Africa is given (with permission) in Table 19-5. This mixture is diffused and/or applied in 1% to 3% dilution (base of sweet almond oil) to the skin.

TABLE 19-4 *Published Studies on Essential Oils and Tuberculosis*

Author	Year	Common Name	Essential Oil	Method	MIC
Başer et al	2009	Caspian carrot	*Daucus littoralis*	Assay	196 µg/mL
Azevedo et al	2013	Sacaca	*Croton cajucara*	Broth dilution	4.88 µg/mL
Pinto et al	2009	Anemia	*Anemia tomentosa var. anthriscifolia*		100 µg/mL
Bueno et al	2011	Columbian Sage	*Salvia aratocensis*	Mammalian cells	125 µg/mL
Zanetti et al	2010	Myrtle	*Myrtus communis*	7H10 agar	0.17% (v/v)
Sherry et al	2004	Tea tree	*Melaleuca alternifolia*	Human ($n = 2$)	inhaled
Machan et al	2006	Indian heliotrope	*Heliotropium indicum*		

Gupta and Viswanathan (1955a) reported on the tuberculostatic activity of *Ocimum sanctum* (holy basil). In a later paper they found that *Ocimum canum* inhibited the growth of TB in a dilution of 1:50,000 (Gupta & Viswanathan 1955a). Siddiqui et al (2012) explored the effects of holy basil *(Ocimum basilicum)* against *M. tuberculosis* H37Rv using MABA assay and found there was a 49% inhibition at 6.25 μg/mL. Kufferath and Mundualgo (1954) found *Eucalyptus globulus* appeared to enhance the activity of streptomycin, isoniazid, and sulfetrone in the treatment of TB. Sherry & Warnke (2002) declared eucalyptus was a new topical antibacterial and an alternative for treatment for TB. Schnaubelt (1993) wrote that *Cupressus sempervirens* (cypress) and *Pinus sylvestris* (Scots pine) are also effective against TB. I could not find any recent studies, but that does not mean they are not effective. Table 19-6 lists essential oils for pulmonary TB.

TABLE 19-5 *Mixture Used for Tuberculosis Patients at Brooklyn Chest Hospital*

Essential Oil	Common Name	%
Melaleuca quinquenervia CT viridiflorol	Niaouli	60
Eucalyptus smithii	Gully gum	5
Myrtus communis CT myrtenyl acetate	Myrtle	10
Abies balsam	Balsam fir	10
Melaleuca alternifolia	Tea tree	10
Pelargonium × *aspermum*	Geranium	4
Mentha × *piperita*	Peppermint	1

TABLE 19-6 *Essential Oils for Pulmonary Tuberculosis*

Common Name	Botanical Name	References
Blue gum	*Eucalyptus globulus*	Kufferath & Mundualgo 1954 Sadlon & Lamson 2010
Klonemax	*Eucalyptus mixture*	Sherry et al 2004
Niaouli	*Melaleuca viridiflora*	Kufferath & Mundualgo 1954
Marjoram	*Origanum majorana*	Valnet 1993
Holy basil	*Ocimum sanctum**	Gupta & Viswanathan 1955 Singh & Agrawal 1991 Siddiqui et al 2012
Juniper	*Juniperus communis*	Duke 1985 Gordien et al 2009

*Low doses: suggested amount below 0.5%.

FORCED VITAL LUNG CAPACITY

Finally, the Forced Vital Lung (FVL) capacity of 20 subjects was evaluated by an R.J. Buckle student, Coon (2007), who is also a chiropractic physician and university assistant professor. The participants were evaluated before and after inhaling peppermint for 5 minutes using an individual personal inhaler. Some of the participants were smokers and some had chest infections. All participants had improved airflow. There was a 5.76% group improvement. One participant was the number one speed skater in the United States for his age group. He felt inhaling peppermint also enhanced his performance (Coon 2007).

For a number of respiratory diseases, clinical aromatherapy is at least a useful adjunct therapy if not mainstay, with substantial benefit to risk when specific essential oils (e.g., peppermint for COPD) are used.

REFERENCES

Akinci A, Zengin N, Yildiz H, Sener E, Gunaydin B. 2011. The complementary and alternative medicine use among asthma and chronic obstructive pulmonary disease patients in the southern region of Turkey. *Int J Nurs Pract.* 17(6):571–82.

Allen-Ramey FC, Gupta S, DiBonaventura MD. 2012. Patient characteristics, treatment patterns, and health outcomes among COPD phenotypes. *Int J Chron Obstruct Pulmon Dis.* 7:779–87.

Azevedo M, Chaves F, Almeida C, Bizzo H, Duarte R. 2013. Antioxidant and antimicrobial activities of 7-hydroxy-calamenene-rich essential oils from Croton cajucara Benth. *Molecules.* 18(1):1128–1137.

Ballenger S. 2002. *Ravansara aromatica and chest infections.* Unpublished dissertation for RJ Buckle Associates.

Bardeau F. 1976. Use of essential aromatic oils to purify and deodorise the air. *Le Chirurgien-Dentiste de France.* 46:53.

Baudoux D. 2007. Aromatology for respiratory pathologies. *Int J of Clinical Aromatherapy.* 4(1):34–39.

Başer K, Kurkcuoğlu M, Askun T, Tumen G. 2009. Antituberculosis activity of Daucus littoralis Sibth. et Sm. (Apiaceae) from Turkey. *J Essential Oil Research.* 21(6):572–575.

Begrow F, Böckenholt C, Ehmen M, Wittig T, Verspohl E. 2012. Effect of myrtol standardized and other substances on the respiratory tract: ciliary beat frequency and mucociliary clearance as parameters. *Adv Ther.* 29(4):350–8.

Ben-Ayre E, Dudai N, Eini A, Torem M, Schiff E, Rakover Y. 2011. Treatment of upper respiratory tract infections in primary care: a randomized study using aromatic herbs. *Evid Based Complement Alternat Med.* 2011:690346.

Berger H, Jarosch E, Madreiter H. 1978. Effect of Vaporub and petrolatum on frequency and amplitude of breathing in children with acute bronchitis. *J Int Med Res.* 6(6):483–6.

Borgatti M, Mancini I, Bianchi N, Guerrini A, Lampronti I et al. 2011. Bergamot (*Citrus bergamia Risso*) fruit extracts and identified components alter expression of interleukin 8 gene in cystic fibrosis bronchial epithelial cell lines. *BMC Biochemistry.* 12. 12:15.

Boskabady M, Khatami A. 2003. Relaxant effect of *Foeniculunl vulgare* on isolated guinea pig tracheal chains. *Pharmaceutical Biology.* 41(3):211–215.

Boyd E. 1954. Expectorants and respiratory tract fluid. *Pharmacological Review.* 6:521–542.

Brooker C. 2008 *Medical Dictionary.* 16th edition. Churchill Livingstone, Edinburgh.

Bryant J, McDonald VM, Boyes A, Sanson-Fisher R, Paul C, Melville J. 2013. Improving medication adherence in chronic obstructive pulmonary disease: a systematic review. *Respir Res.* 14(1):109.

Bueno J, Escobar P, Martinez J, Leal S, Stashenko E. 2011. Composition of three essential oils, and their mammalian cell toxicity and antimycobacterial activity against drug resistant-tuberculosis and non-tuberculous mycobacteria strains. *Nat Prod Commun.* 6(11):1743–8.

Buhner S. 2012. *Herbal Antibiotics: Natural alternatives to treating drug-resistant bacteria.* Storey Publishing. MA.

Camporese A. 2013. (Le infezioni in medicina : rivista periodica di eziologia, epidemiologia, diagnostica, clinica e terapia delle patologie infettive). In vitro activity of *Eucalyptus smithii* and *Juniperus communis* essential oils against bacterial biofilms and efficacy perspectives of complementary inhalation therapy in chronic and recurrent upper respiratory tract infections. *Infez Med.* 21(2):117–24.

Centers for Disease Control and Prevention. 2013. Chronic obstructive disease among adults – USA, 2011. *Morbidity and Mortality Weekly Report.* 61(46):938–843.

Charron J. 1997. Use of *Lavandula latifolia* as an expectorant. *J Alt Complementary Medicine.* 3(3):211.

Christoph, F, Kaulfers, P-M and Stahl-Biskup, E. 2001. In vitro evaluation of the antibacterial activity of β-triketones admixed to Melaleuca oils. *Planta Medica.* 67(8):768–771.

Coon S. 2007. *The effect of peppermint on Forced Vital Lung Capacity.* Unpublished dissertation for RJ Buckle Associates.

Crawford N. 2003. *Eucalyptus globulus* and sinusitis. Unpublished dissertation for RJ Buckle Associates.

Duke J. 1985. *Handbook of Medicinal Herbs.* Boca Raton, FL: CRC Press.

Dunster C. 2007. *The use of three inhaled essential oils for rhinitis.* Unpublished dissertation for RJ Buckle Associates.

Dye S. 2007. Letter from South Africa: Community outreach on a tuberculosis (TB) ward. *Int J Clinical Aromatherapy.* 4(1):43–45.

Dykewicz M, Hamilos D. 2010. Rhinitis and sinusitis. *J Allergy & Clin Immunology.* 125(2):S103–S115.

El Gazzar M, El Mezayen R, Nicolls M, Marecki J, Dreskin S. 2006. Downregulation of leukotriene biosynthesis by thymoquinone attenuates airway inflammation in a mouse model of allergic asthma. *Biochimica et Biophysica Acta.* 1760(7):1088–1095.

Elshoff R. 2001. *The use of inhaled peppermint for sinusitis.* Unpublished dissertation for RJ Buckle Associates.

European Medicines Agency. 2013. *Assessment Report of* Eucalyptus globulus, *Eucalyptus polybractea and Eucalyptus smithii.* EMA/HMPC/307782/2011.

Falk A, Gullstrand E, Lof A. 1990. Liquid/air partition coefficients of four terpenes. *British Journal of Industrial Medicine.* 47(1):62–64.

Fathy Balaha M, Tanaka H, Yamashita H, Rahman M, Inagaki N. 2012. Oral *Nigella sativa* oil ameliorates ovalbumin-induced bronchial asthma in mice. *International Immunopharmacology.* 14(2):224–231.

Fedeles R, Butje A. 2007. Asthma, allergies and aromatherapy. *Int J Clinical Aromatherapy.* 4(1):9–15.

Fenu G, Foddai M, Carai A, Pirino A, Usai M. 2008. Therapeutic properties of myrtle essential oil: an in vitro study on human nasal mucosa cells. *Int J Essential Oil Therapeutics.* 2(1):21–25.

Filipsson A. 1996. Short term inhalation exposure to turpentine, toxicokinetics and acute effects in men. *Occupational and Environmental Medicine.* 53(2):100–105.

Forey BA, Thornton AJ, Lee PN. 2011. Systematic review with meta-analysis of the epidemiological evidence relating smoking to COPD, chronic bronchitis and emphysema. *BMC Pulm Med.* 11:36.

Gilani A, Shah A, Zubair A, Khalid S, Kiani J et al. 2009. Chemical composition and mechanisms underlying the spasmolytic and bronchodilatory properties of the essential oil of *Nepeta cataria*. *Journal of Ethnopharmacology.* 121(3):405–4011.

Gillissen A, Wittig T, Ehmen M, Krezdorn HG, de Mey C. 2013. A multi-centre, randomised, double-blind, placebo-controlled clinical trial on the efficacy and tolerability of GeloMyrtol® forte in acute bronchitis. *Drug Res (Stuttg).* 63(1):19–27.

Gordien A, Gray A, Franzblau S, Seidel V. 2009. Antimycobacterial terpenoids from Juniperus communis L. (Cuppressaceae). *J Ethnopharmacology.* 126(3):500–505.

Görnemann T, Nayal R, Pertz H, Melzig M. 2008. Antispasmodic activity of essential oil from *Lippia dulcis* Trev. *Journal of Ethnopharmacology.* 117(1):166–169.

Grisk A, Fischer W. 1969. On the pulmonar excretion of cineole, menthol and thymol in rats following rectal application. *Zeitschrift fur Arztliche Fortbildung.* 63(4):233–236.

Guarneri F, Barbuzza O, Vaccaro M, Galtieri G. 2008. Allergic contact dermatitis and asthma caused by limonene in a labourer handling citrus fruits. *Contact Dermatitis.* 58(5):315–316.

Gupta K, Viswanathan R. 1955a. A short note on antitubercular substance from *Occimum sanctum*. *Antibiotics and Chemotherapy*. 6(3):247.

Hamoud R, Sporer F, Reichling J, Wink M. 2012. Antimicrobial activity of a traditionally used complex essential oil distillate (Olbas(®) Tropfen) in comparison to its individual essential oil ingredients. *Phytomedicine*. 19(11):969–76.

Harris B. 2007. 1,8 cineole – a component of choice for respiratory pathologies. *Int J Clin Aromatherapy*. 4(1):3–8.

Hasani A, Pavia D, Toms N, Dilworth P, Agnew J. 2003. Effect of aromatics on lung mucociliary clearance in patients with chronic airways obstruction. *J Altern Complement Medicine*. 9(2):243–9.

Holm M, Kim J, Lillienberg L, Storaas T, Jögi R et al. 2012. Incidence and prevalence of chronic bronchitis: impact of smoking and welding. The RHINE study. *Int J Tuberc Lung Dis*. 16(4):553–7.

Juergens U, Stöber M, Schmidt-Schilling L, Kleuver T, Vetter H. 1998. Anti-inflammatory effects of eucalyptol (1,8-cineole) in bronchial asthma: Inhibition of arachidonic acid metabolism in human blood monocytes ex vivo. *European Journal of Medical Research*. 3(9):407–412.

Juergens U, Dethlefsen U, Steinkamp G, Gillissen A, Repges R, Vetter H. 2003. Antiinflammatory activity of 1,8 -cineole (eucalyptol) in bronchial asthma: A double-blind placebo-controlled trial. *Respiratory Medicine*. 97(3):250–256.

Kamin W, Kieser M. 2007. Pinimenthol ointment in patients suffering from upper respiratory tract infections – a postmarketing observational study. *Phytomedicine*. 14(12):787–91.

Kehrl W, Sonnemann U, Dethlefsen U. 2004. Therapy for acute nonpurulent rhinosinusitis with cineole: results of a double-blind, randomised, placebo-controlled trial. *Laryngoscope*. 114(4):738–742.

Kerr P. 2013. Plants and tuberculosis: phytochemicals potentially useful in the treatment of tuberculosis. *Fighting multiple drug resistance with herbal extracts, essential oils and their components*. Academic Press: 45–64.

Khan M, Kuiantseva L, Rassulova M, Bykova H. 2011. The efficacy of health improvement measures for sickly children in a children's health promotion facility. *Vopr Kurortol Fizioter Lech Fiz Kult*. 5:21–4.

Kilina A, Kolesnikova M. 2011. The efficacy of the application of essential oils for the prevention of acute respiratory diseases in organized groups of children. *Vestn Otorinolaringol*. 5:51–4.

Kufferath F, Mundualgo G. 1954. The activity of some preparations containing essential oils in TB. *Fitoterapia*. 25:483–485.

Kumar P, Mishra S, Malik A, Satya S. 2012. Compositional analysis and insecticidal activity of *Eucalyptus globulus* (family: *Myrtaceae*) essential oil against housefly (*Musca domestica*). *Acta Trop*. 122(2):212–8.

Lall N, Meyer J. 1999. In vitro inhibition of drug-resistant and drug-sensitive strains of *Mycobacterium tuberculosis* by ethnobotanically selected South African plants. *J Ethnopharmacology*. 66(3):347–354.

Lancet Respiratory Medicine. 2013. 1(8):585.

Latimer K. 2012. *A mixture of four inhaled essential oils for seasonal rhinitis*. Unpublished dissertation for RJ Buckle Associates.

Lawal T, Adeniyi B, Adegoke A, Franzblau S, Mahady G. 2012. In vitro susceptibility of Mycobacterium tuberculosis to extracts of *Eucalyptus camaldulensis* and *Eucalyptus torelliana* and isolated compounds. *Pharm Biol*. 50(1):92–8.

Latimer K. 2012. *Frankincense, Spike lavender, Eucalyptus globulus and peppermint for seasonal rhinitis*. Unpublished dissertation for RJ Buckle Associates.

Laurence J. 2012. *Teatree and Lemon Eucalyptus for respiratory congestion*. Unpublished dissertation for RJ Buckle Associates.

Lee, H-Y, Kim K-R, Kang, S-M. 2010. The effect of nebulized frankincense essential oil in an OVA-induced allergic asthma mouse model. *Korean Journal Microbiology & Biotechnology*. 38(1):93–104.

Lima F, Brito T, Freire W, Costa R, Linhares M et al. 2010. The essential oil of *Eucalyptus tereticornis*, and its constituents alpha- and beta-pinene, potentiate acetylcholine-induced contractions in isolated rat trachea. *Fitoterapia*. 81(6):649–55.

Lockhart N. 2000. *Inhalation of frankincense and its affect on asthmatics*. Unpublished dissertation. RJ Buckle Associates.

Machan T, Korth J, Liawruangrath B, Liawruangrath S, Pyne S. 2006. Composition and antituberculosis activity of the volatile oil of *Heliotropium indicum* Linn. growing in Phitsanulok, Thailand. *Flav Frag Journal*. 21(2):265–267.

Machon L. 2000. Eucalyputus, ravansara and Scotch pine for sinusitis. Unpublished dissertation for RJ Buckle Associates.

Machon L. 2001. *Use of four essential oils in the treatment of sinus infections*. Unpublished dissertation. R J Buckle Associates.

MacSween R, Whaley K (eds.). 1992. *Muir's Textbook of Pathology*. London: Edward Arnold.

Masoko P, Nxumalo K. 2013. Validation of antimycobacterial plants used by traditional healers in three districts of the Limpopo Province (South Africa). *Evid Based Complement Alt Med*. PMCID: PMC3728536.

Massie J, Curnow L, Gaffney L, Carlin J, Francis I. 2010. Declining prevalence of cystic fibrosis since the introduction of newborn screening. *Arch Dis Child*. 95(7):531–3.

Mattys H, de Mey C, Carls C et al. 2000. Efficacy and tolerability of myrtol. Standardized in acute bronchitis. A multi-centre, randomised, double-blind, placebo-controlled parallel group clinical trial vs. cefuroxime and ambroxol. *Arzneimittel-Forschung Drug Research*. 50(8):700–711.

May J. 2003. *Peppermint for sinusitis*. Unpublished dissertation for RJ Buckle Associates.

Melis K, Bochner A, Hanssens G. 1989. Accidental nasal eucalyptol and menthol instillation. *European Journal of Pediatrics*. 148(8):786–788.

McCormick J, Mehta G, Olesen H, Viviani L, Macek M Jr, Mehta A. 2010. Comparative demographics of the European cystic fibrosis population: a cross-sectional database analysis. *Lancet*. 375(9719):1007–13.

Millqvist E, Ternesten-Hasséus E, Bende M. 2013. Inhalation of menthol reduces capsaicin cough sensitivity and influences inspiratory flows in chronic cough. *Respir Med*. 107(3):433–8.

Misra A, Hickey A, Rossi C, Borchard G, Terada H et al. 2011. Inhaled drug therapy for treatment for tuberculosis. *Tuberculosis*. 91(1):71–81.

Morise M, Ito Y, Matsuno T, Hibino Y, Mizutani T et al. 2010. Heterologous regulation of anion transporters by menthol in human airway epithelial cells. *European J Pharmacology*. 635:1–3.

NIAID 2013. National Institute of Allergy and Infectious Diseases.

Nicolato E, Boschi F, Marzola P, Sbarbati A., 2009. Secretory response induced by essential oils on airway surface fluid: a pharmacological MRI study. *J Ethnopharmacology*. 124(3):630–634.

Ogunlesi M, Okiei W, Odor E, Osibote A. 2009. Analysis of the essential oil from the dried leaves of *Euphorbia hirta* Linn (*Euphorbiaceae*), a potential medication for asthma. *African Journal of Biotechnology*. 8(24):7042–7050.

Pereira E, Sim L, Driver H, Parker C, Fitzpatrick M. 2013. The effect of inhaled menthol on upper airway resistance in humans: a randomized controlled crossover study. *Can Respir J*. 20(1):e1–4.

Petrosian F, L'vov S, Levchenko G. 1999. The methods of traditional medicine in the treatment of tuberculosis. *Voenno-Meditsinskii Zhurnal*. 320(10):45–48.

Pinto S, Leitão G, de Oliveira D, Bizzo H, Ramos D. 2009. Chemical composition and antimycobacterial activity of the essential oil from *Anemia tomentosa* var. *anthriscifolia*. *Natural Product Communications*. 4(12):1675–1678.

Pitcher L. 2000. Peppermint for sinusitis. Unpublished dissertation for RJ Buckle Associates.

Pitcher L. 2001. *The Effects of Mentha piperita on chronic upper respiratory symptoms in adults*. Unpublished dissertation. RJ Buckle Associates.

Podlogar J, Verspohl E. 2012. Antiinflammatory effects of ginger and some of its components in human bronchial epithelial (BEAS-2B) cells. *Phytotherapy Research*. 26(3):333–336.

Rantzsch U, Vacca G, Dück R, Gillissen A. 2009. Antiinflammatory effects of Myrtol standardized and other essential oils on alveolar macrophages from patients with chronic obstructive pulmonary disease. *Eur J Med Res*. 14 (Suppl 4):205–9.

Razvi S, Quittell L, Sewall A, Quinton H, Marshall B, Saiman L. 2009. Respiratory microbiology of patients with cystic fibrosis in the United States, 1995 to 2005. *Chest*. 136(6):1554–60.

Reh D, Higgins T, Smith T. 2012. Impact of tobacco smoke on chronic rhinosinusitis: a review of the literature. *Int Forum Allergy Rhinol*. 2(5):362–9.

Ren C, Desai H, Platt M, Dixon M. 2011. Clinical outcomes in infants with cystic fibrosis transmembrane conductance regulator (CFTR) related metabolic syndrome. *Pediatr Pulmonol.* 46(11):1079–84.

Roche N, Chavannes NH, Miravitlles M. 2013. COPD symptoms in the morning: impact, evaluation and management. *Respir Res.* 14(1):112.

Rohr AC, Wilkins CK, Clausen PA, Hammer M, Nielsen GD et al. 2002. Upper airway and pulmonary effects of oxidation products of (+)-alpha-pinene, d-limonene, and isoprene in BALB/c mice. *Inhal Toxicol.* 14(7):663–84.

Rosenfeld R, Andes D, Battacharyya N, Dickson C, Eisenberg S et al. 2007. Clinical Practice Guidelines: Adult sinusitis. *Otolaryngology-Head & Neck Surgery.* 137 (3): suppl S1–S31.

Rudansky R. 2000. *Eucalyptus globulus and cystic fibrosis: a case-study.* Unpublished dissertation. RJ Buckle Associates.

Sadlon A, Lamson D. 2010. Immune-modifying and antimicrobial effects of Eucalyptus oil and simple inhalation devices. *Altern Med Rev.* 15(1):33–47.

Schnaubelt K. 1993. *Aromatherapy Course, Part 3.* San Rafael, CA: Pacific Institute of Aromatherapy.

Scholar E. 2007. Menthol in *xPharm: The Comprehensive Pharmacology Reference.* Elsevier, 1-3.

Shah A, Gilani A-H, Abbas K, Rasheed M, Ahmed A, Ahmad V. 2011. Studies on the chemical composition and possible mechanisms underlying the antispasmodic and bronchodilatory activities of the essential oil of *Artemisia maritima L. Archives Pharmacal Research.* 34(8):1227–1238.

Sherry E, Reynolds M, Sivananthan S, Mainawalala S, Warnke P. 2004. Inhalational phytochemicals as possible treatment for pulmonary tuberculosis: Two case reports. *American Journal of Infection Control.* 32(6):369–370.

Sherry E, Warnke P. 2002. Alternative for MRSA and tuberculosis (TB): Eucalyptus and tea tree oils as new topical antibacterials. *American Academy of Orthopaedic Surgeons,* Annual Meeting, February 13–17, Dallas, TX, United States.

Siddiqui B, Bhatti H, Begum S, Perwaiz S. 2012. Evaluation of the antimycobacterium activity of the constituents from *Ocimum basilicum* against *Mycobacterium tuberculosis. J Ethnopharmacology.* 144(1):220–222.

Singh S, Agrawal S. 1991. Antiasthmatic and antiinflammatory activity of *Ocimum sanctum. International Journal of Pharmacognosy.* 29(4):306–310.

Slavin R, Spector S, Bernstein L. 2005. The diagnosis and management of sinusitis: A practice parameter update. *J Allergy & Clin Immunology.* 116(6):S13–S47.

Smith A, Boden C. 2012. Effects of chewing menthol gum on the alertness of healthy volunteers and those with an upper respiratory tract illness. *Stress Health.* 29(2):138–42.

Spear B. 1999. *Essential oils and their effectiveness in the relief of symptoms of asthma.* Unpublished dissertation. RJ Buckle Associates.

Stevenson C. 1995. Aromatherapy. In Rankin-Box D (ed.), *The Nurses' Handbook of Complementary Therapies.* London: Churchill Livingstone, 52–58.

Stewart D. 2005. *The Chemistry of Essential Oils Made Simple.* Care Publications. Marble Hill MO. USA.

Straif K, Cohen A, Samet J. 2013. *Air Pollution & Cancer.* IARC scientific publication. No 161.

Takaishi M, Fujita F, Uchida K, Yamamoto S, Sawada Shimizu M et al. 2012. 1,8-cineole, a TRPM8 agonist, is a novel natural antagonist of human TRPA1. *Mol Pain.* 29(8):86.

Tamaoki J, Chiyotani A, Sakai A, Takemura H, Konno K. 1995. Effect of menthol vapour on airway hyperresponsiveness in patients with mild asthma. *Respiratory Medicine.* 89(7):503–504.

Tilert T, Dillon C, Paulose-Ram R, Hnizdo E, Doney B. 2013. Estimating the US prevalence of chronic obstructive pulmonary disease using pre- and post-bronchodilator spirometry: the National Health and Nutrition Examination Survey (NHANES) 2007-2010. *Respir Res.* 14(1):103.

Tisserand R, Young R. 2013. *Essential Oils Safety.* 2nd edition. Elsevier, 108–109.

Valnet J. 1990. *The Practice of Aromatherapy.* Saffron Walden, UK: CW Daniels.

Vij N, Amoako M, Mazur S, Zeitlin P. 2008. CHOP transcription factor mediates IL-8 signaling in cystic fibrosis bronchial epithelial cells. *Am J Respir Cell Mol Biol.* 38(2):176–84.

Wolkoff P, Clausen P, Larsen K, Hammer M, Larsen S, Nielsen G. 2008. Acute airway effects of ozone-initiated d-limonene chemistry: importance of gaseous products. *Toxicol Lett.* 181(3):171–6.

Worth H, Dethlefsen U. 2012. Patients with asthma benefit from concomitant therapy with cineole: A placebo-controlled, double-blind trial. *J Asthma.* 49(8):849–853.

World Health Organization. 2013. http://www.afro.who.int/en/clusters-a-programmes/dpc/non-communicable-diseases-managementndm/programme-components/chronic-respiratory-diseases.html.

World Health Organization. 2011. Asthma factsheet 2011. http://www.who.int/mediacentre/factsheets/fs307/en/.

World Health Organization. 2007. Global Alliance against Chronic Respiratory Diseases (GARD). June. 2007.

Zanetti S, Cannas S, Molicotti P, Bua A, Cubeddu M et al. 2010. Evaluation of the Antimicrobial Properties of the Essential Oil of *Myrtus communis L.* against Clinical Strains of *Mycobacterium spp. Interdiscip Perspect Infect Dis.* 2010. doi:pii: 931530.

Chapter 20

Women's Health

"When all the trappings and affections of civilization are stripped away, we are merely scented apes."

Michael Soddart, 1990

CHAPTER ASSETS

DYSMENORRHEA

The menstrual cycle is delicately balanced and can easily be thrown out of equilibrium by stress, illness, or a poor diet. Dysmenorrhea is defined as painful menstruation that includes low abdominal pains (menstrual cramps) and can also be accompanied by nausea and fatigue. Dysmenorrhea is very common. Studies suggest that 25% to 95% of women experience menstrual cramps and that 10% to 26% of women experience severe pain (Hur et al 2006, Gagua et al 2012, Sultan et al 2012). Hur's 2006 study found that in the most severe cases, women rated their pain as 7.9 on a 10-point visual analog scale (VAS). Milsom et al (1988) showed that the intrauterine pressure (IUP) of a patient with dysmenorrhea was 55.3 mm Hg in the relaxation phase and 175 mm Hg in the contraction phase. This means the IUP during contraction is greater than in labor. Despite dysmenorrhea being severe enough to affect daily activities, menstrual cramps are not acknowledged as a serious problem or one requiring nursing intervention.

TABLE 20-1 *Antispasmodic Essential Oils for Dysmenorrhea*

Common Name	Botanical Name	Reference
Roman chamomile	*Chamaemelum nobile*	Pollard 2008
Peppermint	*Mentha piperita*	De Sousa et al 2010
Rosemary	*Rosmarinus officinalis*	Taddei et al 1988
Clary sage	*Salvia sclaria*	Hur et al 2012
Lavender	*Lavandula angustifolia*	Hadi & Hanid 2011

Primary dysmenorrhea is related to an overproduction of uterine prostaglandins. These cause myometrium hypercontractility and arteriolar vasoconstriction, both involved in painful menstrual cramps. Primary dysmenorrhea manifests symptoms such as low abdominal cramping that starts just before or with the menstrual flow. This is often associated with nausea, vomiting, headache, and faintness. Secondary dysmenorrhea usually affects older women who have symptoms of congestion and aching associated with low abdominal cramps that typically start up to 1 week before menstruation (McFerren 1996).

The most common way to treat period pain is with nonsteroidal antiinflammatory drugs (NSAIDs) (Harel 2008). A loading dose of NSAIDs (typically twice the regular dose) is used initially for dysmenorrhea in adolescents, followed by a regular dose until symptoms abate. Adolescents with symptoms that do not respond to treatment with NSAIDs for three consecutive menstrual cycles are often offered hormonal treatment. This is usually the combined estrogen/progestin oral contraceptive pill. A large metaanalysis published in *The Lancet* (Bhala et al 2013) showed that NSAIDs increase the risk of cardiovascular disease (CVD) (naproxen the least) and upper gastrointestinal (GI) complications. Surprisingly, CVD caused by NSAIDs was independent of a person's individual risk for CVD.

AROMATHERAPY FOR DYSMENORRHEA

Applying a 5% to 20% mix of antispasmodic, hormonal balancing and analgesic essential oils to the lower abdomen can be useful. Many essential oils such as Roman chamomile, lavender, clary sage, and rosemary have antispasmodic properties (Table 20-1). For essential oils with possible hormonal effects, choose from clary sage, sage, rose, geranium, and fennel. For analgesic essential oils, choose from lemongrass, lavender, sweet marjoram, ginger, and peppermint (Table 20-2). Han et al (2006) carried out a placebo-controlled study on 85 nurses with dysmenorrhea using rose, clary sage, and lavender in 3% dilution applied to the abdomen. The mixture reduced the severity of symptoms significantly. Hur et al (2006) used lavender, clary sage, and rose. In her later study (Hur et al 2012), she used clary sage, marjoram, cinnamon, ginger, and geranium. Ou et al (2012) used lavender, clary sage, and marjoram. An Iranian study looked at the effects of fennel essential oil taken orally for dysmenorrhea (Khorshidi et al 2003) (Table 20-3). Sixty students with dysmenorrhea took 1% or 2% fennel by mouth at the commencement of pain

TABLE 20-2 *Analgesic Essential Oils That Could Be Useful for Dysmenorrhea*

Common Name	Botanical Name	Reference
Lavender	*Lavandula angustifolia*	Ghelardini et al 1999, Sheikhan et al 2012
Lemongrass	*Cymbopogon citratus*	Viana et al 2000, Brito et al 2012
Peppermint	*Mentha piperita*	Kim et al 2005
Sweet marjoram	*Origanum majorana*	Deans & Svoboda 2006
Ginger	*Zingiber officinalis*	Yip & Tam 2008

TABLE 20-3 *Published Research on Aromatherapy and Dysmenorrhea*

Hur et al	2006	67	Dysmenorrhea	Lavender, clary sage, rose	Topical
Hur et al	2012	55	Dysmenorrhea	Clary sage, marjoram, cinnamon, ginger, geranium	Topical
Ou et al	2012	48	Dysmenorrhea	Lavender, clary sage, marjoram	Topical
Darsareh et al	2012	90	Dysmenorrhea	Lavender, geranium, rose, rosemary	Topical
Khorshidi et al	2003	60	Dysmenorrhea	Fennel	Oral

and thereafter at 4-hour intervals. Results showed that the 2% fennel group had a much greater reduction of pain and bleeding.

Between 2004 and 2008, RJBA students carried out six studies on aromatherapy and dysmenorrhea. Please see Table 20-4. The first three studies each chose one essential oil—clary sage; the next three studies chose mixtures, but each mixture included clary sage. All had positive effects. For one of the RJBA studies, Clark (2007) chose geranium, Roman chamomile, fennel, and clary sage—her mixture appeared to help premenstrual syndrome (as well as dysmenorrhea) more than the control group.

Compresses can give comfort when applied to the lower abdomen. A hot water bottle has been an effective remedy for period pains for eons. Placed on top of an essential oil compress, it will encourage more rapid absorption of the essential oils, as well as give the added comfort of heat. This can really help painful cramps. A soap-scented skin patch was tested by Ough et al (2008) on 11 women with menstrual cramps. In this study, a crushed bar of conventional soap (Ivory by Proctor and Gamble) was put onto gauze swabs and held in place with an elastic bandage. In some instances, the patch was in place for 20 hours. The study concludes that the

TABLE 20-4 *RJBA Student Studies on Aromatherapy for Dysmenorrhea, Labor, and Menopause*

Name	Year	State	Number	Condition	Essential Oil
Cavallo	2004	AZ	27	Dysmenorrhea	Clary sage
Rodriques	2005	WI	14	Dysmenorrhea	Clary sage
Reimer	2005	WI	12	Dysmenorrhea	Clary sage
Nichols	2006	NC	7	Dysmenorrhea	Lavender/clary sage/petitgrain
Clark	2007	NE	10	Dysmenorrhea	Mixture*
Tibljas	2008	TX	11	Dysmenorrhea	Clary sage/geranium
Adams	2000	AZ	23	Labor	Lavender
Swingle	2001	NY	25	Labor	Clary sage/frankincense
Marino	2004	AZ	11	Labor	Sweet marjoram
Bowles	2004	AZ	9	Labor	Frankincense
Ryan	2010	MA	20	Postpartum anxiety	Lavender
Brown	2002	PA	12	Hot flashes	Clary sage or lemon
Maher	2005	MN	8	Hot flashes	Cypress
Bilton	2005	MA	9	Hot flashes	Clary sage, cypress, and geranium
Meske	2005	WI	10	Hot flashes	Clary sage and cypress
Johnson	2006	MN	10	Hot flashes	Geranium and cypress

*Geranium, Roman chamomile, fennel, clary sage.

application of "concentrated scents to the skin…may represent a new method of medicinal delivery."

The whole process of tending a painful area topically brings with it strong placebo and mind–body links that can enhance the efficacy of the therapy. Of course some of the essential oil will also be inhaled, producing a psychological effect. Severe dysmenorrhea sometimes presents with nausea. Inhaling a little essential oil of peppermint or spearmint will help alleviate this. Aromatherapy, used in this way, works along with the body's own self-regulating mechanisms.

PREGNANCY AND LABOR

Evidence-based practice (EBP) or practice-based evidence (PBE)? This can be a dilemma because sometimes the latter has to come first. This has certainly been the

TABLE 20-5 *Essential Oils Used in the Burns et al (2000) Study*

Common Name	Botanical Name
Rose	*Rosa centifolia*
Lavender	*Lavandula angustifolia*
Jasmine	*Jasminum grandiflorum*
Roman chamomile	*Chamaemelum nobile*
Blue gum	*Eucalyptus globulus*
Mandarin	*Citrus reticulata*
Clary sage	*Salvia sclarea*
Frankincense	*Boswellia carteri*
Peppermint	*Mentha piperita*
Lemon	*Citrus limonum*

case with aromatherapy in pregnancy and labor, where the PBE of Ethel Burns and her team in Oxford led to EBP. She collected evidence of 8058 women in labor during the 1990s and then published her findings (Burns et al 2000). The essential oils she used are listed in Table 20-5. She did a repeat study several years later (Burns 2007). It would be excellent if midwives would replicate this! However, only a few studies have been published. Despite this, essential oils have been used by midwives, doulas, nurses, and mothers-to-be all over the world for several years (Buckle et al 2014, Fanner 2005, Mousley 2005, Zwelling et al 2006) without causing harm to the woman, fetus, or infant (Tillett & Ames 2010). Many labor units use essential oils during and after delivery (Imura et al 2006), and there are guidelines and protocols in place for the use of essential oils in pregnancy and delivery (Dunning 2005, Pollard 2008).

PREGNANCY

The use of essential oils during pregnancy remains slightly controversial. Expectant mothers and their physicians are extremely cautious of using anything that could have an adverse effect on the unborn child or the security of the pregnancy. However, most fears are unfounded (Guba 2002). To be on the safe side, aromatherapy schools suggest not using essential oils during the first trimester. However, not every woman knows she is pregnant until about the third trimester and most women use some form of perfume, bath essence, or scented soap.

There are no records of abnormal fetuses or aborted fetuses as a result of the "normal" use of essential oils, either by inhalation or by topical application. There are no records of a few drops of essential oil taken by mouth causing any problems either. However, there are a handful of records that link two specific essential oils, pennyroyal and parsley seed, both taken orally, to abortion. The amount of essential oil (taken by mouth) was extremely high—several milliliters at one time—which caused hepatotoxicity. This meant the body was unable to maintain the pregnancy. However, there were two other cases recorded where the same amount of

SECTION III | Aromatherapy in Clinical Specialties

pennyroyal taken by mouth did not result in the fetus being aborted, and the mothers recovered. The amounts taken varied from 10 mL (in the case of pennyroyal) and 1.5 to 6 mL for 8 consecutive days (parsley seed). This is between 100 and 200 times greater than the normal amount of essential oil used in aromatherapy. (Usually only one to five drops are applied topically to the skin or inhaled.) For internal use, the normal amount is between 10 and 20 drops per day (Brinker 2000). However, Price suggests it is lower at nine drops a day (Price & Price 2007, p 151) (Schnaubelt suggests one drop at a time repeated throughout the day (Schnaubelt 2011, p 133).) There is only one essential oil compound, sabinyl acetate, that has been shown to have a teratogenic effect in laboratory animals (Guba 2002). Sabinyl acetate comprises 20% savin *(Juniperus sabina)* and less than 10% Spanish sage *(Salvia lavandulifolia)*. Both essential oils should be avoided in pregnancy and have no aromatherapeutic use. More information on these oils is given in Chapter 4.1 on toxicity.

Several excellent articles and books have been written by British midwife Denise Tiran (1996, 2011, 2012). Tiran is a lecturer at the University of Greenwich and founder and Educational Director for Expectancy. Expectancy won a special award in 2010 for its unique contribution to education in maternity. Her kindle version of *Safety of Essential Oils in Pregnancy and Childbirth* is a must-read for anyone wanting to use essential oils in this category (Tiran 2012). Another helpful article is by Williams (2005) about aromatherapy use during labor in Australia.

In the UK, essential oils have been used during pregnancy and delivery at many hospitals for approximately 25 years, and expectant mothers often appear at the delivery suite with their own box of essential oils especially chosen for the birth of their child. Essential oils have been used at Hinchingbrooke Hospital, Huntingdon, St. John's, and St. Elizabeth's Hospitals in London and at the Radcliffe Infirmary in Oxford, England, since 1987. It would be expected that any adverse effects would have been reported by now.

When used correctly, essential oils are very safe in pregnancy and can give the expectant mother a sense of empowerment, reduce the annoying side effects of pregnancy, and can help make her feel beautiful. If there is a choice between a synthetic chemical (with no studies on long-term effects) or an essential oil (with hundreds of years of use), it would be judicious to choose the latter. Aromatherapy can be helpful for many symptoms of pregnancy: general tiredness, aches and pains, nausea, insomnia, and backache.

Some essential oils are thought to have emmenagogic actions, meaning they cause tiny uterine contractions and can bring on a menstrual period early. However, the hormonal and physical effects of pregnancy are quite different from those of the menstrual cycle, and Guba (2002) suggests that the topical or inhaled effect of emmenagogic essential oils will not compromise a stable pregnancy (Bastard & Tiran 2005). It is extremely unlikely that a secure pregnancy will be compromised because a mother has used an emmenagogic essential oil. Babies are difficult to dislodge in a secure pregnancy. However, if the mother has had a previous miscarriage, it would be prudent to avoid aromatherapy. However, I have many friends and colleagues who have used aromatherapy throughout their pregnancies and they have given birth to healthy babies.

One of the most significant medical events for a pregnant woman is the development of pregnancy-induced hypertension (PIH) and its more severe complications—preeclampsia and HELLP syndrome (hemolysis, elevated liver enzymes, and low platelets). The patient usually presents with epigastric pain and blood pressure may (or may not) be elevated. HELLP is a variant of preeclampsia and eclampsia.

PIH

This condition occurs in 7% to 10% of all pregnancies and causes 15% of maternal deaths. Women who have a history of hypertension before pregnancy are twice as likely to develop PIH. PIH can also lead to intrauterine fetal death through placental insufficiency. Orthodox treatment is bed rest with the feet elevated and intravenous magnesium sulfate. If the blood pressure does not come down to levels below 150-110/110 mm Hg, labetalol, an alpha- and beta-adrenergic blocking agent, is given. A blood pressure of 150-160/100-110 mm Hg constitutes severe preeclampsia, calling for antihypertensives (hydralazine or labetalol). Common side effects are drowsiness, fatigue, pulse slower than 50 beats per minute, and nausea. The mother is kept quiet in a darkened room. However, her mind is unlikely to be quiet! At such a terrifying time, smell and touch can do much to help reassure a woman, and reassurance can play an important role in this situation.

Nathan (2000), a midwife on Long Island, New York, used aromatherapy to help a mother whose blood pressure remained above 200/100 mm Hg despite intravenous medication. The patient was continuously monitored for blood pressure and pulse. Unable to control the hypertension, the attending physician asked Nathan if she would try aromatherapy. After verbal consent from the patient, Nathan used a 2% solution of *Lavandula angustifolia* in a hand 'M' Technique. Slowly the blood pressure began to come down. After 15 minutes it was 150/85 mm Hg. The fetal heart rate also improved, from mid 150s to mid 130s (beats per minute). Within 1 hour, the mother's blood pressure was 140/85 mm Hg. The patient was given 5 minutes of 'M' Technique with diluted lavender every hour during the night, and her blood pressure was maintained at 140/85 mm Hg. The mother was discharged 2 days later and the pregnancy proceeded to full term. Following on from this case study, Nathan carried out a small project on eight hypertensive patients in her maternity unit in 2000. Each patient chose rose or lavender essential oil and received a 5-minute 'M' Technique on the hand. This resulted in a measurable drop in blood pressure for each patient. It would be good to see more research in this area, either inhaling lavender and/or rose, or applying them as a hand 'M' Technique or hand massage. Rose is an excellent essential oil to use for all women's complaints—although research has concentrated on identifying components, the whole rose oil has a synergy of its own that is especially helpful to women.

LABOR

Aromatherapy has come a long way since Burn's study, and today aromatherapy is welcomed in many labor units throughout the world (Allright & Pidgeon 2003,

TABLE 20-6 *Published Research on Aromatherapy in Labor and Postpartum*

Name	Year	Number	Condition	Essential Oil	Method
Hur et al	2005	48	Labor	Mixture	Topical
Conrad & Adams	2012	28	Postpartum depression	Lavender/rose	Topical
Lane et al	2012	35	Post-C-section pain	Peppermint	Inhaled
Hur & Han	2004	74	Perineal healing	Lavender, myrrh, neroli, rose, grapefruit, mandarin, orange, and Roman chamomile	Sitz bath and soap
Sheikhan et al	2012	60	Episiotomy pain	Lavender	Topical
Hadi & Hanid	2011	200	Post-C-section pain	Lavender	Inhaled
Imura et al	2006	36	Postpartum	Mixture	Topical
Melli et al	2007	216	Sore nipples	Peppermint	Topical

Conrad 2012, Tiran 2012). There was even a Cochrane systemic review (Smith et al 2011). During early labor, soothing essential oils such as rose, lavender, geranium, and mandarin can relax the woman and reduce anxiety (Pollard 2008, Conrad 2012, Tillett and Ames 2010). When the mother is transitioning to the more active stage of labor, frankincense, jasmine, and peppermint may be useful—either as a back massage, or inhaled (Pollard 2008, Horowitz 2011). Nausea can be a problem in the transition stage and peppermint is especially useful then. During active labor, clary sage may help increase uterine contractility and also act as a stress reducer and antidepressant (Coleman-Smith 2012), much like the action of dopamine (Seol et al 2010) (Table 20-6).

Burns et al (2000) evaluated the effect of aromatherapy on 8058 mothers during an 8-year period (see Table 20-5 for a list of the essential oils used). Mothers in labor were offered aromatherapy to relieve pain, anxiety, or nausea or to strengthen contractions. Data from the unit audit were used to provide a comparison group of mothers not given aromatherapy (*n* = 15.799). Aromatherapy was offered by a core group of midwives who followed guidelines laid down by a qualified aromatherapist.

More than 50% of the mothers found aromatherapy useful. Only 14% of mothers found it unhelpful. The number of adverse symptoms reported was low (1%) and included symptoms commonly found in labor such as headache, nausea, and itchy rash. Aromatherapy was typically used by mothers in established labor (60%) or in the latent stage (29%). Of the women who used aromatherapy, 32% had their labor induced. Fewer women needed pain relief in the aromatherapy group than the control group, and fewer epidurals were given. During the 8 years of the study, the use of pethidine declined—in 1990, 13% of mothers used pethidine; by 1997, use had dropped to less than 0.2%. Frankincense was found to be the most effective essential oil for pain. Rose was found to be the most helpful for anxiety (71%). Peppermint was found to be the most effective for nausea (96%). Aromatherapy did not appear to augment contractions. However, 70% of multigravidae in dysfunctional labor did not require an oxytocin infusion, and 92% of the mothers went on to spontaneous vaginal delivery. This is an unusually high figure. Only 36% of women said they found aromatherapy helped strengthen their contractions, and the most commonly offered essential oil for this was clary sage (87%).

Burns' later study (2007) reassessed the effects of aromatherapy on laboring women. This study had 252 mothers in the aromatherapy group and 262 in the control group. The findings showed no significant differences in the number of cesarean sections (C-sections), ventouse, or Kristeller maneuver. However, fewer babies ($N = 0.0017$) in the aromatherapy group were transferred to the neonatal intensive care unit (NICU) and first-time mothers in the aromatherapy group had reduced pain perception. Dhany et al (2012) explored how the use of an aromatherapy and massage service (AMIS) impacted the use of analgesia and anesthesia in women in labor. Women who had given birth in the hospital and received AMIS ($n = 1079$) were compared to women receiving standard care. General anesthesia and epidurals were reduced (P = 0.033 and 0.001, respectively). However, there was little difference in the use of pethidine and more women in the AMIS group chose to use transcutaneous electrical stimulation (TENs; P= 0.001). The most commonly chosen essential oils in this study were bergamot and frankincense.

INDUCED LABOR

Adams (2000), an RJBA student, carried out a controlled study on the use of lavender to reduce patient anxiety when labor was induced at Desert Samaritan Hospital in Mesa, Arizona. One or two drops of lavender were inhaled continuously, or at will, from a cotton ball. Each of the 23 patients self-evaluated her anxiety level before the lavender and 30 minutes after the lavender. The levels of evaluation were as follows: very nervous, nervous, OK, calm, and very calm. The lavender group had a greater perception of reduced anxiety than the control group. Two subjects commented that their headaches went away when they inhaled lavender. All had positive comments. The attending nurses' comments ranged from "patient slept after lavender," to "more calm, much more mellow," to "less anxious, physician very pleased with effects of lavender." Direct inhalation using an aromastick or patch could be really helpful here.

Another RJBA student, Swingle (2001), carried out a study at the Newborn Family Center in Chenango Memorial Hospital in Norwich, New York, on 25 laboring mothers. Four essential oils, lavender, geranium, frankincense, and clary sage, were used in 1% dilution. The oils were used from early labor through delivery. Each essential oil was used for specific reasons. Lavender was used for relaxation, to relieve backache, and to help expel the placenta, and was successful on all counts.

Geranium was used to decrease perineal swelling and to relieve hemorrhoids; it was also successful. Clary sage was used to stimulate contractions but was not found successful. Frankincense was used successfully for extreme anxiety between transition and the second stage of labor. There were no side effects from any of the essential oils used and everyone commented on their nice aromas.

POSTPARTUM CARE

BABY BLUES

There have been several articles on the use of complementary and alternative medicine (CAM) in postpartum depression (Mantle 2003, Weier & Beal 2004, Gossler 2010). Imura et al (2006) explored the effect of a 30-minute aromatherapy massage on first-time mothers with vaginal delivery of a full-term healthy infant. Sixteen mothers were randomly allocated to the aromatherapy massage group and 20 mothers to the control group. Maternity Blues, Feeling Towards Baby Scale, Profile of Mood States (POMS), and State–Anxiety Inventory all improved more for the aromatherapy group than the control group. Conrad and Adams (2012) explored the effect of inhaled aromatherapy and topically applied essential oils (in a hand 'M' Technique) on 28 women with high-risk postpartum depression. The essential oils used were rose and lavender. Both aromatherapy groups (inhaled and topical) had greater improvements in their outcomes (Edinburgh Postnatal Depression Scale and Generalized Anxiety Disorder Scale) than the control group.

EPISIOTOMY

Hur & Han (2004) explored the use of an aromatherapy sitz bath for episiotomy. Both the bath lotion and soap used contained essential oils of lavender, myrrh, neroli, rose, grapefruit, mandarin, orange, and Roman chamomile. The outcome measure used was the REEDA scale (redness, edema, ecchymosis, drainage, approximation). The aromatherapy group had a significantly lower score on days 5 and 7 postpartum (P = 0.009 and P = 0.003) than the control group. Sheikhan et al (2012) explored the use of lavender essential oil on postepisiotomy pain. Outcome measure was REEDA and VAS. Pain was evaluated 4 and 12 hours after episiotomy and after 5 days. Hadi & Hanid (2011) explored the effect of inhaled lavender on post-C-section pain. The lavender was diffused through an oxygen mask to 100 mothers following C-section who were randomly allocated to the aromatherapy group. The control group received a "clinically neutral aromatic" smell. VAS was taken after 30 minutes, then 8 hours and 16 hours later. The aromatherapy group had less pain (P = 0.001).

CRACKED NIPPLES

Sore nipples are common during breastfeeding and are the major reason for failing to establish successful breastfeeding. Melli et al (2007) conducted a randomized, placebo-controlled study on 216 breastfeeding women to explore the effects of peppermint gel on preventing nipple cracks. There were 72 mothers (primiparous) in each group. Each mother had a maximum of four follow-up visits within 2 weeks, and a final visit at week 6. The rates of nipple and areola cracks and pain were evaluated. Prophylactic peppermint gel in breastfeeding lactating women produced fewer nipple cracks and was more effective than lanolin and placebo (P = 0.01). In an Iranian study by Sayyah et al (2007), 196 primiparous breastfeeding women were randomized to receive either peppermint water or expressed breast milk EBM. Each woman received three visits or telephone calls within the first 2 weeks and then telephone contact until the sixth week postpartum. The mothers who used peppermint water had fewer nipple and areola cracks (9%) compared to women using EBM (27%; P < 0.01). Nipple pain was also lower (P < 0.005).

Finally, inhaled peppermint reduced nausea in women following C-section in a study by Lane et al (2012). In this randomized, controlled study of 35 nauseated women post-C-section, the level of nausea in the peppermint group was reduced more than either the placebo or the control groups.

MENOPAUSE

MENOPAUSAL PROBLEMS

The menopause is the natural cessation of a woman's fertility. Estrogen levels fall to between 40% and 60% of the premenopausal level, and progesterone levels fall to almost zero (Moskowitz 2001). Once looked upon with secret delight as the end of menstruation and its accompanying problems, menopause now seems to be viewed by many women with dismay and despair and by orthodox medicine as a condition to be fixed. Hot flashes, night sweats, sleep disturbance, depression, loss of energy, and loss of concentration are all common symptoms of the menopause (Schmid & Rubinow 1991). Menopausal women seek hormone replacement therapy (HRT) mainly for night sweats and hot flashes (Ettinger & Pressman 1999). However, between one- and two-thirds of woman discontinue HRT during the first 2 years because of weight gain and unwanted side effects such as bloating and breakthrough bleeding (Den Tonkelaar & Oddens 2000). Following the Women's Health Initiative (WHI) study, there were concerns about HRT being linked to an increase in strokes in women taking HRT. However, these concerns have been moderated (Dessapt & Gourdy 2012). HRT or SERMS (selective estrogen receptor modulators) can be very helpful to reduce osteoporosis (Eriksen 2012) although frequent trips to the gym for intensive weight bearing exercises are also good for building bone density (Mosti et al 2013).

Plant estrogens are becoming increasingly accepted for menopausal symptoms (Bedell et al 2012).

AROMATHERAPY

Most published aromatherapy studies concerning the menopause have been on topically applied essential oils—usually in the form of a massage. In most published research, mixtures of essential oils have been used, such as lavender, rose, geranium, and jasmine (Hur et al 2007, Hur et al 2008). Murakami et al (2005)

TABLE 20-7 *Published Research on Aromatherapy and Menopause*

Hur et al	2007	86	Menopause: lipid level and blood pressure	Lavender, rose, geranium, jasmine	Topical
Hur et al	2008	52	Menopause: hot flashes, depression	Lavender, rose, geranium, jasmine	Topical
Murakami et al	2005	15	Menopause: Kupperman's Index	18 different EOs*	Topical
Darsareh et al	2012	90	Menopause: Menopause Rating Scale	18 different EOs*	Topical

*Essential oils (EOs) = ylang ylang, clary sage, geranium, rose, Roman chamomile, gettou, neroli, petitgrain, yuzu, melissa, sandalwood, marjoram, lavender, bergamot, cypress, juniper, peppermint, and lavender.

also used aromatherapy massage. In her study, participants saw a gynecologist and then received a 30-minute aromatherapy consultation that included a short aromatherapy massage session (to the back, leg, chest, head, and neck using a 1% mixture chosen from 18 essential oils). The 15 participants were given the same aromatherapy mixture to rub on their skin after bathing or before sleeping three to four times a week. After they carried out approximately 1 month of home care, they received a second consultation with the gynecologist. In 13 out of 15 women, menopausal symptoms were reduced by the second consultation. It was clever methodology to involve the participants in their own treatment. Darsareh et al (2012) chose a biweekly 30-minute massage with essential oils for 4 weeks to explore the effects on menopausal symptoms on 90 women (Table 20-7). Although both massage and aromatherapy massage produced a reduction in severity of symptoms more than the placebo group, the aromatherapy group had a greater effect than plain massage (P = 0.001).

Another method to use is a spritzer. Essential oils such as rose (Belaiche 1979), cypress (Valnet 1993), or clary sage can be helpful when used in a hydrosol spray or spritzer sprayed around the face, neck, and shoulders during a hot flash. A few drops of peppermint added to the mixture is wonderfully cooling. Essential oils that could be used for estrogen support in a massage, patch, or personal inhaler include fennel (Marini-Bettolo 1979), sage (Franchomme & Penoel 1991), and aniseed (Albert-Puleo 1980). Geranium (Holmes 1993) and rose give added support. Adding a mixture of essential oils to a daily bath and body lotion can also be very beneficial. I used menopausal oils in this way for many years with no ill effect. Rotating the mix of calming and estrogen-supportive essential oils helps prevent the body from becoming inured to the essential oils. The combinations and permutations of some 20 essential oils can be very therapeutic for menopausal symptoms (Table 20-8).

TABLE 20-8 *Essential Oils with Possible Estrogen Effect*

Common Name	Botanical Name	Reference
Fennel	*Foeniculum vulgare*	Khorshidi et al 2003
Geranium	*Pelargonium graveolens*	Murakami et al 2005
Rose	*Rosa damascena*	Han et al 2006
Chasteberry	*Vitex agnes*	Lucks 2003

For night sweats, cypress, with its recognized deodorant effect and hormonal properties, is comforting (Valnet 1993). For insomnia, any of the gently relaxing and sedative oils could be added, but try also root of *Angelica archangelica* (Duke 1985). Adding or increasing soy in the diet and taking daily food supplements such as red clover and black cohosh (phytoestrogens) will also help. In particular, red clover was a great success for me. Lucks et al (2002) and Lucks (2003) explored the effects of a less known essential oil, chasteberry *(Vitex agnus)*, in two separate survey studies. The results were encouraging and suggest that this would be a good essential oil to consider for menopausal symptoms.

Kozlowski (2000), an RJBA student, explored the use of clary sage and geranium on 11 menopausal women aged between 47 and 56 years using a 5% solution applied to the reflexology point for ovaries and uterus on the feet. Clary sage produced some useful changes in hot flash intensity. One subject wrote that two nights after stopping clary sage, the hot flashes returned to their original intensity.

VAGINAL INFECTIONS

Vaginal infections are one of the leading reasons that women visit their healthcare provider. The three most common vaginal infections are vulvovaginal candida, bacterial vaginosis (BV), and trichomoniasis (Mashburn 2012). Although these can be treated with conventional medicines, essential oils offer a pleasant alternative.

THRUSH *(Candida albicans)*

Vaginal yeast infection, caused mainly by *Candida albicans* (and to some extent by *Candida glabrata*), is a common nuisance factor in many women's lives. It thrives in an acid environment and is often the side effect of antibiotics, or it may occur during pregnancy or when a woman is immune compromised or diabetic. Thrush is messy, uncomfortable, embarrassing, and can reappear with depressing regularity. Approximately 75% of U.S. women have vaginal thrush at least once during their reproductive years. Between 40% and 50% of these women will have recurrent episodes, and 5% to 8% will experience chronic candida infections. This means that approximately 3 million women in the United States alone have recurrent candidial infections (Wilson 2005). The prevalence of vulvovaginitis candidiasis is expected to rise as a result of the growing number of non-*Candida albicans* species (which are immune to most antifungal medications) and as a result of more widespread antifungal resistance. Common drugs for treatment of thrush include flucytosine, fluconazole, voriconazole, posaconazole, itraconazole, ketoconazole, clotrimazole, miconazole, ciclopirox olamine, amphotericin B, and caspofungin. However, sometimes both systemic and topical azole antifungal agents do not work (Danby et al 2012).

There is at least one essential oil that may eradicate this fungal infection permanently and within only a few days (Belaiche 1985)—the oil in question is tea tree. Belaiche (1985) first wrote about its positive effect on vaginal infections 25 years ago. Since that time there have been many studies on essential oils and the effects of their components on candida. Please see Table 20-9. Duarte et al (2005) found that *Aloysia triphylla, Anthemis nobilis, Cymbopogon martini, Cymbopogon winterianus, Cyperus articulatus, Cyperus rotundus, Lippia alba, Mentha arvensis, Mikania glomerata, Mentha piperita, Mentha* sp., *Stachys byzantina,* and *Solidago chilensis* all had anticandida activity. However, in my opinion, tea tree reigns supreme—I have used and recommended it for many years, so I know that it is safe. If the correct tea tree is used, it has little if any side effects.

Tea tree is the common name used for all species of *Melaleuca, Leptospermum, Kunzea,* and *Baeckea* plants (Guenther 1972). In other words, specifying tea tree is not enough because it covers several hundred different plants. In New Zealand, *Leptospermum flavescens* is also sometimes called "tea tree," but this plant has a completely different genus to the real "tea tree." The tea tree needed to treat vaginal infections is *Melaleuca alternifolia* and it comes from Australia. The Australian government has set standards for the amount of terpineol (an alcohol) and 1,8-cineole (an oxide) in tea tree. Some tea tree imitations are available that contain high levels of 1,8-cineole. Essential oils high in oxides can be uncomfortable when applied to irritated or abraded vaginal tissue. To avoid this, make sure the bottle of essential oil includes the botanical name, and purchase it from a reliable source. The functional group alcohol is kinder on abraded vaginal tissue. The levels of 1,8-cineole and terpineol will show up on a gas chromatograph/mass spectrometer.

Mix two to three drops of *Melaleuca alternifolia* in 5 mL of cold-pressed vegetable oil, such as oil of evening primrose or sweet almond oil. The simplest method is to mix the essential oil and vegetable oil on a saucer. Then roll a tampon in the mixture until it is saturated, then insert into the vagina. Use the remainder on your fingers to spread the mixture over the labia. Then wash your hands. The tampon should be changed three times a day for a new tampon with a fresh dilution of carrier oil and tea tree. A tea tree tampon needs to remain in situ overnight. It will not lead to toxic shock syndrome. Tea tree tampons are a very safe and effective method of eradicating candidiasis (and many other vaginal infections) and there appear to be no adverse side effects.

However, a word of caution should be given. If the yeast infection has exposed raw areas in the vaginal wall or on the labia, *Lavandula angustifolia* diluted in vegetable oil should be used first. This can be applied in exactly the same way, on a tampon, for 1 or 2 days until the excoriated area has healed. Alternatively, use lavender in a sitz bath. The tea tree tampon method has been used successfully in pregnancy with no adverse effects to the mother or baby. Having suggested this

TABLE 20-9 *Published Studies on Essential Oils for Candida albicans*

Common Name	Botanical Name	Reference
Tea tree	*Melaleuca alternifolia*	Belaiche 1985, Pena 1962, Hammer & Carson 2000, D'Auria et al 2001, Ergin & Arikan 2002, Oliva et al 2003, Mondello et al 2003, Mondello et al 2005, Carson et al 2006, Maruyama & Abe 2012
Peppermint	*Mentha piperita*	Carson & Riley 1994, Sahakhiz et al 2012
Palma rosa	*Cymbopogon martinii*	Pattnaik et al 1996, Kahn et al 2012
Eucalyptus	*Eucalyptus globulus*	Pattnaik et al 1996, Argawal et al 2010
Lemongrass	*Cymbopogon citratus*	Pattnaik et al 1996, Abe et al 2003
Geranium	*Pelargonium graveolens*	Pattnaik et al 1996, Maruyama et al 2008
Melissa	*Melissa officinalis*	Suresh et al 1997, Hăncianu et al 2008
Rosemary	*Rosmarinus officinalis*	Larrondo & Calvo 1991, Hofling et al 2008
Lippia	*Lippia alba*	Soliman et al 1994, Funari et al 2012
Austrian pine	*Picea albies*	Stiles et al 1995, Kartnig et al 1991
Coriander	*Coriandrum sativum*	Furletti et al 2011
Mugwort Japanese	*Artemesium princeps*	Trinh et al 2011
Bergamot	*Citrus bergamia*	Romano et al 2005
Apple mint	*Mentha suaveolens*	Pietrella et al 2011
Clove	*Syzygium aromaticum*	Ahmad et al 2005
Lavender	*Lavandula angustifolia* (high linalool)	D'Auria et al 2005

treatment to many patients and colleagues over the last 20 years, I am confident *Melaleuca alternifolia* will remove the infection within 3 days, regardless of how long the woman has had the infection, or if the infection is resistant to conventional antifungals. Table 20-9 lists other essential oils that have been shown to be effective against *Candida albicans* in vitro. However, if you want to use an essential oil other than tea tree, please choose to use an essential oil that will be kind to such a sensitive area. Please see the chemistry chapter. If in a sexual relationship, your partner also needs to use tea tree so the infection does not pass back and forth between the two of you.

Bacterial Vaginosis

BV is a very common polymicrobial vaginal infection that affects women of reproductive age (Cook et al 1992). Although it has never been proven to be a sexually transmitted disease, some suggest that the epidemiologic evidence is quite robust (Muzny & Schwebke 2013). BV has also been linked to an increased susceptibility to the human papillomavirus (King et al 2011). Many of the bacteria causing BV, such as *Peptostreptococcus*, are anaerobic and appear to replace the normally predominant *Lactobacilli*. One of the main symptoms is copious, smelly discharge, often reducing a woman to tears of frustration. The fishy smell is from the amine compounds produced by anaerobes. There is no inflammatory reaction, so there are no white blood cells in the discharge. Orthodox treatment is oral metronidazole, but this often produces unpleasant side effects such as GI upsets or an unpleasant taste in the mouth. These can lead to patients stopping the 7-day course of treatment (Armstrong & Wilson 2010). Recent research has shown a slightly higher success rate if probiotics are given orally with metronidazole (Ling et al 2012) or intravaginally for 1 week after oral metronidazole (Coste et al 2012). Tinidazole is another orthodox treatment, thought to be as effective as metronidazole but with fewer side effects. However, it is much more expensive (Armstrong & Wilson 2010). In the United States, 500 mg metronidazole costs about 30 cents, whereas 2 mg tinidazole costs $18.

Walsh and Longstaff (1987), Shapiro et al (1994), Carson and Riley (1993), Carson and Riley (1999), and Carson et al (2006) tested tea tree against the bacteria causing BV and all came up with comparable data. Blackwell (1991) published a letter in *The Lancet* detailing how she treated a patient with BV using *Melaleuca alternifolia* vaginal pessaries with good results. A 5 mL bottle of tea tree *(Melaleuca alternifolia)* from a reputable essential oil supplier compares very favorably with the cost of metronidazole. There are 20 drops in 1 mL and therefore 100 drops of tea tree in one 5 mL bottle. This is sufficient for many treatments. Solsto and Benvenuti (2011) compared a daily douche (containing essential oil components thymol and eugenol) to one metronidazole vaginal suppository per night for 1 week and one econazole vaginal suppository per night for 3 days. The extracted components came from essential oils *Thymus vulgaris* and *Eugenia caryophyllus* and the mixture is marketed under the trade name Saugella. In Salso's research, Saugella was found to be "an effective prescription drug in minor recurrent vaginal infectious episodes and its use can reduce the repeated exposure to antibiotics."

However, pessaries can be messy and tea tree tampons are not. So, it is worth trying 2% to 5% diluted tea tree in cold-pressed carrier oil on a tampon. Diluted tea tree is easy to use—it smells pleasantly antiseptic, and the tampon application makes the vagina feel fresh. Usually, symptoms will disappear within 1 week. It is interesting how little research appears to be done on BV and tea tree.

Trichomoniasis

Trichomonas vaginalis is a bacterial infection that causes inflammation of the vaginal mucosa accompanied by an unpleasant, pungent discharge. The sufferer is embarrassed and frequently complains of "feeling dirty." Conventional treatment is with systemic metronidazole. Metronidazole can cause nausea and vomiting and leaves a metallic taste in the mouth. Drinking alcohol is not allowed while taking metronidazole and for at least 48 hours after finishing the course of antibiotics. Drinking alcohol while taking metronidzole increases the severity of the side effects.

According to the World Health Organization (WHO), trichomoniasis is a sexually transmitted infection (STI) (Sherrard et al 2011). Humphrey suggested tea tree for trichomoniasis as long ago as 1930, and it was found effective by Pena (1962). Azimi et al (2011) found that tea tree and many of its isolated components had antibacterial, antifungal, and antiprotozoal properties against trichomonas. Tea tree (5%) in cold-pressed carrier oil (olive oil is suitable) on a tampon is an effective treatment. Use every 4 hours for 3 to 5 days. and leave the tampon in overnight (up to 8 hours). Usually, the infection will be gone within 1 week. Because this is a sexually transmitted disease, the partner(s) need to be treated also.

REFERENCES

Abe S, Sato Y, Inoue, S, Ishibashi, H, Maruyama, N et al. 2003. Anti-*Candida albicans* activity of essential oils including lemongrass (*Cymbopogon citratus*) oil and its component, citral. *Jpn J Med Mycol.* 44(4):286-91.

Adams A. 2000. Does *Lavandula angustifolia* reduce patient anxiety during induced labor? Unpublished dissertation. RJ Buckle Associates.

Agarwal V, Lal P, Pruthi V. 2010. Effect of plant oils on *Candida albicans*. *Microbiol Immunol Infect.* 43(5):447-51.

Ahmad N, Alam M, Shehbaz A, Khan A, Mannan A et al. 2005. Antimicrobial activity of clove oil and its potential in the treatment of vaginal candidiasis. *J Drug Target.* 13(10):555–61.

Albert-Puleo M. 1980. Fennel and anise as estrogenic agents. *Journal of Ethnopharmacology.* 2(4): 337-344.

Allright K, Pidgeon K. 2003. Supporting mothers and midwives with aromatherapy: a relaxing dream come true. *Midwifery Matters.* 99(4-9).

Armstrong N, Wilson J. 2010. Tinidazole in the treatment of bacterial vaginosis. *Int J Womens Health.* 9(1):59-65.

Azimi H, Fallah-Tafti M, Karimi-Darmiyan M, Abdollahi M. 2011. A comprehensive review of vaginitis phytotherapy. *Pak J Biol Sci.* 1;14(21):960-6.

Bastard J, Tiran D. 2005. Aromatherapy and massage for antenatal anxiety: its effect on the fetus. *Complement Ther Clin Pract.* 12:48-54.

Bedell S, Nachtigall M, Naftolin F. 2012. The pros and cons of plant estrogens for menopause. *J Steroid Biochem Mol Biol.* doi: pii: S0960–0760(12)00256-7. Accessed February 3, 2013.

Belaiche P. 1979. *Traite de Phytotherapie et d'Aromatherapie*, Vol. 1. Paris: Maloine SA.

Belaiche P. 1985. Treatment of vaginal infections of *Candida albicans* with essential oil of *Melaleuca alternifolia*. *Phytotherapie.* 15:13-15.

Bhala N, Emberson J, Mehri A, Abramson S, Arber N et al. 2013. Vascular and upper gastrointestinal effects of non-steroidal anti-inflammatory drugs: meta-analyses of individual participant data from randomised trials. *Lancet.* 382(9894):769-79.

Bilton C. 2005. Aromatherapy spritzers for menopausal hot flashes. Unpublished dissertation for RJBA.

Blackwell R. 1991. Teatree oil and anaerobic (bacterial) vaginosis (letter). *Lancet.* 337(8736):300.

Bowles V. 2004. Lavender for laboring women. Unpublished dissertation for RJBA.

Brinker F. 2000. *The Toxicology of Botanical Medicine,* 3rd edn. Sandy, OR: Eclectic Medical Publications.

Brito R, Santos P, Prado D, Santana M, Araújo A. 2012. Citronellol reduces orofacial nociceptive behaviour in mice – evidence of involvement of retrosplenial cortex and periaqueductal grey areas. *Basic Clin Pharmacol Toxicol.* doi:10.1111/bcpt.12018. Accessed February 3, 2013.

Brown D. 2002. Clay sage or lemon to reduce hot flushes in menopause? Unpublished dissertation for RJBA.

Buckle J, Ryan K, Chin K. 2014. Clinical Aromatherapy for pregnancy, labor and post partum. *Int J Childbirth Education.* 19(4):21-28.

Burns E, Blamey C, Ersser S, et al. 2000. An investigation into the use of aromatherapy in intrapartum midwifery practice. *J Altern Complement Med.* 6(2):141-7.

Burns E, Zobbbi V, Panzeri D, Oskrochi R, Regalia A. 2007. Aromatherapy in childbirth: a pilot randomized controlled trial. *BJOG.* 114(7):838-44.

Carson C, Riley T. 1993. Antimicrobial activity of the essential oil of *Melaleuca alternifolia. Lett Appl Microbiol.* 16:49-55.

Carson C, Riley T. 1994. The antimicrobial activity of teatree. *Med J Australia.* 160:236.

Carson C, Riley T. 1999. In vitro susceptibilities of lactobacilli and organisms associated with bacterial vaginosis to *Melaleuca alternifolia* (tea tree) oil. *Antimicrob Agents Chemother.* 43(1):196.

Carson C, Hammer K, Riley T. 2006. *Melaleuca alternifolia* (tea tree) oil: a review of antimicrobial and other medicinal properties. *Clin Microbiol Rev.* 19:50-62.

Cavallo D. 2004. Clary sage for dysmenorrheal. Unpublished dissertation for RJBA

Clark M. 2007. Aromatherapy for dysmenorrhea. Unpublished dissertation for RJBA.

Coleman-Smith V. 2012. Aromatherapy as a comfort measure during the childbearing year. *Int J Childbirth Education.* 27(3):26-30.

Conrad P, Adams C. 2012. The effects of clinical aromatherapy for anxiety and depression in the high risk postpartum woman – a pilot study. *Complement Ther Clin Pract.* 18(3):164-8.

Cook R, Redondo-Lopez V, Schmitt C et al. 1992. Clinical, microbiological and biochemical factors in recurrent bacterial vaginosis. *J Clin Microbiol.* 30(4):870-7.

Coste I, Judlin P, Lepargneur JP, Bou-Antoun S. 2012. Safety and efficacy of an intravaginal prebiotic gel in the prevention of recurrent bacterial vaginosis: a randomized double-blind study. *Obstet Gynecol Int.* 147867. doi: 10.1155/2012/147867.

Danby C, Boikov D, Rautemaa-Richardson R, Sobel J. 2012. Effect of pH on in vitro susceptibility of *Candida glabrata* and *Candida albicans* to 11 antifungal agents and implications for clinical use. *Antimicrob Agents Chemother.* 56(3):1403-6.

Darsareh F, Taavoni S, Joolaee S, Haghani H. 2012. Effect of aromatherapy massage on menopausal symptoms: a randomized placebo-controlled clinical trial. *Menopause.* 19(9):995-9.

D'Auria F, Laino L, Strippoli V, Tecca M, Salvatore G, Battinelli L, Mazzanti G. 2001. *In vitro* activity of tea tree oil against *Candida albicans* mycelial conversion and other pathogenic fungi. *J Chemother.* 13:377-83.

D'Auria FD, Tecca M, Strippoli V, Salvatore G, Battinelli L, Mazzanti G. 2005. Antifungal activity of *Lavandula angustifolia* essential oil against *Candida albicans* yeast and mycelial form. *Med Mycol.* 43(5):391-6.

Deans S, Svoboda K. 2006. The antimicrobial properties of marjoram (*Origanum majorana* L.) volatile oil. *Flavour Fragrance J.* 5(3):187-90.

Den Tonkelaar I, Oddens B. 2000. Determinants of long-term hormone replacement therapy and reasons for eary discontinuation. *Obstetrics & Gynecology.* 95(4):507-512.

Dessapt A, Gourdy P. 2012. Menopause and cardiovascular risk. *J Gynecol Obstet Biol Reprod (Paris).* 41(7 Suppl.):F13-9.

De Sousa A, Soares P, de Almeida A, Maia A, de Souza E, Assreuy A. 2010. Antispasmodic effect of *Mentha piperita* essential oil on tracheal smooth muscle of rats. *J Ethnopharmacol.* 130(2):433-6.

Dhany A, Mitchell T, Foy C. 2012. Aromatherapy and massage intrapartum service impact on use of analgesia and anesthesia in women in labor: a retrospective case note analysis. *J Alt Complement Med.* 18(10):932-8.

Duarte M, Figueira G, Sartoratto A, Rehder V, Delarmelina C. 2005. Anti-candida activity of Brazilian medicinal plants. *J Ethnopharmacol.* 97(2):305-11.

Duke J. 1985. *The Handbook of Phytochemical Constituents of GRAS Herbs and Other Economic Plants.* CRC Press. Boca Raton, FL, USA.

Dunning, T. 2005. Applying a quality use of medicines framework to using essential oils in nursing practice. *Complement Ther Clin Practice.* 11:172-81.

Ergin A, Arikan S. 2002. Comparison of microdilution and disc diffusion methods in assessing the in vitro activity of fluconazole and *Melaleuca alternifolia* (tea tree) oil against vaginal *Candida* isolates. *J Chemother.* 14(5):465-72.

Eriksen E. 2012. Hormone replacement therapy or SERMS in the long term treatment of osteoporosis. *Minerva Ginecol.* 64(3):207-21.

Ettinger B, Pressman A. 1999. Continuation of postmenopausal hormone replacement therapy in a large health maintenance organization: transdermal matric patch versus oral estrogen therapy. *American Journal of Managed Care.* 6(6):779-875

Evans W. 1994. *Trease and Evans' Pharmacognosy*, 13th ed. London: Bailliere Tindall.

Fanner F. 2005. The use of aromatherapy for pain management in labour. *Int J Clin Aroma.* 2(1):10-14.

Franchomme P, Penoel D. 1991. *Aromatherapie Exactement.* Limoges, France: Jollois.

Funari CS, Gullo FP, Napolitano A, Carneiro RL, Mendes-Giannini MJ et al. 2012. Chemical and antifungal investigations of six *Lippia* species (Verbenaceae) from Brazil. *Food Chem.* 135(3):2086-94.

Furletti V, Teixeira I, Obando-Pereda G, Mardegan R, Sartoratto A. 2011. Action of *Coriandrum sativum* L. essential oil upon oral *Candida albicans* biofilm formation. *Evid Based Complement Altern Med.* Article ID 985832, http://dx.doi.org/10.1155/2011/985832. Accessed August 25, 2014.

Gagua T, Tkeshelashvili B, Gagua D. 2012. Primary dysmenorrhea – leading problem of adolescent gynecology. *Georgian Med New.* 207:7-14.

Ghelardini C, Galeotti N, Salvatore G, and Mazzanti, G. 1999. Local anesthetic activity of essential oil of Lavandula angustifolia. *Planta Medica.* 65(8):700-703.

Gossler S. 2010. Use of complementary and alternative therapies during pregnancy, postpartum, and lactation. *J Psychosoc Nurse Ment Health.* 48(11):30-6.

Guba R. 2002. *Toxicity Myths.* International Society of Professional Aromatherapists. London: Regents College. (Handout from conference presentation, March 2002).

Guenther E. 1972. *The Essential Oils.* Melbourne, FL: Krieger Publishing.

Hadi N, Hanid A. 2011. Lavender essence for post-cesarean pain. *Pakistan J Biol Sci.* 14(11):664-7.

Hammer K, Carson C. 2000. *Melaleuca alternifolia* (tea tree) oil inhibits germ tube formation by *Candida albicans. Med Mycol.* 38(5):355-62.

Han S, Hur M-H, Buckle J. 2006. Effect of aromatherapy on symptoms of dysmenorrhea in college students. A randomized, placebo-controlled clinical trial. *J Alt Complement Med.* 12(6):535-41.

Hăncianu M, Aprotosoaie A, Gille E, Poiată A, Tuchiluş C et al. 2008. Chemical composition and in vitro antimicrobial activity of essential oil of *Melissa officinalis* L. from Romania. *Rev Med Chir Soc Med Nat Iasi.* 112(3):843-7.

Harel Z. 2008. Dysmenorrhea in adolescents. *Exp Opin Pharmacother.* 13(15):2157-70.

Höfling J, Anibal P, Obando-Pereda G, Peixoto I, Furletti V et al. 2008. Antimicrobial potential of some plant extracts against *Candida* species. *Braz J Biol.* 70(4):1065-8.

Holmes P. 1993. *The Energetics of Western Herbs.* Berkeley, CA: NatTrop.

Horowitz S. 2011. Aromatherapy: current and emerging applications. *Altern Complement Ther.* 17(1):26-31.

Hur M, Han S. 2004. Clinical trial of aromatherapy on postpartum mother's perineal healing. *Taehan Kanho Hakhoe Chi.* 34(1):53-62.

Hur M, Cheong N, Yun H, Lee M, Song Y. 2005 Effects of delivery nursing care using essential oils on delivery stress response, anxiety during labour and postpartum status anxiety. *Taehan Kanho Hakhoe Chi.* 35(7):1277-84.

Hur S, Hur M, Buckle J, Choi J, Lee M. 2006. Effect of aromatherapy on symptoms of dysmenorrhea in college students: a randomized, placebo-controlled clinical trial. *J Altern Complement Med.* 12(6):535-41.

Hur M, Oh H, Lee M, Kim C, Choi A, Shin G. 2007. Effects of aromatherapy massage on blood pressure and lipid profile in Korean climacteric women. *Int J Neurosci.* 117(9):1281-7.

Hur M, Yang Y, Soo Lee M, 2008. Aromatherapy massage affects menopause symptoms in Korean climacteric women: a pilot-controlled trial. *Evid Based Complement Altern Med.* 5(3):325-8.

Hur M, Lee M, Seong K, Lee M. 2012. Aromatherapy massage on the abdomen for alleviating menstrual pain in high school girls: a preliminary controlled clinical study. *Evid Based Complement Alternat Med.* 187163.

Imura M, Misao H, Ushijima H. 2006. The psychological effects of aromatherapy massage in healthy postpartum mothers. *J Midwifery Women's Health.* 51(2):e21-e27.

Johnson B. 2006. Geranium and cypress for female nurses with menopausal hot flashes. Unpublished dissertation for RJBA.

Kartnig T, Still F, Reinthaler F. 1991. Antimicrobial activity of the essential oil of young pine shoots *(Picea albies). J Ethnopharmacol.* 35(92):155-7.

Khan MS, Malik A, Ahmad I. 2012. Anti-candidal activity of essential oils alone and in combination with amphotericin B or fluconazole against multi-drug resistant isolates of *Candida albicans. Med Mycol.* 50(1):33-42.

Kim M, Nam E, Paik S. 2005. The effects of aromatherapy on pain, depression, and life satisfaction of arthritis patients. *Taehan Kanho Hakhoe Chi.* 35(1):186-94.

Khorshidi N, Ostad N, Mosaddegh M, Soodi M. 2003. Clinical effects of fennel essential oil on primary dysmenorrhea. *Iranian J Pharm Res.* 1177:89-93.

King C, Jamieson D, Wiener J, Cu-Uvin S, Klein R et al. 2011. Bacterial vaginosis and the natural history of human papillomavirus. *Infect Dis Obstet Gynecol.* doi:10.1155/2011/319460.

Kozlowski G. 2000. Clary sage and geranium for menopause. RJBA unpublished dissertation.

Lane B, Cannella K, Bowen C, Copelan D, Nteff G et al. 2012. Examination of the effectiveness of peppermint aromatherapy on nausea in women post C-section. *J Holistic Nursing.* 30(2):90-104.

Larrondo J, Calvo M. 1991. Effect of essential oils on *Candida albicans*: a scanning electron microscope study. *Biomed Lett.* 46(184):269-72.

Ling Z, Liu X, Chen W, Luo Y, Yuan L et al. 2012. The restoration of the vaginal microbiota after treatment for bacterial vaginosis with metronidazole or probiotics. *Microb Ecol.* [Epub ahead of print]. PMID:23250116. Accessed February 2, 2013.

Lucks B, Sorensen J, Veal L. 2002. Vitex agnus castus essential oil and menopausal balance: self-care survey. *Complement Ther Nursing Midwifery.* 8(3):148-154.

Lucks B. 2003. Vitex agnus castus essential oil and menopausal balance: a research update. *Complement Ther Nursing Midwifery.* 9(3):157-60.

Maher K. 2005. Cypress for hot flushes of menopause. Unpublished dissertation for RJBA.

Mantle F. 2003. The role of alternative medicine in treating postnatal depression. *Comp Ther Nursing Midwifery.* 8(4):197-203.

Marini-Bettolo G. 1979. Plants in traditional medicine. *Journal of Ethnopharmacology.* 1(3):303-306.

Marino D. 2004. 2% lavender applied topically to laboring women. Unpublished dissertation for RJBA.

Maruyama N, Takizawa T, Ishibashi H, Hisajima T, Inouye S et al. 2008. Protective activity of geranium oil and its component, geraniol, in combination with vaginal washing against vaginal candidiasis in mice. *Biol Pharm Bull.* 31(8):1501-6.

Maruyama N, Abe S. 2012. Development of anti-infectious aromatherapy against candida infections. Conference Proceedings Kyoto Japan. ICA (International Congress of Aromatherapy). August 31–September 2.

Mashburn J. 2012. Vaginal infections update. *J Midwifery Womens Health.* 57(6):629-34.

McFerren T, ed. 1996. *Oxford Dictionary of Nursing*, 2nd ed. Oxford, UK: Oxford University Press.

Melli M, Rashidi M, Nokhoodchi A, Tagavi S, Farzardi L et al. 2007. A randomized trial of peppermint gel, lanolin ointment, and placebo gel to prevent nipple crack in primiparous breastfeeding women. *Med Sci Monit.* 13(9):CR406-411.

Meske D. 2005. Clary sage and cypress for hot flushes. Unpublished dissertation for RJBA.

Milsom I, Andersch B, Sundell G. 1988. The effect of flurbiprofen and naproxen sodium on intra-uterine pressure and menstrual pain in patients with primary dysmenorrhea. *Acta Obstet Gynecol Scand.* 67:711-6.

Mondello F, De Bernardis F, Girolamo A, Cassone A, Salvatore G. 2005. In vivo activity of terpinen-4-ol, the main bioactive component of *Melaleuca alternifolia* Cheel (tea tree) oil against azole-susceptible and -resistant human pathogenic *Candida* species. *BMC Infectious Diseases.* 6:158.

Mondello F, De Bernardis F, Girolamo A, Salvatore G, Cassone A. 2003. In vitro and in vivo activity of tea tree oil against azole-susceptible and -resistant human pathogenic yeasts. *J Antimicrob Chemother.* 51(5):1223-9.

Moskowitz D. 2001. Hormones and Balance. In Wilson K, Moskowitx D, Thomas D (eds.), *A Woman's Health Resource.* Portland OR. Transitions for Health, Inc., 3-37.

Mosti M, Kaehler N, Stunes A, Hoff J, Syversen U. 2013. Maximal strength training in postmenopausal women with osteoporosis or osteopenia. *J Strength Cond Res.* 2013 Jan 2. [Epub ahead of print]. PMID:23287836. Accessed February 3, 2013.

Mousley S. 2005. Audit of an aromatherapy service in a maternity unit. *Complement Ther Clin Pract.* 11(1):205-10.

Murakami S, Shirota T, Hayashi S, Ishizuka B. 2005. Aromatherapy for outpatients with menopausal symptoms in obstetrics and gynecology. *J Altern Complement Med.* 11(3):491-4.

Muzny C, Schwebke J. 2013. Gardnerella vaginalis: still a prime suspect in the pathogenesis of bacterial vaginosis. *Curr Infect Dis Rep.* Feb 1. [Epub ahead of print]. PMID:23371405.

Nathan E. 2000. Aromatherapy for pregnancy induced hypertension. Unpublished dissertation. RJ Buckle Associates.

Nichols A. 2006. Do topically applied essential oils reduce menstrual cramps? Unpublished dissertation for RJBA.

Oliva B, Piccirilli E, Ceddia T, Pontieri E, Aureli P, Ferrini AM. 2003. Antimycotic activity of *Melaleuca alternifolia* essential oil and its major components. *Lett Appl Microbiol.* 37:185-7. doi: 10.1046/j.1472-765X.2003.01375.x.

Ou M, Tsu T, Lai A, Lin Y, Lin C. 2012. Pain relief assessment by aromatic essential oil massage on outpatients with primary dysmenorrhea: a randomized, double-blind clinical trial. *J Obstet Gynaecol Res.* 38(5):817-22.

Ough Y, Albert R, Bhaskar D, Jones G, Loftus K. 2008. Soap-scented skin patch for menstrual cramps: a case-series. *J Altern Complement Medicine.* 14(6):618.

Pattnaik S, Subramanyam V, Kole C. 1996. Antibacterial and antifungal activity of essential oils in vitro. *Microbios.* 86(349):237-46.

Pena E. 1962. *Melaleuca alternifolia* oil. Its use for trichomonal vaginitis and other vaginal infections. *Obstet Gynecol.* 19(6):793-5.

Pietrella D, Angiolella L, Vavala E, Rachini A, Mondello F et al. 2011. Beneficial effect of *Mentha suaveolens* essential oil in the treatment of vaginal candidiasis assessed by real-time monitoring of infection. *BMC Complement Altern Med.* 11:18. doi: 10.1186/1472-6882-11-18. Accessed February 1, 2013.

Pollard K. 2008. Introducing aromatherapy as a form of pain management into a delivery suite. *J Assoc Chartered Physiother Womens Health.* 103:12-16.

Price S, Price L. 2007. *Aromatherapy for Health Professionals.* 3rd edition. Churchill Livingstone, London, p 151.

Reimer J. 2005. Clary sage for dysmenorrhea. Unpublished dissertation for RJBA

Rodrigues D. 2005. Clary sage for dysmenorrhea. Unpublished dissertation for RJBA

Romano L, Battaglia F, Masucci L, Sanguinetti M, Posteraro B et al 2005. In vitro activity of bergamot natural essence and furocoumarin-free and distilled extracts, and their associations with boric acid, against clinical yeast isolates. *J Antimicrobial Chemother.* 55(1):110-4.

Ryan K. 2010. Lavender for post partum anxiety. Unpublished dissertation for RJBA.

Saharkhiz MJ, Motamedi M, Zomorodian K, Pakshir K, Miri R, Hemyari K. 2012. Chemical composition, antifungal and antibiofilm activities of the essential oil of *Mentha piperita. ISRN Pharm.*:718645. doi: 10.5402/2012/718645. Accessed February 2, 2013.

Sayyah M, Rashidi M, Delazar A, Madarek E, Kargar Maher M. 2007. Effect of peppermint water on nipple cracks in lactating primiparous women: a randomized, controlled trial. *I Int Breastfeed Journal.* 2(1):7.PMCID: PMC1865372. Accessed Aug 23, 2014.

Schmid P, Rubinow D. 1991. Menopausal related affective disorders: a justification for further study. *American Journal of Psychiatry.* 148(1): 844-852.

Schnaubelt K. 2011. *The Healing Intelligence of Essential Oils.* Healing Arts Press. Rochester, VT, USA. P 133.

Seol G, Shim H, Kim P, Moon H, Lee K et al. 2010. Antidepressant-like effect of *Salvia sclaria* is explained by modulation of dopamine activity in rats. *J Ethnopharmacol.* 130(1):187-90.

Shapiro S, Meier A, Guggenheim B. 1994. The antimicrobial activity of essential oils and essential oil components towards oral bacteria. *Oral Microbiol Immunol.* 9:202-8.

Sheikhan F, Jahdi F, Khoei E, Shamsalizadeh N, Sheikhan M, Haghani H. 2012. Episiotomy pain relief: use of lavender oil essence in primiparous Iranian women. *Complement Ther Clin Pract.* 18(1):66-70.

Sherrard J, Donders G, White D, Jensen J. 2011. IUSTI/WHO guideline on the management of vaginal discharge. *Int J STD AIDS.* 22(8):421-9.

Smith C, Collins C, Crowther C. 2011. Aromatherapy for pain management in labour. *Cochrane Database of Systematic Reviews,* 7.

Soliman F, El-Kashoury E, Fathy M et al. 1994. Analysis and biological activity of the essential oil of *Rosmarinus officinalis* from Egypt. *Flavour Fragrance J.* 9:29-33.

Solsto F, Benvenuti C. 2011. Controlled study on thymol + eugenol vaginal douche versus econazole in vaginal candidiasis and metronidazole in bacterial vaginosis. *Arzneimittelforschung.* 61(2):126-31.

Stiles J, Sparks M, Ronzio B et al. 1995. The inhibition of *Candida albicans* by oregano. *J Appl Nutrition.* 47(4):96-102.

Sultan C, Gaspari L, Paris F. 2012. Adolescent dysmenorrhea. *Endocr Dev.* 2012;22:171-80. doi: 10.1159/000331775. Epub 2012 Jul 25. Accessed January 26, 2013.

Suresh B, Siram S, Dhanarj S et al. 1997. Anticandidal activity of *Santolina chamaecyparisus* volatile oil. *J Ethnopharmacol.* 55:151-9.

Swingle J. 2001. Use of essential oils in intrapartum care. Unpublished dissertation. RJ Buckle Associates.

Taddei I, Giachetti D, Taddei E, Mantovani P. 1988. Spasmolytic activity of peppermint, sage and rosemary essences and their major constituents. *Fitoterapia.* 59(6): 463-468.

Tibljas T. Clary sage and geranium to reduce menstrual cramping. Unpublished dissertation.

Tillett J, Ames A. 2010. The uses of aromatherapy in women's health. *J Perinat Neonat Nurse.* 24(3): 238-45.

Tiran D. 1996. *Aromatherapy in Midwifery Practice.* London: Bailliere Tindall.

Tiran, D. 2011. Smell's good! Aromatherapy in midwifery. *Practising Midwife.* 14(10):11-5.

Tiran D. 2012. *Safety of Essential Oils in Pregnancy and Childbirth.* Available from www.expectancy.co.uk.

Trinh H, Lee I, Hyun Y, Kim D. 2011. *Artemisia princeps* Pamp. essential oil and its constituents eucalyptol and -terpineol ameliorate bacterial vaginosis and vulvovaginal candidiasis in mice by inhibiting bacterial growth and NF-kB activation. *Planta Medica.* 77(18):1996-2002.

Valnet J. 1993. *The Practice of Aromatherapy.* CW Daniel. Saffron Walden, UK.

Viana G, Vale T, Pinho R, Matos F 2000. Antinociceptive effect of the essential oil from Cymbopogon citratus in mice. *Journal of Ethnopharmacology.* 70(3): 323-327.

Walsh L, Longstaff J. 1987. The antimicrobial activity of an essential oil on selected oral pathogens. *Periodontology.* 8:11-15.

Weier K, Beal M. 2004. Complementary therapies as adjuncts in the treatment of postpartum depression. *J Midwifery Women's Health.* 49(2):96-104.

Williams W. 2005. Preconception care and aromatherapy in pregnancy. *Int J Clin Aromather.* 2(1):15-19.

Wilson C. 2005. Recurrent vulvovaginitis candidiasis: an overview of traditional and alternative therapies. *Advance for Nurse Practitioners.* 13(5):24-9.

Yip Y, Tam A. 2008. An experimental study on the effectiveness of massage with aromatic ginger and orange essential oil for moderate-to-severe knee pain among the elderly in Hong Kong. *Comp Ther Med.* 16(3):131-8.

Zwelling E, Johnson K, Allen K. 2006. How to implement complementary therapies for laboring women. *Matern Child Nurs.* 31(6):364-70.

Appendix

Recommended Essential Oil Distributors and Resources

There are many essential oil distributors that sell good essential oils, and it would be impossible to list them all. Instead I have listed a few companies I have used for many years. The four companies I use for the USA programs are listed first, followed by a list of other companies that I use regularly.

Suppliers for USA Courses
Nature's Gift
316 Old Hickory Blvd. East, Madison, TN 37115
Tel: (615) 612-4270; Fax: (615) 860-9171
www.naturesgift.com

SunRose Aromatics, LLC
1120 Dean Avenue, Bronx, NY 10465
Tel: (718) 794-0391; Fax: (718) 792-3276
www.SunRoseAromatics.com

Applachian Valley Natural Products
260 Maple Street, P.O. Box 515, Friendsville, MD 21531
Tel: 301-746-4630: Fax: (301) 746-4633
www.av-at.com

Florihana
Les Grands Prés, 06460 Caussols, France
Tel: +33 (0) 493-09-06-09
www.florihana.com

Other Recommended Distributors
Oshadi Ltd
Oshadi House, Unit 6 Sycamore Close
Cambridge, CB1 8PG, UK
Tel: +44 (01223) 242242; Fax: +44 (0871) 2476628
www.oshadi.co.uk

Quinessence Aromatherapy Ltd
Forest Court, Linden Way, Coalville
Leicestershire LE67 3JY, UK
Tel: +44 (01530) 835918; Fax: +44 (01530) 519771
www.quinessence.com

Chemistry Notes
Ian Smith, www.fragrantearth.com

Diffusers
Plant Extracts International Inc.
600 11th Avenue, Hopkins, MN 55343-7840
Tel: (952) 935-9903; Fax: (952) 935-9903
www.plantextractsinc.com

Aromapatches
Bioesse Technologies
13040 Woodbridge Trail, Minnetonka, MN 55305
Tel: (952) 221-8610; Fax: (952) 797-0133
www.bioessetech.com

Aromapackets
Aeroscena
10000 Cedar Road Cleveland, OH 44106
Phone: 800-671-1890
Info@aeroscena.com

Recommended Essential Oil Journals
Europe
International Journal of Clinical Aromatherapy. Editor: Rhiannon Lewis
    (formerly Harris)
www.ijca.net

UK
In Essence. Editor: Pat Herbert
Journal of International Federation of Professional Aromatherapists
www.ifparoma.org

Australia
Aromatherapy Today. Editor: Deby Atterby
www.aromatherapytoday.com

USA

International Journal of Professional Holistic Aromatherapy. Editor: Lora Cantele
www.ijpha.com

Essential Oil Research Database

Bob Harris's database (excellent resource)
http://www.quintessential.uk.com
Finally, my favourite perfume blends (that I have worn for many years) are from
    Australia:
Goddess and Spirit of Woman
Springfields Health Care Group PTY Ltd
www.healthyskin.com.au

Index

Page numbers followed by f indicate figures; t, tables; b, boxes.